Nutrition and HIV

Nutrition and HIV

Edited by

Vivian Pribram

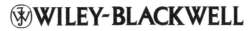

A John Wiley & Sons, Ltd., Publication

This edition first published 2011
© 2011 Blackwell Publishing Ltd

Blackwell Publishing was acquired by John Wiley & Sons in February 2007. Blackwell's publishing programme has been merged with Wiley's global Scientific, Technical, and Medical business to form Wiley-Blackwell.

Registered office
John Wiley & Sons Ltd, The Atrium, Southern Gate, Chichester, West Sussex, PO19 8SQ, United Kingdom

Editorial offices
9600 Garsington Road, Oxford, OX4 2DQ, United Kingdom
2121 State Avenue, Ames, Iowa 50014-8300, USA

For details of our global editorial offices, for customer services and for information about how to apply for permission to reuse the copyright material in this book please see our website at www.wiley.com/wiley-blackwell.

The right of the author to be identified as the author of this work has been asserted in accordance with the Copyright, Designs and Patents Act 1988.

Library of Congress Cataloging-in-Publication Data

Nutrition and HIV / edited by Vivian Pribram.
     p. ; cm.
  Includes bibliographical references and index.
  ISBN 978-1-4051-8270-6 (pbk. : alk. paper)
  1. AIDS (Disease)–Diet therapy.   I. Pribram, Vivian.
  [DNLM: 1. HIV Infections–prevention & control.   2. Health Behavior.   3. Nutritional Physiological Phenomena. WC 503.6 N976 2011]
  RC606.6.N877 2011
  362.196′9792–dc22

                                                                                    2010007738

A catalogue record for this book is available from the British Library.

Set in 10/12 pt Sabon by Aptara® Inc., New Delhi, India

1   2011

Contents

SECTION 6:   PALLIATIVE, END OF LIFE CARE AND NUTRITION

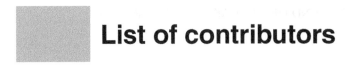

List of contributors

Paul Archer, Registered Nurse (Child) BSc (Hons) in Community Children's Nursing
Specialist Community Children's Nurse, Community Children's Nursing Team – Lewisham PCT, London, UK

Angela C Bailey, BM ChB, MRCP(UK), DTM&H, DipHIVMed, DipGUMed
Consultant Physician in Genitourinary Medicine, Jefferiss Wing, St Mary's Hospital, Imperial College Healthcare NHS Trust, London, UK

Theresa W. Banda, Msc, Bsc (Agric)
Africa Regional Manager, Valid International, VALID, Lilongwe, Malawi

Tim Barnes, Medical Officer, MB, BS
Albion Street Centre, 150-154 Albion Street Centre, Sydney, Australia

Rachel Barrett, BSc (Hons), RD
Principal Haematology / Oncology Dietitian, Department of Nutrition and Dietetics, Guy's & St Thomas' NHS Foundation Trust, London, UK

Joanna Lucy Bowtell, PhD, BSc
Head of Sport and Exercise Science Research, Academy of Sport, London South Bank University, London, UK

Sharon Byrne, BSc Pharm (Hons), MRPharmS
Principal HIV and Sexual Health Pharmacist, Wolverton Centre and Pharmacy Department, Kingston Hospital NHS Trust, London, UK

Sarah Cassimjee, BSc (Diet), PG Dip (Diet), RD
Senior Specialist Dietitian HIV/CHD, Department of Nutrition and Dietetics, University Hospital Lewisham, Lewisham, London, UK

Emily Cheserem, MBChB, MRCP
Specialist Trainee, Genito-urinary Medicine and HIV, Department of Sexual Health and HIV, King's College Hospital NHS Foundation Trust, London UK

Lisa Cooke, MA BSc, RD
Head of Paediatric Dietetics, Department of Nutrition and Dietetics, Bristol Royal Hospital for Children, Bristol, UK

Claire de Menezes, RSCN (GOS), MSc Public Health Developing countries (LSHTM)
Independent consultant for INGOs in the field of Nutrition and HIV, Formerly Health and Nutrition Adviser, ACF-International, UK

Rachael Donnelly, BSc (Hons), RD
Principal Macmillan Head & Neck Dietitian, Department of Nutrition and Dietetics, Guy's & St Thomas' NHS Foundation Trust, London, UK

Shema Doshi, Pharm (Hons) MRPharmS
Principal Pharmacist Sexual Health, Department of Sexual Health and HIV, Kings College Hospital NHS Foundation Trust, London, UK

Alastair Duncan, BSc (Hons) MSc PGDipD, RD
Principal Dietitian, HIV, Guy's and St. Thomas' Hospital NHS Foundation Trust, London, UK

Kirsten Foster, BSc (Hons) Applied Human Nutrition, PG Dip Dietetics
Health Improvement Practioner Advanced (Sexual Health and Tobacco Control), Public Health Directorate, NHS Kirklees. Formerly Community Dietitian (HIV Service), Leeds Community Nutrition and Dietetic Services, Leeds, UK

Shirley Hamilton, Registered Mental Health Nurse, PG Dips in Person Centred Therapy and Family Therapy
Clinical Nurse Consultant HIV/Mental Health, Sydney South West Area Health Service, Sydney, NSW, Australia

Lisa Hamzah, MA, MBBS, DTM&H, MRCP, DFSRH
Specialist Registrar, Department of Sexual Health and HIV, King's College Hospital NHS Foundation Trust, London, UK

Louise Houtzager, BSc, MSc (Nutrition and Dietetics), Accredited Practising Dietitian (APD)
Honorary Associate Lecturer in the School of Molecular and Microbial Biosciences, University of Sydney, Australia. Manager, Nutrition Development Division, Albion Street Centre, Sydney, Australia

Deepa Kariyawasam, BSc, RD
Senior Renal Dietitian, Department of Nutrition and Dietetics, King's College Hospital NHS Foundation Trust, London, UK

Karen Klassen, BHEc (Hons), RD, HIV Specialist Dietitian
Imperial College Healthcare NHS Trust, Honorary Research Associate, Imperial College, London, UK

Julie Lanigan, Bsc, RD
MRC-Childhood Nutrition Research Centre, Institute of Child Health and HIV Family Clinic Dietitian, Great Ormond Street Children's Hospital, London, UK

Margaret Lawson, MSc, PhD, Cert Ed, FBDA
Honorary Senior Research Fellow, Childhood Nutrition Research Centre, Institute of Child Health, University College, London

Christian Lee, BSc (Hons), MSc, RD, MBDA, Specialist Clinical Lead Eating Disorders Dietitian
Team Leader, The Phoenix Wing – Eating Disorder Unit, Barnet, Enfield, Haringey Mental Health Trust (BEH-MHT), London, UK

Charlé Maritz, BSc Dietetics, MSc Human Nutrition
Senior Specialist Metabolic Dietitian, Department of Nutrition and Dietetics, University College London Hospital, London, UK

Kirilee Matters, MSc, RD
Senior Specialist Dietitian, Nutrition and Dietetics, University College London Hospital, London, UK

Amy McDonald, BCApSC, PGDip Diet, RD
Formerly Specialist HIV Dietitian, University Hospital Birmingham NHS Foundation Trust

Catherine Mkangama, Msc, Bsc (Agric)
Director, Nutrition, HIV and AIDS, Office of President and Cabinet, The Government of Malawi, Lilongwe, Malawi

Bavithra Nathan, MBBS, MRCP, DipGUM
Specialist Registrar, Caldecot Clinic, King's College Hospital NHS Foundation Trust, London, UK

Daya Nayagam, MBBS, DCH, LRCP, MRCS, MSc in Community Paediatrics
Community Paeditrician for Specialist Services, Community Child Health, Childrens' and Young Peoples' Development Centre, Southwark PCT, London, UK

Gertrude M. Nyirenda, BSc (Community Nursing), SRN, Dip (Nursing)
Community Therapeutic Care (CTC) Advisor, Valid International, VALID, Lilongwe, Malawi

Kate Ogden, MSc Human Nutrition, Food Security and Nutrition Specialist, World Food Programme
Food Security Analysis Unit, formerly Head of Food Security Service, ACF-International, France

Vivian Pribram, BA (Hons), Bsc (Hons), MSc, RD
Senior Specialist Dietitian, Department of Sexual Health and HIV, King's College Hospital NHS Foundation Trust, London, UK

Tracy Russell, BSc Nutrition and Dietetics
Specialist Dietitian, Department Nutrition & Dietetics – Regional Infectious Diseases Unit, Western General Hospital, Edinburgh, UK

Susheela Sababady, BSc (Hons), PG Dip Dietetics
Specialist Paediatric Dietitian, Department of Nutrition and Dietetics, King's College Hospital NHS Foundation Trust, London, UK

Amanda Samarawickrama, BSc, MB BS, MRCP, DipGUM, DTMH, DFRSH, CTH®
Specialist Registrar in HIV and Genitourinary Medicine, Department of Sexual Health and HIV, King's College Hospital NHS Foundation Trust, London, UK

Ella Sherlock, Doctorate in Clinical Psychology, BSc Clinical Psychologist
CASCAID Child and Family Psychology Service. South London and the Maudsley NHS Trust, London, UK

Michelle Sutcliffe, BSc (Hons), RD
Community Team Lead Dietitian, Department of Nutrition and Dietetics, Southampton University Hospitals NHS Trust, Royal South Hants Hospital, Brintons Terrace, Southampton, SO14 0YD

Rebecca Weissbort, BA (Hons) and PGCert
Independent Fitness Expert, Register of Exercise Professionals, 3rd Floor, 8-10 Crown Hill, Croydon, CR0 1RZ, UK

Tanya Welz, MRCP, MSc, DTMH, DipHIV
Specialist Registrar in Genitourinary Medicine and HIV, Caldecot Centre, Department of Sexual Health and HIV, King's College Hospital NHS Foundation Trust, London, UK

Ruth Westwood, BSc (Hons), Food Science and Health Studies, PGdip in Dietetics 2000
Royal Free Hampstead NHS Trust, London, UK

Sarah Woodman, BSc (Hons), RD, Dip ADP
Diabetes Lead Dietitian, Department of Nutrition and Dietetics, Southampton University Hospitals NHS Trust, Royal South Hants Hospital, Brintons Terrace, Southampton, SO14 0YD

Preface

The aim of this publication is to provide health professionals with a source of comprehensive information on the nutritional care and treatment of people living with HIV (PLHIV). This includes people of different age groups and varying states of health and in a wide range of settings. While the main geographical focus of the publication, in terms of content, is the UK, attempts have been made to provide information which is relevant internationally, as much as is possible, given the differences in infrastructures, access to medication, and health care facilities in diverse regions of the globe in which the tens of millions of people living with HIV reside. This publication is intended for use by trained professionals in accordance with local care pathways and local, national, and international guidelines for nutritional screening, assessment, monitoring, and interventions.

This book originated as a chapter in the *Manual of Dietetic Practice* (edited by Briony Thomas and Jacki Bishop) first published in 1988 by Wiley-Blackwell.

While many books about HIV and AIDS are available on a range of topics, including medical treatment, epidemiology, and the social and political impact of the disease, surprisingly few books about the nutritional care of patients with HIV and AIDS have been published. Such a publication is long overdue.

Nutritional screening, assessment and treatment have been essential aspects of HIV care and treatment since the early days of the pandemic. Nutritional experts now see HIV patients with conditions as diverse as advanced wasting, obesity, cancers, renal failure, metabolic disorders, and many other illnesses. Serious non-AIDS conditions have become a leading cause of morbidity and mortality in this populations group A reference work addressing these issues is needed to help practitioners, in various clinical and community settings, understand and provide high quality and comprehensive care and treatment for the diverse population groups affected by HIV.

This book is divided into the following sections:

1. Introduction to HIV and nutritional care for HIV
2. Paediatric nutrition, maternal and child health
3. Nutritional management of HIV disease
4. Healthy eating, and the promotion of well-being and longevity
5. The nutritional management of HIV and co-morbidities
6. Palliative, end of life care and nutrition

It is not within the scope of this book to provide an in-depth description of the social, economic and political factors that impact greatly of the nutritional status of people living with HIV.

Chapter authors include practicing dietitians, nutrition experts, doctors, academics, pharmacists and other health professionals with specialist knowledge of the field. The content has been based on best evidence and practice guidelines available.

Acknowledgements

I would like to thank the contributors for their hard work in completing the chapters and making this publication possible. I would also like to thank the reviewers for their helpful suggestions and alterations, the team at Wiley-Blackwell for giving me the opportunity to edit this book, the Department of Sexual Health at King's College Hospital NHS Foundation Trust, individuals who gave permission for photographs and other materials to be used, and the many friends and colleagues who helped along the way.

Section 1
INTRODUCTION

1 Introduction to Human Immunodeficiency Virus

Tanya Welz, Amanda Samarawickrama, Vivian Pribram, Bavithra Nathan, Lisa Hamzah and Emily Cheserem

Key Points

- The HIV pandemic is one of the greatest threats to human health in history.
- Seventy per cent of worldwide deaths from AIDS occur in sub-Saharan Africa.
- Without treatment for HIV, worsening immunocompromise leads to the development of opportunistic infections and certain cancers.
- Factors associated with more rapid HIV disease progression include older age, poor nutrition and co-infection with tuberculosis and hepatitis C.
- Preventative strategies, such as behaviour change, screening of blood products, post-exposure prophylaxis and treatment of HIV during pregnancy, help decrease rates of HIV transmission.
- Improved access to treatment worldwide has reduced the annual number of HIV-associated deaths and may also reduce the number of new HIV infections globally.

1.1 Introduction

HIV-1 and HIV-2 are related viruses, both of which gradually destroy the body's immune system. Since 1981, more than 25 million people have died from the complications of HIV infection, making the HIV pandemic one of the greatest threats to human health in history.

HIV-1 is found throughout the world and is responsible for the global epidemic (UNAIDS, 2009). It is more infectious than HIV-2 and causes a more rapid decline in the immune system resulting in a shorter time between infection and death. HIV-2 is less easily transmitted than HIV-1 and is found primarily in West Africa (Jaffar *et al.*, 2004). HIV-1 is responsible for the global epidemic and will be the focus of this book.

There is evidence that HIV originated as Simian Immunodeficiency Virus (SIV) in non-human primates in West-Central Africa and transferred to humans early in the twentieth century (Worobey *et al.*, 2008). AIDS was first recognised as a clinical syndrome in 1981 and the HIV-1 virus was first identified in a French laboratory in 1983. HIV-1 is classified into three groups (M, N and O), each of which arose from a separate transmission of SIV into humans. Whilst N and O are extremely rare, M (major) is further divided into 11 subtypes (A to K) which differ from one another in their genetic make-up and their geographic distribution. The commonest subtype worldwide is subtype C, whereas subtype B is the predominant subtype in the USA and Western Europe (Lynch *et al.*, 2009). There is evidence that untreated subtype D has a worse prognosis than other subtypes (Baeten *et al.*, 2007) but the response to treatment between subtypes is similar (Geretti *et al.*, 2009).

1.2 Current state of the epidemic

1.2.1 Worldwide

Globally, an estimated 33.4 million [31.1 million–35.8 million] people were living with HIV as at December 2008. This number has increased from around 8 million in 1990.

Sub-Saharan Africa remains the worst affected region globally with 22.4 million [20.8 million–24.1 million] adults and children living with HIV. This compares with 850 000 [710 000–970 000] adults in Western and Central Europe and 1.4 million [1.2 million–1.6 million] in North America. Overall, 5.2% [4.9%–5.4%] of sub-Saharan African adults between 15 and 49 years old are HIV-infected (UNAIDS, 2009).

Sixty-one per cent of people infected with HIV in sub-Saharan Africa are women and several population-based surveys in Africa have found extremely high rates of infection amongst young women – for example, HIV infection rates of 51% among women between 25 and 29 years in rural South Africa (Welz *et al.*, 2007).

During 2008 alone, 2.7 million people [2.4–3.0 million] were newly infected with HIV and 2.0 million people [1.7–2.4 million] people died from AIDS. Since new cases outnumber deaths, the number of people living with HIV therefore continues to increase (see Figure 1.1, UNAIDS, 2009).

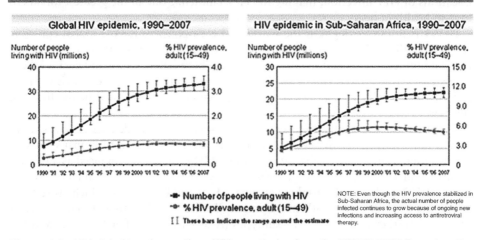

Figure 1.1 HIV global trends over time. With permission from the UNAID 2008 Report on the global AIDS epidemic.

1.2.2   UK and USA

An estimated 83 000 people are living with HIV in the UK. An estimated 58% of people newly diagnosed in 2007 acquired their infection through heterosexual contact and 38% from sex between men. Three quarters of those infected heterosexually probably acquired their infection outside the UK. In 2007, an estimated 6% of UK men who have sex with men (33 300 individuals) aged 15 to 44 years were HIV-infected (Health Protection Agency, 2009).

The HIV prevalence rate in the USA is considerably higher than in the UK at 448 per 100 000 population (1.1 million adults and adolescents). In 2006 Black Americans accounted for 49% of HIV cases diagnosed. The HIV prevalence rate among black people (1715.1 per 100 000) is 7.6 times that of white people (224.3 per 100 000), demonstrating the association between social marginalisation and HIV risk. Seventy-five per cent of prevalent cases were men with the greatest risk factor being sex with men (Centers for Disease Control, 2008).

According to anonymous HIV testing data, around 1 in 4 people with HIV in the UK remain undiagnosed. In 2008, 32% of adults newly diagnosed with HIV in the UK were diagnosed late with a CD4 cell count below 200 cells/mm^3 (Health Protection Agency, 2009).

Late diagnosis is the most important factor associated with HIV-related morbidity and mortality in the UK. At least a quarter of the deaths reported in HIV-positive individuals in the UK between 2004 and 2005 may have been prevented if HIV diagnosis had occurred earlier. Late presentation also means that opportunities to reduce HIV transmission by reducing high-risk behaviours or by reducing HIV viral load (and hence infectivity) through treatment are missed (Girardi *et al.*, 2007).

1.2.3   AIDS-related mortality

HIV remains the single greatest cause of death in sub-Saharan Africa – responsible for more than 20% of deaths in the region. In 2008, 70% of all deaths worldwide from AIDS occurred in sub-Saharan Africa (UNAIDS, 2009). Since the start of the epidemic, HIV/AIDS has more than reversed gains in life expectancy made in many African countries since the 1960s. For example, in Lesotho, where 1 in 4 adults are estimated to be living with HIV, life expectancy at birth between 1990 and 1995 was nearly 60 years. This fell to 34 years by 2005 to 2010 as a result of AIDS-related mortality (United Nations Population Division, 2005).

As many as 14.1 million (11.5–17.1 million) children in sub-Saharan Africa have lost at least one parent due to AIDS. This has devastating effects on communities and on the economy of affected countries (UNAIDS, 2009).

With the advent of effective antiretroviral therapy (ART), the crude mortality rate among HIV-infected persons in the UK declined from 4.7% in 1997 to 0.95% in 2006. Due to co-morbidities, such as hepatitis C, the mortality rate among injecting drug users in the UK remained considerably higher at 2.9% per year in 2006 (May *et al.*, 2007).

1.3   HIV transmission

The commonest route of HIV transmission is through unprotected sexual intercourse and contact with infected genital secretions. HIV may be transmitted vertically (from mother to child) either in utero, during labour or through breast-feeding. HIV is also transmitted via contaminated blood and blood products, for example through sharing contaminated needles for injection of drugs and via transfusions of unscreened blood products.

Receptive anal intercourse is associated with a 10- to 20-fold greater risk of HIV transmission than vaginal intercourse. This is at least partly attributable to the immunology of the rectal mucosa. Only a single layer of columnar epithelium separates the rectal lumen from the lamina propria, a layer of immunologically active cells which contain a broad range of HIV target cells expressing CD4 co-receptors (see below) (Royce *et al.*, 1997; Boily *et al.*, 2009).

Studies have identified several specific, biological risk factors for infection: The presence of other sexually transmitted infections increases the risk both of becoming infected and of infecting a partner with HIV (Cohen, 2004). Circumcised men are less likely to become infected with HIV (Mills *et al.*, 2008).

A high HIV viral load in body fluids also increases the risk of HIV transmission. In a study of couples in Uganda where one partner was HIV-infected and the other was not, an HIV-1 viral load above 50 000 copies/ml in the HIV-positive partner was associated with a rate of HIV transmission of 23 infections per 100 person years, whereas no infections occurred in couples where the HIV-positive partner had a viral load below 1500 copies/ml (Quinn *et al.*, 2003).

Despite the high rates of infection amongst women in Africa, women do not have an intrinsic biological vulnerability to HIV infection. At any given viral load, women are as likely to become infected with HIV as men (Boily *et al.*, 2009). Rather, the increased vulnerability of young women is due to societal structures and unequal gender roles which render women unable to negotiate safe sexual relations or force them to have sex to survive (Chersich and Rees, 2008; Jukes *et al.*, 2008; MacLachlan *et al.*, 2009).

1.4 About the virus

HIV (human immunodeficiency virus) is a retrovirus that uses the enzyme reverse transcriptase to produce proviral deoxyribonucleic acid (DNA) from ribonucleic acid (RNA). HIV primarily attacks white blood cells, particularly T-helper lymphocytes containing the CD4 receptor. It also infects other cells expressing CD4 receptors, including macrophages, Langerhans' cells, monocytes and microglial cells (Wang *et al.*, 2000) T-helper cells have an essential role in cell-mediated immune responses. As a result of this selective destruction of the immune system, people infected with HIV are more susceptible to illnesses and opportunistic infections. (Munier and Kelleher, 2007)

1.4.1 Structure of HIV

The HIV particle contains three components: the core, the surrounding protein matrix and the outer lipid envelope. The core contains the viral genetic material, RNA, encapsulated by the capsid protein p24, which contains enzymes (reverse transcriptase, integrase and protease) involved in viral replication. The glycoproteins gp41 and gp120, which are attached to the envelope, enable HIV to bind and fuse with target host cells (Wang *et al.*, 2000).

1.4.2 HIV life cycle

Recognition, binding, fusion and entry

HIV can only replicate inside human cells. The HIV particle binds to a host cell containing protein receptors (Figure 1.2), of which CD4 is the most important. The binding of the HIV enables the viral envelope to fuse with the host cell. The viral RNA contents are released into the cell, leaving the envelope behind (Figure 1.2) (Nisole and Saïb, 2004).

Reverse transcription and integration

Inside the host cell, the enzyme reverse transcriptase converts the viral RNA into DNA (Figure 1.2). This DNA is transported to the nucleus, where it is incorporated into the human genome by the enzyme integrase (Figure 1.2). Once integrated, the HIV DNA is called a provirus (Nisole and Saïb, 2004).

Transcription and translation

The HIV provirus can lie dormant within the cell for a long period. Once activated, the DNA is converted back to RNA, is transported outside the nucleus and is translated into new HIV proteins and enzymes (Wang *et al.*, 2000).

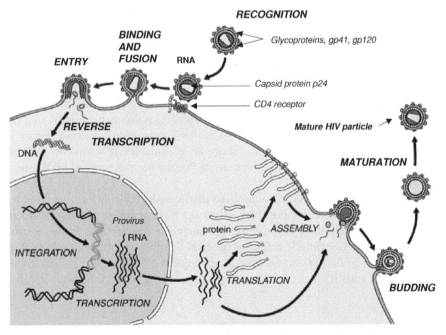

Figure 1.2 The HIV life (Source: http://media.wiley.com/CurrentProtocols/PH/ph1205/ph1205-fig-0001-1-full.gif).

Assembly, budding and maturation

The enzyme protease is involved in cleaving long protein strands into smaller ones that are incorporated into the HIV particle (Figure 1.2). At the host cell surface, the new HIV proteins and enzymes combine with viral RNA to form new HIV particles. These newly matured HIV particles are released from the host cell. They are ready to infect new cells and restart the replication cycle. The entire process is very active and large numbers of HIV particles are released daily (Gomez and Hope, 2005).

1.5   Diagnosis of HIV

1.5.1   The HIV test

Until recently, HIV tests detected only antibodies produced by the infected host in response to infection with HIV. Most people develop detectable HIV antibodies within 6 to 12 weeks of infection. This meant that the 'window period', i.e. the time from HIV infection until these tests become positive, was around 3 months.

The HIV test currently recommended by the British HIV Association and widely used internationally is a 'fourth generation HIV test' which detects both HIV antibodies and the p24 antigen. These are very accurate tests with sensitivities and specificities greater than 99%. Because the test can detect the p24 antigen (i.e. a part of the virus itself) the fourth generation HIV test has reduced the window period to around one month (Weber *et al.*, 2002; BHIVA, 2008b).

The rapid HIV test, also known as the point of care test (POCT), can give results either from a finger prick or from an oral swab sample in 15 minutes. Rapid tests do not require laboratory facilities and are useful in resource limited settings and other clinical scenarios where routine blood testing is not possible or where the rate of return for results is low. However, as with most screening tests there is a relatively high rate of false positive results particularly in areas of low HIV prevalence. Therefore all positive results should be confirmed by a conventional test.

It is generally recommended that HIV testing is performed in a health care setting and pretest discussion should establish informed consent for the test. Specific guidance regarding pretest discussion is available from the British HIV Association. These guidelines also suggest routine HIV testing of all patients presenting to a range of hospital departments with so-called 'indicator conditions', i.e. conditions which may be caused or worsened by HIV. Examples include severe psoriasis and seborrheic dermatitis which may be the first manifestations of undiagnosed HIV infection (BHIVA, 2008b).

Conventional tests for HIV are unable to distinguish recent infections from longstanding infections. Recent laboratory advances have made it possible to identify HIV infections which have been acquired during a recent time frame – usually around 6 months. The generic term 'Serological Testing Algorithm for Recent HIV Seroconversion' (STARHS) covers several serological methods (also called 'detuned' or sensitive/less sensitive assays (S/LS)) which can identify recent infections (UNAIDS, 2001).

1.6   Measurement of CD4 cells

Because HIV infects CD4 cells and uses them to produce more HIV copies, HIV infection is characterised by a progressive fall in the number of T-helper/inducer

CD4 positive cells. Assessment of the degree of immunosuppression in HIV may be done in a number of ways.

The absolute CD4 count is the measurement of the number of CD4 cells per cubic millimetre of blood (CD4 cells/mm^3). The normal absolute CD4 count in adolescents and adults ranges from 500 to 1500 cells/mm^3 of blood (Laurence, 1993). The CD4 count can vary slightly due to other factors such as infections, stress, smoking, exercise, the menstrual cycle and the contraceptive pill.

The threshold marking a substantially increased risk of clinical disease progression is a CD4 cell count of 200 cells/mm^3. UK, USA and European guidelines recommend that antiretroviral medication is started at any CD4 count below 350 cells/mm^3 to prevent the development of AIDS-related illnesses and for optimal long-term outcomes (BHIVA, 2008a; EACS, 2009; Panel on Antiretroviral Guidelines, 2009). In resource-constrained settings, guidelines recommend starting antiretroviral treatment before the CD4 count falls below 200 cells/mm^3 (WHO, 2006b).

CD4 percentage (the percentage of all white blood cells that are CD4 cells) is another useful clinical indicator of disease progression and of response to treatment (UK Collaborative HIV Cohort (CHIC), 2007). Compared to the CD4 count, the CD4 percentage tends to vary less due to other factors. A typical CD4 percentage in a person without HIV infection is around 40%. A CD4 percentage below 14% in a person infected with HIV is thought to reflect the same degree of immunosuppression as an absolute CD4 count of <200 cells/mm^3.

A third approach is the CD4:CD8 ratio, in which the number of CD4 cells in a sample of blood is compared with the number of CD8 cells. The CD4/CD8 ratio is rarely less than 1.0 in HIV-negative individuals, but may drop as low as 0.1 in patients with very advanced HIV infection. The lower the CD4/CD8 ratio, the worse the level of immune suppression.

Both the CD4 percentage and the CD4:CD8 ratio are affected by changes in the number of CD8 cells, which tends to rise through the course of HIV infection (Taylor et al., 1989).

1.6.1 Measurement of viral load

The number of HIV particles in the blood is measured by a viral load test. Commonly used tests measure HIV RNA and report the results as the number of HIV RNA copies per millilitre (mL) of blood. The amount of HIV RNA in the blood correlates strongly with progression to AIDS (Mellors et al., 1996).

The results of the viral load test may range from undetectable to millions of copies per mL of blood. Depending on the assay used, the lower limit of detection is either below 40 copies or below 25 copies in developed world settings. In some countries, older assays only measuring as low as 400 copies/ml are still commonly used.

Due to high numbers, a logarithmic scale with a factor of 10 is often used to express changes in viral load. For example, if the viral load test detects 500 000 copies of virus and treatment reduces this by 1 log, this means that the level has fallen by 10 times to 50 000 copies per mL. Similarly, an increase in the viral load of 2 logs equates to a 100-fold increase and a half a log increase to approximately a threefold increase (Pattman et al., 2005).

Only about 2% of the total virus in an infected person's body is in circulating blood. The rest is in the lymphatic tissue and other body tissues, sometimes referred to as sanctuary sites. Changes in viral load in the blood are usually mirrored in the tissues, but complete elimination of HIV from sanctuary sites is not possible with current therapies (Saksena and Potter, 2003).

Antiretroviral treatment is discussed in depth in Chapter 12 'Medications, Adherence and Interactions with Food'.

1.7   Natural history of untreated HIV infection and AIDS

HIV disease is a term broadly used to describe the illness caused by infection with the human immunodeficiency virus. If untreated, the disease typically progresses slowly from asymptomatic infection. Worsening immunocompromise finally results in the Acquired Immune Deficiency Syndrome (AIDS). This process may take many years. The median time from HIV-1 infection to death in the absence of antiretroviral treatment is 9.4 years, i.e. 50% of infected individuals die within 10 years of becoming infected (Morgan et al., 2002).

As HIV progressively damages the body's ability to protect itself from infectious organisms, HIV-infected individuals become susceptible to opportunistic infections (so called because they take advantage of the body's weakened immune system), including certain types of cancers caused by viruses which rarely occur in people with healthy immune systems.

Since the depressed immune system renders the individual vulnerable to many illnesses, almost any symptom may occur in HIV infection. Specific conditions and opportunistic infections occur at more or less predictable levels of immune suppression as reflected in the CD4 cell count (see Table 1.1). Most complications occur with increased frequency at lower CD4 cell counts. The commonest AIDS-associated conditions are candidiasis (thrush), pneumonia, tuberculosis, Kaposi's sarcoma (cancer of the lining of the blood vessels), toxoplasmosis (a parasitic infection affecting the central nervous system), cryptococcal meninigitis (an indolent fungal meningitis) and cytomegalovirus (CMV) infection (a common viral infection that can cause retinitis and blindness).

The rate of CD4 cell decline and of HIV disease progression varies among individuals (Pantaleo et al., 1995; UK Collaborative HIV Cohort (CHIC), 2007) and depends on interactions between the human host and viral and environmental factors.

Factors associated with more rapid HIV disease progression include older age, poor nutrition and co-infection with tuberculosis and hepatitis C. Psychological factors such as depression, impaired intellectual functioning, drug use and social deprivation may also adversely affect health-seeking behaviour and adherence to antiretroviral medication and may therefore be associated with more rapid progression to AIDS.

A small number of HIV-infected individuals (5–10%) remain well for many years with virtually normal immune systems. These so-called 'long-term non-progressors' have certain genetic characteristics which are protective against progression of HIV (Pantaleo et al., 1995; Stewart et al., 1997).

1.8   Staging and classification of HIV disease

HIV staging and classification systems provide clinicians and patients with important information about HIV disease stage and clinical management. They are also vital tools used in clinical and epidemiologic research – particularly in settings where CD4 monitoring is not available (CDC, 1993, WHO, 2006a).

Table 1.1 Natural history of untreated HIV infection.

Stage	CD4 cell count/mm^3	Potential complications
Primary HIV infection	>500	Asymptomatic – high viral load and a decrease in CD4 cells
Early	>500	Usually asymptomatic or • Persistent generalised lymphadenopathy (PGL) • Acute retroviral syndrome (a flu-like illness which occurs soon after infection) • Candidal vaginitis (thrush) • Skin disorders, e.g. dermatitis and apthous ulcers
Middle	200–500	Asymptomatic/mildly symptomatic or • Recurrent herpes simplex infection • Varicella zoster (shingles) • Bacterial pneumonia • Pulmonary tuberculosis • Diarrhoea, weight loss and fever may develop • Lymphomas (Hodgkins/B Cell) • Kaposis's sarcoma • Oral hairy leukoplakia (white plaques in the mouth caused by Ebstein Barr virus) • Cervical cancer
Advanced	50–200	Manifestations of AIDS • Wasting • Pneumocystis jirovecii pneumonia • Kaposi's sarcoma • Lymphomas • Mycobacterium avium complex (MAC) • Progressive multifocal leukoencephalopathy (PML) • Peripheral neuropathy • HIV-associated dementia • Toxoplasmosis
Late	<50	Very high viral load • Wasting • Disseminated cytomegalovirus (CMV) • Disseminated MAC • Neurological manifestations/central nervous system lymphoma

Adapted from Pattman *et al.*, 2005. *Oxford Handbook of Genitourinary Medicine, HIV and AIDS.*

Two main staging systems are currently in use: the U.S. Centers for Disease Control and Prevention (CDC) classification system and the World Health Organization (WHO) Clinical Staging and Disease Classification System (CDC, 1993; WHO, 2006a). Both staging systems reflect the fact that specific opportunistic infections and HIV-related conditions occur at particular levels of immune suppression as shown in Table 1.1.

The CDC disease staging system classifies the severity of HIV disease by CD4 cell counts and by the presence of specific HIV-related conditions. The definition of AIDS

Table 1.2 Classification system for HIV infection and AIDS in adults and adolescents.

	Clinical categories/symptoms		
CD4 Cell Categories	A	B	C
≥500 cells/μL	A1	B1	C1
200–499 cells/μL	A2	B2	C2
<200 cells/μL	A3	B3	C3

Adapted from centers for disease control (CDC, 1993).

includes all HIV-infected individuals with CD4 counts below 200 cells/μL (or CD4 percentage below 14%) as well as those with specific HIV-related conditions and symptoms.

The CDC classification recognizes three stages (Table 1.2). Stage A represents 'Acute retroviral syndrome', i.e. generalised lymph node enlargement or asymptomatic infection.

Stage B ('Symptoms of AIDS-related complex') includes specific symptoms suggestive of immunosuppression but which may also occur in individuals without HIV, e.g. candidiasis and shingles.

Stage C ('AIDS-defining conditions') includes cancers, e.g. lymphomas and Kaposi's sarcoma, opportunistic infections, e.g. cryptosporidiosis and specific HIV-related syndromes, i.e. HIV wasting syndrome, HIV encephalopathy and progressive multifocal leukoencephalopathy (a form of dementia caused by JC virus)(CDC, 1993).

All patients in categories A3, B3, C1, C2 and C3 have an AIDS diagnosis. This definition has been used for finding and reporting AIDS in the United States. It is less useful since the advent of ART, because, where possible, patients are treated before these problems arise.

In contrast to the CDC system, the World Health Organisation Clinical Staging and Disease Classification System (developed in 1990 and last revised in 2005) can be readily used in resource-constrained settings without access to CD4 cell count measurements or other laboratory testing methods (WHO, 2006a).

The WHO Staging (see Appendix 1) is based on clinical findings that guide the diagnosis, evaluation and management of HIV/AIDS. This staging system is used in many countries to determine eligibility for ART (WHO, 2006b).

WHO stages are categorized as 1 to 4 and are defined by specific clinical conditions or symptoms which cover a continuum from asymptomatic infection to advanced AIDS. For example, whilst Stage 1 represents primary HIV infection (i.e. acute seroconversion illness – flu-like symptoms which may occur a few weeks after HIV infection), Stage 2 includes moderate unexplained weight loss (<10% of presumed or measured body weight). Stage 3 has progressed to severe weight loss (>10% of presumed or measured body weight) and Stage 4 to HIV wasting syndrome (WHO, 2006a).

1.9   Monitoring the HIV pandemic

HIV *prevalence* refers to all HIV infections regardless of duration. HIV *incidence* refers only to recent infections – usually those acquired in the previous year. Whilst successful prevention efforts which reduce the number of new HIV infections *reduce* the prevalence of the infection slowly over time, continuing new infections and fewer deaths of HIV-infected persons on ART *increase* the prevalence of HIV – as does migration of HIV-infected individuals into a particular area.

To be able to understand the contribution of all these factors to the HIV prevalence in every country, sophisticated HIV/AIDS surveillance systems have been set up to better understand the global HIV epidemic and to monitor trends (UNAIDS, 2001). This includes anonymous HIV testing of pregnant women attending antenatal clinics and HIV surveys of vulnerable groups, e.g. sex workers. In the last 5 years, approximately 20 countries have conducted national, household HIV surveys, producing more accurate estimates of global HIV prevalence (UNAIDS, 2009).

Historically, HIV epidemics have been regarded as 'concentrated' if the prevalence in the general population is below 1% and generalised if the prevalence is greater than 1%. In a 'concentrated epidemic', HIV transmission is primarily attributable to HIV vulnerable groups, e.g. men who have sex with men, sex workers and injecting drug users. In contrast, HIV in a generalised epidemic is firmly established in the general population and protecting high-risk groups would not impact on HIV transmission (UNAIDS, 2001).

An understanding of the epidemiology of HIV in a particular country offers opportunities for more effective control measures. An example is Accra in Ghana, where the HIV prevalence in the general population is 2% but that among sex workers is 80%. An estimated 75% of HIV infections among young adult men are attributable to sex work (Cote *et al.*, 2004). In such a concentrated epidemic, interventions aimed at protecting sex workers and their clients would dramatically reduce the number of new HIV infections.

In contrast, only between 1 and 9% of HIV infections can be attributed to sex workers and their clients and other so-called 'bridging populations' such as soldiers and truck drivers in African countries with generalised epidemics (Leclerc and Garenne, 2008). Widespread change in community norms and sexual practices are required to change the course of such generalised epidemics.

The long time period between HIV infection and the onset of symptoms (typically between 8 and 11 years) makes the interpretation of trends in the prevalence of HIV difficult. Conventional tests for HIV are unable to distinguish recent infections from long-standing infections. The use of STARHS testing (discussed above) for surveillance purposes allows monitoring of HIV incidence as an indicator of HIV transmission. Increasing or decreasing numbers of recent infections provide important information about the impact of HIV prevention programmes (UNAIDS, 2001).

1.10 Prevention

Blood and blood products have been screened for HIV within the UK since 1985. For prevention of sexual transmission, condoms can be up to 95% effective (Pinkerton and Abramson, 1997). Condoms were a mainstay of some of the earliest prevention strategies such as the 'ABC' approach: 'Abstain', 'Be faithful' and 'Consistent and correct use of condoms' (Green *et al.*, 2006) continue to be important for prevention, particularly within high-risk groups such as sex workers or in sero-discordant relationships (i.e. where only one partner has HIV).

Prevention of mother to child HIV transmission (MTCT) with Zidovudine (AZT) was shown in 1994 to reduce the MTCT rate by two-thirds (Connor *et al.*, 1994).

MTCT rates within the UK are now less than 2% (Townsend *et al.*, 2008) and, with the use of ART, mothers who maintain undetectable viral loads can now choose to deliver vaginally. For sero-discordant couples with a positive male partner, the use of sperm washing to remove viral particles and artificial insemination of virus-free sperm has been used successfully (Bujan *et al.*, 2007).

Post-exposure prophylaxis for needlestick injuries has been used for many years. Current recommendations are to take three antiretroviral drugs for 4 weeks following an accidental exposure. Post-exposure prophylaxis for sexual exposure (PEPSE) is also now routinely offered following high-risk sexual exposures (European AIDS Clinical Society, 2009). Trials of pre-exposure prophylaxis (PreP) (i.e. taking antiretroviral drugs prior to an anticipated high-risk exposure) are underway (Derdelinckx *et al.*, 2006).

Other strategies such as treatment of intercurrent sexually transmitted infections have been shown to reduce HIV risk and circumcision decreases HIV transmission rates among heterosexual males (Cohen, 2004; Mills *et al.*, 2008).

Several countries in Africa reported reduced HIV prevalence rates by 2005. Whilst this reduction was partly due to improved surveillance and HIV-related deaths, there was also evidence that behaviour change was starting to occur. In Uganda, where HIV prevalence has declined dramatically in the past 10 years, population-based surveys of sexual behaviour have provided evidence for behaviour change (Green *et al.*, 2006). This has been mirrored in several African countries (UNAIDS, 2009).

Despite the devastating effects of the pandemic, the 2009 UNAIDS epidemiological update showed some encouraging trends: a reduction in the number of annual new HIV infections globally and a reduction in HIV-associated deaths, partly attributable to improved access to treatment (UNAIDS, 2009).

1.11   Effect of antiretroviral therapy on the HIV epidemic

Seventy five percent of HIV-infected persons who accessed care in the UK in 2008 received ART (Health Protection Agency, 2009).

In developing and transitional countries, 6.7 million people are in immediate need of ART. Although there has been a dramatic scale-up of antiretroviral treatment programmes outside of industrialised countries, only 31% of the 9.7 million people needing HIV treatment worldwide were receiving it at the end of 2007 (UNAIDS, 2009).

Apart from the humanitarian imperatives for increasing access to ART globally, there is also a public health argument that treatment of infected individuals reduces their HIV viral load and therefore their infectiousness and the number of new HIV infections (Castilla *et al.*, 2005). The availability of treatment also encourages more people to test for HIV with the opportunity for behaviour change and reduced onward transmission by those who are infected.

1.12   Stigma

The stigma of HIV is often added to the stigma already experienced by vulnerable individuals – sex workers, drug users, the homeless and men who have sex with men. Stigma includes both the individual internalized feelings regarding HIV status and external experiences of discrimination. There is an increasing body of research on interventions to reduce HIV-related stigma and on the direct, negative effects of stigma on HIV prevention and treatment behaviours (Doherty *et al.*, 2006; Rintamaki *et al.*, 2006). This includes evidence of stigmatizing behaviours brought to bear by health care workers – even in industrialized settings (Mahendra *et al.*, 2007).

Stigma may result in the rejection of HIV-infected individuals by their families, partners and communities. The fear or experience of stigmatisation has been shown to reduce the likelihood of having an HIV test, of disclosing HIV status to relatives and sexual partners, of engaging with HIV treatment services and of adhering to ART. Stigma therefore directly results in the continued spread of HIV and in preventable HIV-related deaths.

Stigma is increasingly recognised as a significant contributor to the success or failure of HIV interventions and many HIV programmes now have stigma-reduction components (Mahajan *et al.*, 2008). Interventions to reduce stigma will increase in importance as other obstacles to testing and treatment for HIV are addressed worldwide.

Acknowledgements

The authors would like to thank Melinda Tenant-Flowers, Consultant HIV/GUM Physician, Department of Sexual Health and HIV, King's College Hospital NHS Foundation Trust, London.

References

Baeten JM, Chohan B, Lavreys L *et al*. HIV-1 subtype D infection is associated with faster disease progression than subtype A in spite of similar plasma HIV-1 loads. *J Infect Dis* 2007; **195**:1177–80.

British HIV Association (BHIVA). British Association of Sexual Health and HIV (BASHH) and British Infections Society (BIS). UK National Guidelines for HIV Testing. 2008a. http://www.bhiva.org/files/file1031097.pdf. Accessed 13 June 2009.

British HIV Association (BHIVA). Treatment guidelines writing group. BHIVA guidelines for the treatment of HIV-1-infected adults with antiretroviral therapy. 2008b. http://www.bhiva.org/files/file1030835.pdf. Accessed 13 June 2009.

Boily MC, Baggaley RF, Wang L *et al*. Heterosexual risk of HIV-1 infection per sexual act: systematic review and meta-analysis of observational studies. *Lancet Infect Dis* 2009; **9**:118–29.

Bujan L, Hollander L, Coudert M *et al*. Safety and efficacy of sperm washing in HIV-1-serodiscordant couples where the male is infected: results from the European CREAThE network. *AIDS* 2007; **21**:1909–14.

Castilla J, Del Romero J, Hernando V *et al*. Effectiveness of highly active antiretroviral therapy in reducing heterosexual transmission of HIV. *J Acquir Immune Defic Syndr* 2005; **40**:96–101.

Centers for Disease Control (CDC). HIV and AIDS in the United States: a picture of today's epidemic. http://www.cdc.gov/hiv/topics/surveillance/pdf/us_media.pdf. Accessed 9 June 2009. March 2008.

Centers for Disease Control and Prevention (CDC). Revised classification system for HIV infection and expanded surveillance case definition for AIDS among adolescents and adults. *MMWR Morb Mortal Wkly Rep* 1993; **41**:1–19. (http://www.cdc.gov/mmwr/preview/mmwrhtml/00018871.htm. Accessed 9 June 2009.

Chersich MF, Rees HV. Vulnerability of women in southern Africa to infection with HIV: biological determinants and priority health sector interventions. *AIDS* 2008; **22** Suppl 4:S27–40.

Cohen MS. HIV and sexually transmitted diseases: lethal synergy. *Top HIV Med* 2004; **12**:104–7.

Connor EM, Sperling RS, Gelber R *et al*. Reduction of maternal-infant transmission of human immunodeficiency virus type 1 with zidovudine treatment. Pediatric AIDS Clinical Trials Group Protocol 076 Study Group. *N Engl J Med* 1994; **331**:1173–80.

Cote AM, Sobela F, Dzokoto A, Nzambi K *et al*. Transactional sex is the driving force in the dynamics of HIV in Accra, Ghana. *AIDS* 2004; **18**:917–25.

Derdelinckx I, Wainberg MA, Lange JM *et al.* Criteria for drugs used in pre-exposure prophylaxis trials against HIV infection. *PLoS Med* 2006; 3:e454.

de Silva TI, Cotten M, Rowland-Jones SL. HIV-2: the forgotten AIDS virus. *Trends Microbiol* 2008; 16(12):588–95.

Doherty T, Chopra M, Nkonki L *et al.* Effect of the HIV epidemic on infant feeding in South Africa: 'When they see me coming with the tins they laugh at me'. *Bull World Health Organ* 2006; 84:90–6.

European AIDS Clinical Society (EACS). Guidelines for the clinical management and treatment of HIV infected adults in Europe. November 2009. Available at http://www.europeanaids clinicalsociety.org/Guidelines/G1.htm Accessed 28 June 2010.

Geretti AM, Harrison L, Green H *et al.* Effect of HIV-1 subtype on virologic and immunologic response to starting highly active antiretroviral therapy. *Clin Infect Dis* 2009; 48:1296–305.

Girardi E, Sabin CA, Monforte AD. Late diagnosis of HIV infection: epidemiological features, consequences and strategies to encourage earlier testing. *J Acquir Immune Defic Syndr* 2007; 46 Suppl 1:S3–8.

Gomez C, Hope TJ. The ins and outs of HIV replication. *Cell Microbiol* 2005; 7:621–6.

Green EC, Halperin DT, Nantulya V, Hogle JA. Uganda's HIV prevention success: the role of sexual behavior change and the national response. *AIDS Behav* 2006; 10:335–46; discussion 347–50.

Health Protection Agency. HIV in the United Kingdom: 2009 Report. Available at http://www.hpa. org.uk/web/HPAwebFile/HPAweb_C/1259151891830. September 2009. Accessed 28 June 2010.

Jaffar S, Grant AD, Whitworth J *et al.* The natural history of HIV-1 and HIV-2 infections in adults in Africa: a literature review. *Bull World Health Organ* 2004; 82:462–9.

Jukes M, Simmons S, Bundy D. Education and vulnerability: the role of schools in protecting young women and girls from HIV in southern Africa. *AIDS* 2008; 22:Suppl 4:S41–56.

Laurence J. T-cell subsets in health, infectious disease, and idiopathic CD4+ T lymphocytopenia. *Ann Intern Med* 1993; 119:55–62.

Leclerc PM, Garenne M. Commercial sex and HIV transmission in mature epidemics: a study of five African countries. *Int J STD AIDS* 2008; 19:660–4.

Lynch RM, Shen T, Gnanakaran S, Derdeyn CA. Appreciating HIV type 1 diversity: subtype differences in Env. *AIDS Res Hum Retroviruses* 2009; 25:237–48.

MacLachlan E, Neema S, Luyirika E *et al.* Women, economic hardship and the path of survival: HIV/AIDS risk behavior among women receiving HIV/AIDS treatment in Uganda. *AIDS Care* 2009; 21:355–67.

Mahajan AP, Sayles JN, Patel VA *et al.* Stigma in the HIV/AIDS epidemic: a review of the literature and recommendations for the way forward. *AIDS* 2008; 22 Suppl 2:S67–79.

Mahendra VS, Gilborn L, Bharat S *et al.* Understanding and measuring AIDS-related stigma in health care settings: a developing country perspective. *SAHARA J* 2007; 4:616–25.

May M, Sterne JA, Sabin C *et al.* Prognosis of HIV-1-infected patients up to 5 years after initiation of HAART: collaborative analysis of prospective studies. *AIDS* 2007; 21:1185–97.

Mellors JW, Rinaldo CR, Jr., Gupta P *et al.* Prognosis in HIV-1 infection predicted by the quantity of virus in plasma. *Science* 1996; 272:1167–70.

Mills E, Cooper C, Anema A, Guyatt G. Male circumcision for the prevention of heterosexually acquired HIV infection: a meta-analysis of randomized trials involving 11050 men. *HIV Med* 2008; 9:332–5.

Morgan D, Mahe C, Mayanja B *et al.* HIV-1 infection in rural Africa: Is there a difference in median time to AIDS and survival compared with that in industrialized countries? *AIDS* 2002; 16:597–603.

Munier ML, Kelleher AD. Acutely dysregulated, chronically disabled by the enemy within: T-cell responses to HIV-1 infection. *Immunol Cell Biol* 2007; 85:6–15.

Nisole S, Saïb A. Early steps of retrovirus replicative cycle. *Retrovirology* 2004; 1:9.

Panel on antiretroviral guidelines for adult and adolescents. Guidelines for the use of antiretroviral agents in HIV-1-infected adults and adolescents. Department of Health and Human Services. November 3, 2008; pp. 1–139. Available at http://www.aidsinfo.nih.gov/ContentFiles/ Adultan-dAdolescentGL.pdf. Accessed 9 June 2009.

Pantaleo G, Menzo S, Vaccarezza M *et al.* Studies in subjects with long-term nonprogressive human immunodeficiency virus infection. *N Engl J Med* 1995; 332:209–16.

Pinkerton SD, Abramson PR. Effectiveness of condoms in preventing HIV transmission. *Soc Sci Med* 1997; **44**:1303–12.

Pattman R, Snow M, Handy P, Sankar KN, Elawad B, eds. *Oxford Handbook of Genitourinary Medicine, HIV and AIDS.* Oxford: Oxford University Press, 2005.

Quinn TC, Wawer MJ, Sewankambo N *et al.* Viral load and heterosexual transmission of human immunodeficiency virus type 1. Rakai Project Study Group. *N Engl J Med* 2003; **42**:921–9.

Rintamaki LS, Davis TC, Skripkauskas S *et al.* Social stigma concerns and HIV medication adherence. *AIDS Patient Care STDS* 2006; **20**:359–68.

Royce RA, Sena A, Cates W, Jr., Cohen MS. Sexual transmission of HIV. *N Engl J Med* 1997; **336**:1072–8.

Saksena NK, Potter SJ. Reservoirs of HIV-1 in vivo: implications for antiretroviral therapy. *AIDS Rev* 2003; **5**:3–18.

Stewart GJ, Ashton LJ, Biti RA *et al.* Increased frequency of CCR-5 delta 32 heterozygotes among long-term non-progressors with HIV-1 infection. The Australian long-term non-progressor study group. *AIDS* 1997; **11**:1833–8.

Taylor JM, Fahey JL, Detels R, Giorgi JV. CD4 percentage, CD4 number, and CD4:CD8 ratio in HIV infection: which to choose and how to use. *J Acquir Immune Defic Syndr* 1989; **2**:114–24.

Townsend CL, Cortina-Borja M, Peckham CS *et al.* Low rates of mother-to-child transmission of HIV following effective pregnancy interventions in the United Kingdom and Ireland, 2000–2006. *AIDS* 2008; **22**:973–81.

UK Collaborative HIV Cohort (CHIC). Study Steering Committee. *J Acquir Immune Defic Syndr* 2007; **46**:275–8.

UNAIDS. Guidelines for using HIV testing technologies in surveillance. Selection, evaluation, and implementation. 'Second generation surveillance.' http://data.unaids.org/Publications/IRC-pub02/JC602-HIVSurvGuidel_en.pdf. Accessed 13 June 2009. 2001.

UNAIDS. Report on the global AIDS epidemic, UNAIDS/08.25E/JC1510E (English original, August 2008) © Joint United Nations Programme on HIV/AIDS (UNAIDS) 2008. Available at: http://www.unaids.org/en/KnowledgeCentre/HIVData/GlobalReport/2008/2008_Global_report.asp.

UNAIDS. AIDS epidemic update: November 2009. UNAIDS/09.36E/JC1700E. © Joint United Nations Programme on HIV/AIDS (UNAIDS) and World Health Organization (WHO) 2009. Available at: http://www.unaids.org/en/KnowledgeCentre/HIVData/EpiUpdate/EpiUpdArchive/2009/default.asp. Accessed 28 June 2010.

United Nations Population Division. World population prospects: the 2004 revision. February 2005 http://www.un.org/esa/population/publications/WPP2004/2004Highlights_finalrevised.pdf. Accessed 13 June 2009.

Wang WK, Chen MY, Chuang CY *et al.* Molecular biology of human immunodeficiency virus type 1. *J Microbiol Immunol Infect* 2000; **33**:131–40.

Weber B, Gurtler L, Thorstensson R *et al.* Multicenter evaluation of a new automated fourth-generation human immunodeficiency virus screening assay with a sensitive antigen detection module and high specificity. *J Clin Microbiol* 2002; **40**:1938–46.

Welz T, Hosegood V, Jaffar S *et al.* Continued very high prevalence of HIV infection in rural KwaZulu-Natal, South Africa: a population-based longitudinal study. *AIDS* 2007; **21**:1467–72.

WHO (World Health Organisation). Antiretroviral therapy for HIV infection in adults and adolescents: recommendations for a public health approach (2006 revision). 2006a.http://www.who.int/hiv/art/ARTadultsaddendum.pdf. Accessed 9 June 2009.

WHO (World Health Organisation) WHO case definitions of HIV for surveillance and revised clinical staging and immunological classification of HIV-related disease in adults and children. 2006b Available at http://www.who.int/hiv/pub/guidelines/hivstaging/en/index.html.

Worobey M, Gemmel M, Teuwen DE *et al.* Direct evidence of extensive diversity of HIV-1 in Kinshasa by 1960. *Nature* 2008; **455**:661–4.

2 Introduction to Nutrition and HIV

Vivian Pribram

Key Points

- Nutritional care for HIV and related conditions involves interventions for both acute and chronic conditions.
- Malnutrition and HIV may cause similar changes in immune function and have a negative effect on each other.
- Some adverse effects are known to occur with greater frequency among people with HIV compared to the general population. These include hyperlipidaemia, alterations in glucose metabolism, decreased bone mineral density, and body shape changes.
- Nutritional interventions for infectious diseases among people living with HIV include optimising nutritional intake, attaining and maintaining ideal body weight, restoring lean body mass, preventing further nutrient deficiencies and food-borne infections and symptom management.
- Treatment of HIV infection should include optimum nutrition and healthy lifestyle interventions to help people lead long and healthy lives.

2.1 Introduction

Nutrition has always been an important aspect of HIV care. In the early days of the pandemic, clinical nutrition was, of necessity, experimental and required urgent responses to extreme and often fatal weight loss and wasting associated with disease progression. While severe malnutrition resulting from acute, life-threatening complications is still a major problem, for many people HIV has become a long-term chronic condition and the knowledge and skills required to manage this have changed rapidly and profoundly. It is increasingly apparent that treatment of HIV infection should include optimum nutrition and healthy lifestyle interventions to help people lead long and healthy lives. Additionally, with decreased mortality, disease patterns have changed and as a result the requirements of people living with HIV (PLHIV) have also changed. Nutritional experts now see HIV patients with conditions as diverse as advanced wasting, morbid obesity, cancers, renal failure, metabolic disorders and other systemic problems.

While the main focus of this text is the UK, the aim has been to try to address some of the differing needs of diverse population groups affected by HIV in various national and international settings. The chapters have been divided into six sections. The four main sections are: paediatric nutritional care and maternal health; nutritional interventions and care for adults living with HIV; healthy eating and nutritional management to promote well-being and longevity; and the treatment of co-morbidities among PLHIV.

2.2   Malnutrition, infectious disease and immune function

Morbidity and mortality associated with AIDS has had devastating effects on the infrastructure of many countries making survival more difficult due to factors such as reduced food security and access to supplies and medical care. The interaction between HIV/AIDS and food and nutrition security has been described as a vicious cycle in which food insecurity increases susceptibility to HIV exposure and infection and HIV/AIDS, in turn, increases vulnerability to food insecurity (Colecroft, 2008).

Increasing evidence suggests that both protein-energy and essential micronutrient (vitamins, trace minerals, essential amino acids and polyunsaturated fatty acids) malnutrition is the underlying reason for increased susceptibility to infections. PEM is considered to be a critical, yet underestimated factor in susceptibility to infection, including the 'big three' infectious diseases: HIV/AIDS, tuberculosis and malaria (Schaible and Kaufmann, 2007). PEM and advanced HIV infection are associated with similar suppression of antigen-specific and host defence mechanisms of the immune system. Malnutrition and HIV may cause similar changes in immune function and have a negative effect on each other. Malnutrition can weaken the immune system and increase vulnerability to HIV infection (Figure 2.1).

Examples of how infections can contribute to malnutrition are: (1) gastrointestinal infection can lead to diarrhoea; (2) HIV/AIDS, tuberculosis and other chronic infections can cause cachexia and anaemia; and (3) intestinal parasites can cause anaemia and nutrient deprivation. Activation and sustenance of immune responses during infection requires increased energy consumption. Studies have shown that the energy cost of immunity further impairs fitness and, consequently, the nutritive status of the host critically determines the outcome of infection. Infection causes energy loss on the part of the individual, which reduces productivity on the community level and perpetuates the alarming spiral of malnutrition, infection, disease and poverty (Schaible and Kaufmann, 2007) (Figure 2.2).

Infectious diseases are the major causes of death and morbidity in low-income countries, particularly in children (Ambrus and Ambrus, 2004) There is a clear relationship between TB and malnutrition. Malnutrition can predispose people to TB disease and TB can result in secondary malnutrition (Schwenk and Macallan, 2000). Compounding this problem, HIV-infected individuals have a significantly greater risk of developing primary tuberculosis or experiencing a reactivation of a

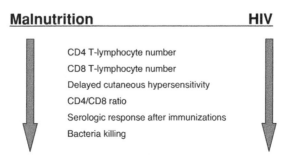

Figure 2.1   Synergistic effects of malnutrition and HIV on the immune system (FANTA, 2003).

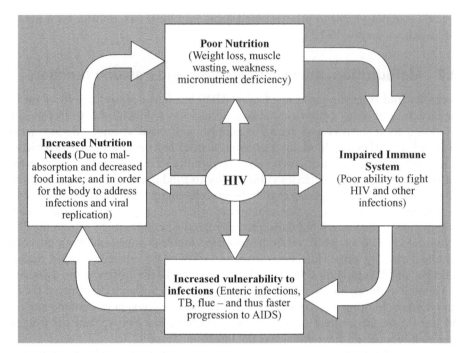

Figure 2.2 Cycle of malnutrition and infection in the context of HIV/AIDS (Source: FANTA, 2003).

previous tuberculosis infection. They are also likely to have a more severe and more progressive disease experience (Pratt, 2003). Nutritional considerations and care for people with HIV and TB co-infection are discussed in Chapter 18. This includes optimising nutritional intake, attaining and maintaining ideal body weight, restoring lean body mass and preventing further nutrient deficiencies.

2.2.1 Opportunistic infection

Infections may develop from (1) reactivation of an infection acquired earlier in life (as the immune system becomes less effective, the infection flares up and causes disease) or (2) newly acquired infections from the environment. These infections may be caused by bacteria, viruses, fungi, or parasites (American Cancer Society, 2008) (see Table 1.1, Chapter 1).

Where possible, it is best to prevent infection from occurring. PLHIV may have an increased risk of contracting food- and water-borne diseases if they are immune-compromised and therefore need to take additional precautions with food and water safety. Food and water safety advice given at an early stage is extremely helpful in order to aid the prevention of food- and water-borne infection. This is discussed in detail in Chapter 17.

However, many opportunistic infections (OIs) cannot be prevented by lifestyle changes. PLHIV may be taking medication (such as the antibiotic Co-trimoxazole (septrin)) to prevent or treat opportunistic infections (as pneumocystis pneumonia (PCP)), in addition to medication to treat the HIV (see Table 12.3, Chapter 12). Advances in preventing and treating these infections have led to longer survival and improved quality of life for HIV-positive persons, although these infections remain a leading cause of death among people with HIV disease (American Cancer Society, 2008).

A large number of symptoms may occur as a result of OIs and the effects of HIV that affect a person's nutritional status, requirements and oral intake. Generally, symptoms may increase in severity with advanced disease. Common symptoms and conditions that impact on nutritional status include:

- fever
- anorexia
- cachexia
- weight loss and wasting
- candidiasis (thrush)
- oral/GI ulcers/lesions/inflammations
- loss of appetite
- night sweats
- diarrhoea / malabsorption of nutrients
- nausea and vomiting
- anaemia
- neutropenia
- pain on swallowing food
- dysphagia
- taste changes
- changes in mental condition and behaviour including dementia (WHO, 2006).

The nutritional management of symptoms related to HIV disease and OIs is discussed in Chapter 9, 'Symptom Control and Management'.

With the majority of the estimated 33 million (UNAIDS, 2008) PLHIV residing in regions where there may be limited access to adequate medication, food, clean drinking water and shelter, key aims of global nutritional interventions remain the prevention and treatment of malnutrition in children and adults, and AIDS-associated weight loss and wasting. Many resource-limited settings affected by HIV are also high on the global hunger and poverty indices. Chapter 11 describes community nutritional interventions that can be applied in resource-limited settings affected by HIV, and some of the social and financial constraints which make nutrition and HIV a challenging priority requiring maximum input and political support.

2.3   HIV infection and decreased nutritional status

In regions with good access to anti-HIV medications, malnutrition and wasting associated with HIV disease are still highly prevalent and various forms of nutrition support are routinely required (see Chapter 7). Resource constraints often exist in these regions at household level where PLHIV are often affected by unstable immigration and poor socio-economic status.

The impact of HIV and malnutrition may result in the following:

- weight loss reported in 95–100% of PLHIV with advanced disease
- loss of muscle tissue and body fat
- vitamin and mineral deficiencies

- increased susceptibility to secondary infections
- increased nutritional needs due to reduced food intake and increased loss of nutrients, leading to rapid HIV disease progression (RCQHC, 2003).

Wasting is a defining criteria of AIDS and it has been cited as one of the most common AIDS-associated conditions, throughout the course of the disease (Mangili *et al.*, 2006).

Increased risk of morbidity and mortality can occur with as little as 5% weight loss in PLHIV.

Wasting can be secondary to HIV infection itself, but is also commonly associated with opportunistic infections and HIV-related cancers. Not all pathogenetic mechanisms of wasting in HIV have been fully elucidated, but many factors that promote progressive weight loss are understood. These include disturbances of metabolism and resting energy expenditure characterised by catabolism, preferential loss of lean body mass over fat, and, conversely, preferential gain of fat over lean mass when enteral or parenteral therapy is used. This continuous loss of cell mass and negative nitrogen balance promotes progression of advanced disease and can hasten death (Reiter, 1996).

Three key factors contribute to malnutrition in patients with HIV: inadequate intake, malabsorption and increased energy expenditure. Management of weight loss and wasting may include nutritional interventions, resistance exercise training and, if necessary, pharmacological treatment such as hormone therapy, and cytokine treatments. More detailed consideration of this subject can be found in Chapters 3, 4 and 7.

2.4 Nutritional screening and assessment

Screening and assessment of nutritional status should be made at the outset and repeated at regular intervals (Pribram and Lanigan, 2007). Nutritional screening is a quick process used to detect those with malnutrition. Nutritional assessment includes anthropometric, biochemical, clinical and dietary parameters. At a minimum, basic anthropometry should include weight and skinfold measurements (reflecting regional adiposity and lipodystrophy to obtain some appreciation of lean body mass and adiposity), and height and length measurements in infants and children. Assessment of food frequency to assess normal dietary constituents and patterns is informative as is documentation of dietary supplement use, including use of herbal and botanical therapies, and participation in government-sponsored micronutrient supplementation programs (Raiten *et al.*, 2005).

Among children, measurement of weight and height should be monitored in children (Hsu *et al.*, 2005) (please refer to Chapters 3 and 4).

Repeat nutritional assessment and screening can help to identify individual trends and can highlight the need for timely and effective nutritional intervention. This is particularly important for PLHIV given the wide range of conditions and differences in nutritional status commonly encountered. Awareness of the effects of a chronic condition like HIV and its potential impact on a child's growth is required to inform the dietary treatment options. Nutritional screening and assessment are discussed in detail in Chapter 4 (paediatrics) and Chapter 8 (adults).

2.5 Metabolic and morphological complications

Although highly successful in controlling the virus, antiretroviral medications have been linked to many potential side effects and metabolic complications such as bone demineralisation, raised cholesterol and triglycerides and fat redistribution. Fat redistribution and metabolic disturbances have been described in conjunction with the broad availability of potent antiretroviral regimens, shifting the emphasis from prevention and treatment of opportunistic infections and malignancies to management of the metabolic and related complications associated with HIV infection and its treatment (Morse and Kovacs, 2006).

The condition is often referred to as lipodystrophy. There is still disagreement on how to classify lipodystrophy but it characteristically may include loss of fat from the cheeks producing a clinically striking gaunt facial appearance, accumulation of fat around the neck (the buffalo hump), waist, viscera and shoulders (Hsu *et al.*, 2005) and loss of subcutaneous limb fat. Added to this are the wide range of symptoms associated with derangements in intermediary metabolism, potentially secondary to ART, which include dyslipidaemia (elevated circulating concentrations of total cholesterol and triglycerides and disadvantageous shifts in the ratio of high- to low-density lipoprotein cholesterol), insulin resistance, glucose intolerance and diabetes in people with HIV infection. Numerous reviews of these conditions were published (Raiten *et al.*, 2005). Metabolic disorders, including lipodystrophy, dyslipidemia and insulin resistance, occur at a high rate in HIV-infected individuals receiving highly active antiretroviral therapy (HAART) (Morse and Kovacs, 2006). These disorders are associated with increased risk of cardiovascular disease and have become an important cause of morbidity and mortality in HIV-infected patients (Morse and Kovacs, 2006). Among HIV-infected adults, in addition to antiretroviral drug exposures, being overweight and having a low income level were associated with increased predicted coronary heart disease (CHD) risk. This suggests a need to target HIV-infected men and women with these characteristics for vascular risk factor screening (Kaplan *et al.*, 2007). Dietary advice for metabolic disturbances is the most common intervention in the clinical setting, while anthropometry and/or bioelectric impedance analysis (BIA) are/is often used to monitor alterations in body composition.

A range of bone-related conditions from osteonecrosis to osteopaenia and osteoporosis have been reported in HIV-infected adults and children. In addition to the traditional risk factors for these bone-related conditions (i.e., age, gender and weight), the relative contribution of HIV and/or treatments has emerged as an additional risk factor. Evidence indicates that HIV per se causes problems with bone mineralisation. What is less clear is the relative contribution of ART to these problems. This lack of clarity is in part due to the complexity of bone mineralisation processes and the nature and the range in quality of the studies that examined these relationships in HIV-positive people. In addition, the effect of ART on bone may vary between classes of drugs as well as among drugs within the same class (Raiten *et al.*, 2005). Consequently, study results have been inconsistent.

Nonetheless, bone loss is a potentially serious problem that affects the long-term health and quality of life of PLHIV, and assessment of bone health should become part of the clinical care of PLHIV. Of particular concern are the implications for perinatally infected children who experience years of exposure to both HIV and ART. To prevent these complications and to ensure an enhanced quality of life, strategies will be needed for the incorporation of assessment of not only bone health but also risk factors that can be controlled – including diet – into clinical care (Raiten *et al.*, 2005).

See Chapters 6 and 10 for further details including nutritional management of long-term metabolic complications associated with HIV and ART in children and adults living with HIV.

2.6   Paediatric undernutrition and maternal and child health

2.6.1   Effect of HIV infection on infants and children

Malnutrition is responsible, directly or indirectly, for 54% of the 10.8 million deaths per year in children under 5 and contributes to every second death (53%) associated with infectious diseases among children under 5 years of age in developing countries (Schaible and Kaufmann, 2007). This provides the baseline setting on which the HIV pandemic has been imposed in many areas of sub-Saharan Africa (Raiten *et al.*, 2005), contributing further to the cycle of ill health, infection and malnutrition.

While childhood HIV infection has decreased in some parts of the world, with successful Prevention of Mother to Child Transmission (PMTCT) Programmes, there has been an increase in global juvenile infections in 2007 and, currently, 90% of all juvenile HIV infections occur in sub-Saharan Africa (UNAIDS, 2008). HIV remains the single most important cause of the death of infants and young children in Southern and East Africa, the only regions of the world with increasing rates of childhood undernutrition (Rollins and Mphatswe, 2008).

2.6.2   Maternal undernutrition and the effects on the child

Limited studies comparing HIV-positive and HIV-negative pregnant women suggest anthropometric measures decline with increasing viral load and decreasing CD4+ cell count, less weight gain on average in each trimester and on average throughout pregnancy and a higher prevalence of anaemia, low albumin, foliate and vitamin A deficiency among women infected with HIV (Rollins and Papadakos, 2005).

Higher viral load and lower CD4+ in maternal HIV infection during pregnancy is associated with increased prevalence of adverse birth outcomes, including increases in the prevalence of intrauterine growth retardation in small-for-gestational age infants and premature births. Children infected prenatally and intra-partum have deceleration of growth that is detectable by ages 3 to 4 months (Raiten *et al.*, 2005).

In children the course of the disease has a more rapid progression to AIDS than in adults. Children under 5 years of age have higher viral loads and are susceptible to more frequent recurrent bacterial infections than usual. Due to immature immune systems, opportunistic infections such as PCP and CMV are common in children and can be life-threatening (Lanigan, 2007).

Paediatric HIV infection often presents as growth faltering diagnosed by a downward crossing of growth centiles and frequent recurrent infections (Lanigan, 2007). High rates of stunting are reported throughout childhood in the US and European studies. Limited data support the existence of stunting in HIV-positive children in Africa, albeit with more pronounced wasting. Poor growth in children is associated with increased mortality. Supplemental feeding is efficacious in improving weight and fat losses but there are no apparent compensatory gains in height or lean body mass (Raiten *et al.*, 2005). In the era of successful ART many trials have shown improvements in markers of disease progression and infected children may remain healthy for many years. Cohort studies have reported that 40–50% of vertically infected children now survive to around 10 years of age without antiretroviral therapy (Lanigan, 2007). During opportunistic infections, requirements for energy and protein are likely to increase to about 30–50% above the usual requirements, but it is unlikely that an unwell child will be able to achieve increased intake above 10%. However, once acute infection is resolved further intake can be encouraged to aid nutritional recovery (Lanigan, 2007).

Children of HIV-infected mothers are more likely to die, irrespective of their own HIV status, if the mother has advanced disease (odds ratio 3.5) or dies (3.8–4.0) (Rollins and Mphatswe, 2008). The most striking opportunity for intervening to save HIV-infected women and their infants is to identify those with advance disease (CD4 cell counts < 200 cells/ml) and start them on antiretroviral drugs for life; these women represent approximately 9–15% of the HIV-infected pregnant population (Rollins and Mphatswe, 2008).

2.6.3   Infant feeding and the prevention of mother-to-child transmission of HIV

HIV transmission through breastfeeding is not a major issue in well-resourced regions of the world where there is usually easy access to safe, clean water and where milk substitutes are affordable. In resource-limited settings, the health risks of not breast-feeding are heavier than those of breastfeeding in cases of maternal HIV positivity. This is due to the high mortality rate from diarrhoeal diseases as a consequence of lack of water sanity, reduced resistance to gastrointestinal infections in formula-fed babies and lack of enough resources for supply of milk substitutes. Breastfeeding by HIV-infected mothers is not without risk for the infant. The risk of HIV infection for the infant must be balanced with risks associated with artificial feeding and this must be done for each HIV-infected woman on an individual basis. The dilemma to breastfeed or not in resource-limited countries should be dealt with on an individual basis considering the financial circumstances of HIV parents, their level of understanding of the risks to HIV transmission through breast milk and their role in the prevention of gastrointestinal infections (please see Chapter 3 for more detailed information on this subject).

2.6.4   Maternal health and lactation

While few studies have specifically addressed issues pertaining to nutritional needs of HIV-positive women before, during or after pregnancy or during lactation (Raiten *et al.*, 2005), two reports highlight the nutritional cost of breastfeeding for HIV-infected mothers (Papathakis *et al.*, 2006; Otieno *et al.*, 2007). The implication of existing data is that nutritional support is warranted for HIV-infected women who choose to breastfeed. Such interventions should improve the well-being of the mother and her ability to care for her child (see Chapter 3).

2.7   Healthy eating and management of HIV for well-being and longevity

Nutritional care in HIV infection involves more than treatment of disease states. It has become increasingly apparent that optimum nutrition and healthy lifestyle interventions are essential to help enable people with HIV to lead long and healthy lives. This is particularly important for people with HIV compared to the general population for a number of reasons. At the outset, when someone receives news that they are HIV positive, healthy eating and exercise are activities people can control in their lives and this often helps to maintain a positive state of mind. Because predicted lifespan has increased substantially in the era of antiretroviral therapy, good dietary intake and healthy lifestyle measures, including smoking cessation, may help mitigate against risk of serious non-AIDS conditions (such as cancer, CVD, liver and renal failure) linked to immunodeficiency, adverse effects of antiretroviral treatment and HIV itself. Subgroups of people with HIV infection have high rates of certain conditions such as obesity, high blood pressure, hepatitis B and/or C and dietary and lifestyle measures are also important to prevent further complications, ill health and early mortality. (For more detailed consideration of this subject, see Chapter 6, 'Healthy Eating, Prevention and Management of Obesity and Long-Term Complications in Children' for children and Chapter 13, 'Healthy Eating and Well-Being' for adults.)

Exercise has been used by many HIV-positive people to improve fitness, well-being and body image. With the increased chronicity of HIV it is also used as a strategy to reduce disabling consequences from chronic health problems caused by HIV infection (Nixon et al., 2005). A Cochrane review found that certain exercise programmes appear safe and may be able to improve cardiopulmonary fitness and especially psychological well-being for adults living with HIV/AIDS, although quality studies are limited and more research is warranted (Nixon et al., 2005) (see Chapter 14, 'Exercise and Physical Activity and Long-Term Management of HIV').

High rates of depression and mental ill health among people with HIV is known, which can be due to organic or inorganic causes. The importance of good oral intake is well documented and some of the medical treatments for these conditions can promote weight gain or loss and other GI disturbances which can affect consumption of food and fluids (McQuire, 2007). Poverty, poor housing, uncertain immigration status, lack of hygienic living conditions and limited income are other major factors in this population group that could impact on oral intake. This is discussed further in Chapter 15 on Mental Health.

Although anti-HIV medications are highly effective, they are not a cure, so lifelong medication is the reality for people with HIV and dietary advice may help promote the high levels of adherence required. There are many food and drug interactions, and people taking antiretrovirals need to be aware of food requirements and restrictions. Nutrients are also required for the metabolism of medication. For detailed information on this subject, see Chapter 12, 'Medications, Adherence and Interactions with Food'.

Use of complementary/alternative products such as medicines, treatments and dietary supplements, including herbal and botanical substances, is common in the general population and likewise among people with HIV infection. There is some concern over this due to the potential for adverse interactions with therapeutic drugs.

This highlights the importance of better understanding of the effects of herbal/botanical treatments on the metabolism of therapeutic drugs when both are being used concomitantly (Raiten *et al.*, 2005).

Use of complementary therapies should be addressed in the clinical setting to help people living with HIV maximise potential benefits and avoid or minimise harmful and adverse effects. Please refer to Chapter 16, 'Complementary and Alternative Therapy', for further information on this subject.

2.8   Management of co-morbidities and serious non-HIV conditions

With potent anti-HIV medication mortality rates among HIV-infected patients continued to show impressive declines. At the same time, causes of death in this population shifted from traditional AIDS-related illnesses to non-AIDS events, the most common being atherosclerotic cardiovascular disease, liver disease, end-stage renal disease and non-AIDS–defining malignancies (Baker and Henry, 2007). As a result, nutritional interventions for patients with HIV are often required for a wide range of complex conditions.

Initially, the premature development of non-AIDS conditions during HIV infection was attributed to metabolic complications of ART and other drug-related toxicities. However, additional analysis from various studies also highlights the potential role of immunodeficiency in the development of non-AIDS diseases: The lower the latest CD4 cell count, the greater the risks for non-AIDS–related death in general and, more specifically, for fatal liver disease and fatal non-AIDS–related malignancies (Baker and Henry, 2007).

Many inflammatory biomarkers that are elevated during HIV infection are also associated with progression of renal disease and with risk for cardiovascular events and certain cancers. Co-infection with other viruses, such as human papilloma virus and hepatitis B or C, in the setting of long-standing impaired immune function, may also facilitate a pro-oncogenic state or contribute to the progression of end-organ diseases.

For patients with access to potent ART, non-AIDS conditions are likely to dominate the HIV landscape for the foreseeable future, creating a need for treatment approaches that minimize the risk for both AIDS and non-AIDS diseases. Given that median survival after HIV diagnosis is now estimated to be more than 30 years, the rate of many non-AIDS conditions in this population will continue to increase (Baker and Henry, 2007).

2.8.1   Renal disease

Renal disease has long been recognised as a common complication associated with HIV infection. There are several renal syndromes and diseases associated with HIV infection. HIV-associated renal disease and metabolic complications overlap in that conditions such as diabetes, obesity and hypertension predispose towards chronic renal failure in the general population and, in turn, chronic kidney diseases are at increased risk of cardiovascular disease (CVD). Nutritional care of people with

HIV and renal disease should be holistic in that it includes ways to prevent or treat conditions such as hypertension and abnormalities in blood glucose which can impact on the progression of renal disease. Other main nutritional interventions and considerations include modifications in protein, salt, potassium and phosphate intake, depending on the stage of renal disease, and there are particular issues for those undergoing renal replacement treatments (see Chapter 19, 'The Nutritional Management of Patients Living with HIV and Renal Disease').

2.8.2 Liver disease

Because of shared modes of transmission, HIV and viral hepatitis infections often coexist. Since therapies have made HIV a manageable condition, clinicians are seeing more infected patients with complex liver issues. The prospective D:A:D study of 23 441 HIV patients showed that liver-related disease was the most frequent cause of non-AIDS–related death and 90% of those in the study had HBV and/or HCV infection. HIV and HCV co-infection may mean a greater likelihood of developing liver disease, mother-to-child transmission of HCV and metabolic abnormalities associated with anti-HIV therapy (such as insulin resistance and diabetes) (Carter, 2005). Malnutrition is a complication of chronic liver disease and there is a direct correlation between the severity of malnutrition and the progression of liver disease (Weber *et al.*, 2006). Additionally, some anti-HIV drugs can cause abnormal liver function. Liver transplants are now commonly performed in HIV and HBV/HCV co-infected patients and malnutrition could be an exclusion criterion for liver transplant in HIV-infected patients (O'Grady *et al.*, 2005).

As with renal disease, a holistic approach is also desirable when it comes to the nutritional care of people living with HIV and liver disease, as both undernutrition and overnutrition could impact greatly on severity and progression of liver disease. (see Chapter 20 for more information on the nutritional care of PLHIV with liver disease.)

2.8.3 Cancers

It has been known for a considerable time that a wide range of cancers occurs at increased rates in people with AIDS. A range of mainly infection-related cancers occurs at increased rates (e.g. Epstein–Barr virus [non-Hodgkin lymphoma (NHL), Hodgkin disease], human herpes virus (Kaposi sarcoma), human papillomavirus (anogenital and head and neck cancers)), as well as a limited number of other cancers with no known infectious cause (Grulich, 2009). See Chapter 22 for further details and nutritional management of PLHIV and cancer.

2.8.4 Multi-organ failure, respiratory conditions and critical care

The number of HIV-infected patients admitted to hospital has decreased significantly with the advent of HAART, but the number admitted to intensive care units (ICUs) has largely remained the same as has the main reason for admission: respiratory failure due to opportunistic infection. Other common reasons for critical care admissions for HIV patients include sepsis, CNS dysfunction, gastrointestinal bleeding and cardiovascular disease. Immune Reconstitution Inflammatory Syndrome (IRIS) may be responsible for respiratory failure or worsening of the central nervous system (CNS) disease (Crothers and Huang, 2006). Many HIV patients with HIV infection admitted to intensive care units are unaware of their HIV status, may have wasting and failure of one or more organs. These factors complicate nutritional care and special considerations apply although evidence is lacking. Weight loss and wasting are of particular concern as critically ill patients have an increased risk of undernutrition due to the metabolic response to stress. For further information on this subject, see Chapter 21, 'Critical Care, Respiratory and Multi-organ Failure'. For further details of these conditions and nutritional management, see Section 4 on Co-morbidites.

2.9   End-of-life care and ethical issues

Even with the widespread availability of ART, a small number of infected people will die of HIV-related conditions such as non-Hodgkin's lymphoma or other tumours, conditions and complications related to weakened immune systems and treatment failures. High-quality end-of-life care will always be required for these patients (Cox, 2006). In Chapter 23, particular attention is devoted to nutritional aspects involved in end-of-life care, including multidisciplinary decisions about provision and withdrawal of nutritional support.

Access to palliative care allows for a holistic assessment and includes management of physical symptoms and pain control. If not addressed, these symptoms could affect quality of life and ability to adhere to medication. Nutritional aspects of symptom management for PLHIV are discussed in Chapter 9.

The management of multiple aspects of HIV infection and nutrition-related complications of HIV, such as medication interactions, co-infection with other infections and diseases, wasting and lipodystrophy remain challenges for patients and for those involved with HIV/AIDS prevention, care and treatment efforts. Nutrition and dietetic professionals, other health care professionals and people infected with HIV will need to understand and address multiple complex aspects of HIV infection and treatment to improve survival, body functions and overall quality of life. Nutrition interventions can increase quality of life, assist in symptom management, support medication therapy and improve resistance against infection and complications. Research is required to identify best practices and to develop guidelines to achieve desired outcomes on health status, disease management and quality of life (ADA, 2004).

References

Ambrus JL Sr, Ambrus JL Jr. Nutrition and infectious diseases in developing countries and problems of acquired immunodeficiency syndrome. *Exp Biol Med (Maywood)* 2004; **229**:464–72.

American Cancer Society. Detailed Guide: HIV Infection and AIDS Prevention and Treatment of Opportunistic Infections, 2008. Available at http://www.cancer.org/docroot/CRI/content/CRI_2_4_4x_Treatment_and_Prevention_of_Opportunistic_Infections.asp. Last revised 09/10/2009. Accessed 28 April 2010.

(ADA) American Dietetic Association / Dietitians of Canada. Position of the American Dietetic Association and Dietitians of Canada: nutrition intervention in the care of persons with human immunodeficiency virus infection. (Expires 2009). *J Am Diet Assoc* 2004; **104**:1425–41.

Baker J, Henry K. Serious Non-AIDS conditions: redefining the spectrum of HIV-related disease. *AIDS Clin Care* 2007. Available at http://aids-clinical-care.jwatch.org/cgi/content/full/2007/730/1.

Carter M. HIV and hepatitis. Information series for HIV-positive people, *National AIDS Manual*, 3rd ed., London 2005. Available at (www.aidsmap.com).

Colecroft E. HIV/AIDS: nutritional implications and impact on human development. *Proc Nutr Soc* 2008; **67**:109–113.

Cox S. Palliative Care and HIV management, id21 Insights, UK Government Department for International Development (DFID)/Institute of Development Studies at the University of Sussex, 2006. http://www.id21.org/insights/insights-h08/art06.html. Accessed 26 July 2009.

Crothers K, Huang L. Critical care of patients with HIV. In: HIV InSite Knowledge Base [online], 2006. Available at http://hivinsite.ucsf.edu/InSite?page=kb-03-03-01. Accessed 20 June 2007.

Fanta Project. Nutrition and HIV/AIDS: a training manual nutritional management of HIV/AIDS related symptoms, 2003. FANTA, RCQHC and The Linkages Project. Available at http://www.fantaproject.org/focus/preservice.shtml. Accessed 26 September 2009.

Grulich AE. Living Longer with HIV: what does it mean for cancer risk? *Curr Opin HIV and AIDS* 2009; **4**(1):1–2.

Hsu J W-C, Pencharz PB, Macallan D, Tomkins A. Macronutrients and HIV/AIDS: a review of current evidence. *Consultation on Nutrition and HIV/AIDS in Africa: Evidence, Lessons and Recommendations for Action*. Durban, South Africa: Department of Nutrition for Health and Development World Health Organization, 2005.

Kaplan RC, Lawrence AKA, Sharrett AR *et al*. Ten-year predicted coronary heart disease risk in HIV-infected men and women. *Clin Infect Dis* 2007; **45**:1074–1081.

Lanigan J. In: Shaw V, Lawson M, eds. *Clinical Paediatric Dietetics*, 3rd ed., (London: Institute of Child Health), Oxford: Blackwell, 2007.

Mangili A, Murman DH, Zampini AM, Wanke CA. Nutrition and HIV infection: review of weight loss and wasting in the era of highly active antiretroviral therapy from the nutrition for healthy living cohort. *Clin Infect Dis* 2006; **42**:836–42.

McQuire S. In: Thomas B, Bishop J, eds. *Mental Illness, Manual of Dietetic Practice*. 4th ed., Oxford: Blackwell, 2007.

Morse CG, Kovacs JA. Metabolic and skeletal complications of HIV infection, the price of success. *JAMA* 2006; **296**:844–54.

Nixon S, O'Brien K, Glazier RH, Tynan AM. Aerobic exercise interventions for adults living with HIV/AIDS. *Cochrane Database Syst Rev* 2005, Issue 2. Art. No.: CD001796. DOI: 10.1002/14651858.CD001796.pub2.

O'Grady J, Taylor C, Brook G. Guidelines for liver transplantation in patients with HIV infection: British HIV association. *HIV Med* 2005; **6**(Suppl 2):149–53.

Otieno PA, Brown ER, Mbori-Ngacha DA, Nduati RW, Farquhar C. HIV-1 disease progression in breast-feeding and formula-feeding mothers. *J Infect Dis* 2007; **195**:220–9. Epub 2006 Dec 13.

Papathakis P, Loan MD, Rollins N, Chantry C, Bennish ML, Brown KH. Body Composition Changes During Lactation in HIV-Infected and HIV-Uninfected. South African Women. *JAIDS J Acquir Immune Defic Syndr* 2006; **43**:467–74.

Pratt RJ. (2003). *HIV and AIDS: A Foundation for Nursing and Healthcare Practice*. 5th ed., London: Arnold.

Pribram V, Lanigan J. Nutrition and HIV. In: Thomas B, Bishop J, eds. *Manual of Dietetic Practice*. 4th ed., Oxford: Blackwell, 2007.

Raiten DJ, Grinspoon S, Arpadi S. Nutritional considerations in the use of ART in resource-limited settings. *Consultation on Nutrition and HIV/AIDS in Africa: Evidence, Lessons and Recommendations for Action*. Durban South Africa: Department of Nutrition for Health and Development, World Health Organization, 2005.

RCQHC (Regional Centre for Quality of Healthcare). Nutrition and HIV: A Training Manual, RCQHC, FANTA. 2003. http://www.aidsalliance.org/graphics/OVC/documents/0000520e00.pdf.

Reiter G. Available at http://aids-clinical-care.jwatch.org/cgi/content/full/1996/1101/1. 1996.

Rollins N, Mphatswe W. From prevention of mother-to-child transmission to child survival... and back. *Curr Opin HIV and AIDS* 2008; **3**:180–85.

Rollins N, Papathakis P. HIV and nutrition: pregnant and lactating women. *Consultation on Nutrition and HIV/AIDS in Africa: Evidence, Lessons and Recommendations for Action*. Duban, South Africa: Department of Nutrition for Health and Development, World Health Organization, 2005.

Schaible UE, Kaufmann SHE. Malnutrition and infection: complex mechanisms and global impacts. *PLoS Med* 2007; 4:e115 doi:10.1371/journal.pmed.004011.

Schwenk A, Macallan D. Tuberculosis, malnutrition and wasting. *Curr Opin Clin Nutr Metab Care* 2000; 3:285–91.

UNAIDS. Report on the global AIDS epidemic. 2008. Geneva, UNAIDS. Available at http://data.unaids.org/pub/GlobalReport/2008/jc1510_2008_global_report_pp325_358_en.pdf.

Weber R, Sabin CA, Friis-Møller N *et al.* Liver-related deaths in persons infected with the human immunodeficiency virus: the D:A:D study. *Arch Intern Med* 2006; **166**:1632–41.

WHO. The Management of Opportunistic Infections and General Symptoms of HIV/AIDS, 2006. Clinical Protocol for the WHO European Region, WHO Regional Office for Europe. Available at http://www.euro.who.int/document/SHA/Chap_2_IOs_for_web.pdf.

Section 2
PAEDIATRIC NUTRITION, MATERNAL AND CHILD HEALTH

3 Malnutrition, Infant Feeding, Maternal and Child Health

Theresa Banda, Vivian Pribram,
Margaret Lawson, Catherine Mkangama
and Gertrude Nyirenda

Key Points

- Most children become infected with HIV through mother-to-child transmission (MTCT) during pregnancy, delivery or breastfeeding.
- Prevention of mother-to-child transmission (PMTCT) programmes have significantly reduced MTCT of HIV by up to <1%.
- HIV counselling and testing should be routinely offered to women and their partners to help empower them to make informed choices about their reproductive life, access to PMTCT services, and appropriate infant feeding practices.
- Current infant feeding options are exclusive breastfeeding or replacement feeding, providing specific conditions are met.
- There is a high prevalence of HIV among children with severe acute malnutrition (SAM) and mortality rates are very high.
- There is a need to generate new standards for quality of care in nutrition rehabilitation of children with complicated SAM.

3.1 Introduction

The global HIV epidemic continues to be a challenge for both males and females, old and young, with women and children being particularly vulnerable to HIV infection due to a variety of factors. The vast majority of people living with HIV (PLHIV) are in the developing world, with more than two-thirds in sub-Saharan Africa. Seventy-two per cent of all deaths from AIDS in 2007 occurred in this region.

In some parts of the world, females (aged 15–24 years) are more likely to be infected than men of the same age (UNAIDS, 2008). Reports show that women constitute half of the people living with HIV worldwide and that their share of infection is increasing in several countries (UNAIDS, 2008).

Reports indicate that the number of children less than 15 years of age living with HIV increased from 1.6 million to 2 million from 2001 to 2007 and almost 90% of these live in sub-Saharan Africa (UNAIDS, 2008). Most children become infected with HIV through mother-to-child transmission (MTCT). Programmes for prevention of MTCT (PMTCT) have been developed, introduced and rolled out in different countries to reduce prevalence of paediatric HIV infection. Global reports show that provision of antiretroviral therapy (ART) through PMTCT programmes to pregnant women living with HIV in low- and middle-income countries increased from 9% in 2004 to 33% in 2007 (UNAIDS, 2008). According to UNAIDS estimates, the annual incidence of children newly infected with HIV has declined worldwide since 2002 due to expansion of PMTCT services in different countries. Annual AIDS-related deaths are also reported to be falling due to scale up of treatment and PMTCT services (UNAIDS, 2008). In high-income countries, such as the UK and the USA, wide implementation of PMTCT interventions has virtually eliminated HIV infections amongst children. By contrast, in the hardest hit countries of sub-Saharan Africa such as South Africa, Zimbabwe, Botswana, Namibia, Uganda, Tanzania, Rwanda and Kenya, where 61% of all women living with HIV reside, and where most of the HIV infections in children occur through MTCT, scaling up of PMTCT programmes began at a much later stage (UNAIDS, 2008).

Undernutrition is the largely preventable cause of over a third (3.5 million) of all child deaths. Stunting, severe wasting, and intrauterine growth restriction are among the most important problems. The golden interval for intervention is from pregnancy to 2 years of age, after which undernutrition will have caused irreversible damage for future development towards adulthood (Horton, 2008). There are proven effective interventions to reduce stunting and micronutrient deficiencies: breastfeeding counselling, vitamin A supplementation, and zinc fortification have the greatest benefits. Attention to maternal nutrition through adequate dietary intake in pregnancy and supplementation with iron, folic acid and, possibly, other micronutrients and calcium are likely to provide value (Horton, 2008).

Although the importance of nutrition in the treatment and care of people living with HIV/AIDS is now widely recognised, it has been a neglected aspect of treatment programmes.

3.2   Maternal health and nutrition

3.2.1   Undernutrition and maternal health: prevalence and consequences

Globally, some 10–19% of women of reproductive age are undernourished (defined as a body mass index (BMI) of less than 18.5 kg/m^2. A serious problem of maternal undernutrition is evident in most countries in sub-Saharan Africa, south-central and southeastern Asia, and in Yemen, where more than 20% of women have a body-mass index of less than 18.5 kg/m^2. Maternal short stature and low body-mass index have independent adverse effects on pregnancy outcomes (Black et al., 2008).

3.2.2   Maternal health and nutritional status during pregnancy

The nutritional status of a woman before and during pregnancy is important for a healthy pregnancy outcome. Low maternal body-mass index is associated with intrauterine growth retardation. Macronutrients (protein, fatty acids and energy) are important for foetal growth and development. Adequate maternal nutrition supports the growth of both maternal and foetal tissues and helps to ensure the birth of a healthy infant. It reduces the likelihood of miscarriage, stillbirth and low birthweight babies (Black et al., 2008).

The amount of weight gained by the mother during pregnancy depends on various factors such as pre-pregnancy weight, activity level and body size. Teenage mothers need extra nutrients to support their own growth as well as the baby's and are urged to gain enough weight despite their body type and size to support the growth of both themselves and the baby. Dieting to reduce weight during pregnancy and lactation is not recommended (USAID/AED, 1999).

Specific micronutrients such as vitamin A, zinc, iodine, iron and folate are also required for the healthy development of the foetus and maternal health. In developed countries, most of these micronutrient requirements, with the exception of iron, can be met from a normal diet. However, in many developing countries, diets are often deficient in micronutrients so supplementation is required, especially of iron and folate.

3.2.3 Nutritional status and HIV infection: pregnancy and lactation

Women infected with HIV, particularly in limited resource settings who have high levels of background poverty, malnutrition and food insecurity, may be particularly at risk when they are pregnant or lactating due to increased energy needs which, in many cases are not met unless supplemented. Many women are already energy deficient prior to becoming pregnant. The increased metabolic and nutrient demands of pregnancy and lactation, in conjunction with poor nutritional status compounded by HIV infection, will increase the risk of maternal depletion of nutrient stores (Bentley et al., 2005) and also the risk of mortality.

In a review of nutrition in pregnant and lactating women with HIV, the rates of weight gain reported in HIV-positive mothers were found to be consistent with weight gains in undernourished pregnant women in developing countries. A high proportion of women were found with low or deficient folate or with low vitamin A status. Rates of anaemia also suggest that many pregnant women living with HIV (WLHIV) in developing countries do not consume a varied diet rich in micronutrients and do not have access to prenatal supplements. Some evidence shows that low or deficient levels of folate, albumin and vitamin A are associated with an increased viral load and decreased CD4$^+$ cell counts (Papathakis and Rollins, 2005). Micronutrient deficiencies develop early in the course of the HIV infection and are often complicated by poor absorption, reduced oral intake, increased utilisation and loss of nutrients contributing to increased needs among individuals infected with HIV (Friis, 2002).

Breastfeeding does not seem to increase the mortality of WLHIV but there may be an increased risk of weight loss during breastfeeding compared to those without HIV infection (Papathakis and Rollins, 2005). This should be balanced against the risk to the infant of diarrhoeal disease if the infant is not breastfed. Nutrition supplementation for the mother should be the primary line of intervention and not cessation of breastfeeding.

Maternal undernutrition has little effect on the volume or composition of breast milk unless malnutrition is very severe. The concentration of some micronutrients (vitamin A, iodine, thiamin, riboflavin, pyridoxine and cobalamin) in breast milk is dependent on maternal status and intake, so the risk of infant depletion is increased by maternal deficiency (Friis, 2002). This factor is most evident in the case of vitamin A, where the content in breast milk is the main determinant of an infant's status because stores are low at birth. Maternal supplementation with these micronutrients increases the amount secreted in breast milk, which can improve infant status (Black *et al.*, 2008).

3.2.4 Pregnancy and micronutrient supplementation

Micronutrients that may be important for maternal, infant and child outcomes include iron, vitamin B_{12}, folic acid, vitamin A, vitamin D and selenium (Bhutta and Haider, 2009). There is a need for close monitoring of iron supplementation in HIV infection due to concerns that this may increase replication of HIV and lead to adverse outcomes (McDermid *et al.*, 2007).

Care should be taken not to exceed an intake of 3000 μg daily of vitamin A as this can be harmful to the foetus (WHO, 1998). Micronutrient supplementation and fortification have been identified as among the most cost-effective interventions to address infant and child undernutrition globally (Deolalikar and Martonell, 2008). Studies are ongoing in the general population, but if proven effective and safe, multiple micronutrient supplementation may replace supplementation with iron and folate only, in future (Bhutta and Haider, 2009). Women with dark skin living in the Northern Hemisphere are at particular risk of vitamin D deficiency due to limited sunlight and levels should be monitored. There are no specific recommendations for micronutrient supplementation for WLHIV during pregnancy and lactation. Local/national guidelines for the general population should also be followed by WLHIV.

UK health departments recommend:

- 10 micrograms of vitamin D each day for pregnant and breastfeeding women
- 400 micrograms of folic acid for women who may become pregnant and up until the 12th week of pregnancy.

A daily dose of vitamins A, C and D for:

- breastfed infants from 6 months (or from 1 month if there is any doubt about the mother's vitamin status during pregnancy)
- formula-fed infants who are over 6 months and taking less than 500 ml infant formula per day
- children under 5 years of age (Healthy Start, 2009).

In areas where vitamin A deficiency is endemic, a supplement is recommended during pregnancy with a bolus at delivery, plus a bolus dose at age 6 months for all infants (WHO, 1998)

3.2.5 Maternal energy and protein requirements

Pregnant and lactating women without HIV have increased energy requirements of between 200 and 500 kcal per day, according to USAID data (USAID/AED, 1999). For people living with HIV (PLHIV) who are not pregnant or lactating, WHO recommends an increase in energy intake by 10% in asymptomatic cases and by 20–30% for those displaying symptoms (WHO, 2003b). This suggests that pregnant and lactating WLHIV have substantially increased energy requirements compared to women without HIV and PLHIV without pregnancy and infant feeding concerns (WHO/FAO/UNU, 2007).

Specific nutrient requirements for pregnant and lactating HIV-positive women need to be developed and disseminated. Careful monitoring during the antenatal period will support the mother and the foetus in the meantime.

3.2.6 Maternal nutritional assessment

Estimation of body composition and nutritional assessment (including clinical and biochemical parameters and an assessment of dietary intake) are important to determine appropriate nutritional interventions (see Chapters 4 and 8). Simple anthropometric measurements of height, weight and MUAC are generally useful to monitor adiposity during pregnancy and lactation (Papathakis and Rollins, 2005).

- Mid-upper arm circumference (MUAC) (see Chapters 4 and 8) recommended for screening and management of identified malnutrition in both pregnant and lactating women. The measurement is independent of gestational age in pregnant women and has been investigated as a screening tool for low birthweight, late foetal and infant mortality (Gibson, 2005). The following criteria are used for pregnant and lactating women based on SPHERE standards (The Sphere Project, 2004):
  - **MUAC <230 mm** in the mother is associated with moderate risk and growth retardation of the foetus. Using this cut-off for feeding programmes would help identify malnutrition for both the foetus and the mother and interventions could potentially improve birth outcomes.
  - In most interventions in developing countries <220 mm is used for inclusion in nutrition programmes.
  - A MUAC of <190 mm is used as a criterion for severe acute malnutrition (SAM) (Ministry of Health and Population. Malawi, 2003).

Regular body weight monitoring

Pregnant women should be encouraged to attend antenatal clinics to benefit from PMTCT services. A pregnant woman is expected to gain weight about 1–2 kg by the end of the first trimester and about 0.5 kg each week until delivery. Mothers that do not gain 1 kg per month in the second and third trimester should be referred to a health facility for assessment, counselling and appropriate care (Shetty et al., 2003). Any loss of weight or static weight needs discussion with the mother to identify the causes and agree on a plan of action to promote weight gain (unless the mother had a high BMI to start with). Weight loss might indicate medical problems such as TB or HIV or inappropriate energy intake and or household food insecurity (Ministry of Health, Uganda, 2004).

Oedema as a marker of malnutrition

- Oedema is a non-specific sign of health and nutrition and may be associated with pre-eclampsia or other problems of pregnancy. It is important to ascertain if oedema is associated with signs of malnutrition such as:
  - MUAC <220 mm
  - shiny skin or discoloured skin and hair
  - thinning of arms, legs and waist

Anaemia

Follow local guidelines for nutritional screening and assessment as these may vary. Not all anaemia is due to dietary deficiency: parasites and the presence of haemoglobinopathies may also cause iron deficiency and require different treatment:

- Paleness of inner lids and palms may be a sign of anaemia.
- Individuals displaying any signs of anaemia should have their haemoglobin level checked. A result of <11 mg/dl should be referred for treatment, which may include food-based supplementation.

3.2.7   Nutrition counselling

Nutrition counselling, care and support are integral to comprehensive HIV care and should ideally already be in place before pregnancy. However, many women are tested for HIV for the first time at an antenatal clinic and may not be part of any HIV programme.

Nutritional counselling has been found to improve energy intake and certain aspects of cognitive function in PLHIV (Rabeneck et al., 1998) and better nutrition status is associated with improved birth outcomes for both mother and child. Nutrition counselling includes the management of nutrition-related symptoms of common HIV-related illnesses/opportunistic infections, and management of drug side effects impeding oral intake such as nausea and diarrhoea (Ministry of Health Malawi, 2007) (see Chapter 9, 'Symptom Control and Management') and support for appropriate infant feeding choices starting in pregnancy.

3.2.8   Moderate and severe acute malnutrition

Following diagnosis of malnutrition in pregnancy, WHO or local nutrition rehabilitation protocols for moderate or severe acute malnutrition can be followed.

3.2.9   Management of symptoms associated with HIV and pregnancy

Nausea and vomiting usually occurs in pregnancy, in the first trimester, due to hormonal imbalances, but in HIV it is also a common condition occurring due to frequent infections or as a side effect for people who are on ART. Therefore, if a woman is both pregnant and HIV positive, it is likely that she will experience a heightened degree of nausea and vomiting and may require special advice to help maintain oral intake. For management of nausea, vomiting and other conditions including mouth pain (e.g. due to oral thrush), change or loss of taste, swallowing difficulties, loss of appetite, diarrhoea and fatigue (including fatigue related to anaemia), please see Chapter 9, 'Symptom Control and Management').

Heartburn (indigestion) is also common in pregnancy. Women are advised to eat small frequent meals, avoid spicy food and to avoid lying down after meals.

3.2.10   Food safety

Foods that should be avoided during pregnancy include:

- some types of cheeses: Camembert, Brie or chèvre (a type of goat's cheese), or others that have a similar rind; soft blue cheeses
- pate including vegetarian pate
- raw or lightly cooked eggs
- raw or undercooked meat
- liver products and supplements containing vitamin A
- undercooked ready meals
- some types of fish: avoid swordfish, marlin, shark; have no more than two portions of oily fish per week, and no more than 140 g of tuna per week (FSA, 2009).

Refer to local/national guidelines (see Chapter 17, 'Food and Water Safety').

3.2.11   Summary

Good nutrition is essential during pregnancy to provide adequate nutrients to maintain normal body functions, to support immune function in HIV infection, to prevent premature and /low birthweight babies and to support lactation (where this is advised). The role of nutrition support in treatment regimens should be investigated as a matter of priority in order to develop treatment and care programmes that deliver effective nutrition support to pregnant and lactating women living with HIV. Nutrition counselling care, support and assessment are crucial processes during this period and should be an integral part of PMTCT, ART and other HIV and pre- and post-natal care services.

3.3   Mother-to-child transmission

Mother-to-child transmission (MTCT) occurs when an infected mother passes the virus directly to her baby either during pregnancy, labour and delivery, or during breastfeeding. Without treatment, it is estimated that around 15–30% of babies born to WLHIV would become infected with HIV during pregnancy and delivery, and a further 5–20% would become infected through breastfeeding (De Cock *et al.*, 2000).

WHO guidelines *(WHO, 2009a – Rapid advice: use of antiretroviral drugs for treating pregnant women and preventing HIV infection in infants. WHO Switzerland, 2009b)* now recommend that all HIV-positive pregnant women, whether they show symptoms or not, should receive ART from 14 weeks of pregnancy at least until the end of breastfeeding. Women with severe or advanced disease, or those who present with a CD4 count of less than 350 cells/mm^2 should receive lifelong ART.

Antiretroviral therapy (ART) should be administered during pregnancy and labour to: reduce viral replication, lower maternal plasma viral load to reduce transmission in utero and during delivery, and also as post-exposure prophylaxis for HIV-exposed infants whether breastfeeding or not (Volmink *et al.*, 2007). It is estimated that ART for all HIV-positive pregnant women, irrespective of clinical status, could prevent 75% of all MTCT (WHO, 2009b).

Implementation of PMTCT interventions such as pre-labour Caesarean section, formula feeding and ART has been shown to reduce transmission to less than 1% for pregnant women in developed countries.

In developing countries, similar trends in reduction of MTCT have been reported. For example, the government of Botswana reported reduction of MTCT of HIV to less than 4% (William, 2009). However prevention of mother-to-child transmission (PMTCT) interventions must always be balanced against other risks to mortality in the local environment. In developing countries this particularly applies to elective Caesarean and infant feeding choices.

While there is inconclusive evidence for the role of micronutrient supplementation in MTCT, Fawzi et al. concluded that although multivitamin and vitamin A supplementation did not influence rates of MTCT, micronutrient supplementation improved CD4 lymphocyte counts and infant weight as well as decreasing the risk of growth restriction and severe prematurity (Fawzi et al., 2002).

3.3.1 Prevention of mother-to-child transmission

Prevention of mother-to-child transmission in resource-limited settings is the biggest challenge that health workers, pregnant women, families and governments face in their efforts to reduce prevalence of HIV in children. MTCT has been associated with several factors including advanced maternal HIV disease, a high maternal plasma viral load, vaginal delivery, prematurity and breastfeeding, particularly if the mother has cracked nipples or mastitis (Foster and Lyall, 2003). Prevention of MTCT strategies include HIV testing and counselling, provision of ART during pregnancy and throughout breastfeeding, choosing delivery methods that reduce risk of transmission such as elective Caesarean and choice of feeding practices that are suitable for the physical and socio-economic environment of the family.

PMTCT programmes aim to deliver healthy infants and to maintain the health of the mother. In order to benefit, individuals must be aware of their HIV status and the general public should be encouraged to be HIV tested and counselled in order to enable them to make informed choices on their reproductive lives. The health care provider has a moral, legal and ethical responsibility to help ensure that pregnant women and their families understand available options.

Most women preparing to parent a newborn are concerned about their baby's health and safety and therefore are receptive to the information that health care professionals can provide. Unfortunately, in many cases pre-conception discussion between WLHIV and health care providers does not take place. The management of HIV infection in pregnancy requires careful consideration of the balance between the mother's health needs, locally available prevention and treatment options and the need to reduce mother-to-child transmission.

3.3.2 Summary

WLHIV with children face the additional challenges of complex medication regimens, infant feeding choices, greater risk of infections and poor wound healing due to compromised immunity. Good adherence to drug regimens for themselves and their infants must be encouraged and supported. Women and their infants should be monitored closely for general health and development to ensure optimal maternal and child health. Prevention of mother-to-child transmission (PMTCT) services are crucial to reduce HIV transmission and mortality and should form an integrated part of maternal and child health service (WHO, 2009a).

3.4   Infant feeding in the context of HIV

3.4.1   Overview

Without any intervention, it is estimated that 5–20% of infants born to HIV-infected women would acquire the virus from breastfeeding. Transmission occurs at any time the infant is breastfeeding; however, exclusive breastfeeding for the first few months carries a relatively low risk of transmission (Coovadia *et al.*, 2007). Provision of ART for the mother and her infant throughout the entire period of breastfeeding should reduce the risk of MTCT through breast milk to <5% (WHO, 2009a).

Regardless of HIV status, infant and young child feeding practices have a direct impact on child nutrition which is essential for growth, health and development. Poor nutritional status increases the risk of illness, contributes to mortality and can lead to long-term health problems such as obesity (WHO, 2003a) Optimal infant feeding for the first 2 years of life provides an opportunity for ensuring ideal growth and development (World Bank, 2006).

Evidence shows that universal optimal breastfeeding could prevent 13% of deaths occurring worldwide in children under 5 years of age and appropriate complementary feeding practices could lead to an additional 6% reduction in under-5 mortality rates (WHO, 2003a).

The World Health Assembly (WHA) and UNICEF adopted the Global Strategy for Infant and Young Child Feeding to focus world attention on the impact of feeding practices on nutritional status, growth, development, health and survival.

3.4.2   Recommended feeding options of infants at risk of HIV infection

According to the 2009 consensus statement (WHO, 2009b Rapid Advice: HIV and Infant Feeding; revised principles and recommendations November 2009):

- ART given to pregnant women or to the infant should continue for 1 week after all breastfeeding has ceased.
- Exclusive breastfeeding is recommended for infants born to WLHIV for the first 6 months of life.
- Complementary foods should be introduced at age 6 months and breastfeeding should continue for 12 months in environments where replacement feeding is not appropriate.
- Breastfeeding should only stop when a nutritionally adequate and safe diet can be provided without breast milk.
- When replacement feeding is appropriate, avoidance of all breastfeeding by HIV-infected women is recommended.
- The most appropriate infant feeding option for an HIV-infected mother should continue to depend on her individual circumstances and resources.

3.4.3   Situations where replacement feeding may be appropriate

a. Safe water and sanitation are assured at the household level and in the community
b. the mother or other caregiver can reliably provide sufficient infant formula milk to support normal growth and development of the infant
c. the mother or caregiver can prepare it cleanly and frequently enough so that it is safe and carries a low risk of diarrhoea and malnutrition
d. the mother or caregiver can, in the first 6 months, exclusively give infant formula milk
e. the family is supportive of this practice, and
f. the mother or caregiver can access health care that offers comprehensive child health services.

These definitions of specific conditions where replacement feeding may be considered replace the earlier conditions described as AFASS (acceptable, feasible, affordable, sustainable and safe) detailed by the 2006 WHO recommendations on feeding infants of WLHIV (WHO, 2006a).

HIV transmission through breastfeeding is a rare issue in the developed world where there is access to safe, clean water and where milk substitutes are affordable and easily available. In the UK and other well-resourced countries, avoidance of breastfeeding by WLHIV is recommended to prevent transmission of HIV via this route, in accordance with the 2006 consensus statement (WHO, 2006a). In this situation the risk of HIV transmission is far greater than the risks associated with replacement feeding (DH, 2004). This advice does not apply in countries without uninterrupted access to infant formula milk and clean water. WHO reviewed recommendations in 2009 to reflect the needs of breastfeeding populations in under-resourced settings (WHO, 2009b).

In the developing world the health risks of WLHIV breastfeeding are smaller than those of replacement feeding, even without ART backup. This is due to the high mortality rate from diarrhoeal diseases as a consequence of lack of safe water, reduced resistance to gastrointestinal infections in formula-fed babies and lack of resources for the supply and preparation of breast milk substitutes (Birahinduka, 2007). Although HIV can be transmitted through breastfeeding, there is no doubt that an infant's chances of survival when living in a poor or rural community are greatly decreased by not breastfeeding (Rollins, 2007). Exclusive breastfeeding for up to 6 months has been associated with substantially decreased risk of transmission of HIV compared to non-exclusive breastfeeding in three large cohort studies (WHO, 2007). Breastfeeding of HIV-infected infants beyond 6 months was associated with improved survival compared to those who stopped breastfeeding (WHO, 2007) and in resource-poor settings breastfeeding should continue until age 1 year or until a safe and adequate diet is available without breast milk.

Counselling about infant feeding options for the HIV-positive women and their partners needs to start during pregnancy and should include the risks of MTCT of the virus through breastfeeding with and without ART backup; appropriate feeding options that are feasible in the local context considering national policies; and advantages and disadvantages of each option (WHO, 2002; WHO, UNICEF, UNFPA & UNAIDS, 2007; WHO, 2009b).

Once a decision about infant feeding has been made, ideally a home visit to confirm the appropriateness of the choice should be made. If there is doubt about the choice made, counselling should be offered to review feeding choices.

Counselling and support for infant feeding should continue during pregnancy, delivery and the post-natal period. The risk of transmission of HIV from mother to child increases greatly if the infant is mixed-fed with both breast and formula milk. Mothers who choose to breastfeed should be supported to breastfeed exclusively to ensure an adequate milk supply and to prevent breast problems such as mastitis, cracked and sore nipples.

During counselling, all HIV-positive mothers should be encouraged to receive medication appropriate both for their own health and for reasons of PMTCT.

3.4.4 Breastfeeding

Breastfeeding is the most natural and best way of feeding infants. The benefits of breastfeeding related to infant health, survival, growth and development, and maternal health are well known and widely reported in the literature (USAID/AED, 1999) This includes nutritional, anti-infective, contraceptive, psychological, economic and long-term health benefits.

However, breastfeeding poses an ongoing transmission risk for WLHIV. Without ART medication it is known to double the rate of mother-to-child transmission of HIV compared to replacement feeding with transmission highest during the first few months of life (De Cock *et al.*, 2000). A number of factors are associated with increased transmission of HIV through breastfeeding (WHO, UNICEF & USAID, 2008):

- a high maternal viral load
- severity of the disease as indicated by low CD4 count and high RNA viral load
- severe clinical symptoms
- poor breast health, including mastitis, subclinical mastitis and fissured nipples
- poor maternal nutritional status
- infant oral infection (thrush and herpes)
- mixed feeding
- duration of breastfeeding beyond 6 months.

3.4.5 Exclusive breastfeeding

Exclusive breastfeeding on demand for the first 6 months of life meets all the energy and nutrient requirements of the majority of infants (WHO, UNICEF & UNFPA, 2006, WHO, 2009b). It is defined as feeding only breast milk (from the mother or a wet nurse), or expressed breast milk and no other liquids. All other liquids, even water, are excluded. Oral dehydration solution, drops or syrups consisting of vitamins, minerals supplements or medicine can be included. Studies have shown that healthy infants that are exclusively breastfed do not need additional water even in hot climates as breast milk contains sufficient water to satisfy the infant's thirst (WHO, 2002). Many mothers and family members do not believe this and give the baby water and other fluids as early as the first week. This practice constitutes mixed feeding and is associated with a twofold increased risk of diarrhoea (Butte *et al.*, 2002). Exclusive breastfeeding for up to 6 months was associated with a three- to fourfold decrease in risk of transmission of HIV compared to mixed breastfeeding in three large cohort studies conducted in Cote d'Ivoire, South Africa and Zimbabwe. Other studies have found, that with exclusive breastfeeding, deaths due to diarrhoea and pneumonia could be reduced by a third compared to mix-fed infants for the first 4 months (WHO, 2007). It is recommended that all mothers whether they are infected with HIV or not should *exclusively* breastfeed their infants for the first 6 months unless replacement feeding meets specific conditions (see Section 3.4.2).

3.4.6   Replacement feeding

Replacement feeding is defined as a process whereby a non-breastfed child is given foods that provide all nutrients normally obtained from breast milk; the process continues until the child is fully established on family foods (Shetty *et al.*, 2003; WHO, UNICEF, UNFPA & UNAIDS, 2007). *This feeding option is recommended only* if it meets specific conditions (see above Section 3.4.2). In the UK, infant formula milk is advised as an alternative to breast milk for the first 12 months of life until cow's milk can be introduced (DH, 2004). In regions where the specific conditions can be met, support and advice on replacement feeding are still needed: it can be difficult to implement in an environment where breastfeeding is encouraged by health care professionals. There may be pressure to breastfeed from family and friends who are unaware of the mother's HIV status and many women think people will become aware of their HIV status if replacement feeding is used. The advantage of replacement feeding is that there is a reduced risk of transmission of HIV from mother to infant and the mother's body reserves are not depleted. However, problems associated with replacement feeding include a higher risk of other infections to the child as breast milk substitutes do not transfer mother's protective antibodies, and poorer nutritional status if the replacement feed is not designed for infants or is misused.

3.4.7   Types of replacement feeding

Heat-treated expressed breast milk

Expressed breast milk (EBM) can be heated to kill HIV virus in milk. Heat-treated expressed breast milk can be considered as an interim strategy in specific circumstances (WHO, 2009b):

- where an infant is born with low birthweight or is ill during the neonatal period and unable to breastfeed
- where the mother is unwell or has temporary breast health problems and is unable to breastfeed
- where ARV drugs are temporarily unavailable
- to assist mothers to stop breastfeeding.

Methods of home treatment of EBM (Israel-Ballard *et al.*, 2007) include:

- a covered container of milk is placed in a pan of water so that the water level is above the milk; water is brought to the boil and the milk is removed and allowed to cool
- water is brought to the boil, removed from the heat and a covered container of milk is placed into the pan and left for 20 minutes.

The use of heat-treated expressed breast milk is not recommended as a long-term feeding strategy for HIV infected mothers who wish to breastfeed (WHO, 2009b). Heat treatment of EBM requires time and organisation and needs significant support. Where this method is used training should be given on the correct method to express milk, heat treatment, cup feeding and appropriate quantities of EBM (Shetty *et al.*, 2003; WHO, UNICEF, UNFPA & UNAIDS, 2007). Heat-treated EBM carries with it a risk of food-borne infection and advice on safe preparation and storage should be included in training.

Wet nursing

Wet nursing describes the process where a lactating woman breastfeeds an infant who is not her own. If the family decides on a wet nurse, she will need all the support that a breastfeeding mother needs, including counselling about avoiding any risk of HIV infection for the duration of breastfeeding and good breast health (WHO, UNICEF, UNFPA & UNAIDS, 2003a, b).

Modified animal milk

Unmodified and home-modified animal milk is no longer recommended as a replacement feed for infants less than 6 months of age because it does not provide all the nutrients that the infant needs (Sidley, 2005; WHO, 2009b). According to WHO Guidelines, undiluted animal milks can be added to the diet and served as a suitable substitute for breast milk for children 6 months of age and older. The recommended volumes are 200–400 ml per day if adequate amounts of other sources of foods are consumed regularly, otherwise it is 300–500 ml per day (WHO, 2006b). However, in the UK it is recommended that cow's milk, as a drink, should not be introduced before the infant is 1 year old (FSA, 2009).

Infant formula

There are two main types of infant formulas: starter formulas suitable for use from birth, and follow-on milks, suitable for use after the age of 6 months. They should comply with WHO recommendations (Codex, 1987) and provide all nutrients necessary for normal growth and development. Powdered infant formulas are likely to be expensive and beyond the reach of families in resource-poor environments. The high cost of infant formula often means that they are given in small quantities, over-diluted or mixed with less nutritious foods such as porridge, resulting in severe malnutrition in young infants. They should only be recommended where the family can afford to provide them in adequate quantities for at least 6 months.

3.4.8 Preparation of feeds

Preparation of feeds requires soap, water, fuel and utensils, time to make feeds and knowledge of how to prepare them accurately and hygienically. They need detailed guidelines on how to measure milk, water and other ingredients and how to clean utensils. Commercial infant formula must be prepared according to the instructions on the label and given in quantities appropriate for the child's weight and age.

Information about the volume of feeds is also included on the label. Powdered infant feeds are not microbiologically safe and it is important to make up the feed with water at a temperature of about 70°C. In practice this means boiling the water and leaving it to cool for no longer than 30 minutes. After preparation the feed needs to be further cooled so that the milk should not feel hot when dropped onto the back of the wrist before giving to the baby. Feeds should be made up as required and not stored (DH, 2007; WHO, 2007). Safe preparation, storage and handling of powdered infant formula). Because of the difficulty of adequately cleaning baby bottles and teats (nipples), cup feeding rather than bottle-feeding is recommended in environments where adequate hygiene is in doubt.

3.4.9   Management of transition from breastfeeding to replacement feeding

Mothers or infants who have been receiving ARV prophylaxis should continue with medication for 1 week after breastfeeding is fully stopped (WHO, 2009a, b).

Mothers who choose to stop breastfeeding should be assisted when changing to replacement feeding if appropriate or if the infant is old enough to get all nutritional requirements from family foods.

Mothers are supported to gradually stop breastfeeding over a period a period of about 1 month. Abrupt cessation of breastfeeding is no longer recommended (WHO, 2009b). The mother may need to express breast milk and heat it (see Section 3.4.7) to accustom the baby to cup feeding of EBM. She can then gradually reduce breastfeeds (express and discard milk in between feeds to keep breasts healthy until the end of the process) and replace EBM, changing from EBM to replacement feeds given by cup. This process of separation is emotionally difficult for both mother and baby and should be discussed in counselling beforehand and maximum support given when the decision is made to go ahead. Cup feeding should be attempted, prior to the 6-month deadline, to aid the transition.

3.4.10   Complementary feeding

Complementary feeding is defined as the process of introducing other foods and liquids when breast milk or replacement feeding is no longer adequate to satisfy the nutritional requirements of the infant. At 6 months of age complementary foods should be introduced and the child should continue to be fed the same amounts of milk feeds, although there might be variation due to availability of milk and other foods the child demands. This is recommended from the age of 6–23 months, even though breastfeeding may continue beyond 2 years (WHO, UNICEF, UNFPA & UNAIDS, 2007; WHO, 2009b). It is important to refer to national policies for PMTCT as these may differ between countries.

Mothers living with HIV should continue to breastfeed their infants until the age of 1 year and give complementary foods in addition. All breastfeeding should stop once an adequate diet without breast milk can be provided (Shetty et al., 2003; WHO, UNICEF, UNFPA & UNAIDS, 2007). For children who do not breastfeed and do not have adequate breast milk substitutes, there is a need to provide nutrients, through extra meals and snacks, that would otherwise be met by breast milk or breast milk substitute.

If infants and young children are known to be HIV-infected, mothers are strongly encouraged to exclusively breastfeed for the first 6 months of life and continue breastfeeding as per the recommendations for the general population, that is up to 2 years or beyond (WHO, 2009b).

3.4.11   Follow-up and support

All HIV-exposed infants should receive regular follow-up care and periodic re-assessment of infant feeding practices choices, particularly at the time of infant diagnosis and at 6 months. Infant diagnosis should not change the decision to breastfeed or not. Mothers should be discouraged from stopping breastfeeding on a negative infant diagnosis if they do not meet the conditions for replacement feeding. Care and support should continue for all mothers and caregivers for at least 2 years to ensure that the child is adequately fed and growing. Weight and growth monitoring is essential (see Chapter 4, 'Paediatric Nutritional Screening, Assessment and Support').

3.5   Malnutrition in children with HIV

3.5.1   Malnutrition

Malnutrition encompasses stunting, wasting and deficiencies of essential vitamins and minerals as one form of the condition known as malnutrition, with obesity or over-consumption of specific nutrients as another form (Black *et al.*, 2008).

3.5.2   Maternal and child undernutrition

Maternal and child undernutrition remains a pervasive and damaging condition in low- and middle-income countries. A framework developed by UNICEF recognises the basic and underlying causes of undernutrition, including the environmental, economic and socio-political contextual factors, with poverty playing a central role (Black *et al.*, 2008).

Maternal and child undernutrition is the underlying cause of 3.5 million deaths, 35% of the disease burden in children younger than 5 years and 11% of total global disability-adjusted life years (DALYs) (Black *et al.*, 2008). Deficiencies of vitamin A and zinc, sub-optimal breastfeeding and maternal iron deficiency are responsible for many of these deaths and DALYs (Black *et al.*, 2008).

3.5.3   Prevalence wasting and severe wasting

The global estimate of wasting (weight-for-height Z score below minus two (-2)) is 10% (55 million children). South-central Asia is estimated to have the highest prevalence (16%) and numbers affected (29 million). Most children with severe wasting (weight-for-height Z score below minus 3 (-3)), live in South Asia and Central Africa, where such malnutrition accounts for a large number of deaths in children aged under 5 years (Black *et al.*, 2008; Bhutta, 2009). The prevalence of Severe acute Malnutrition (SAM), is 3·5% or 19 million children. SAM is often used

Table 3.1 Recommendation for diagnostic criteria for SAM in children aged 6–60 months.

Indicator	Measure	Cut-off
Severe wasting*	Weight-for-height†	≤ 3 SD
Severe wasting*	MUAC	< 115 mm
Bilateral oedema*	Clinical sign	

*Independent indications of SAM that require urgent action.
†Based on WHO Standards (www.who.int/childgrowth/standards) (see Appendices 2–4).
Source: WHO and UNICEF, 2009. Note: At the time of going to press the changeover of reference standards being used was in process. It was recommended therefore that both the WHO standards and the older NCHS standards continue to be used as independent criteria for admission, pending further investigation as each method selected different cases using weight-for-height and MUAC.

as a criterion for therapeutic feeding interventions (Black *et al.*, 2008). Children with severe acute malnutrition have almost a tenfold higher risk of dying compared with their non-malnourished counterparts (Bhutta, 2009) and the disorder is associated with 1–2 million preventable child deaths each year (Collins *et al.*, 2006).

While some of this wasting is due to strife and displacement, many populations face chronic poverty and food insecurity and high disease burdens; in particular, the combination of SAM with HIV/AIDS (Bhutta, 2009); see Table 3.1 for the classification of severe acute malnutrition.

By contrast, chronic malnutrition (termed 'stunting') is defined by low height-for-age while composite forms of malnutrition, including elements of both stunting and wasting, is defined using weight-for age (Collins *et al.*, 2006).

3.5.4 Prevalence of HIV and SAM

In a systematic review it was found that, overall, 29.2% of children presenting with SAM were HIV-infected (Fergusson and Tomkins, 2009). Prevalence varied widely between studies and in some study populations it was not possible to confirm HIV test results (Fergusson and Tomkins, 2009). In a Southern African study, prevalence of HIV among children treated for SAM was reported to range from 22 to 54% while case-fatality rates ranged from 20 to 50%, despite the use of WHO guidelines (Chinkhumba *et al.*, 2008). Children with HIV and SAM commonly present with the marasmus presentation of SAM (Collins *et al.*, 2006; Chinkhumba *et al.*, 2008).

3.5.5 Clinical presentation of SAM and HIV

The clinical presentation of SAM has become increasingly complex. SAM and HIV infection often occur in regions with extreme poverty, food insecurity and inadequate health care. Children without HIV infection are also affected due to their mothers' or caretakers' chronic disease and increased orphan status. In Zambia and Malawi, more than half of the patients admitted to nutrition rehabilitation units are HIV positive, with case-fatality rates of 40% or higher within the HIV positive group.

The HIV-uninfected and HIV-infected children both present with severe malnutrition and similar morbidities but have different patho-physiology, case-management and referral pathways, including palliative care. Severe erosion of health systems means that guidelines are difficult to apply (Heikens *et al.*, 2008).

Infants present with multiple pathologies including persistent diarrhoea, *Pneumocystis jirovecii* and other forms of pneumonia, extensive skin infections and oral thrush. Young children aged 3–6 years often present with persistent diarrhoea and, in such children, case fatality is high and response to management as set out in current guidelines is poor. Extremely wasted and stunted young adolescents, previously rarely admitted outside the setting of famine, are now admitted for nutritional recovery and present with chronic HIV-related multi-system disease (Heikens *et al.*, 2008). Severe wasting makes clinical assessment of dehydration difficult, so the presence of metabolic acidosis and lethargy often require resuscitation (Heikens *et al.*, 2008).

3.5.6   Mortality HIV and SAM

In Rwanda, over a 2-year follow-up period following recovery from SAM, 75% of children with HIV died compared with 23% of HIV-negative children. In a Burkina Faso study, it was reported that mortality ranged from 38.4 to 92.3% in seropositive children and from 32.1 to 37.1% in sero-negative children (Fergusson and Tomkins, 2009). This systematic review reported that HIV-infected children were significantly more likely to die than HIV-uninfected children (30.4% vs. 8.4%; $P < 0.001$; relative risk (RR) = 2.81, 95% CI 2.04–3.87). The review authors concluded that higher mortality among HIV-infected children from the same facilities as negative children with SAM is indicative of complex clinical case management issues and a high prevalence of complicated SAM rather than poor quality of care. HIV-infected children with SAM and low CD4 counts are especially vulnerable to complicating opportunistic infections. A 2008 review reported that a low CD4 count was found to be the most important predictor of mortality in untreated HIV-infected children (Cross Continents Collaboration for Kids, 2008; Ferguson and Tomkins, 2009).

3.5.7   Management of SAM

Previously, an exclusive in-patient approach to the clinical care of SAM was recommended. The core of accepted WHO management protocols is the 10-step protocol in two phases (stabilisation and rehabilitation) requiring many trained staff and substantial in-patient bed capacity (Collins *et al.*, 2006; WHO, 1999). This approach has been criticised as it has failed to decrease fatality rates in most hospitals in developing countries. Many hospitals do not have sufficient resources to implement the protocols and there is a lack of control trials looking at the effect of the use of WHO protocols in operational settings (Collins *et al.*, 2006). Added to this, TB and HIV co-infection has increased the workload of hospitals with an increased prevalence of SAM and case fatality rate (Collins *et al.*, 2006). In-patient facility-based treatment of SAM with medical protocols is still necessary for complicated cases, but this is now used in conjunction with community-based management resulting in lower demand on in-patient facilities, and a much wider coverage with the ability to treat uncomplicated cases at home (Figure 3.1).

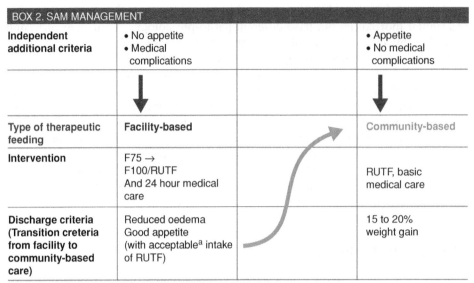

BOX 2. SAM MANAGEMENT			
Independent additional criteria	• No appetite • Medical complications		• Appetite • No medical complications
	↓		↓
Type of therapeutic feeding	**Facility-based**		Community-based
Intervention	F75 → F100/RUTF And 24 hour medical care		RUTF, basic medical care
Discharge criteria (Transition creteria from facility to community-based care)	Reduced oedema Good appetite (with acceptable[a] intake of RUTF)		15 to 20% weight gain

[a] Child eats at least 75% of their calculated RUTF ration for the day

Figure 3.1   SAM Management. With permission from WHO and UNICEF.

3.5.8   Community management of SAM

A major improvement in the management of SAM has been the large-scale community-based management with the introduction of ready-to-use therapeutic foods (Bhutta and Haider, 2009, Heiken *et al.*, 2008) with therapeutic diets and appropriate rehydration fluids are reserved for more severe cases under in-patient care. Community management of acute malnutrition (CMAM) has resulted in recovery rates for uncomplicated severe malnutrition of more than 90%, reported case-fatality rates of less than 5%; and improvements in micronutrient and macronutrient deficiencies (Black *et al.*, 2008; Heikens *et al.*, 2008). CMAM has been widely shown to achieve good rates of nutritional recovery for children with SAM through increased coverage, decreased mortality and increased recovery rates (Ferguuson and Tomkins, 2009).

Box 3.1

Ready-to-use therapeutic food (RUTF) is an energy-dense food enriched with minerals and vitamins, with a similar nutrient profile but greater energy and nutrient density than F100, the diet recommended by WHO for the in-patient treatment of complicated SAM. In contrast to the water-based F100, RUTF is an oil-based paste with an extremely low water activity so that RUTF does not support bacterial growth, even when accidentally contaminated, allowing it to be kept unrefrigerated in simple packaging for several months. As the food is eaten uncooked, heat-labile vitamins are not destroyed during preparation and there are no fuel demands on poor households. The production process is simple, and RUTF can be made from local crops (Collins *et al.*, 2006). The RUTF should be soft or crushable and easy for children to eat without any preparation (WHO, 2009b).

3.5.9   Identifying SAM in children

Community health workers or volunteers can identify children affected by SAM using simple, coloured plastic strips that are designed to measure mid-upper arm circumference (MUAC). The children can then be referred for treatment. Community health workers can also be trained to recognise nutritional oedema of the feet, a sign of kwashiorkor, also a severe form of acute malnutrition (WHO, 2007).

Once children are identified as having SAM, they should be seen by a health worker who has the skills to fully assess them following the Integrated Management of Childhood Illness (IMCI) approach. The health worker should determine whether they can be treated in the community with regular visits to the health centre (if their condition is not complicated by life-threatening illness), or whether referral to an in-patient facility is required (if they have complications). Early detection, coupled with decentralised treatment, makes it possible to start management of SAM before the onset of life-threatening conditions but is dependent on community awareness and early referral (WHO, 2007).

In some community-based therapeutic programmes, children receive 837 kJ/kg/day (200 kcal/kg/day) as a take-home ration of RUTF, a course of oral broad-spectrum antibiotics, vitamin A, folic acid, anthelminthics and, if required, antimalarials (Collins *et al.*, 2006).

3.5.10   Outcomes of community management of HIV and SAM

CMAM has been suggested as being beneficial for HIV-infected children. However, a systematic review in Malawi showed that there was no significant difference in mortality for HIV-infected children with SAM treated in the community (30.0%) or in in-patient facilities (31.3%) (Ferguson and Tomkins, 2009). While CMAM was beneficial in reducing mortality among HIV-uninfected children, these benefits are more likely to be seen in children presenting with uncomplicated malnutrition (Ferguson and Tomkins, 2009). This can include children with HIV as long as early referrals are made.

3.5.11   HIV-related SAM – resources and developments required

Advances have been made initially by improving treatment protocols and more recently with community-focused programmes but challenges persist. In particular, mortality within 4–6 weeks of diagnosis remains unacceptably high (38%, Heikens *et al.*, 2008).

Key issues in the community management of acute malnutrition include scaling up interventions in existing health systems and effectiveness trials to address additional factors that could determine success or failure (Bhutta, 2009). Current issues include:

- New approaches to diagnosis and treatment of childhood tuberculosis are urgently needed in order to prevent complicated SAM. In South Africa, among children with lower respiratory tract infection, tuberculosis was identified 22 times more often among HIV-infected children than in HIV-uninfected children; (WHO, 2003b)

- Moderately and severely malnourished children must be promptly recognised and receive essential life-saving interventions in addition to food. There is little to gain from supply of RUTF alone if effective and timely treatment for malaria, pneumonia and diarrhoea is not available (Bhutta, 2009).
- Rapid and continued access to ART and ancillary support strategies for children with severe acute malnutrition are key to ensuring that HIV-positive children survive and benefit from nutrition interventions (Bhutta, 2009).
- There is an urgent need to integrate HIV testing and treatment into care for children with SAM in regions of high HIV prevalence (Ferguson and Tomkins, 2009). When available, CD4 cell count would help to identify those requiring treatment, since up to a quarter of severely malnourished children in food insecure settings will be above the threshold for initiation of ART (Heikens *et al.*, 2008).

3.5.12   HIV and SAM research recommendations

- International minimum standards for nutrition rehabilitation developed in the emergency context do not reflect the case mix seen in high HIV prevalence settings (Ferguson and Tomkins, 2009). Improvements in initial treatment strategies will depend upon improved knowledge of the cause of infection and antimicrobial susceptibilities (USAID/AED, 1999); pharmacokinetics in malnourished children with HIV; and complex drug interactions and toxicities (e.g. ART and therapy for tuberculosis) (Heikens *et al.*, 2008).

Research recommendations include:

- Areas that require further research:
  - the optimum timing and dosing of ART for children with SAM
  - the definition of the best therapeutic feeding regimens
  - better understanding of acute and chronic infection and the metabolic changes in HIV-infected severely malnourished children
  - improved understanding and development of evidence-based guidelines for the management of severely malnourished children in areas of high HIV prevalence (Heikens *et al.*, 2008)
  - the prevention of severe acute malnutrition (Bhutta, 2009).

3.5.13   Summary

Optimum infant feeding practices in the context of HIV play a very significant role in the prevention of mother-to-child transmission and provide a key component in the prevention of childhood malnutrition and mortality.

The health of the child depends on the health of the mother, so maternal health and effective management of maternal HIV in pregnancy and beyond is paramount to child survival.

SAM in children in high HIV prevalence areas should be seen as a potential clinical indication of HIV and all children with SAM should be tested for HIV status.

High mortality rates in nutrition rehabilitation programmes in regions with high HIV prevalence are not only related to quality of care but are also caused by low CD4 counts and the associated complex case management issues.

Effective and timely HIV and TB treatment as a part of nutrition care is crucial.

There is a need to generate new standards for quality of care in nutrition rehabilitation of children with complicated SAM.

Acknowledgements

This chapter was reviewed by:

Lisa Cooke MA BSc RD, Head of Paediatric Dietetics, Department of Nutrition and Dietetics, Bristol Royal Hospital for Children, Bristol.

Claire de Menezes, RSCN (GOS), MSc Public Health Developing countries (LSHTM), Independent consultant for INGOs in the field of Nutrition and HIV, formerly Health and Nutrition Adviser, ACF-International, UK.

Julie Lanigan, Bsc, RD, MRC-Childhood Nutrition Research Centre, Institute of Child Health and HIV Family Clinic Dietitian, Great Ormond Street Children's Hospital, London.

Further reading

For detailed information on management of SAM in the acute setting, please refer to: WHO. Management of severe malnutrition: a manual for physicians and other senior health workers, 1999. http://www.who.int/nutrition/publications/en/manage_severe_malnutrition_eng.pdf.

References

Bentley ME, Corneli AL, Piwoz E *et al*. Perceptions of the role of maternal nutrition in HIV-positive breast-feeding women in Malawi. *J Nutr* 2005; **135**:945–9.

Bhutta ZA. Addressing severe acute malnutrition where it matters. *Lancet* 2009; **374**:9684.

Bhutta ZA, Haider BA. Prenatal micronutrient supplementation: are we there yet? *Can Med Assoc, CMAJ* 2009; **180**(12):E99–E108.

Birahinduka D. Infant feeding and HIV. *BMJ* 2007; **334**:487–8.

Black RE, Allen LH, Bhutta ZA *et al*. and for the Maternal and Child Undernutrition Study Group. Maternal and child undernutrition: global and regional exposures and health consequences. *Lancet* 2008; **371**:243–60.

Butte N, Lopez-Alarcon MG, Garza C. *Nutrient Adequacy of Exclusive Breastfeeding for the Term Infant During the First Six Months of Life*. Geneva: World Health Organisation, 2002.

Chinkhumba J, Tomkins A, Banda T, Mkangama C, Fergusson P. The impact of HIV on mortality during in-patient rehabilitation of severely malnourished children in Malawi. *Trans R Soc Trop Med Hyg* 2008; **102**:639–44.

Codex Alimentarius. *Codex standard 72 on infant formula* 1987;1–7. www.codexalimentarius.net/download/standards/288/CXS_072e.pdf. Accessed 1 March 2006.

Collins S, Dent N, Binns P, Bahwere P, Sadler K, Hallam A. Management of severe acute malnutrition in children. *Lancet* 2006; **368**:1992–2000.

Coovadia HM, Rollins NC, Bland RM, Little K *et al*. Mother-to-child transmission of HIV-1 infection during exclusive breastfeeding in the first 6 months of life: an intervention cohort study. *Lancet* 2007; **369**:1107–16.

Cross Continents Collaboration for Kids (3Cs4kids) Analysis and Writing Committee. Markers for predicting mortality in untreated HIV-infected children in resource-limited settings: a meta-analysis. *AIDS* 2008; **22**:97–105.

De Cock K, Fowler MG, Mercier E, de Vincenzi I *et al*. Prevention of mother-to-child HIV transmission in resource-poor countries: translating research into policy and practice. *JAMA* 2000; **283**:1175–82.

Deolalikar A, Martonell R. Malnutrition and Hunger, The Copenhagen Consensus, Copenhagen Business School, 2008. Available at http://www.copenhagenconsensus.com/The 10 Challenges OLD/Malnutrition and hunger.aspx. Accessed 27 November 2009. http://www.copenhagen consensus.com/The%2010%20challenges%20OLD/Malnutrition%20and%20hunger.aspx.

DH (Department of Health). *Bottle Feeding*. London: Central Office of Information, 2007. Available at www.dh.gov.uk/publications.

DH (Department of Health). *HIV and Infant Feeding: Guidance from the UK Chief Medical Officers' Expert Advisory Group on AIDS*. London: Central Office of Information, 2004. Available at www.dh.gov.uk/publications.

Fawzi WW, Msamanga GI, Hunter D, Renjifo B *et al.* Randomized trial of vitamin supplements in relation to vertical transmission of HIV-1 in Tanzania. *J Acquir Immune Defic Syndr* 2002; **23**:246–54.

Fergusson P, Tomkins A. HIV prevalence and mortality among children undergoing treatment for severe acute malnutrition in sub-Saharan Africa: a systematic review and meta-analysis. *Trans R Soc Trop Med Hyg* 2009; **103**:541–8.

FSA (Food Standards Agency, UK), Weaning your baby. www.fsa.gov.uk, 2009. Available at http://www.eatwell.gov.uk/agesandstages/baby/weaning/. Accessed 28 July 2009.

Foster C, Lyall EG. Preventing mother to-child transmission of HIV-1. *Paedriatr Child Health* 2003; **17**(4):126–31.

Friis H *et al.* Does the first pregnancy precipitate age-related fat deposition? *Int J Obes Relat Metab Disord* 2002; **26**:1274–6.

Gibson RS. *Principles of Nutritional Assessment*, 2nd ed., New York: Oxford University Press, 2005.

Heikens GT, Bunn J, Amadi B *et al.* and for the Blantyre Working Group. Case management of HIV-infected severely malnourished children: challenges in the area of highest prevalence. *Lancet* 2008; **371**:1305–7.

Horton. Maternal and child under nutrition. *Lancet* 2008; **371**(9608):179.

Israel-Ballard K, Donovan R, Chantry C *et al.* Flash-heat inactivation of HIV-1 in Human milk: a potential method to reduce postnatal transmission in developing countries. *J Acquir Immune Defic Syndr* 2007; **45**(3):318–23.

McDermid JM, Jaye A, Schim Van Der Loeff MF *et al.* Elevated iron status strongly predicts mortality in West African adults with HIV infection. *J Acquir Immune Defic Syndr* 2007; **46**(4):498–507.

Ministry of Health. *National Nutrition Guidelines for Malawi*. Lilongwe, Malawi: Government of Malawi. 2007.

Ministry of Health. *Nutritional Care and Support for People Living with HIV/AIDS in Uganda: Guidelines for Service Providers*. Uganda Ministry of Health STD/AIDS Control Programme, Uganda Action for Nutrition, Food and Nutrition Technical Assistance Project (FANTA), 2004.

Ministry of Health and Population. *Manual for the Management of Acute Severe Malnutrition*. Lilongwe, Malawi: Government of Malawi, 2003.

NHS, Healthy Start. Vitamin supplement recommendations, 2009. Available at http://www.healthystart.nhs.uk/en/fe/page.asp?n1=1&n2=8&n3=97&n4=100. Accessed 19 August 2009.

Papathakis P, Rollins N. HIV and nutrition, pregnant and lactating women, World Health Organization, Geneva, 2005. Available at http://www.who.int/nutrition/topics/Paper_3_Pregnant_and_Lactation_bangkok.pdf. Accessed 28 July 2009.

Rabeneck L, Palmer A, Knowles JB, Seidehamel RJ *et al.* A randomized controlled trial evaluating nutrition counseling with or without oral supplementation in malnourished HIV-infected patients. *J Am Diet Assoc* 1998; **98**:434–8.

Rollins N. Infant feeding and HIV, Avoiding transmission is not enough. *BMJ* 2007; **334**:487–8.

Shetty AK, Coovadia HM, Mirochnick MM, Maldonado Y, Mofenson LM, Eshleman SH, Fleming T, Emel L, George K, Katzenstein DA, Wells J, Maponga CC, Mwatha A, Jones SA, Abdool Karim SS, and Bassett MT. Safety and trough concentrations of nevirapine prophylaxis given daily, twice weekly, or weekly in breast-feeding infants from birth to 6 months. *J Acquir Immune Defic Syndr* 2003; **34**:482–90.

Sidley P. Wet nursing increases risk of HIV infection among babies. *BMJ* 2005; **330**:862.

The Sphere Project. *Humanitarian Charter and Minimum Standards in Disaster Response*. Geneva: Sphere, 2004.

UNAIDS. Report on the global AIDS epidemic, 2008. UNAIDS/08.25E/JC1510E (English original, August 2008) © Joint United Nations Programme on HIV/AIDS (UNAIDS) 2008. Available at http://www.unaids.org/en/KnowledgeCentre/HIVData/GlobalReport/2008/2008_Global_report.asp.

USAID/AED. The Linkages Project. Recommended Feeding and Dietary Practices to Improve Infant and Maternal Nutrition. 1999.

Volmink J, Siegfried NL, van der ML, Brocklehurst P. Antiretrovirals for reducing the risk of mother-to-child transmission of HIV infection. *Cochrane Database Syst Rev* 2007; CD003510.

WHO. *Safe Dose of Vitamin A during Pregnancy and Lactation WHO/NUT/98.4.* Geneva: World Health Organization, 1998.

WHO. Management of severe malnutrition: a manual for physicians and other senior health workers, 1999. http://www.who.int/nutrition/publications/en/manage_severe_malnutrition_eng.pdf. Accessed 22 July 2009.

WHO (World Health Organization). *Global Strategy for Infant and Young Child Feeding.* Geneva, Switzerland: World Health Organization, 2003a, reviewed 2009.

WHO. *Nutrient Requirements for People Living with HIV/AIDS: Report of a Technical Consultation.* Geneva: World Health Organization, 13–15 May 2003b.

WHO. Consensus statement. WHO HIV and infant feeding technical consultation held on behalf of the inter-agency task team (IATT) on prevention of HIV infections in pregnant women, mothers and their infants. Geneva, 25–27 October 2006a. http://www.who.int/nutrition/publications/infantfeeding/en/index.html (WHO 2007).

WHO. Home-modified animal milk for replacement feeding: is it feasible and safe? *Discussion Paper for Technical Consultation on HIV and Infant Feeding.* Geneva: World Health Organisation, 2006b.

WHO. *Rapid Advice: Use of Antiretroviral Drugs for Treating Pregnant Women and Preventing HIV Infection in Infants.* Geneva: World Health Organization, November 2009a. Available at http://www.who.int/hiv/pub/mtct/advice/en/index.html. Accessed 4 January 2010.

WHO (World Health Organization). HIV and infant feeding. Revised Principles and Recommendations, RAPID ADVICE, Geneva, Switzerland, November 2009b. Available at http://www.who.int/hiv/pub/paediatric/advice/en/index.html. Accessed 4 January 2010.

WHO/FAO/UNU. Protein and Amino Acid Requirements in Human Nutrition, Report of a Joint WHO/FAO/UNU Expert Consultation, Technical Report Series, No. 935, World Health Organization, 2007.

WHO and UNICEF, WHO child growth standards and the identification of severe acute malnutrition in infants and children, 2009. http://www.who.int/nutrition/publications/severemalnutrition/9789241598163/en/index.html. Accessed 23 May 2009.

WHO, UNICEF & UNFPA. *HIV and Infant Feeding Technical Consultation Held on Behalf of the Inter-agency Task Team (IATT) on Prevention of HIV Infection in Pregnant Women, Mothers and Their Infants: Consensus Statement.* Geneva: World Health Organisation, 2006.

WHO, UNICEF, UNFPA & UNAIDS. *HIV and Infant Feeding: Guidelines for Decision-makers (revised).* Geneva: Wold Health Organisation, 2003a.

WHO, UNICEF, UNFPA & UNAIDS. *HIV and Infant Feeding: A Guide for Health-Care Managers and Supervisors.* Geneva: Wold Health Organisation, 2003b.

WHO, UNICEF, UNFPA & UNAIDS. *HIV and Infant Feeding Update.* Geneva: World Health Organisation, 2007.

WHO, UNICEF & USAID. *Indicators for Assessing Infant and young Child Feeding Practices.* Geneva, 2008.

WHO World Health Organization. LINKAGES. *52.* Exclusive breastfeeding: The only water source young infants need. *FAQ Sheet 5 Frequently Asked Questions.* Geneva: World Health Organization, 2002.

WHO. World Food Programme, UN System Standing Committee on Nutrition and UNICEF, Community-based management of severe acute malnutrition, 2007. http://www.who.int/nutrition/topics/statement_commbased_malnutrition/en/index.html. Accessed 23 May 2009.

World Bank. *Reposition Nutrition as Central to Development: A Strategy for Large Scale Action.* Washington DC, 2006.

4 Paediatric Nutritional Screening, Assessment and Support

Lisa Cooke

Key Points

- Nutritional assessment is vital in the diagnosis and treatment of children with HIV.
- Growth monitoring using calibrated equipment, trained staff and growth reference curves is essential care in this group.
- Dietary assessment and supporting the psychosocial needs of the child with HIV are also important aspects of care.
- Good dietary habits should be instilled at an early age and, when well, children should follow a healthy diet similar to the rest of the UK population.
- If appetite is affected or there are gastrointestinal complications due to AIDS-related illness, this needs to be addressed and managed by an experienced nutritional practitioner.
- Excess weight gain should be avoided to help prevent the development of cardiovascular problems.

4.1 Introduction

The principles of nutritional assessment for the infant, child or adolescent with HIV are similar to the assessment of any other child with a chronic condition. What is important is that the assessor has a comprehensive understanding of how a healthy child grows and develops and how to assess this. An understanding of growth and development, and the limitations of the tools used to assess this, will allow for an informed and comprehensive approach to the nutritional management of a child with HIV. Additionally, the physical, environmental and social effects of HIV on the child's health and well-being should be taken into account when devising a long-term treatment plan for them. This chapter will give an overview of how and what to include when nutritionally assessing a child with HIV, what is currently being used in the UK to screen and assess a child's nutritional status, and how to provide nutritional support for a child who is not growing and developing.

4.2 Nutritional assessment and screening

There are many methods available for the nutritional assessment of children, but no one method should be used in isolation. Awareness of the effects of a chronic condition like HIV, and its potential impact on a child's growth is required to inform the dietary treatment options.

4.2.1   Clinical signs

Unfortunately, illness, nutritional intake and environmental factors can have a detrimental affect on a child's growth and this also needs to be taken into account. Therefore a good knowledge of a child's social circumstances is vital when supporting the nutritional management of a child with a chronic condition. It is essential that the clinician is aware of the clinical signs which will affect the treatment of a child with HIV and understands their implications on the success of a treatment plan.

4.2.2   Growth

Growth is measured by obtaining measurements of weight, height, head circumference (in children under 2 years) and Body Mass Index (BMI kg/m^2). These measurements should then be accurately plotted against a reference growth curve, if one is available, to allow the practitioner to accurately assess the individual child.

4.2.3   Weight

Weight should be measured routinely (e.g. weekly) and ideally on the same digital scales, to reduce the risk of inaccuracy. Scales should be calibrated regularly as standards dictate (UK Weighing Federation, 2002). Errors can occur if these standards are not maintained. This can have dramatic effects on a child's care, e.g. if the practitioners involved in the care misinterpret measurements, a child's faltering growth may not be identified. If the same practitioner measures serial weights and uses the same set of scales the risk of inaccuracy will be reduced.

4.2.4   Height/length

Supine length (lying down) should be measured (quarterly) using a length mat until a child is able to stand unsupported; this is usually around 2 years of age. Then a stadiometer should be used, (it is important to remember that at this point there will be a difference in height/length). When the change from supine to upright height is made it should be noted on the growth chart.

4.2.5   Head circumference

This is a useful measurement for children in early infancy and up to the age of 2 years, and sometimes when isolated due to prenatal and early post-natal effects. Children with untreated HIV can show signs of neuro-developmental delay (Newton, 2005) and this can be influenced by poor growth and/or motility during infancy. Head circumference is a slower indicator of growth, but is an important measure at this crucial time in development and will support the practitioner in their global growth assessment.

4.2.6   Body mass index

This is useful in assessing and monitoring overweight and obesity (Gilbert and Fleming, 2007), but not so useful when assessing faltering growth, so it should not be used in isolation. HIV may increase the long-term risk of developing coronary vascular disease (CVD). This is due to the HIV metabolic complication associated lipodystrophy syndrome (HIV-LDS) and will be discussed in a later chapter (see Chapter 6, 'Healthy Eating, Prevention and Management of Obesity and Long-Term Complications in Children'). It is therefore important that a child's weight or BMI is maintained within the normal range to reduce long-term health risks.

4.2.7   Growth charts

'Growth charts' or 'Growth centile charts' allow the practitioner to plot sequential weights and lengths/heights for an individual child against a reference growth curve, based on a healthy population. Different countries use different growth charts and it is important the practitioner is aware of the charts used within their setting. There are World Health Organization (WHO) charts for children under 5 years of age, which have been based on measurements of a large sample of children exclusively breastfed, from different countries around the world. The sample population included a diverse ethnic mix of children (WHO, 2007a) and the results suggest that most children from all ethnic groups grow in the same exponential manner. It is recommended that these charts can be used as a global standard.

Accurately plotted growth charts indicate whether a child is growing appropriately, faltering or inappropriately gaining weight. Individual weights will not always allow for an accurate interpretation of a child's growth and a series of measurements over time must be used to make a solid judgement. Whenever possible, both weight and height should be measured and plotted, along with head circumference for the younger infant.

Every child has a genetic potential to reach optimum height and this should be maximised wherever possible. By calculating the mid-parental centile it is possible to assess the height range that might be expected for that child's height potential as an adult.

When a child crosses over two centile channels in a downward direction, this indicates growth faltering and appropriate support should be implemented immediately. Conversely, when a child crosses two centile channels in an upward direction, (when the practitioner is confident they were growing to their optimal potential previously) this is indicative of inappropriate weight gain and steps should be taken to help stabilise weight gain without compromising growth and development.

Growth charts like any other assessment tool are only as good as the practitioner who plots and then interprets them.

4.2.8   Mid upper arm circumference

This is a useful measurement for the assessment of body mass and can help to determine whether weight gain is from fat or lean muscle mass. It is especially helpful in the under 5 years age group as in this age group mid upper arm circumference (MUAC) increases rapidly. Oedema is less likely to affect this area of the body and therefore distort readings.

To differentiate between levels of lean body mass and fat, Tricep Skinfold (TSF) measurements need to be measured in conjunction with MUAC. This is not a particularly pleasant experience for children and a good relationship needs to be built up with the practitioner and child. Currently there are no published charts to plot results against. Time constraints and lack of practitioner training, along with inter and intra operator variation and inaccuracies has informed practice in paediatric units within the UK, to not (routinely) include this as an assessment tool. This may change in future clinical practice when appropriate charts are available.

4.2.9   Waist circumference

This is a useful measurement, although not precise, which can support the identification of central adiposity in children with HIV. As we see signs of lipodystrophy in both children and adults receiving antiretroviral treatment (ART), it is important we screen for signs. Additionally, a high waist circumference, along with a high BMI, is indicative of obesity. Children who are fit and potentially weigh more due to larger stores of lean body tissue tend to have a smaller waist circumference. Therefore, it is important that this measurement is not looked at in isolation and conclusions are made when the whole anthropometric picture is viewed.

4.2.10   In summary

Accuracy in recording the relevant anthropometric data using calibrated equipment, plotting and interpreting the results accurately can provide comprehensive information and help the practitioner to make an informed assessment of growth status and onset of complications associated with HIV and ART. Therefore, it is essential that staff are trained in all aspects of growth assessment and able to make an informed decision on treatment options in conjunction with the other members of the multidisciplinary team.

4.3   Dietary assessment – what to do

The dietary assessment of a child will vary depending on the age of the child.

4.3.1   The first six months of life

Within the first 6 months of life a child requires a diet consisting solely of breast or formula milk. In the UK setting, breastfeeding an infant born to an HIV-positive mother is not advised as discussed in Chapter 3.

It is relatively straightforward to assess the intake of a bottle-fed child by using a straightforward dietary recall which can be used to ascertain; feed volume, timing of feeds, history of any positing/vomiting and stool output. It is also very important to check which formula the infant is taking and to assess the formula preparation practice. Advice in the UK is that each bottle is made up individually (One scoop of formula powder added to 1 oz/30 ml) using boiled water which has been cooled to between 70 and 90°C (British Dietetic Association, 2007). WHO guidelines advise no introduction of complementary food until the age of 6 months (World Health Organization, 2007b). The guidelines are part of a global consensus strategy that includes areas of the world where food hygiene can be a problem. It is important infants are as fit and as well developed as possible before potential antigens are introduced into the body in the form of solid food. In the UK we advise the introduction of solids at 6 months, but earlier (not before 17 weeks) if the infant is showing developmental signs of being ready for solid food. An infant's iron stores have been laid down in utero. These iron stores last for the first 6 months and then iron must be provided by the diet. Milk is not a good source of iron, although it is well absorbed from breast milk and formula milks are fortified. Sometimes, late weaning and breastfeeding can cause a delay in getting adequate iron-containing foods into the diet as good sources, e.g. red meat, are difficult to puree down into a smooth consistency – some cultures do not eat meat and it can be cost prohibitive. For the infant with HIV it is important to monitor growth and development, delay weaning until the child is physically ready for solids, whilst monitoring their immune system to support the introduction of new foods, without leaving them at risk of acquiring a food-borne infection. Good food hygiene is imperative with this age group, but especially HIV-infected infants who are at increased risk.

4.3.2   Six months to two years of age

During this age range, good eating habits for life need to be established. Between the ages of 6 and 18 months a child should have as much exposure to different tastes and textures of food as possible. This is an important time and limited exposure will lead to poor choice and variety of foods eaten throughout childhood and life, leading to potential nutritional deficiencies.

Between 6 months to 1 year, an infant should still receive a large amount of nutrition from breast or formula milk, but this should be less than during the first 6 months of life. By the age of 1 year, providing the child is growing well, 350 ml in the form of milk plus other calcium-containing foods like diary products should be included in the diet, alongside three small meals and three nutrient-dense snacks in between. By 1 year of age an infant should be eating chopped up solids in the form of family food. It is important that no salt or sugar is used in cooking.

It is important to note here that many of the HIV-positive infants living in the UK are from a diverse ethnic and cultural background. Therefore, weaning practice may vary between individuals. It is, therefore, very important to understand the feeding practices of the mother and to provide the necessary support. Resources to support weaning are currently limited and it is the responsibility of the dietitian managing the infant's care to spend time with the mother and assess and understand her dietary knowledge and practices.

In the UK there has been a recent increase in the number of children presenting with micronutrient deficiencies. Therefore, population-wide supplementation continues to be recommended.

In the UK, a daily dose of vitamins A and D is recommended for all breast fed infants and for formula-fed infants who are over six months of age and taking less than 500 ml infant formula per day. If vitamin supplementation is necessary, they should receive the 'Healthy Start' vitamins obtained through the health visitor (Department of Health, 1994). These include vitamins A, D and C. However, vitamins are not always offered routinely and many children with HIV do not have a Health Visitor. In such cases, the well-baby clinics should ensure these vitamins are available locally.

When carrying out a dietary assessment it is important the practitioner is aware of the differing needs of this age group, the importance of assessing the psychosocial factors influencing feeding practice and the need for supplementation. Careful questioning regarding these issues can be extremely informative. A diet history alone will not give the wider picture necessary to understand the family dynamics. Advice should be given about best feeding practice to support the family and child. This advice needs to be given in conjunction with background information gathered through the other members of the multidisciplinary team to help ensure that it is tailored to meet the needs of individual circumstances.

4.3.3   Over two years of age

For this age group a diet recall history, i.e. habitual intake rather than a snapshot of 1 day would be the normal tool used in a clinical setting. Additionally, it is important to discuss feeding practices within the home setting and how they fit in with the rest of family life.

For the child under 5 years of age, healthy eating advice for the adult population is not appropriate as the child is still growing at a fast rate, although slower than in the first year of life. Therefore, energy requirements are high in proportion to their size. This equates to the need for a diet which has a higher fat content compared to that of an older child or adult. The advice for this age group is to avoid use of low-fat products including milk (if the child is growing well, semi-skimmed milk is suitable for use from 2 years), unless their growth and development as well as knowledge of their diet is adequate to continue to promote normal growth and development. The fat-soluble vitamins are also very important for this age group and, therefore, the 'Healthy start' vitamins should continue until the age of 5, if there is any doubt surrounding the quality of the diet.

4.3.4   Over five years of age

Again, a diet history recall should be used with this age group. Healthy eating advice should now be given, and the diet gradually changed towards the 'Eat well plate model' (FSA, 2007). (see Chapter 6 'Healthy Eating, Prevention and Management of Obesity and Long-Term Complications in Children')

4.3.5   Adolescents

Adolescence is the transition period from childhood to independent adulthood. This is a challenging age to manage any behaviour change. Without any health care needs it can be a 'tricky time', with the complexities of HIV on top, it can put added strain and worry around those caring for a child with HIV. It is vital that the process of preparation for adulthood is started at a young age and that all the multidisciplinary team are working towards and through this process together and in a structured and well communicated way. Food may be the one area that the young person rebels against. As a dietitian, it is important to be aware of all the issues surrounding the young person's life and direct any dietary advice necessary, with these issues in mind. It might be that some things have to be reinforced but not pushed during this stage, and reliance on previous advice and education is reintroduced at a later stage. Support for the young person around working towards independence through food choice and cooking practice can be a useful way of relaying healthy messages.

4.3.6 In summary

When managing a child with HIV and their diet, it is essential that the other family members, their health and attitudes to food are understood. This enables the practitioner to support and tailor change behaviour around food for the child through the carers. Questions surrounding supplements and vitamin and mineral prophylaxis, which carers may have introduced, should be discussed and discouraged if the diet is adequate and there are no other clinical requirements for them. Some nutrient deficiencies can be at a subclinical level and will not always present as a physical symptom. A detailed history of food intake, impact of illness and the psychosocial environment adds to a clearer and fuller picture supporting a detailed assessment. It is therefore vital that a multidisciplinary setting is provided as a gold standard when caring for a child with HIV. Additionally, the child's nutritional assessment must be communicated to the team in the wider context to support long-term treatment therapy. Where possible, it is preferable to have the same nutrition practitioner involved with the child and family's care over time so that a relationship can be built upon.

Good nutritional foundations at this age support long-term health benefits for the child with HIV.

4.3.7 Biochemistry and haematology

No extra blood tests are necessary on a routine basis for a child with HIV who is growing well and is medically and nutritionally stable, unless the diet history reveals concerns around potential missing nutrients. Should the diet history highlight potential deficits, the child should have these specific biochemical markers checked for during their routine blood tests and, where possible, additional blood tests should be avoided as this causes stress for the child.

Regular haemoglobin tests are good markers of iron status and should be part of the routine biochemical assessment. The results can be assessed by the dietitian.

4.3.8 Global nutritional assessment

Due to the nature of HIV, there is potential for side effects of the drugs to cause symptoms which may affect the interpretation of a physical nutritional assessment. The presence of lipodystrophy (see Chapter 6, 'Healthy Eating, Prevention and Management of Obesity and Long-Term Complications in Children') can confound measurements like MUAC, and waist circumference. It is therefore important that these measurements are recorded routinely and it is suggested this should be done on an annual basis, for all children, even those who are naive to treatment or on drug regimens which are less likely to cause lipodystrophy. Due to the potential long-term effects of HIV treatment on the growth and development of children, it is important to have a full and thorough picture of each child. In a resource-deprived setting this can be unrealistic and problematic so, as a minimum, serial weight and height should be recorded on a regular basis.

Within the UK setting, an annual assessment form (Figure 4.1) has been designed specifically for the use of dietitians working within the multidisciplinary paediatric setting. This enables the practitioner to collect appropriate dietary growth and biochemical data on an annual basis. As discussed previously within this chapter, it directs the collection of appropriate data which is evidence and best practice based. This annual assessment form is under development and has been in limited use in the UK since January 2006. Once audited, if found useful, the aim is to use the tool countrywide to inform practice.

Name:		DOB:			Date:			
Decimal DOB:		Decimal Age:			Start Time:			
Hospital No:				Current Treatment: Start Date:				
Ht (cm):	Wt (kg):	BMI (kg/m²):	MUAC (cm):	Waist (cm):	Hip (cm):	Calf (cm):	Thigh (cm):	
Centile:	Centile:	Centile:	Centile:	Centile:	Centile:	Centile:	Centile:	

Skinfolds (mm)	Triceps SFT	Biceps SFT	Subscapular SFT	Suprailiac SFT
1				
2				
3				
Mean				

Lipids (1 = latest; 2 = previous)	Date	Result	Blood Results	Date	Result
TC 1			Glucose		
TC 2 Ref (≥4.4 -≤5.2)			Ref		
HDL 1			Insulin		
HDL 2 Ref (≥0.9)			Ref		
LDL 1			CD₄ No. (%)		
LDL 2 Ref (≤3.4) ≥3.4 (lipid advice) ≥4.9 (refer lipid clinic)			Viral load		
TAG 1			Anthropometric/metabolic/nutritional concerns		
TAG 2 Ref (≤2.2)					
HDL:LDL					
Ref					
Comments/actions					

Figure 4.1 Family clinic dietetic annual assessment form.

Diet history		Diet Summary
Breakfast		Meat/ Fish/Pulses
		Milk/dairy
AM		Fruit/vegetables
		Butter/margarine/oil
Lunch		Drinks
		Checklist: Snacks Nuts Crisps Cakes Sweets Choc Biscuits
PM		Out of home e.g. friends/relatives/school Weekends/holidays
EM		Exercise
		Omega 3 sources
		Vitamins/minerals/supplements
Advice/goals		
Dietitian's Signature:		**Time Completed:** **Time taken:**

Figure 4.1 (*Continued*)

4.3.9 Nutritional deficiencies

There are many physical signs of nutritional deficiencies (see Table 4.1, Shaw and Lawson, 2007). These signs can be the result of other clinical problems and should not be assessed in isolation, although an indication from a diet history, blood results and physical symptoms together can give a dietary deficiency diagnosis.

Table 4.1 Physical signs of nutritional problems.

Assessment	Clinical sign	Possible nutrients
Hair	Thin, sparse Colour change 'Flag sign' Easily plucked	Protein and energy, zinc, copper
Skin	Dry, Flaky Rough, 'sandpaper' Texture Petechiae, bruising	Essential fatty acids, B vitamins Vitamin A Vitamin C
Eyes	Pale conjunctiva Xerosis Keratomalacia	Iron Vitamin A
Lips	Angular stomatitis Cheilosis	B vitamins
Tongue	Colour changes	B vitamins
Teeth	Mottling of enamel	Fluorosis (excess Fluoride)
Gums	Spongy, bleed easily	Vitamin C
Face	Thyroid enlargement	Iodine
Nails	Spoon shape, koilonchyia	Iron, zinc, copper
Subcutaneous tissue	Oedema, Over-hydration, depleted subcutaneous fat	Protein, sodium Energy
Muscles	Wasting	Protein, energy, zinc
Bones	Craniotabes Parietal and frontal bossing Epiphyseal enlargement Beading of ribs	Vitamin D

From Shaw and Lawson (2007).

Global nutritional assessment is a useful procedure and combines various measurements which allow the practitioner to make an informed diagnosis of potential nutritional deficiencies and their affect on health. (Secker and Jeejeebhoy, 2007)

4.3.10 In summary

Nutritional status should be assessed at regular intervals as part of the management of HIV-infected children. This should ideally be performed by an experienced nutritional practitioner who understands the effects of growth and development in childhood and the effects HIV can have on a child. (Knox *et al.*, 2003) The use of a standardised assessment tool like the annual assessment form (Figure 4.1) enables a full assessment to be performed on a child, and allows for monitoring of any adverse effects from drug therapy and HIV in a proactive rather than a reactive way. Additional dietetic input may be required and this should be made through referrals by the multidisciplinary team and requested to the dietitian.

4.4 Nutritional support

With the introduction of new and superior drug therapies, antenatal screening policies and better screening in the clinical management of HIV in regions with a high standard of living, the presentation of children living with HIV today is very different from that seen in the 1990s when children often presented with high rates of infection, morbidity and mortality.

4.4.1 Energy

Studies of healthy children with HIV show that the resting metabolic rate (RMR) is much the same as that in the general population, although the RMR becomes raised when these children are exposed to opportunistic infections (Arpadi *et al.*, 2000). The child's diet should therefore be fortified with additional calories during this period.

4.4.2 Protein

Insufficient evidence is available to say whether a child with HIV has an increased requirement for protein, when well.

4.4.3 Vitamins and minerals

There is no evidence to say that a child with HIV should be routinely supplemented with vitamins or minerals. Although, in line with standard UK guidance, the infant and child under 5 years of age should be supported with the 'Healthy Start' vitamins, unless the dietitian managing the care of the child feels this is inappropriate. Should the diet show inadequacies, then the child should be supported with any missing or depleted vitamins and minerals following a detailed assessment and relevant biochemical markers as a check.

Nutritional support is the cornerstone to optimise antiretroviral therapy (ART) in the treatment of HIV infection in children. The combination of a good quality, adequately balanced diet, a healthy lifestyle and appropriate drug therapy helps support a child to achieve a healthy childhood while optimising growth potential, minimising long-term complications and building healthy foundations for adult life.

Historically, nutritional support for children with HIV was viewed as an increase in calories and the necessity for a complex feeding regimen to combat malabsorption and other side effects of AIDS-related illnesses. As successful drug therapies for HIV have been instrumental in reversing growth failure, they are a vital tool in treatment of the condition. There are times when children do not meet the diagnostic criteria for treatment with ART and, therefore, nutritional intervention is vital in their treatment plan.

Once growth assessment has taken place, as discussed previously, the practitioner must make a clinical judgement on how to dietetically manage the child.

Complications requiring nutritional support associated with HIV infection are as follows.

4.4.4 Growth faltering

There is little evidence to support the treatment needs of a child with HIV and faltering growth, although it is thought that the loss of lean body tissue during severe infection is increased (Polsky *et al.*, 2001).

Evidence suggests that protein should be increased by 10% during a period of chronic illness. It is important to increase the non-protein energy content of the diet as well to a total of 30–40% (Polsky *et al.*, 2001).

In reality, it is very difficult to achieve this percentage increase in intake, when a child is unwell, without artificial nutritional support. It is important that when the child is well following illness, the diet is increased to allow for catch up following any growth faltering due to illness.

Poor weight gain and growth are the most common symptoms of HIV which manifest in infancy, often before other symptoms. It is, therefore, vital that children within this age group are assessed frequently, including a detailed assessment of growth and diet. Knowledge of the child's environment is also important in order to support good growth and development (Scott, 2006).

In most cases, a child who has access to good food and drug treatment will not suffer with progressive growth failure. Opportunistic infections should be managed by the medical team, while appropriate nutritional support should be provided during and after any course of illness.

4.4.5   Gastrointestinal complications

Side effects from drug therapy along with presentation of enteropathies in undiagnosed children can cause a full range of gastrointestinal symptoms such as intolerance, diarrhoea, constipation and malabsorption.

Some of these symptoms can be transitory and side effects of common childhood illness. Whereas others can be more sinister and show signs of poorly managed or untreated AIDS-defining illness.

4.4.6   Food intolerances

Food intolerances can be due to a post-infection enteropathy and are often transient. Once health has returned the enteropathy is usually reversed. One of the naturally occurring food intolerances in the Black African population is lactose intolerance. Therefore, if a child presents with persistent diarrhoea following the ingestion of lactose, then a diet either low or exclusive of lactose should be advised on a permanent basis. The diet may need to be supplemented with calcium, as a diet low in dairy produce can lead to deficiencies.

4.4.7   Diarrhoea

If this is not related to an enteropathy, it could be due to poor hygiene at home and this should be considered. Whilst monitoring the child's immune status and checking hygienic practice around food preparation at home, advice should be given supporting this.

4.4.8   Constipation

This can be a common side effect following an illness where toilet habits have been compromised. Always, check the diet for fluid adequacy and the possibility of excessive fibre intake in the younger age groups. In the under 5 years age group, children can have an aversion to going to the toilet when using unfamiliar toilets; this can lead to them holding onto their stools and becoming constipated. Following assessment, the dietitian can advise according to cause and symptoms.

4.4.9   Malabsorption

A child who presents with unmanaged HIV and AIDS-defining illness caused by opportunistic infections, such as Cytomegalovirus (CMV), may suffer with gastrointestinal complications. This may subject the child to malabsorption problems which should be managed by using age-appropriate semi-elemental/elemental feeds. The needs for these feeds are usually temporary and once the infection has been treated a standard regimen using a whole protein feed can be resumed. In the rare event, this should continue and artificial feeding via a nasogastric feed is required, then a gastrostomy followed by the fitting of a skin-level device should be considered and planned for.

4.4.10   Lipodystrophy syndrome

The features of this metabolic syndrome are characterized by insulin resistance, impaired glucose intolerance, dyslipidaemia and the physical signs of body fat redistribution. These factors known as HIV-associated lipodystrophic syndrome (HIV-LDS) are important considerations in the treatment of children who already have an increased risk of cardiovascular disease (Charakida et al., 2005). Hence, supporting nutritionally with a Mediterranean-style diet is important in the prevention and treatment of this syndrome (see Chapter 6, 'Healthy Eating, Prevention and Management of Obesity and Long-Term Complications in Children').

4.4.11   Overweight and obesity

As discussed in Sections 4.4.3 and 4.4.4, the incidence and severity of growth faltering has declined since the advent of effective ART. Children who are well managed live a full and active life and often have a good appetite. This means that they are exposed to the same problems in the UK and other resource-rich settings, as other children. Overweight and obesity are fast becoming an epidemic (Butland, 2007) in the UK in both children and adults. Due to the potential long-term effects of HIV drug therapy and the potential metabolic effects of the condition, it is especially important to avoid overweight and obesity in this group of children. The majority of children managed within the UK are from sub-Saharan Africa and perceptions of body image and concepts of an ideal body weight are known to vary between cultures. For this reason, it is important to explain the rationale for advice given about maintaining or achieving an ideal body weight in terms of potential benefits to health and well-being (see Chapter 6, 'Healthy Eating, Prevention and Management of Obesity and Long-Term Complications in Children')

4.4.12   Summary

Nutritional support in the management of a child with HIV covers the full spectrum of symptoms. Age will dictate the main areas of concern and the child should be managed ideally by an experienced dietitian who understands growth and development and the impact HIV can have on a child nutritionally.

Acknowledgements

This chapter was reviewed by:

Julie Lanigan, Bsc, RD, MRC-Childhood Nutrition Research Centre, Institute of Child Health and HIV Family Clinic Dietitian, Great Ormond Street Children's Hospital, London, UK.

Margaret Lawson, MSc, PhD, Cert Ed, FBDA. Honorary Senior Research Fellow, Childhood Nutrition Research Centre, Institute of Child Health, University College, London.

References

Arpadi SM, Cuff PA, Kotler DP *et al*. Growth velocity, fat-free mass and energy intake are inversely related to viral load in HIV-infected children. *J Nutr* 2000; **130**:2498–502.

British Dietetic Association. *The Special Feed Working Group of the Paediatric Group of the BDA, Guidelines for Making Up Special Feeds for Infants and Children in Hospital.* London: Food Standards Agency, 2007.

Butland B. *Foresight Tackling Obesities; Future Choices, Project Report*, 2nd edn. Department Government Office for Science, Department of Innovation, Universities and Skills, Oct 2007.

Charakida M, Donald AE, Green H *et al*. Early structural and functional changes of the vasculature in HIV-infected children: impact of disease and antiretroviral therapy. *Circulation* July 2005; **112**:103–9.

Food Standards Agency. *The Eatwell Plate Model*. London: Food Standards Agency, 2007.

Gilbert MJ, Fleming MF. Use of enhanced body mass index charts during the pediatric health supervision visit increases physician recognition of overweight patients. *Clin Pediatr* Oct 2007; **46**(8):689–97.

Knox TA, Zafonte-Sanders M, Fields-Gardner C, Moen K, Johansen D, Paton N. Assessment of nutritional status, body composition and human immunodeficiency virus-associated morphologic changes. *Clin Infect Dis* 2003; **36**(Suppl 2):S63–8.

Newton Charles R.J.C. Interaction between plasmodium falciparum and human immunodeficiency virus type 1 on the central nervous system of African children. *J Neurovirol* 2005; **11**(Suppl 3):45–51.

Department of Health. Weaning and the Weaning Diet. Report on the Working Group on the Weaning Diet of the Committee on Medical Aspects of Food Policy (COMA). Report on Health and Social Subjects No. 45. London: HMSO, 1994.

Polsky B, Kotler D, Steinheart C. HIV-associated wasting in the HAART ers: guidelines for assessment, diagnosis and treatment. *AIDS Patient Care STDS* Aug 2001; **15**:411–23.

Scott GB. Supportive care for HIV infected children and their families. In: *HIV/Aids: Primary Care Guide*, Bethel, CT: Crown House Publishing, 2006, pp. 477–84, p. xxii.

Secker DJ, Jeejeebhoy KN. Subjective Global Nutritional Assessment for Children. *Am J Clin Nutr* Apr 2007; **85**(4):1083–9.

Shaw V, Lawson M. *Clinical Paediatric Dietetics*, 3rd edn. Oxford: Blackwell Publishing, 2007.

UK Weighing Federation. Guidance notes relating to the legal prescription of medical weighing scales. June 2002.

World Health Organization. Growth reference data for 5–19 years, WHO Reference 2007, Geneva: WHO. 2007a. Available at www.who.int/growthref/en.

World Health Organization. Promoting proper feeding for infants and young children, Genevay WHO. 2007b, Available at www.who.int/nutrition/topics/infantfeeding.

5 Adherence, Symptom Management, Psychological Aspects and Multidisciplinary Care of Children with HIV

Daya Nayagam, Paul Archer, Susheela Sababady, Shema Doshi, and Ella Sherlock

Key Points

Although there are many similarities between paediatric and adult HIV, there are a few differences in children which will influence treatment and management:

- Most paediatric HIV infections occur via vertical transmission (mother to child).
- There are age-specific differences in children's immunology (T-cells/CD4 count).
- Due to continuous growth of their organs, drug doses need to be adjusted according to their metabolism and clearance.
- Adherence to antiretroviral therapy in children can be challenging due to drug formulations, the child's understanding, social issues and outside influences.
- Due to the complexity of adhering to medications in both children and adolescents, a high level of continued support is needed.
- Nutritional status of children living with HIV may vary greatly between individuals. Due to this, nutritional assessments will help identify children who may need dietetic interventions.
- Psychological input may be needed for the family as well as the child due to the complexities of HIV infection.

5.1 Transmission of HIV in children and young people

Most children are infected with HIV through vertical transmission either in utero, during delivery or whilst breastfeeding. Children and young persons may also acquire the infection in the following ways:

- Through unprotected sex with an infected person or by sexual assault.
- By sharing contaminated needles, syringes or other equipment during intravenous drug abuse.

- From transfusion of infected blood, blood products or organ transplantation. This mode of transmission is very rare in the UK since the blood and blood products are screened routinely.

The overall estimated risk of vertical transmission of HIV infection in the UK and Europe in the absence of antiretroviral therapy (ART) and non-breastfeeding is between 15 and 30% (Peckham and Gibb, 1995).

5.2   Prevention of mother-to-child transmission (vertical transmission)

In the UK, transmission rates of HIV from the mother to the unborn child have been reduced to less than 1% (De Ruiter et al., 2008) since the introduction of ART to mothers, delivery by caesarian section, avoidance of breast feeding, and zidovudine treatment to neonates. The voluntary confidential HIV testing of all pregnant women is a routine part of antenatal care (Royal college of Paediatrics and Child Health, 1998). As a result, HIV infection among pregnant women is identified in the majority of cases. This has resulted in better management of women with HIV during pregnancy and childbirth and better post-natal care of both mother and child.

A study (ACTG 076) showed that the administration of zidovudine during pregnancy, labour and early infancy reduced the chance of vertical transmission by two-thirds (Conner et al., 1994). The estimated rate of mother-to-child transmission in the UK and the rest of Europe is between 15 and 30% in non-breastfeeding populations without antiretroviral therapy (Peckham and Gibb, 1995).

It is the current practice (in most parts of the UK) for pregnant women with HIV to be managed by a multidisciplinary team, including obstetricians, midwives, adult HIV physicians, paediatric team, pharmacists and nurses. In most cases a dietician is involved as required. The multidisciplinary team will plan antenatal/post-natal care of the pregnant woman, birth plan and care of the new born baby.

5.3   Clinical presentation of paediatric HIV infection

Children infected with HIV or any form of immunodeficiency present with recurrent infections usually within the first 6 to 12 months of age. They may present with poor appetite, weight loss and wasting.

Respiratory tract infection is the most common presentation in infancy and childhood. Primary *Pneumocystis jeroverci* (previously known as *Pneumocystis carinii* pneumonia or PCP) is most common in immuno suppression, although concurrent infections with other organisms can occur (e.g. Respiratory Syncytial Virus (RSV)/Cytomegalovirus (CMV)). It is characterised by progressive dry cough, dyspnoea on exertion and minimal chest signs. It is not possible to differentiate clinically or radiologically from other severe pulmonary interstitial infections in infants. The bronchio-alveolar lavage will help to make a definitive diagnosis.

5.4   Failure to thrive

The HIV-infected infant is prone to gastrointestinal infections, but in addition the HIV infection itself may cause an enteropathy with poor absorption of nutrients and chronic diarrhoea. In most cases no specific gastrointestinal pathogens are identified and the symptoms only improve once the HIV infection is treated with antiretroviral therapy (ART). The older children will have problems with growth and puberty. Oral thrush is also a frequent finding.

5.5   Central nervous system

Up to 10% of infants presenting with HIV infection have developmental delay and encephalopathy. Infants with HIV infection and encephalopathy have signs of motor dysfunctions resembling those of children with other causes of cerebral palsy.

5.6   Hepatosplenomegaly

Majority of infants presenting with HIV have significantly enlarged liver and spleen. They also present with enlarged lymph nodes and parotid glands.

5.7   Older children

Many children who present with HIV infection may have had mild symptoms for many years, prior to diagnosis of HIV infection. Up to 70% may have had some minor symptoms in the first year of life. Children may present with recurrent mild infections (upper respiratory tract infections, otitis media, sinusitis and skin sepsis) or more serious infections (e.g. pneumonia, meningitis and osteomyelitis).

Bilateral painless enlargement of parotids for more than 1 month in children is most likely to be due to HIV infection. Children may present with more severe episodes of common childhood infections such as chicken pox or may take longer to recover from such infections. Older children may also have problems with pubertal delay. Central nervous system manifestations include subtle cognitive dysfunction, short concentration span and language delay, and poor school performances.

5.8   HIV disease and opportunistic infections

When the immune system is affected by HIV replication, the CD4 count goes down, which makes the individual susceptible to opportunistic infections and chronic diarrhoea. Bone marrow failure may be the consequence of HIV infection with or without other infections. HIV-related malignancy is less common in children than in adults but it does occur rarely.

5.9   Prophylaxis

All infants with HIV infection should receive prophylaxis against PCP from 6 weeks of age. Older children should be given prophylaxis according to the CD4 count or CD4 percentage (Sharland et al., 2004). Co-trimoxazole is highly effective against PCP and prevention of other bacterial infections in children with HIV infection (Dunn et al., 1994).

Children living with HIV infection should be given routine vaccinations that are given to children without HIV infection according to national immunisation schedules, with the exception of BCG (Bacillus Calmette-Guérin) for tuberculosis and live vaccines (D.O.H., 2006).

5.10   Antiretroviral treatment for children

When antiretroviral treatment (ART) is initiated, it is hoped that this will reduce viral load to undetectable levels (less than 40 copies/mL). Viral suppression will help to regain normal immune functions and prevent progression of HIV infection.

In all infants (under 12 months of age) ART should be started as soon as the diagnosis of HIV infection is confirmed, irrespective of the clinical or immunological stage. A fourfold decrease in HIV progression/mortality was observed in children starting ART earlier (Goetghebuer *et al.*, 2008).

In children over 12 months of age, the clinical stage of HIV infection (CDC classification), age-specific CD4 count and CD4 count percentage are taken into consideration before starting treatment with ART.

The choice of ART depends on the availability of suitable formulations for the infants and children (see Box 5.1). Other antiretroviral agents are used, but complete dosing schedules have not been established. Off label use of antiretrovirals should only be used in collaboration with a specialist in paediatric HIV who may have access to unpublished data regarding dosing.

Drug usage in children has not been studied widely. Generally, dosing schedules have been outside of licence and based on little data. Some medicines have been studied more than others. Recent changes to applications for drug licensing require more data on use of drugs in children.

Children are not just little adults when it comes to handling medicines.

The major principles to consider are how children process medicines, i.e. what are the pharmacokinetic mechanisms in children?

Pharmacokinetics refers to what drugs are doing to the body. This is generally broken down into the following:

- absorption
- distribution
- metabolism
- excretion.

5.10.1   Absorption

Children under 2 years old have a higher gastric pH than adults at between 6 and 8. This can result in oral medicines not dissolving in gut fluid and reduced absorption.

Also peristalsis is reduced in young infants, resulting in slower gastric emptying.

5.10.2   Distribution

Neonates have a very high water content, both intra- and extracellular. This leads to neonates having a higher volume of distribution, and therefore requiring higher dosing to achieve adequate drug levels.

5.10.3   Metabolism

Metabolism generally takes place in the liver via phase 1 and 2 metabolism.

Box 5.1   Common antiretroviral agents used in children.

Nucleoside Reverse Transcriptase Inhibitors (NRTIs)
Abacavir (Ziagen®) 300 mg tablet; oral solution. Ages 3 months to 12 years –
8 mg/kg twice a day (max 600 mg daily)

   Lamivudine (3TC or Epivir®) 150 mg and 300 mg tablets; oral solution. Ages
3 months upwards – 4 mg/kg twice a day (max 300 mg daily)

   Didanosine (ddi or Videx®) 25 mg and 200 mg chewable or dispersable tablet.
Ages 3 months upwards. Initially 240 mg/m^2 or 180 mg/m^2 daily

   Stavudine (D4 T or Zerit®) 20 mg, 30 mg and 40 mg capsules; oral solution.
Ages 3 months upwards: <30 kg – 1 mg/kg twice a day; 30 to 60 kg – 30 mg
twice a day; >60 kg – 40 mg twice a day.

   Emtricitabine (FTC or Emtriva®) 200 mg capsule; oral solution. Ages 4 months
upwards – 6 mg/kg up to a maximum of 240 mg per day.

   Zidovudine (AZT or Retrovir®) 100 mg and 250 mg capsule; oral solution)
Ages 3 months to 12 years – 360–480 mg/m^2 taken in three or four divided doses
per day.

Non-Nucleoside Reverse Transcriptase Inhibitors (NNRTIs)
Efavirenz (Sustiva®) 50 mg, 200 mg and 600 mg capsule; oral solution. Ages
3 years upwards and >13 kg. Once-a-day dose: 13–15 kg – 200 mg; 15–20 kg
– 250 mg; 20–25 kg – 300 mg; 25–32.5 kg – 350 mg; 32.5–40 kg – 400 mg;
>40 kg – 600 mg (dosage for capsules – oral solution is not bioequivalent and
therefore dosed differently).

   Nevirapine (Viramune®) 200 mg tablet; oral solution. Ages 2 months upwards:
2 months to 8 years – 4 mg/kg once a day for 2 weeks, then 7 mg/kg twice a day;
8 to 16 years – 4 mg/kg once a day for 2 weeks, then 4 mg/kg twice a day (max
400 mg daily)

Protease Inhibitors (PIs)
Ritonavir (Norvir®) 100 mg capsule; oral solution. Ages 2 years upwards. Initially
250 mg/m^2 twice a day. Increase by 50 mg/m^2 twice a day every 2–3 days, to
350 mg/m^2 twice a day (max 600 mg twice a day), but now most commonly used
as a pharmacokinetic booster.

   Lopinavir/ritonavir (Kaletra®) 200 mg/50 mg or 100 mg/25 mg; oral solution.
Ages 2 years upwards – 230/57.5 mg/m^2 twice a day (max 400/100 mg twice a
day).

   Indinavir (Crixivan®) 200 mg and 400 mg capsule. Ages 4 to 17 years –
500 mg/m^2 every 8 hours (max 800 mg every 8 hours).

   Adapted from: Plusve (2007).

   Plusve (2007) *UK daily dosing of paediatric antiretroviral agents.* Plusve.

With permission from Plusve (How's That Publishing Limited).

Phase 1 metabolism is reduced in neonates and increases to adult levels by 6
months. Because of the way medication is metabolised in children, higher doses may
be required (sometimes exceeding adult levels) in order to treat at a therapeutic level.
Phase 2 metabolism varies by the substrate involved. In neonates some pathways of
phase 2 metabolism have not matured and therefore metabolism is reduced and a
different pathway to adults may be used.

5.10.4   Excretion

Renal excretion is reduced in children under 1 year old in comparison to adults. Therefore, lower dosing and/or increased dosing frequency may be required.

As all of these processes are involved in drug metabolism, trying to take all the above factors into consideration is complex. There is limited data to guide usage of medicines. Regular measurement of heights and weights is essential and, where possible, use of therapeutic drug monitoring (TDM) can guide usage and help individualise treatment strategies (see PENTA treatment guidelines (password required) or US guidelines for the use of antiretroviral agents in pediatric HIV infection (www.aidsinfo.nih.gov).

5.11   Monitoring of paediatric HIV infection

5.11.1   Laboratory

CD4 counts and percentage values in healthy infants who are not infected with HIV are considerably higher than those observed in uninfected adults and slowly decline to adult values by the age of 5 years (CDC, 1994).

In children under 5 years the absolute CD4 count tends to vary more with the age within an individual child compared to CD4 percentage. Therefore, in HIV infected children under 5 years of age, CD4 percentage is preferred for monitoring immune status, whereas absolute CD4 count can be used in older children (The European Collaborative Study, 1992).

5.11.2   Viral load

Viral burden in peripheral blood can be determined by using quantitative HIV RNA assays. HIV RNA copy numbers should be assessed as soon as possible after a child has a positive virological confirmatory test.

5.11.3   Disease progression

With the advent of effective combination antiretroviral therapy (AART), HIV infection has become a treatable chronic disease. Increased use of a combination of antiretroviral medications has resulted in a substantial decrease in morbidity, mortality (Resino, 2006) and rates in hospitalisation (Bertolli et al., 2006).

5.12   Caring for children and their families in the community

In the UK the great majority of children living with HIV are cared for in the community in outpatient clinics, not in acute centres due to the availability of effective ART. As a result of this treatment, children are living longer, attending mainstream schools, achieving good academic grades in many cases and are transitioning to adult services. Living full, active lives raises the medical and social issues of disclosure (discussing the confidential diagnoses), adolescence issues, sexual relationships, sexual health, as well as long term exposure to ART which may lead to multiple drug resistance and side effects.

The majority of children and families attending HIV clinics in the U.K are from sub-Saharan Africa. Many of the families have experienced immigration, financial, housing and language problems. Due to stigma attached to a child with HIV infection many of the families are socially isolated. Often a considerable amount of support is needed from social services, voluntary agencies and psychological services. The care for these children and families should be provided by a multidisciplinary team, including statutory and voluntary organisations.

HIV infection in itself may be the last in the list of concerns for the families. Their priorities may be to solve their immigration status, financial burden or housing issues. The health care professionals should be able to assess and address the families in a very sensitive manner.

The services in the community should be well coordinated to avoid duplication. The issues faced by the families are complex, thus the care for these families are best addressed in multidisciplinary settings. The health professionals need to develop mutual trust. The role of health care professionals in the community is made up of three main areas, i.e. liaison, provision of care and education of the families and their carers.

5.13   Adherence, symptom management, psychological aspects and multidisciplinary care of children with HIV and AIDS

5.13.1   Why adherence is important in paediatric HIV care

When treating HIV infection, great emphasis is placed on adhering to the antiretroviral medication as prescribed, and to the consequences of non-adherence. There are good reasons for this. First, this is because of the risk of building up resistance to the medication. In order to achieve virological suppression, a constant level of medication is required in the bloodstream. If this is not achieved, HIV will multiply and also develop resistant strains of the virus. This will result in the current combination of ART being ineffective in suppressing the virus. The implication of this is that the combination will have to be changed to a new drug regimen (Kalichman and Rompa, 2003). Adults have a wide choice of drugs to choose from but unfortunately, because of drug restrictions in children, the available range of paediatric medications is more limited.

If virological suppression is achieved through good adherence, not only will it ensure that HIV is kept under control, but it will also ensure that the patient's immune system has time to recover and repair itself. By doing this, the patient is at less risk of developing opportunistic infections and becoming seriously ill (Welch, 2008).

Adherence is key to the long-term survival of patients. Before the advent of ART, children living with HIV had a life expectancy of approximately one decade. Since then, with the introduction of a variety of ART combinations, patients can look forward to a relatively normal life expectancy. This, however, will only be achieved with good adherence to ART and by ensuring that each combination of ART lasts as long as possible (Welch, 2008).

5.13.2   How to support adherence

Adherence to medication is easy to achieve theoretically but in practice it is a complicated and multifaceted concept that few people manage to achieve in the long term. It is even more complicated in children as they often have to manage a large pill burden, foul-tasting drug formulations, while they are often not fully aware of why they are taking the medication (Goode *et al.*, 2004)

One of the key methods of achieving good adherence in children is to ensure that the child is fully supported by their parents. In the past there has been a lot of misinformation regarding ART, coupled with the parents' own negative experiences of taking the medication. In such cases, it is important to work alongside the parents to address these issues rather than work against them. It is best to work with the parents and gain their trust as they will then be more likely to accept information provided by health professionals about the ART and, therefore, more willing to allow their children to take these drugs.

5.13.3   Cultural and religious beliefs

The cultural and religious beliefs of children and parents can have an impact on a child's adherence to their ART (Bruton, 2005). For some people, using modern medicine can go against the very basis of religious belief which includes the use of traditional remedies. It is also not uncommon for people to refuse treatment on the basis that they believe that they will be healed through prayer or meditation. It would be very easy for the health care professional to be drawn into an argument around these issues. However, by engaging with different cultural groups and religious leaders it is possible to understand belief systems, which, in turn, makes it possible to adapt the approach taken and reach some kind of compromise about starting treatment. Some religious leaders are very supportive of the use of ART and it is important to identify and engage with influential individuals, at an early stage, to avoid problems later on.

5.13.4   Taking the medications

Newly diagnosed adults in the UK have a very small pill burden compared with children. Fixed-dose combination tablets such as Atripla® make it possible to take as little as one tablet, once a day (see Chapter 12, 'Medications, Adherence and Interactions with Food'). Unfortunately, because of paediatric drug dosing and restrictions on tablet strength, children tend to be on a greater amount of pills. This has a huge impact on adherence as many children struggle to swallow tablets. Also, many of the tablets cannot be crushed or dissolved. If swallowing tablets is not an option for these children, another option is suspensions or liquids. The problem with these is that many of them have a bitter taste and/or high alcohol content. Therefore, children struggle to take them, may vomit the dose, or refuse point-blank to take them.

There are steps that can be taken to encourage children to take their medication. The unpleasant taste of many liquid suspensions can be disguised using foods. For example, Kaletra® suspension has a very bitter taste and can not be disguised by sweet food. Mixing the Kaletra® with something that is slightly bitter (e.g. marmite or dark chocolate) disguises the taste more effectively (Head, 2009). When it comes to swallowing tablets children tend to struggle with the size of the tablet rather than the amount. Certain drug formulations come with smaller half strength tablets that can be used in children e.g. Kaletra® and zidovudine (AZT) 100 mg capsules. This greatly improves children's adherence to the ART as they find the smaller tablets easier to swallow.

Some children also have a mechanical problem in swallowing tablets. They are either physically unable to swallow tablets or they have never been shown how to take tablets without chewing them. This can be addressed by using placebo tablets of different sizes and showing children the correct technique to swallow tablets (Head, 2009).These techniques can be effective in children as young as 5 years of age to enable them to swallow tablet formulations of ARTs.

For many children HIV isn't a major focus of their lives. They tend to be more focused on friends, family and schoolwork. Because of this, medication tends to fit around their hectic daily routines. If children struggle to fit in taking their medication twice a day due to, for example, catching the bus to school, it may be possible to switch them onto a once-daily (OD) regimen where they only take their ART during the evening. If a once-daily regimen is possible, care has to be taken to ensure that adherence is as near 100% as possible, as the risk of resistance may increase with OD regimens. Care also has to be taken with which drugs are taken and when they are taken. For example, an OD regimen containing Efavirenz is possible but a common side effect of this drug is drowsiness, so it is not recommended to be taken in the morning.

As children reach the age of puberty adherence tends to become more of a problem. This may be due to a variety of reasons including body image, peer group pressure, identity issues and not wanting to be reminded of their diagnosis. Some of these issues can be addressed jointly with the young person using a variety of supportive parties including family, psychology and the voluntary. Adolescents often have anxieties and pressures, and they often find it difficult to cope with taking medication. In such times as these it may be possible to offer the young person a structured treatment interruption where they are taken off ART for a period of time and closely monitored. This is not recommended in adults due to the results of the SMART study (SMART, 2008). The study showed that structured treatment interruptions in adults increased the patient mortality rate considerably. However, observations in children and adolescents show that they cope with treatment interruptions very well without generating resistance.

One of the biggest influences on a young person is not their family or culture but their peer group. After all, this is the group of people that the young person will spend most of their school life and beyond with. With this in mind, it is important that children and young people have a supportive peer group around them to achieve good adherence. This does not mean that their peer group will necessarily know their diagnosis. It is well recognised that young people listen to their peers over their parents or health care professionals, so peer support can be key to achieving long-term adherence and long-term survival. As many young people choose not to tell their friends their diagnosis, it may be appropriate for health care professionals to put them in touch with other young people with the same diagnosis. This can be a great form of support, especially where there are adherence issues and they feel that they can't talk to their own friends about it.

Many people, both children and adults, are fearful of starting and staying on ART due to the possible side effects of the medication. Although adults tend to suffer greatly with side effects, this is not generally the case with children and young people. The most common side effects that children tend to suffer are bouts of diarrhoea, stomach cramps, nausea and night sweats. However, these are short-lived and most side effects tend to subside within a couple of weeks. Support is needed to help these young people get through the initial stage of starting treatment as once side effects subside, adherence to medication is both achievable and necessary for long-term survival.

One aspect of paediatric care that is both challenging and difficult is the disclosure of diagnosis to the young person. But it is often necessary in order to achieve adherence. One way of looking at this might be to ask yourself the question, 'would you take medication if you don't know why you have to'. This is what we expect a lot of our young people to do who don't know their diagnosis. Many have been on ART for most of their lives but do not know why they take them. Some will probably have been given some kind of explanation but not in any great detail. It is often found that adherence is greatly improved once people know why they must adhere to their medication. Although some parents are apprehensive about telling their children their diagnosis, there has been a great change in attitudes in recent years and now children are being disclosed to at a younger age with good effects.

Although to achieve good adherence it is important to work with parents, this sometimes may be impossible due to the parents' own belief system or their own physical ability to care for their children. In such instances as these social services may need to be involved. As health care professionals we have a responsibility to act in the best interests of the child. In extreme cases children have been made ward of court due to their parents inability to administer ART. Although this is far from ideal, it is sometimes necessary to ensure long-term survival of children. In cases where parents are physically unable to administer medication due to their own poor health, it may be appropriate for social services to put extra services into the home to enable the parents to meet the child's needs. This may be in the form of a carer going into the family home to administer medication or may be more complex and needs joint parental responsibility with a foster carer, for example. Wherever possible the family should be engaged with and worked with very closely to achieve a positive outcome and the child should be paramount in all decisions made and actions taken.

5.14   Nutritional care in a multidisciplinary team setting

As many of the children in early stages of adolescence are not made aware of their HIV status, it is often difficult for them to relate to discussions about nutrition and medication and how this can affect their general well-being. The focus is mainly on weight and on how well they are feeling.

It is important that nutritional status is assessed on a regular basis as disease state can vary between visits. When discussing nutritional status with a child, the centile chart is a good indicator to use as it brings the focus away from any actual 'disease' and translates well to a child for the need of optimum nutrition, especially as diagnosis cannot be discussed.

As well as diet history, anthropometry and bowel habits, care should be taken to monitor changes in biochemistry (especially cholesterol). Cholesterol may be affected by certain drug therapy regimes. See Chapter 6 ('Healthy Eating, Prevention and Management of Obesity and Long-Term Complications in Children').

Nutrition status of children living with HIV infection may vary greatly between individuals and this can be affected by many things such as disease state and whether they are taking antiretroviral medication. While a small number may have failure to thrive others may be thriving well, overweight, or obese. Nutritional assessment carried out on a regular basis will help detect significant changes in weight and care should be taken when advising on high-calorie, high-protein diets as many children now living with HIV infection in the UK may be at risk of excessive weight gain.

For the few who still do require a high-calorie, high-protein diet, food fortification is the first recommendation and only a few of these children need nutritional sip feeds.

Sip feeds are generally provided in clinic due to confidentiality issues as many general practitioners (GPs) are not aware of the child/family diagnosis. In situations where a patient requires regular sip feeds and lives too far to collect feeds from the clinic, the GP will be contacted for a prescription. In these cases HIV status is still not disclosed but the focus is on the nutritional reason for why sip feeds have been prescribed, e.g. faltering growth and/or poor appetite.

As part of a multidisciplinary team, a paediatric dietitian may be involved with non-nutritional issues such as housing, immigration, schooling, special needs and changes to family set-up, which can all affect nutritional status and intake and should, therefore, be taken into consideration when advising on nutrition goals. When liaising with any professionals or non-professionals, who may or may not be aware of the child's diagnosis, discretion about HIV status is of the utmost importance. This calls for good communication with the team and the parents/carers.

5.15   The psychological effects of HIV on family functioning – key themes which arise in a child setting

5.15.1   Introduction: the role of a psychologist in a paediatric setting

Clinical psychologists who work in a paediatric setting see children individually, with the family or they offer indirect consultation. In dealing with the psychological effects of HIV on family functioning, key emotional issues that arise include challenging stigma, addressing adherence, disclosure, sexual health and issues related to transition.

A key aspect of the psychologist's role involves working in partnership in a multidisciplinary context. Case study 5.1 illustrates how a child's care is often located within multiple systems, involving a large number of professionals. Although Figure 5.1, of the Tayali[1] family, is not based on one true story, it shows how some typical themes can interact to form an individual psychological picture of the impact of HIV. The story illustrates how a psychologist might initially work to engage with a family before starting to assess the presenting difficulty and offering interventions.

---

[1] Note: The name of this family and the main themes have been changed in order to maintain confidentiality. Circles are used to denote females and squares represent male family members.

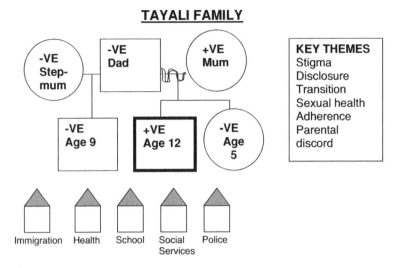

Figure 5.1   Genogram showing typical themes that affect families living with HIV.

Case study 5.1   A child's care

In summary, Margaret is nine; she was born in the UK and her parents came to the UK from Zimbabwe before she was born. They have applied to the Home Office to request leave to remain and are anxiously awaiting a response. Margaret has attended clinic as long as she can remember, and has spoken to the nurse about 'red and white blood cells'. She does not know the name of her health condition, but has to take pills for it. Her brother and sister know that she takes medication, but they are not sure why. Margaret has lots of questions about her medication, and wonders why she should take it when she does not see any changes in her health. Margaret feels confused and alone; she recently ran away. The police and social services were involved because they were concerned about Margaret's well-being and her risk-taking behaviour.

Dad says he does not feel ready to talk to Margaret about her health and he fears the local 'talk' in the community. In his experience, people think you get HIV from having had multiple partners. Margaret is growing up and talks about her favourite music, she is beginning to talk about boys she likes at school. Dad has worries about the future; he trusts the current doctor and is worried about how Margaret will cope when she is older.

The team suggested that the psychologist might speak to dad about Margaret's recent behaviour. Dad was not sure about the idea, as in his experience, psychologists only see crazy people. Like other families, it is not the norm to talk to a stranger about family problems. In dad's experience, talking is not always helpful. The psychologist explained that she can sometimes help make sense of a problem and provide confidential support in thinking about solutions. Margaret and dad then agreed to a brief meeting with the psychologist. Over a series of meetings, Margaret says that she had overheard dad telling an aunty that she has HIV. She is worried that she might die because she saw on the news how HIV kills people in Africa. The family agrees to meet for further sessions in order to think together about ways to make sense of Margaret's health condition and how this fits into her life.

5.15.2   The impact of HIV as a chronic illness on the family

In this section, the 'family' is defined as biologically based and socially chosen. There are different levels of 'family functioning', relating to day-to-day activities, relationships and emotional support, child rearing, management of transitions and economic support (Carr, 2006). The psychological impact of HIV is context driven; it depends on *who, when and where*. A complex and dynamic interaction of factors influence the psychological experience of each family member. The landscape of HIV has changed in recent years with the impact of antiretroviral medication and the health condition is now considered to be a chronic illness within the context of the UK.

There is limited research on the impact of HIV on family functioning, as traditional research has taken a purely individualistic perspective. Much of what we know comes from the body of literature which focuses on the impact of a child's chronic illness on the family (Eiser, 2005). This clearly links the concept of adjustment with family functioning and highlights the importance of helping a child live well when there is no cure. Clearly, there are disadvantages in relying solely on this type of research, as each illness has its own aetiology. However, a non-categorical approach such as this enables thinking about the extent to which the illness and treatment disrupt each family's daily life. A developmental approach is useful in making sense of how a child and family adapt to an illness in different ways at key transition points, such as the infant and toddler years, preschool and early school years, middle school and adolescent periods. Much is yet to be learnt about the impact of HIV on family functioning.

5.15.3   The psychological effects of HIV on family functioning – our current understanding

Perhaps the most important aspect of a paediatric psychologist's role is in re-storying the meaning of 'HIV'. This involves working with the wider system in challenging the social stigma associated with the health condition. Psychologists are trained to work with individuals and are skilled at working with professional and personal narratives in helping address difficulties associated with family functioning as well as individual problems. They consider 'the relationship in focus' and are able to engage in a variety of joining conversations in order to make sense of problems (Goldenberg and Goldenberg, 1980).

Psychological therapies can be useful in helping people explore different meanings of HIV. Acknowledging and creating an alternative understanding of illness can be a powerful tool in reducing people's sense of isolation and can enable them to access resources, such as services provided by the voluntary sector.

Psychological interventions can be offered to people directly on a one-to-one basis, or in groups. An example of some work with a young person around 'adherence' to antiretroviral medication involves jointly examining what this means to the individual, and considering how HIV fits into her wider life. The work involves considering the person as a whole and from working where they are in order to help them take control in making decisions about managing their health. Ideas from Motivational Interviewing (Miller and Rollnick, 2002) can be useful in this type of work.

Another area of work is in helping parents disclose their own and/or the children's diagnosis to the child. Health professionals and the family might think together about who is the best person to talk to the child. Psycho-education can contribute to the process by incorporating a variety of child-friendly materials. Careful consideration is given to the child's current understanding, what they need to know and who else should be informed. This ideally takes place gradually as the child develops. For example, stories can be created about how medicines work and keeping information private. As young people grow into teenagers, there are new conversations and new concerns. These involve helping them navigate life with a chronic health condition, managing medication and thinking about negotiating sex and relationships.

Support for the whole family is paramount, and the needs of affected children (i.e. negative children with positive siblings or positive parents) are easy to overlook. Group work can come in a variety of shapes and sizes. Parent's days, for example, encourage discussion and reflection about concerns such as worries around the disclosure of a person's HIV status, and the dilemmas which arise in considering ways to talk with teenagers about sex and relationships (Wilkins *et al.*, 2007).

Care also needs to be given to preparing the young person for the psychological transition to adult services (Campbell *et al.*, 2009; Campbell *et al.*, 2010).

One group-work approach to transition takes place in the form of 'Looking Forward Days' for young HIV-positive people aged 12–16. This aims to equip young people with the emotional, psychological and behavioural skills necessary to face the challenges of living with HIV, including increased self-management and the development of sexual and romantic relationships.

It is common for a bond to form between health professionals and families, and the conversations to start the process of psychological transition can begin early. There are multiple types of multidisciplinary service delivery and more research is needed to find out the most effective way to help young people with a chronic illness move smoothly into adult care.

Acknowledgements

The authors would like to thank Brigid Hekster, Clinical Psychologist, CASCAID Child and Family Psychology Service, South London and the Maudsley NHS Trust, London.

References

Bertolli J, Hsu HW, Sukalac T *et al*. For the pediatric spectrum of HIV disease. *J Pediatr Infect Dis* July 2006; **25**(7):628–63.

Bruton J. HIV and religion. *HIV Nurs* 2005; **5**(2):4–5.

Campbell T, Beer H, Wilkins R, Parrett N, Jauslin L. 'Sex, love and one-night stands: getting the relationship you want': Evaluation of a sexual health workshop for HIV+ young people. *Education Health* 2009; **27**(2):23–7.

Campbell T, Beer H, Wilkins R, Sherlock E, Merrett A, Griffiths J. 'I look forward. I feel insecure but I am OK with it'. The experience of young HIV+ people attending transition preparation events: a qualitative investigation. *AIDS Care* 2010; **22**(2):263–9.

Carr A. *The Handbook of Child and Adolescent Clinical Psychology: A Contextual Approach*. London: Taylor and Francis, 2006.

Conner EM, Sperling RS, Gelber R *et al*. Reduction of maternal-infant transmission of human immunodeficiency virus type 1 with zidovudine treatment. *N Engl J Med* 1994; **331**:1173–80.

De Ruiter A, Mercey D, Anderson J *et al*. British HIV association and children's HIV association guidelines for the management of HIV infection in pregnant women 2008. *HIV Med* 2008; **9**:452–502.

Department of Health, Welsh Office, Scottish Office Department of Health, DHSS (Northern Ireland). In: Salisbury DM, Begg NT, eds. *Immunisation Against Infectious Disease*. London: HMSO, 2006.

Dunn D, Newell ML, Ades T, Peckham C, Maria AD. European collaborative study. CD4T cell count as predictor of Pneumocystis carinii pneumonia in children born to mother's infection with HIV. *Br Med J* 1994; **308**:437–40.

Eiser C. *Growing Up with a Chronic Disease: The Impact on Children and their Families*. London: Jessica Kingsley Publishers, 2005.

European Collaborative Study. Age-related standards for T lymphocyte subsets based on uninfected children born to human immunodeficiency virus 1-infected women. The European collaborative study. *Pediatr Infect Dis J* 1992; **11**(12):1018–26.

Goetghebuer T, Haelterman E, Le Chenadec J et al. Early vs. deferred highly active antiretroviral therapy in HIV infected infants: a European collaborative cohort study. *Retrovirology* 2008; 5(Suppl 1):O25.

Goldenberg I, Goldenberg H. *Family Therapy: An Overview*, 4th ed. London: Brooks/Cole Publishing Company, 1980.

Goode M, Harrod M, Wales S. The role of the specialist nurses in improving treatment adherence in children with a chronic illness. *Aust J Adv Nurs* 2004; **21**(4):41–5.

Head S. *Pill swallowing protocol*. www.chiva.org. 2009. Available at http://www.chiva.org.uk/health/guidelines/swallowing. Accessed May 2009.

Kalichman SC, Rompa D. HIV treatment adherence and unprotected sex practices in people receiving antiretroviral therapy. *Sex Transm Infect* 2003; **79**:59–61.

Miller WR, Rollnick S. *Motivational Interviewing*, 2nd ed. New York: Guildford Press, 2002.

CDC. Revised classification system for human immunodeficiency virus infection in children less than 13 years of age: official authorized addenda—human immunodeficiency virus infection codes and official guidelines for coding and reporting ICD-9-CM. *MMWR* 1994; **43**(RR-12), 1–19.

Peckham CS, Gibb D. Mother to child transmission of human immunodeficiency virus. *N Engl J Med* 1995; **333**(5):298–302.

Resino S, Bellón JM, Sánchez-Ramón S et al. Impact of antiretroviral protocols on dynamics of AIDS progression markers. *Arch Dis Child* 2002; **86**:119–24. doi:10.1136/adc.86.2.119.

Royal College of Paediatrics and Child Health. Recommendation of an intercollegiate working party of enhancing voluntary confidential HIV testing in pregnancy. In: *Reducing Mother to Child Transmission of HIV Infection in the United Kingdom*. 1998.

Sharland M, Blanche S, Castelli G, Ramos J, Gibb DM. On Behalf of the PENTA Steering Committee. PENTA guidelines for the use of antiretroviral therapy (updated 2008). *HIV Med* 2004; 5(Suppl. 2):61–86.

(SMART) Study Group. The strategies for management of antiretroviral therapy. Inferior clinical outcome of the CD4 cell count-guided antiretroviral treatment interruption strategy in the SMART study: role of CD4 cell counts and HIV RNA levels during follow-up. *J Infect Dis* 2008; **197**:1145–55.

Welch S. *PENTA Guidelines for the Use of Antiretroviral Therapy in Paediatric Infection* (draft revision). PENTA, 2008. Available at http://www.pentatrials.org/guide08.pdf; http://www.pentatrials.org/trials.htm.

Wilkins R, Campbell T, Beer H. Preparing HIV-positive young people for the challenges of adult life: a group work approach. *Aids Hepatitis Digest* 2007; **119**:1–3.

6 Healthy Eating, Prevention and Management of Obesity and Long-Term Complications in Children

Julie Lanigan

Key Points

- Adverse health outcomes, particularly with respect to the cardiovascular system, are associated with obesity and with HIV infection and its treatment. Gaining excess body fat should therefore be avoided in HIV-infected people.
- HIV-infected children are at risk of obesity for several reasons involving physiological and social factors.
- Dyslipidaemia is seen in association with HIV infection in children regardless of treatment and is thought to arise in part secondarily to fat redistribution but also as a result of drug toxicity.
- There is concern that antiretroviral medication use may increase the risk of CVD in adult life.
- Treatment options for management of dyslipidaemia in children include switching antiretroviral medication, dietary management by an experienced practitioner and lipid lowering medication.

6.1 Introduction

The introduction of effective antiretroviral therapy (ART) for the treatment of paediatric HIV infection has improved clinical management markedly. For example, in the UK progression to acquired immune deficiency syndrome (AIDS) has been reduced by 50% and mortality by 80% (Gibb *et al.*, 2003). HIV infection can therefore be considered a chronic rather than an acutely life-threatening condition. However, treatment with ART is associated with metabolic side effects and this is particularly important for children who will usually start treatment during childhood and have greater cumulative exposure to ART. This brings a new set of problems associated with increased longevity; long-term complications both of disease and treatment are now common.

Before the introduction of ART wasting was a common feature of HIV infection and studies reported a survival advantage for patients with the highest body mass index (BMI: weight in kilograms divided by the square of height in metres (kg/m^2)) (Grinspoon and Mulligan, 2003). BMI is positively associated with CD4 counts and inversely related to events marking progression of HIV (Jones *et al.*, 2003), therefore maintenance of body mass is important for survival. Conversely, excess body fat is related to adverse health outcomes, particularly with respect to cardio-vascular disease risk. A healthy body weight and fat distribution is therefore impor-tant for optimal health in HIV-infected children. Both under- and overnutrition can contribute to health problems.

6.2   Metabolic complications

HIV infection is associated with a range of metabolic complications in which both under- and overnutrition are implicated. Undernutrition is characterised by de-creases in anthropometric and biochemical indices and may progress to wasting and cachexia. In children, growth faltering is an early indicator of HIV infection and in untreated children loss of lean body mass and decreased linear growth may occur. Growth faltering is a result of HIV infection rather than a side effect of treatment. On the contrary, initiation of ART in children can reverse adverse effects on growth.

Long-term effects of antiretroviral therapy are a cause for concern, particularly for children who are usually infected from birth or early infancy and will receive treat-ment for much of their life. Nutritional alterations, mainly reported in association with symptomatic HIV or antiretroviral therapy, include micronutrient deficiencies and changes in body composition. In this chapter, nutritional complications associ-ated with disease and treatment of HIV will be discussed and practical advice for dietetic management provided.

6.3   Malnutrition and HIV

HIV infection and malnutrition interact in a vicious cycle where increased nutritional requirements, as a result of infection, are often accompanied by decreased dietary intake (Irlam et al., 2005). Malnutrition takes many forms and, in areas of high poverty and food shortage, is usually characterised by protein energy malnutrition (PEM).

Severe malnutrition and HIV infection coexist and are prevalent in areas of ex-treme deprivation. In some African countries more than half of patients admitted for nutritional rehabilitation are HIV positive and mortality rates are high (Bunn et al., 2007). Clinical signs of PEM such as growth faltering can be detected early with regular growth monitoring and are usually associated with multiple micronu-trient insufficiency. However, unlike PEM, the signs and symptoms of micronutrient deficiency often manifest over a longer time (see Chapter 3 'Malnutrition, Infant Feeding, Maternal and Child Health' and Chapter 4 'Paediatric Nutritional Screen-ing, Assessment and Support').

6.4   Micronutrients and HIV

Micronutrients are implicated in the pathogenesis of HIV disease and contribute to immune dysfunction, infectious morbidity and disease progression. However, data are sparse and mechanisms poorly understood. HIV-infected adults and children have a range of micronutrient deficiencies and these are most severe in advanced disease and malnutrition (Buys et al., 2002). Robust evidence for a beneficial effect of micronutrient supplementation in adults is lacking, however, there is some evidence for a benefit of vitamin A supplementation in children.

6.4.1   Vitamin A

Vitamin A is the most extensively studied vitamin in relation to childhood micronutrient deficiency. Supplementation in HIV-infected children is associated with protection against mortality and morbidity from diseases commonly associated with HIV, similar to that seen in HIV-negative children (Mehta and Fawzi, 2007). In one study, supplementation of children aged 6–59 months achieved a 63% reduction in all cause mortality over a two-year follow-up period. Reductions in morbidity from all causes as well as from respiratory and diarrhoeal infections have also been reported. However, consideration should be given to adverse effects seen in well-nourished and stunted children (Irlam *et al.*, 2005). Vitamin D deficiency is also implicated in HIV pathogenesis.

6.4.2   Vitamin D

People with HIV have increased risk of osteopenia and osteoporosis; a phenomenon that may be attributed both to immune activation and antiretroviral therapy (Stephensen *et al.*, 2006). Initially, bone loss seen in HIV patients was attributed solely to antiretroviral therapy; however, recent studies suggest that factors secondary to HIV infection, including cytokine activation and alterations in vitamin D metabolism, may interact to stimulate bone demineralisation (Soler *et al.*, 2007).

Vitamin D regulates bone metabolism and is central to calcium homeostasis and important for normal immune function. Low serum concentrations have been associated with low CD4 counts, immunological hyperactivity and HIV progression. Prevalence estimates vary widely among studies and are confounded by coexistence of other conditions inducing bone loss including advanced HIV-disease, age, low body weight and drug use. The consensus of current evidence is that prevalence of reduced bone mineral density is higher in HIV-infected subjects, both naive and receiving potent antiretroviral therapy, compared to healthy controls (Bongiovanni and Tincati, 2006)

Few studies have investigated vitamin D status in children which is reported to be insufficient in 47–87% of HIV-infected children and young adults living in the United States (Stephensen *et al.*, 2006; Arpadi *et al.*, 2009). The cut-off for vitamin D deficiency is poorly defined but several experts agree a serum 25-OH D concentration <20 ng/ml represents insufficiency (Holick, 2006). Given its role in skeletal and non-skeletal health, development of interventions to improve vitamin D status in HIV-infected children and adolescents is an important research priority.

There are limited data addressing the management of vitamin D deficiency in a paediatric HIV-infected population. However, a recent trial of supplementation with vitamin D_3 (cholecalciferol) and calcium reported improved vitamin D status in a group of HIV-infected children (Arpadi *et al.*, 2009). In adults, improvements in bone mineral density have also been reported with vitamin D and calcium supplements. Bisphosphanates, a class of drugs that work by decreasing bone turnover rate have also been reported as effective therapy for HIV-associated bone loss (Huang *et al.*, 2009). Additional use of bisphosphonates with calcium/vitamin D supplements resulted in significant improvements in BMD (McComsey *et al.*, 2007). The first report of bisphosphanate therapy in an HIV-positive paediatric patient proved to be successful and safe warranting further investigation (Solar *et al.*, 2007).

6.5   Obesity

Obesity and HIV infection are concurrent epidemics with similar metabolic complications. Adverse health outcomes, particularly with respect to the cardiovascular system, are associated both with obesity and HIV infection and its treatment. Gaining excess body fat should therefore be avoided in HIV-infected people.

6.5.1   Definitions

Obesity is a condition where energy intake above needs for energy output leads to accumulation of excess body fat. Adverse health outcomes are most strongly related to body fat mass and in particular to abdominal or visceral fat mass. Measurement of body fatness (also termed adiposity) provides the most direct measure of obesity but is difficult to measure precisely in clinical settings. BMI is a non-invasive convenient method that is most commonly used in the diagnosis of overweight and obesity.

Adults with BMI > 25 kg/m^2 or > 30 kg/m^2 are classified as overweight or obese respectively; cut-offs which are related to health risks. In children the classification is complicated by effects of age and gender. BMI in children should be calculated and plotted on reference centile charts. Using UK growth charts, overweight and obesity identified by BMI on or above the 91st and 98th BMI centiles respectively. These cut-offs correspond approximately to International Obesity Task Force (IOTF) cut-offs for overweight and obesity in adults. There is no clear relationship between the degree of obesity and increased health risks for children, however, as adverse outcomes may not become apparent until adulthood.

6.5.2   Prevalence

The World Health Organization (WHO) estimates that by 2015, 700 million adults will be obese (WHO, 2006). In the United States, where extensive data from national surveys are available, the national prevalence among adults aged 20 years and above is currently estimated at 34% (CDC, 2008). A similar picture is seen in the UK, where an increase from 22 to 33% for men and 23 to 28% for women is forecast between the years 2003 and 2010 (Zaninotto et al., 2006). Many developing countries are currently affected by high rates of overweight and in some this is a greater problem than underweight (Nishida and Mucavele, 2005). It is uncertain if the pattern of obesity reflects this as survey data are either lacking or out of date (Villamor et al., 2006).

Childhood obesity is a serious problem that affects children from diverse ethnic backgrounds, including both industrialised and developing countries. In recent years prevalence has reached epidemic proportions and is of great public health concern due to associations with adverse short- and long-term health outcomes. For example, many studies have reported relationships between obesity and increased risk of chronic diseases such as cardiovascular disease (CVD) and Type II Diabetes Mellitus. Recent estimates from the IOTF suggest that 155 million school age children worldwide are overweight or obese and the World Health Organization (WHO) reports that at least 20 million children under 5 years are affected. In the UK 17% of boys and 15% of girls, aged 2–15 years were classified as obese in 2006 (UK Health Survey, 2006) and if current trends continue a quarter of all children under 16 could be obese by 2050 (Zaninotto *et al.*, 2006). Data from the USA are similar, where 14–19% of children were classified as obese in 2004.

6.5.3 Aetiology

Obesity is a chronic disease that has many causes and its recent dramatic increase is influenced in part by rapidly changing social profiles and resultant inequalities in health (Law *et al.*, 2007). Increasing wealth is seen to have both positive and negative influences on obesity development. For example, in low income countries it is positively associated with obesity whilst the opposite is true in high income countries. Obesity in the UK follows a similar pattern to other high income countries where the rise in childhood obesity is highest among children from poorer backgrounds (Stamatakis *et al.*, 2005). Reasons put forward to explain this focus on environmental influences. Although genetic susceptibility has a role, adverse environmental conditions are mainly responsible for this rapid increase. An obesogenic environment is proposed by many as the likely cause of recent obesity trends, although the exact mechanisms by which the environment influences obesity are unclear.

Obesity results from an intake of energy that exceeds energy needs and assessments of obesity risk must consider energy needs in relation to growth, metabolism, health status and physical activity as well as dietary energy intake. HIV-infected children are at risk of obesity for several reasons involving physiological and social factors. Furthermore, they may develop lipodystrophy, a syndrome characterised by central fat accumulation or peripheral fat wasting or a combination of both, which shares several features with obesity.

6.6 Lipodystrophy

HIV-associated lipodystrophy was first reported in adults but is also present in children, where prevalence is estimated to be between 13 and 47% (European Paediatric Lipodystrophy Group, 2004; Farley *et al.*, 2005; Carter *et al.*, 2006), a range that reflects the lack of definitive diagnostic criteria. HIV lipodystrophy is also termed 'fat redistribution syndrome' and is associated with dyslipidaemia and insulin resistance, both features of the metabolic syndrome.

Dyslipidaemia is seen in association with HIV infection in children regardless of treatment and is thought to arise, in part, secondarily to fat redistribution but also as a result of drug toxicity (Jaquet *et al.*, 2000). The classical changes observed in the lipid profile of HIV- infected children are elevated serum total cholesterol (TC), low-density lipoprotein cholesterol (LDL-C), triglycerides (TG) and reduced high-density lipoprotein cholesterol (HDL-C). Studies investigating the relationship between ART and the lipid profile in children have reported hypercholesterolaemia (HC) (defined by the American Heart Association as total cholesterol (TC) concentration above the 95th percentile for age and gender ($\geq$200 mg/dl, $\geq$5.2 mM/l)), in 13–47% of treated children (Farley *et al.*, 2005; Carter *et al.*, 2006). Raised plasma TC has been reported in children treated with non-nucleoside reverse transcriptase inhibitors (NNRTI) and protease inhibitors (PI), but the greatest effects have been seen in association with PI use. Synergistic effects have been reported for PI in combination with NNRTI (Rhoades *et al.*, 2006).

The obvious concern of these findings is the implication that ART and particularly PI use may increase the risk of CVD in adult life. This is supported by investigations of vascular function among PI-treated children that have provided evidence for a detrimental effect of ART on CVD risk. Assessment of endothelial dysfunction, an accepted risk factor for development of atherosclerosis, through measurement of brachial artery flow-mediated dilatation, found that children receiving therapy had reduced vascular function compared with those not receiving treatment and children on a PI-inclusive regimen were worst affected (Charakida *et al.*, 2005).

6.6.1   Management of dyslipidaemia

The Cardiovascular Subcommittee of the AIDS Clinical Trials Group recommends that dyslipidaemia in HIV-infected adults should be managed with lipid lowering agents, based on the National Cholesterol Education Programme (NCEP) guidelines (NCEP, 1991). However, the addition of these drugs can further complicate already complex ART regimens. Other strategies such as lifestyle and dietary changes, and switching treatment regimens are therefore advised as first-line treatment (Kannel and Giordano, 2004). There is no evidence to guide treatment of HIV-associated dyslipidaemia in children.

The American Academy of Pediatrics, in its most recent clinical report on lipid screening and cardiovascular health in childhood, provides guidance for identification of hyperlipidaemia and recommendations for treatment (Daniels and Greer, 2008). A treatment protocol for the management of HIV-related paediatric dyslipidaemia, based on AHA guidelines (Williams *et al.*, 2002), is currently being developed by the British Dietetic Association specialist group for dietitians working in HIV/AIDS (DHIVA) (see Figure 6.1).

Dietitians experienced in managing HIV-infected children are essential in any team involved with the management of paediatric HIV, particularly as dietary advice is recommended as first-line intervention. Although there are currently no published data concerning the efficacy of dietary management in children living with HIV, some evidence suggests a beneficial effect in adults (Barrios *et al.*, 2002; Shah *et al.*, 2005).

6.6.2   Dietary interventions

There are currently no evidence-based dietary guidelines specific to prevention or treatment of the HIV-related lipodystrophic syndrome. In the absence of these, the most appropriate dietary advice for children with a normal lipid profile is to follow healthy eating guidelines. Most national guidelines are similar to the recommendations of the American Academy of Pediatrics (1992), which advise the gradual adoption between the ages of 2 and 5 years of a diet containing around 30% energy from fat and consumption of adequate calories to support growth and development.

Saturated fat is generally too high in the modern diet and can be reduced by keeping foods that are highly processed, especially those based on animal fats, to about a third of fat intake. Replacing saturated with polyunsaturated fatty acids, e.g. omega 3 (found in fish, green leafy plants, seeds and nuts) and omega 9 fatty acids (found in olive oil) should be encouraged. These fats have been shown to have beneficial effects on the lipid profile.

There may also be benefits from eating foods rich in soluble fibre. Examples of these include oats, legumes (pulse: lentils, peas and beans), fruits and vegetables. In addition to this, children should be advised to reduce consumption of sugar and high sugar foods such as fruit juice, fizzy drinks and confectionary.

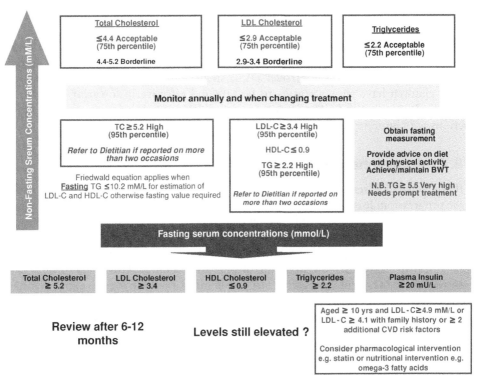

Figure 6.1 A treatment protocol for the management of HIV-related paediatric dyslipidaemia.

HIV and obesity are concurrent epidemics and dietary advice given for the management of dyslipidaemia in HIV is also relevant to obesity.

6.6.3   Obesity prevention and treatment

In the UK, guidance for prevention, management and treatment of childhood obesity has recently been issued from the National Institute for Health and Clinical Excellence (NICE). This body recommends that interventions should include advice on achieving a healthy diet, address lifestyle risk factors within the family and social settings, and incorporate strategies for behavioural change. Importantly, interventions must include at least one other family member. NICE guidelines also recommend that nurseries, schools and childcare facilities should minimise sedentary activities and provide regular opportunities for active play and structured physical activity (NICE, 2006).

6.6.4   Pharmacological interventions

Pharmacological interventions for lipid lowering may be considered as a last resort in refractory cases but should be deferred until the patient is older than 8 years (Daniels and Greer, 2008). However, it is important to consider the extra burden imposed by adding lipid-lowering therapy to complex treatment regimens, which, in turn, may compromise compliance with ART. The possibility of adverse side effects and effects on growth and metabolism in children should also be considered. Pharmacological interventions include statins, fibrates and omega 3 fatty acid supplements.

There are no large-scale studies on the safety and efficacy of statin use in HIV-infected children. Limited data are available in general regarding the use of statins in children and the area is controversial. A small number of short-term clinical trials in children have shown statins to be safe and effective in lowering cholesterol (McCrindle et al., 2007). The use of statins in HIV is further complicated by interactions with antiretrovirals.

6.7   Assessment and monitoring

HIV-infected children should ideally attend outpatient clinics for monitoring of disease progression. It is debatable how frequent this should be, but in the UK appointments are usually three-monthly. Height, weight and blood pressure are routinely measured and a blood sample taken for assessment of immune status, viral load, full blood count and lipid profile. Some centres also assess glucose/insulin status and this can help to identify the need for dietetic intervention. However, in most UK centres where the client caseload is large, it is rarely possible for the clinic dietitian to assess children at each visit and referrals to the dietitian are made on the basis of urgent need. Annual dietary assessment is useful for monitoring nutritional intake and forms the basis for dietary counselling (see Chapter 4 'Paediatric Nutritional Screening, Assessment and Support').

6.8   Dietary intake assessment

Various methods of dietary assessment can be used to estimate a child's food intake (Lanigan et al., 2001). Methods can be both qualitative, providing information on the type of foods usually eaten and meal pattern, or quantitative where additional information about the amounts of foods consumed is provided. Methods range from food frequency questionnaires which are relatively quick and easy to administer to weighed food records that involve the greatest effort for both investigator and subject. The instrument of choice depends on the purpose of the assessment, and in clinical settings the most useful method is the dietary history where either the child or main carer is asked to describe a 'typical' day's diet.

Taking a diet history is a lengthy procedure that requires a skilled assessor; ideally, a dietitian. Assessment should be carried out annually and, additionally, if there is concern about the child's growth or general health. The purpose of assessing dietary intake is usually to compare a child's nutritional intake with what is recommended for their age, size and developmental level.

6.9   Advice for healthy eating

A healthy diet is made up of a variety of foods that collectively provide the nutrients comprising the optimal diet. For infants up to 6 months of age human milk or breast milk substitutes should meet the nutritional requirements of the majority of infants (see Chapter 3, 'Malnutrition, Infant Feeding, Maternal and Child Health'). Complementary foods can be introduced at around 6 months of age. A suggested meal pattern for infancy is given in Table 6.1. Foods from the four main food groups (Table 6.2) should be included in quantities recommended for specific age

Table 6.1 Food groups.

Food groups	Examples of foods	Recommendations
Cereals and starchy foods	Bread, pasta, couscous and semolina Wheat flour Rice, maize, barley, rye, oats potatoes and starchy roots – plantain, yam Breakfast cereals	Infants and young children, 2–4 portions daily Older children, minimum of 5 portions daily, preferably wholegrain varieties
Fruits and vegetables	Green leafy vegetables Salad vegetables and tomatoes Non-starchy root vegetables – carrots and turnip Citrus fruits – oranges and pineapple Berry fruits – blackberry and strawberry Apples and pears Melons, plums, peaches and mango Natural unsweetened fruit juices Dried fruits – raisins, sultanas and dates	Infants and young children, 3–5 portions daily Older children minimum of 5 portions daily
Milk and dairy products	Milk – cow, goat, sheep and buffalo Dried milk powder and evaporated milk Modified and fortified infant formula Soya milk and soya infant formulas Fermented milks and yoghurt Hard and soft cheeses Crème fraiche Soya milks and tofu	Infants – at least 500 ml of breast or formula milk daily until age 1 year Young children – 350 ml milk or equivalent Older children (over 10 years) – 500 ml milk or equivalent
Meat and meat substitutes	Meat, chicken, turkey and goose Bacon, ham, liver, kidney and sausage Fish and shellfish Eggs – hen, duck and goose Meat substitutes, soya products Pulses including dhal, lentils and beans Peas and chick peas Nuts and nut butters Houmous	Infants and children – 1–2 portions daily. Two portions if no animal products (meat, fish and egg) are included in the diet
High energy density, low-nutrient-density foods	Confectionary, sweets (candy) and chocolates Soft drinks – squash and fizzy drinks Cream and ice cream Mayonnaise Sugar, jam and honey Butter, margarine, cooking oil and cooking fat Crisps, chips and packet savoury snacks Biscuits cakes and pastries	Infants – avoid these foods. Children – use sparingly; they should not replace foods in the other 4 groups

Table 6.2 Feeding pattern for infants aged 0–12 months.

Age (months)	Feeding pattern
Up to 4–6 months	Exclusive breastfeeding or 150–180 ml per kg body weight of a modified and fortified infant starter formula. No other foods or fluids (including water)
	Feed about 6 times every 24 hours
6–7	Continue full breast or bottle-feeding. Introduce bland puree foods such as cereals, cooked fruits and vegetables and mashed potato, using a spoon to feed the infant. Initially, introduce at one meal per day, increasing to 2–3 times daily
7–9	When weaning foods are taken three times daily, reduce breast or formula milk by omitting one feed, so that milk is given 4–5 times each day. Maintain fluid intake by giving water using a cup
	Gradually change foods to a soft texture that requires some chewing, e.g. soft mashed vegetables and soft bread. Give some hard foods for infant to hold and bite, e.g. rusks; continue to feed infant with a spoon. Increase the variety of foods offered
9–12	Reduce breast or formula milk to about three times daily. All fluids other than breast milk should be from a cup
	Progress towards a more adult texture with food, continue increasing the variety and continue to feed with a spoon. The infant will begin to self-feed. The meal pattern should be three meals and three snacks or milk drinks each day

groups (Table 6.3). High-energy, low-nutrient-density foods may be included in small quantities but should not displace foods from the other four groups.

In the UK, the Government's Food Standards Agency provides guidance on healthy eating and uses the 'Eatwell' plate model to describe the approximate contribution each food group should make to a healthy balanced diet (Figure 13.3). A more detailed description of the foods in the main groups is given below.

6.9.1 Carbohydrates (starchy foods)

Carbohydrates are found as starch in staples such as bread, rice, potatoes, pasta and other cereals and ideally should provide the base of each main meal. Certain starchy foods contain carbohydrate in a form that is digested more slowly than others. For example, wholegrain varieties of bread and pasta will be broken down more gradually than refined white alternatives.

About one-third of our food and half our daily energy should come from starchy foods and it is recommended that unrefined (wholegrain) types are included regularly. However, because young children have smaller stomachs than adults, high-fibre starches may be too filling and prevent the child from taking adequate nutrients from other essential food groups if given to excess. Therefore, smaller amounts of wholegrain cereals should be given to children.

Children need between 3 and 5 portions of starchy food each day from a variety of sources (Table 6.2). Starches are digested mainly to glucose, which is the body's main energy source. Sugars are more simple carbohydrates and can be found for example in milk (lactose) or fruit (fructose). These can be included as part of a healthy diet

Table 6.3 Meal patterns and portion sizes for children.

Age (years)	1–2	2–3	3–5	5–10
Meal pattern	3 meals + 3 snacks or milk drinks	3 meals + 3 snacks or milk drinks	3 meals + 2–3 snacks or milk drinks	3 meals and 2–3 snacks
Cereals, bread, potato, rice and starchy foods	3–4 portions daily 1 portion bread = $\frac{1}{2}$ slice or 20–30 g mashed potato 30 g breakfast cereal 15 g	4–5 portions daily 1 portion bread = 1 slice or 40 g potato 30–60 g breakfast cereal 15–20 g	5 portions daily 1 portion bread = 1–2 slices or 40–80 g potato 60–80 g breakfast cereal 20–30 g	minimum 5 portions daily 1 portion bread = 2–4 slices or 80–160 g potato 100–150 g breakfast cereal 30–40 g
Fruit and vegetables	3–4 portions daily 1 portion of vegetables (mashed) = 30 g fruit (soft) $\frac{1}{2}$ – 1 banana	3–5 portions daily 1 portion vegetables = 30–60 g fruit 1 piece (e.g.1 apple) 80 g	4–5 portions daily 1 portion vegetables = 60–80 g fruit 1 large fruit 100 g	minimum 5 portions daily 1 portion vegetables = 100–120 g Fruit 1 large fruit 100 g
Milk, cheese and yoghurt	500 ml full-fat cow's milk or infant formula or equivalent 3–4 portions daily 1 portion milk = 120–150 ml yoghurt 60 g grated cheese 20 g	350 ml full-fat or 2.4% fat milk 3 portions daily 1 portion milk = 150 ml Yoghurt 80 g cubed/grated cheese 30 g	350 ml full-fat or 2.4% fat milk 2–3 portions daily 1 portion milk = 150 ml yoghurt 120 g cheese 30–40 g	350 ml full-fat, 2.4% fat or low fat milk 2 portions daily 1 portion milk = 200 ml yoghurt 120–150 g cheese 50–60 g
Meat or fish or egg or >pulses or nuts	1–2 portions daily 1 portion of minced/finely chopped meat = 20–30 g cooked egg $\frac{1}{2}$–1 egg	1–2 portions daily 1 portion chopped meat = 30–40 g egg 1 egg (70 g) pulses 30 g	1–2 portions daily 1 portion meat or fish = 40–60 g pulses 40–60 g	1–2 portions daily 1 portion meat or fish = 80–100 g pulses 80–120 g
General notes	Avoid foods that are high in salt, sugar or are very spicy	Lower fat (2.4%) milk can be used if the child is growing well and has a good appetite. Continued use of a modified and fortified infant formula may be useful if growth or appetite is poor. Use high fat and high sugar foods sparingly	If foods are fried, use an unsaturated fat for cooking and an unsaturated margarine in place of butter Young children still need help and encouragement with feeding until about 5 years	Low (fat-free) milk can be used if the child is growing well. High fat and sugary foods can be included but should not replace foods in the first four food groups

but an excess of simple sugars can be detrimental to health. Carbohydrate provides approximately 4 kcal/g or 16.7 kJ/g.

6.9.2   Fruit and vegetables

Fruit and vegetables are good sources of many vitamins and minerals and in the UK it is recommended that 5 portions are eaten daily. Evidence suggests that people who eat the most fruit and vegetables are less likely to develop chronic diseases such as coronary heart disease and some cancers. The Eatwell plate model shows that roughly one-third of our food intake should come from this group.

As with starches, young children may have difficulty in eating large amounts of fruits and vegetables. Tinned, frozen, dried and juiced fruit can be helpful in achieving recommended levels of intake in young children. However, fruit juices may be high in sugar and should be given only once daily.

As a rough guideline, a child's portion equates approximately to an amount that can fit into the palm of the hand. Giving a variety of fruit and vegetables can help to ensure the optimal complement of vitamins and minerals (see Section 6.9.6).

6.9.3   Meat, fish, eggs and beans (and other non-dairy sources of protein)

Proteins have essential structural and regulatory roles within the human body. The main dietary protein requirement is for growth and repair, but when taken in excess or during times of greater nutritional demand proteins can be used as an energy source. Like carbohydrate proteins provide energy at about 4 kcal/g or 16.7 kJ/g.

Proteins are made up of amino acids, nine of which are essential to humans (i.e. cannot be synthesised from other amino acids): isoleucine, leucine, lysine, methionine, phenylalanine, threonine, tryptophan, valine (and histidine in infancy only). Protein foods vary in their biological value; animal proteins provide a more complete protein source and have a higher biological value, whereas plant foods contain a smaller range of amino acids and it may be necessary to complement the diet with a variety of plant foods to obtain the full range of essential amino acids.

Children need 1–2 portions of protein daily and these should come from a range of sources (Table 6.1). Lower fat versions can be used in children over 2 years, higher fat versions given infrequently or in smaller amounts. Aim for 1–2 portions of fish a week, including a portion of oily fish.

6.9.4   Milk and dairy foods

Milk and dairy products are good sources of protein and vitamins, in particular vitamins A and B12. They are also an important source of calcium, essential for bone health. Calcium in dairy foods is found as cholecalciferol; the most readily absorbed and utilized form.

Milk forms a large part of the diet in many children and whole milk should be taken until they are at least 2 years old. If given to small children, semi-skimmed or fully skimmed milk may provide inadequate energy and nutrients and should only be introduced as a main drink in children over 2 who have access to a varied diet.

Dairy products may be high in saturated fat, which can raise cholesterol and is linked to heart disease. Therefore, in children aged 2 years and above, lower fat options should be used when possible. Recommendations for intake are given in Tables 6.1 and 6.3.

6.9.5   Foods and drinks high in fat and sugar

Foods high in fats, sugar and salt should form the smallest part of the diet. Fats are an essential part of the diet. They provide energy and essential nutrients including vitamins and fatty acids. Fatty acids can be either saturated or unsaturated and a healthy diet should contain a balance of these fats.

Fat is more energy dense than carbohydrate and protein, providing approximately 9 kcal/g or 38 kJ/g and therefore may contribute to excess energy intake and obesity. Saturated fat is found mainly in animal products and a high intake is linked to cardiovascular disease.

The UK government recommends a decrease in saturated fat intake in favour of mono- and poly-unsaturated fats. This can be achieved by reducing intake of foods high in animal fats, e.g. fatty meat and meat products, butter, cheese and processed foods and including more mono-unsaturates, e.g. olive and rapeseed oil, avocados and poly-unsaturates, e.g. oily fish, sunflower and linseed oils and green leafy vegetables.

Fat is also a source of essential fatty acids linoleic (n-6) and alpha-linolenic (n-3) acid and fat-soluble vitamins A, D and E. A healthy balance of fats can be provided by taking care not to give the child an excess of processed foods which contain hidden fats. Infants and toddlers need to obtain a higher percentage of their energy from fat because it is the most energy dense of the macronutrients and less likely to overfill the child's stomach.

6.9.6   Micronutrients

As well as these energy-providing nutrients the body needs small but regular quantities of vitamins and minerals, the micro or 'small' nutrients. These do not provide any dietary energy:

Vitamins

Vitamins are essential nutrients that are required in very small amounts, which, if absent or insufficient in the diet, will lead to general poor health and specific deficiency symptoms. They are found in different foods, i.e. no single food contains the full complement of vitamins. Broadly speaking, they fall into two categories: fat soluble and water soluble.

Fat soluble
Fat-soluble vitamins A, D, E and K are most concentrated in foods of animal origin. Vitamin A as retinol is found only in animal foods but milk and some plant foods, e.g. carrots, green vegetables and apricots contain carotenes which can be converted by the body to retinol. Margarine is also a good source. Vitamin E is found in many foods, the richest sources being vegetable oils, eggs, meat and cereals. Vitamin K is

also widespread in foods and is synthesised in the human body by bacteria. Vitamin D is largely obtained by the action of sunlight on skin but can also be found in the diet, e.g. in margarines or fish and their oils.

Water soluble

Water-soluble vitamins are not stored in the body long-term and regular intake is therefore important. The B vitamins have essential roles as enzyme cofactors and take part in many energy transformation processes. They are found in a variety of foods including wholegrain cereals, green leafy vegetables, pulses and yeast extract e.g. Marmite and Vegemite. Vitamin C is necessary for the maintenance of connective tissue. Deficiency leads to bleeding especially of the gums (scurvy), delayed wound healing and ultimately death. Citrus fruits (oranges and lemons) are good sources as are tomatoes and potatoes.

Minerals

About 15 inorganic elements or minerals are known to be essential to man and have three main functions:

- as constituents of bones and teeth, e.g. calcium, phosphorus and magnesium
- regulatory role as part of extra- and intracellular fluid, e.g. sodium and potassium
- as enzyme cofactors, e.g. iron and phosphorus.

Trace elements

Selections of minerals known as trace elements are required in minute amounts within the human body. These have roles as enzyme cofactors (manganese, selenium, zinc and copper); in energy transformation (cobalt and chromium); hormonal function (iodine); and as structural protection (fluorine).

A balanced healthy diet should provide all minerals and trace elements. However, reports from the National Diet and Nutrition Survey (Gregory *et al.*, 1995) and the Avon Longitudinal Study of Parents and Children (Cowin and Emmett, 2007) suggest that many toddlers in the UK today do not consume a diet that conforms to government recommendations. In particular, iron and zinc were a problem in the younger age group. Meat, in particular red meat, liver and fish are good sources of iron. Vegetable sources such as peas, beans, lentils, cereals and green leafy vegetables are not so well absorbed. Vitamin C can aid the absorption of vegetable iron and foods rich in vitamin C should be given at the same time as plant-based iron. Zinc is found in foods of animal origin and a menu plan providing adequate quantities of these nutrients can be found in Table 6.4.

6.10   Conclusion

HIV is a chronic condition affecting a large number of children globally and is associated with both short and long-term adverse health outcomes. Both under- and overnutrition are implicated in increased disease risk. The concurrent obesity epidemic compounds problems associated with HIV infection and its treatment, in particular cardiovascular disease risk factors are affected. Nutrition has an important

Table 6.4 Portion sizes for 2–3-year-old children, and meal plans adequate in iron, zinc and vitamin D.

Food group	Portion sizes (2–3 years)	Meal plan	Meal plan meeting iron RNI*	Meal plan meeting zinc RNI*	Meal plan meeting vitamin D RNI*
Cereal	1–1½ tablespoons (tbsp) (15–20 g)	Breakfast	Iron-fortified cereal with full-fat, semi-skimmed or iron fortified milk	Porridge with full-fat or semi-skimmed milk and raspberries	Toast with fortified margarine and spread
Bread	1 slice (40 g)		Dilute orange juice		
Vegetables	1–2 tbsp (30–60 g)	Mid-morning snack	Apple or banana	Houmous with carrot sticks	Cheese chunks
Fruit	1 piece (80–100 g)		1 cup milk		
Egg	1 hard cooked egg	Lunch	Boiled egg with wholemeal bread marmite soldiers	Grilled cheese and tomato on wholemeal bread	Canned sardines on wholemeal toast
Cheese	25–30 g cubed/grated		Dilute fruit juice/water		
Vegetables	1–2 tbsp (30–60 g)	Mid-afternoon snack	Houmous with carrot sticks	Sausage chunks and fromage frais dip	Apple or banana
Fruit	1 piece (80–100 g)		1 cup milk	Dilute fruit juice/water	Dilute fruit juice/water
Meat, fish etc.	1½ tbsp (20–30 g)	Dinner	Meatballs (beef or lentil pattie) and tomato dipping sauce	Burger (beef or lentil pattie) with wholemeal buns, tomato relish, and salad.	Fish pie (salmon or tuna) with vegetables and potato topping
Potato	1–2 tbsp (30–60 g)		Dilute orange juice		
Vegetables	1–2 tbsp (30–60 g)				
Yogurt	2 tbsp (60 g)	Dessert	Yoghurt and fruit	Yoghurt and fruit	Yoghurt and fruit
Cheese	25–30 g cubed/grated				
Dessert	2–3 tbsp (60–80 g)				
	2–3 tbsp (60–80 g)				
Drink	1 teacup (150 ml)		1 cup milk or pure juice diluted in 5–10 parts water	1 cup milk or pure juice diluted in 5–10 parts water	1 cup milk or pure juice diluted in 5–10 parts water

*Two- to three-years-old children should consume at least six glasses of fluids per day.
From the Journal of Family Healthcare 17(5), with permission. www.jfhc.co.uk.

role in HIV management. Research is urgently needed to inform management and treatment strategies.

References

American Academy of Pediatrics. National cholesterol education program: report of the expert panel on blood cholesterol levels in children and adolescents. *Pediatrics* 1992; **89**:525–84.

Arpadi SM, McMahon D, Abrams EJ *et al.* Effect of bimonthly supplementation with oral cholecalciferol on serum 25-hydroxyvitamin D concentrations in HIV-infected children and adolescents. *Pediatrics* 2009; **123**:e121–e126.

Barrios A, Blanco F, Garcia-Benayas T *et al.* Effect of dietary intervention on highly active antiretroviral therapy-related dyslipemia. *AIDS* 2002; **16**:2079–81.

Bongiovanni M, Tincati C. Bone diseases associated with human immunodeficiency virus infection: pathogenesis, risk factors and clinical management. *Curr Mol Med* 2006; **6**:395–400.

Bunn JY, Solomon SE, Miller C, Forehand R. Measurement of stigma in people with HIV: a reexamination of the HIV Stigma Scale. *AIDS Educ Prev* 2007; **19**:198–208.

Buys H, Hendricks M, Eley B, Hussey G. The role of nutrition and micronutrients in paediatric HIV infection. *SADJ* 2002; **57**:454–6.

Carter RJ, Wiener J, Abrams EJ *et al.* Dyslipidemia among perinatally HIV-infected children enrolled in the PACTS-HOPE cohort, 1999–2004: a longitudinal analysis. *J Acquir Immune Defic Syndr* 2006; **41**:453–60.

Charakida M, Donald AE, Green H *et al.* Early structural and functional changes of the vasculature in HIV-infected children: impact of disease and antiretroviral therapy. *Circulation* 2005; **112**:103–9.

Cowin I, Emmett P. Diet in a group of 18-month-old children in South West England, and comparison with the results of a national survey. *J Hum Nutr Diet* 2007; **20**:254–67.

Daniels SR, Greer FR. Lipid screening and cardiovascular health in childhood. *Pediatrics* 2008; **122**:198–208.

European Paediatric Lipodystrophy Group. Antiretroviral therapy, fat redistribution and hyperlipidaemia in HIV-infected children in Europe. *AIDS* 2004; **18**:1443–51.

Farley J, Gona P, Crain M *et al.* Prevalence of elevated cholesterol and associated risk factors among perinatally HIV-infected children (4–19 years old) in Pediatric AIDS Clinical Trials Group 219C. *J Acquir Immune Defic Syndr* 2005; **38**:480–7.

Gibb DM, Duong T, Tookey PA *et al.* Decline in mortality, AIDS, and hospital admissions in perinatally HIV-1 infected children in the United Kingdom and Ireland. *BMJ* 2003; **327**:1019.

Gregory J, Collins DL, Davies PSW, Hughes JM, Clarke, PC. *National Diet and Nutrition Survey: Children Aged 1 $^1/_2$ to 4 $^1/_2$ Years.* London: HSMO, 1995.

Grinspoon S, Mulligan K. Weight loss and wasting in patients infected with human immunodeficiency virus. *Clin Infect Dis* 2003; **36**:S69–S78.

Health Survey for England 2006: CVD and risk factors adults, obesity and risk factors children. Jan 31, 2008; March 25, 2009.

Holick MF. High prevalence of vitamin D inadequacy and implications for health. *Mayo Clin Proc* 2006; **81**:353–73.

Huang J, Meixner L, Fernandez S, McCutchan JA. A double-blinded, randomized controlled trial of zoledronate therapy for HIV-associated osteopenia and osteoporosis. *AIDS* 2009; **23**:51–7.

Irlam JH, Visser ME, Rollins N, Siegfried N. Micronutrient supplementation in children and adults with HIV infection. *Cochrane Database Syst Rev* 2005; CD003650.

Jaquet D, Levine M, Ortega-Rodriguez E *et al.* Clinical and metabolic presentation of the lipodystrophic syndrome in HIV-infected children. *AIDS* 2000; **14**:2123–8.

Jones CY, Hogan JW, Snyder B *et al.* Overweight and human immunodeficiency virus (HIV) progression in women: associations HIV disease progression and changes in body mass index in women in the HIV epidemiology research study cohort. *Clin Infect Dis* 2003; **37**(Suppl 2):S69–S80.

Kannel WB, Giordano M. Long-term cardiovascular risk with protease inhibitors and management of the dyslipidemia. *Am J Cardiol* 2004; **94**:901–6.

Lanigan JA, Wells JC, Lawson MS, Lucas A. Validation of food diary method for assessment of dietary energy and macronutrient intake in infants and children aged 6–24 months. *Eur J Clin Nutr* 2001; **55**:124–9.

Law C, Power C, Graham H, Merrick D. Obesity and health inequalities. *Obes Rev* 2007; 8 (Suppl 1):19–22.

McComsey GA, Kendall MA, Tebas P *et al.* Alendronate with calcium and vitamin D supplementation is safe and effective for the treatment of decreased bone mineral density in HIV. *AIDS* 2007; **21**:2473–82.

McCrindle BW, Urbina EM, Dennison BA *et al.* Drug therapy of high-risk lipid abnormalities in children and adolescents: a scientific statement from the American Heart Association Atherosclerosis, Hypertension, and Obesity in Youth Committee, Council of Cardiovascular Disease in the Young, with the Council on Cardiovascular Nursing. *Circulation* 2007; **115**:1948–67.

Mehta S, Fawzi W. Effects of vitamins, including vitamin A, on HIV/AIDS patients. *Vitam Horm* 2007; **75**:355–83.

NCEP: National Cholesterol Education Program. *Report of the Expert Panel on Blood Cholesterol Levels in Children and Adolescents.* National Heart, Lung, and Blood Institute Information Center, Public Health Service, U.S. Department of Health and Human Services, 1991. Bethesda, MD: NIH Publication No. 91-2732.

National Institute for Health and Clinical Excellence. Obesity guidance on the prevention, identification, assessment and management of overweight and obesity in adults and children. 2006; **43**:21–8-2007.

Nishida C, Mucavele P. Monitoring the rapidly emerging public health problem of overweight and obesity: The World Health Organization Global Database on Body Mass Index. *SCN News* 2005; **29**:5–12.

Rhoades MP, Smith CJ, Tudor-Williams G *et al.* Effects of highly active antiretroviral therapy on paediatric metabolite levels. *HIV Med* 2006; **7**:16–24.

Shah M, Tierney K, ms-Huet B *et al.* The role of diet, exercise and smoking in dyslipidaemia in HIV-infected patients with lipodystrophy. *HIV Med* 2005; **6**:291–8.

Soler PP, Torrent A, Rossich R *et al.* Osteoporosis and multiple fractures in an antiretroviral-naive, HIV-positive child. *J Pediatr Endocrinol Metab* 2007; **20**:933–8.

Stamatakis E, Primatesta P, Chinn S, Rona R, Falascheti E. Overweight and obesity trends from 1974 to 2003 in English children: what is the role of socioeconomic factors? *Arch Dis Child* 2005; **90**:999–1004.

Stephensen CB, Marquis GS, Kruzich LA, Douglas SD, Aldrovandi GM, Wilson CM. Vitamin D status in adolescents and young adults with HIV infection. *Am J Clin Nutr* 2006; **83**:1135–41.

U.S. Obesity Trends 1985–2006. Centers for Disease Control and Prevention. July 27, 2007; March 31, 2008.

Villamor E, Msamanga G, Urassa W *et al.* Trends in obesity, underweight, and wasting among women attending prenatal clinics in urban Tanzania, 1995–2004. *Am J Clin Nutr* 2006; **83**:1387–94.

Williams CL, Hayman LL, Daniels SR *et al.* Cardiovascular health in childhood: A statement for health professionals from the Committee on Atherosclerosis, Hypertension, and Obesity in the Young (AHOY) of the Council on Cardiovascular Disease in the Young, American Heart Association. *Circulation* 2002; **106**:143–60.

World Health Organization. Obesity and overweight. *Internet* 2006; **6**: March 25, 2009.

Zaninotto, P, Wardle, H, Stamatakis, E, Mindell, J, and Head, J. Forecasting obesity to 2010. August 25, 2006.

Section 3
NUTRITIONAL MANAGEMENT OF HIV DISEASE

7 Decreased Nutritional Status and Nutritional Interventions for People Living with HIV

Vivian Pribram

Key Points

- HIV-related weight loss and wasting remain common problems.
- Decreased nutritional status in people with HIV infection is associated with disease progression, increased morbidity and reduced survival independent of immunodeficiency and viral load.
- The three main causes of weight loss related to HIV are reduced food intake, malabsorption and hypermetabolism.
- While there is much evidence of severe protein deficiency associated with HIV infection, it is difficult to establish the amount of protein and other nutrients needed to maintain body composition and function in individuals and growth in children.
- Management of weight loss and wasting may include nutritional interventions, resistance exercise training and, if necessary, pharmacological treatment such as hormone therapy, and cytokine treatments.

7.1 Introduction/background

Despite major advances in the treatment and survival of patients infected with human immunodeficiency virus (HIV), weight loss and wasting remain common problems (Mangili *et al.*, 2006) and research on nutritional supplementation, particularly macronutrient supplementation, is limited in the patient group (Koethe *et al.*, 2009). The scope of this chapter includes: definitions, significance and aetiology of weight loss and wasting; macronutrient and micronutrient deficiencies; nutritional and non-nutritional management of malnutrition; and wasting associated with HIV infection.

7.2 Malnutrition, weight loss and wasting

Weight loss may occur at all stages of HIV disease. Weight loss occurs in about one-third of patients in the asymptomatic latent phase and is invariable in the symptomatic and end-stage phases of the disease (Ockenga *et al.*, 2006).

HIV-associated wasting, compared with starvation, preferentially depletes muscle over adipose tissue and reduces muscle phosphate stores necessary to replenish serum phosphate. For patients with wasting and anorexia, a low serum phosphate level may be adequate for the relatively low turnover of metabolic intermediates (e.g. adenosine triphosphate). However, these patients may be particularly at risk of refeeding syndrome when increased oral intake does occur, particularly in areas where staple diets contain a high ratio of carbohydrate compared to protein and fat (Koethe et al., 2009). Decreased lean tissue mass leads to reduced skeletal muscle mass leading to decreased muscular strength, functional performance, and is associated with disease progression (Dudgeon et al., 2006). Several studies have shown that a low BMI at the start of antiretroviral therapy (ART) is an independent predictor of early mortality. The causes for this are poorly understood but a high burden of opportunistic infections may cause rapid weight loss and increase the incidence of immune reconstitution inflammatory syndrome (Koethe et al., 2009). At the time of death, body cell mass (BCM) (intracellular mass of all metabolically active tissues in the body) in persons infected with HIV was found to be only half the ideal values and a progressive depletion of BCM was also shown (Kotler et al., 1989).

However, body weight, body mass index (BMI) and history of weight loss have not been shown to predict prognosis reliably in this patient group. This is possibly because increased extracellular fluid and/or fat mass may mask loss of muscle and visceral mass (Ockenga et al., 2006). Yet, some study results suggest that weight loss in HIV-infected adults is not necessarily a loss of lean body mass (LBM) but is a complex interplay of lean body and fat mass, depending on the baseline body weight and composition and the aetiology of weight loss (Mangili et al., 2006). This may make it difficult, in some cases, to distinguish HIV-related wasting from lipodystrophy, which is a frequent complication of antiretroviral treatment, manifest as fat redistribution with loss of subcutaneous fat, increase in intra-abdominal fat, dorsocervical fat pad, or breast hypertrophy (see Chapter 8 'Nutritional Screening and Assessment' and Chapter 10 'The Nutritional Management of Complications Associated with HIV and Antiretroviral Therapy'). Body weight may increase or decrease depending on the relation between subcutaneous lipoatrophy and intra-abdominal lipohypertrophy (Ockenga et al., 2006).

7.3   Significance of involuntary weight loss

Decreased nutritional status in HIV-infected patients is associated with disease progression, increased morbidity and reduced survival, independent of immunodeficiency and viral load (Hsu et al., 2005; Ockenga et al., 2006), even when ART is not limited (Mangili et al., 2006). Other negative associations of involuntary weight loss include:

- lower CD4$^+$ cell counts (Mangili et al., 2006)
- impaired functional status (Dudgeon et al., 2006)
- HIV RNA correlates positively with weight loss and body mass index (Dudgeon et al., 2006)
- decreased health-related QOL in men but not in women (Mangili et al., 2006).

In the Nutrition for Healthy Living study (NFHL) investigators examined whether ART could completely alleviate weight loss in effectively treated individuals. ART was independently associated with improved survival rates but was neither a confounder nor an effect modifier in the association between weight loss and death. When all wasting definitions were included, there was a significant increase in the risk of death with each 1% increase in weight loss from baseline weight (Mangili et al., 2006). When weight loss was more than 10% from baseline weight, the relative risk of mortality was increased nearly sixfold, while even a 5% weight loss over a 6-month period or weight loss of greater than 3% from baseline were found to be significant predictors of mortality. BMI was inversely associated with risk of death; individuals with a baseline BMI of greater than 25 kg/m^2 had a much lower risk of dying than did those with baseline BMI of less than 25. Weight loss was a stronger predictor of death than loss of LBM (Mangili et al., 2006).

In a cross-sectional analysis including 562 participants with HIV infection enrolled in the NFHL study, BMI was lower in drug users than non-drug users, and was lowest in cocaine users. BMI was also directly associated with CD4 count and inversely related to age greater than 55 years (Quach et al., 2008).

7.4   Definitions of HIV-related weight loss and wasting

The exact point at which progressive weight loss becomes wasting is difficult to define. There is little data to support cut-off points for LBM that correlate to wasting parameters (Mangili et al., 2006). In 1987, the Centers for Disease Control and Prevention (CDC) included HIV-associated wasting as an AIDS-defining condition (ADC) which was revised in 1993. It is defined as an involuntary weight loss of greater than 10% of baseline body weight during the previous 12 months plus either diarrhoea, fever or weakness for more than 30 days in the absence of a concurrent illness (Centers for Disease Control and Prevention, 1993; Dudgeon et al., 2006). Limitations of this definition have been highlighted:

- HIV-associated unintentional weight loss can occur without diarrhoea, fever or weakness and, arguably, this may be more problematic.
- It is assumed that baseline weight, which may have been reported and not measured, represented the patient's usual or ideal weight, whereas HIV-infected patients are seen at varying stages of HIV infection and that 'baseline' values may be less meaningful.
- It does not take into account the rate of weight loss, which may provide valuable information for the assessment of the need for intervention (Mangili et al., 2006).

There is little data to support other definitions but in an attempt to overcome these limitations, capture medically important weight loss, and provide clinical reference points, definitions used in the NFHL study included the following:

- significant weight loss (>10%)
- weight loss that was progressive and advanced
- (BMI, <20 kg/m^2)
- a rapid rate of weight loss (>5% in 6 months).

Rapid, unintentional weight loss and wasting is of particular concern and it is commonly a manifestation of opportunistic infection or malignancy in advanced immunodeficiency (Mangili *et al.*, 2006; Ockenga *et al.*, 2006).

7.5 Prevalence

At the beginning of the pandemic, severe malnutrition and weight loss were common. During the era before the advent of effective antiretroviral treatment, HIV-associated weight loss and wasting were among the most frequently occurring AIDS-defining conditions (ADCs), with wasting once described as one of the three most common ADCs (Mangili *et al.*, 2006). It has been estimated that nearly 20% of those infected with HIV suffer from wasting, even with the widespread implementation of ART (Dudgeon *et al.*, 2006). However, Ockenga *et al.* (2006) report that the introduction of effective antiretroviral treatment in 1996 has decreased the incidence of wasting, and it is now seen mostly in patients who have never been treated or where treatment has failed due to drug intolerance or resistance. However, in resource-limited regions food insecurity may also influence weight gain seen with commencement of ART. Discrepancies in reports of prevalence of HIV-related wasting in the ART era may, in part, be due to shortcomings in definitions of HIV-related wasting. Using the more inclusive NFHL study definition outlined above (see Section 7.4) high incidence (33.5%) and prevalence (38%) were shown among the NFHL cohort studied. The study authors concluded that HIV-associated wasting may have previously been underestimated and under-appreciated and that it occurs as frequently in the post-HAART (Highly Active Anti-retroviral Therapy) era as it did in the pre-HAART era (Mangili *et al.*, 2006).

7.6 Aetiology

The aetiology of HIV-associated wasting is multifactorial and has not been fully elucidated, although changes in whole body protein turnover are now well described (Hsu *et al.*, 2005). During weight loss in HIV, the proportion of body stores that are lost, be they protein, fat or carbohydrate depends on the underlying nutritional state and dietary intake. Thus, the initial level of body protein and fat, together with the dietary intake and the severity of the inflammatory response, will affect the rate of weight loss (Hsu *et al.*, 2005). Patients with advanced immunodeficiency may experience frequent episodes of clinical infection from repeated opportunistic pathogens, in between which they can rebuild nutrient stores. Repeated episodes of weight loss due to loss of fat and lean tissue followed by recovery appear to allow fat to be preferentially repleted, so measurement of body composition is important at this stage (see Chapter 8 'Nutritional Screening and Assessment') Loss of protein mass is markedly accelerated during opportunistic infections. It is not, however, clear why some patients experience a starvation-like metabolic response whereas others, especially those with *Pneumocystis carinii* infection, for example, may experience a hypermetabolic state (Hsu *et al.*, 2005).

The precise relationship between changes in viral load and nutritional status in HIV infection is unclear. In the NFHL study it was shown that changes in both viral load and severity of disease (as measured by CD4$^+$ cell counts) contribute to changes in weight. Changes in viral load were inversely associated with changes in weight for those not on ART or for those starting or stopping ART (Mangili *et al.*, 2006). In this study, it was not possible to explain the role of ADCs due to the low incidence in the era of effective HIV treatment. However, results of longitudinal analysis of 669 participants suggest that

- a diagnosis of one historical AIDS-defining condition (ADC) in the past did not predict wasting-related outcomes
- having had more than one historical ADC predicted a 30% increase in developing a BMI of <20 kg/m^2
- the risk of a 10% weight loss increased 20% with each additional historical ADC
- if an ADC occurred in the 6 months preceding a study visit, the risk of weight loss increased to 2.5–8.0-fold (Mangili *et al.*, 2006).

There are numerous possible causes of weight loss related to HIV and these are usually grouped into three main categories: reduced food intake, malabsorption and hypermetabolism. Weight loss can be affected by a number of factors including:

- socio-economic circumstances
- psychosocial and behavioural factors
- cultural practices
- endocrine abnormalities
- hormonal deficiencies
- hyperlactataemia and lactic acidosis
- metabolic demands and complications of ARV medication
- cytokine dysregulation (Hsu *et al.*, 2005; Mangili *et al.*, 2006; Pribram and Lanigan, 2007).

Effective nutritional therapy, together with medical treatment of any underlying condition, is of prime importance in reversing malnutrition (Grunfeld and Kotler, 1991).

7.6.1   Reduced food intake

Loss of appetite leading to reduced energy intake is the main reason why people lose weight (Macallan *et al.*, 1995; Hsu *et al.*, 2005). Reduction in dietary intake leads to growth failure in HIV-positive children Arpadi *et al.*, 2000 and wasting in HIV-positive adults (Macallan, 1999).

Contributing factors include:

Infection: This includes systematic infections such as TB (which is the leading cause of illness and death among people living with AIDS in developing countries); gastrointestinal infections such as *Cryptosporidium* and oesophageal candidiasis (see section '*Gastrointestinal pathogens*' for further information). Metabolic processes can reduce appetite in many infections (Hsu *et al.*, 2005).

Medication: Many of the medications used to treat HIV and opportunistic infections (OIs) cause anorexia and a variety of GI side effects (Hsu *et al.*, 2005). Conversely, as PLHIV start to improve clinically, once ART is established, they can develop a voracious appetite. Unless food is available the benefits of ART are not achieved (Hsu *et al.*, 2005).

Physical impairment

Effects such as sore mouth, dental caries, missing teeth, oral and oesophageal conditions are common and can cause dysphagia, pain on swallowing and decreased ability to chew and swallow. Fatigue and reduced functional capacity are often found in this population and can affect performance of daily activities related to nutrition and hygiene such as food shopping and meal preparation (Dudgeon *et al.*, 2006) (see Chapter 9 'Symptom Control and Management').

Neurological impairment

HIV/AIDS-related nerve complication occurs throughout the course of the disease, often causing dementia, sensory impairments and neuropathy. Dementia occurs at later stages of the disease in up to 50% of HIV patients, and this decreased mental capacity may result in forgetting to eat and poor medication adherence. Some HIV-infected individuals experience visual and olfactory decrements secondary to cranial nerve damage. Sensory impairments can make foods look, taste and smell different, reducing hunger and placing patients at risk for malnutrition. Neuropathy of the cranial nerves, usually occurring later in the course of the disease and associated with cytomegalovirus (CMV) co-infection, is another potential cause of functional impairment. Loss of cranial nerve function responsible for chewing, taste, swallowing and salivary gland stimulation can prevent complete mastication, cause food to be dry and tasteless and prevent completion of the normal swallowing reflex (Dudgeon *et al.*, 2006).

Lower socio-economic factors, lifestyle (such as injecting drug use) and food insecurity have been shown to be associated with lower calorie and nutrient intake (Mangili *et al.*, 2006).

Psychosocial factors

Different social and cultural norms may have various impacts on an individual living with HIV, e.g. diagnosis and/or stigma and discrimination may lead to depression, anxiety and social isolation. Limited support from family and friends may also affect an individual's ability to access adequate food when ill. Lack of skills in food preparation and meal planning may influence an individual's ability to consume a nutritionally adequate diet for weight maintenance.

- *Personal Beliefs* – religious and cultural beliefs may prohibit the consumption of certain foods and in some instances avoidance of food groups can lead to weight loss if energy intake is reduced.
- *Food Insecurity (including household income, food availability and access)* As HIV disease progresses, an individual's income-generating capacity may decrease and reduce household income. Increasing expenses for medical care may also reduce income available for food. PLHIV may have increased difficulty in accessing adequate food supplies if their health and mobility decline.

7.6.2 Malabsorption

Abnormalities of intestinal absorption have been demonstrated in patients with and without HIV wasting (Ockenga *et al.*, 2006). Fat malabsorption has been shown in many studies and carbohydrate malabsorption is especially severe among children with immune depression. Malabsorption of iron also occurs (Hsu *et al.*, 2005). Eighty-eight per cent of the NFHL cohort had at least one abnormality in gastrointestinal function. Of the participants, 47.7% had abnormal D-xylose absorption, which may serve as a surrogate marker of intestinal absorption while fat malabsorption was observed in 12.8% of the cohort (Mangili *et al.*, 2006). This leads to the possibility of both macro- and micronutrient loss in the stools. Several studies have shown that those with more severe malabsorption have lower body mass index (Arpadi *et al.*, 2000; Hsu *et al.*, 2005). Children living with HIV can have devastating severity of diarrhoea, making it almost impossible to keep pace with rehydration therapy (Hsu *et al.*, 2005) (see Chapters 3, 4 and 11).

Gastrointestinal pathogens

Many secondary infections including tuberculosis (TB), mycobacterium avium complex (MAC), cytomegalovirus (CMV), oesophageal candidiasis and intestinal infections including cryptosporidium, microspora, protozoa and bacterial pathogens cause diarrhoea and secondary malabsorption of nutrients. HIV causes diarrhoea through villous atrophy, crypt hyperplasia, lymphocyte infiltration of bowel epithelium, viral infiltration of the mucosae, and the development of an enteric autonomic neuropathy. Many of the well-known hepatic complications associated with HIV, antiretroviral treatments, CMV, MAC, cryptococcus, toxoplasmosis and TB contribute to diarrhoea and malnutrition. Malnutrition is further exacerbated when patients decrease oral intake in an effort to reduce diarrhoea (Reiter, 2005) (see Chapter 9 'Symptom Control and Management').

Medication-related side effects

Many HIV-infected individuals are on complex antiretroviral drug regimens. While these combinations help keep CD4 cell counts high and decrease viral load, ART may cause gastrointestinal (GI) disturbances and lead to nutritional deficiencies. In fact, the most common side effects reported with HIV medications are diarrhoea, anorexia, vomiting, abdominal pain and cramping, steatorrhoea, and GI upset, all of which affect food consumption and nutrient absorption (Dudgeon *et al.*, 2006).

7.6.3 Hypermetabolism

In the early years before the advent of effective treatment, much research focused on resting energy expenditure (REE) as this was thought to contribute to wasting in HIV infection, but studies produced conflicting results as to whether REE per kilogram of fat-free mass (FFM) is elevated in HIV-infected patients. Studies have shown:

- REE per kilogram of FFM is increased even in asymptomatic HIV-infected patients who are experiencing viral suppression while receiving ART (Chang *et al.*, 2007).
- Patients with AIDS experience greater increases in REE per kilogram of FFM than patients with HIV infection who do not have AIDS (Chang *et al.*, 2007).
- Patients with AIDS and secondary or opportunistic infection experience even greater increases (Hsu *et al.*, 2005; Chang *et al.*, 2007). Conditions such as

infection with *Pneumocystis carinii pneumonia (PCP)*, MAC and CMV can all cause further increases in REE (Williams *et al.*, 2003; Dudgeon *et al.*, 2006).
- Viral load is correlated with REE per kilogram of FFM.
- CD4 cell count may also be associated with changes in REE (Chang *et al.*, 2007).
- Two studies of asymptomatic HIV-infected women have shown that their REE is higher than that of HIV-uninfected women, even after adjusting for body composition (Chang *et al.*, 2007).
- Elevated REE has been shown among patients presenting with lipodystrophy compared to HIV-infected patients with no signs of this syndrome (Kosmiski *et al.*, 2001; Dudgeon *et al.*, 2006).

However, because of the varied complications of HIV infection, there is an extraordinarily wide range in REE, which could accounts for inconsistencies among the results of different metabolic studies (Macallan, 1999; Chang *et al.*, 2007).

Factors associated with increased REE in asymptomatic HIV-infected patients remain unclear:

- Most investigations have focused on men so it is difficult to ascertain if sex has an independent effect on REE.
- There are no reports of differences in REE among HIV-infected patients of different ethnicities.
- Studies investigating the effects of fat redistribution on REE have had varying results.

Studies on the specific contribution of ART to REE have also shown conflicting results but this has been difficult to quantify, because many early studies did not compare asymptomatic patients receiving ART with those not receiving ART. It is possible that various classes of drugs influence REE differently and that duration of HIV treatment may affect REE (Chang *et al.*, 2007).

Many factors may influence anabolic and catabolic processes during infection with HIV and this affects protein metabolism in different tissues in different ways. It is likely that macronutrient requirements are increased due to HIV infection but there has been poor agreement in major reviews as to the nature and quantity of these increases (Hsu *et al.*, 2005; Ockenga *et al.*, 2006).

It has been found that episodes of rapid weight loss associated with opportunistic infections are usually accompanied by fatigue and decreased physical activity, resulting in an overall decrease in total energy expenditure (TEE). This decrease in TEE may help to conserve LBM by counterbalancing increased REE. Diet-induced thermogenesis may not be as important quantitatively, although one study demonstrated that the level of diet-induced thermogenesis in people with HIV infection was elevated, compared with that in HIV-uninfected control subjects (Chang *et al.*, 2007).

Decreased caloric intake, rather than increased REE, significantly correlates with the rate of weight loss. In weight-stable, asymptomatic HIV-infected patients untreated with ART, increased caloric intake compensates for increased REE and accelerated protein turnover (Chang *et al.*, 2007).

The causes of increased REE likely include viral factors, effects of secondary infections or complications and effects of specific antiretroviral drugs (Chang *et al.*, 2007). There is ongoing debate as to if, and to what extent, higher metabolic rates may partially account for the continued weight loss and wasting observed in HIV infection during the era of effective, combination anti-HIV treatment and if this may be associated with the metabolic and body-shape abnormalities seen during the present era (Hsu *et al.*, 2005; Mangili *et al.*, 2006).

Metabolism

A number of anabolic and catabolic factors may play a role in HIV associated weight loss including disturbances in production of testosterone and cytokines, in particular tumour necrosis factor (TNF). These are summarized in Table 7.1.

Table 7.1   Anabolic and catabolic factors associated with HIV/AIDS wasting.

Agent	Action	Implications in HIV/AIDS wasting
Anabolic agents Testosterone	↑developmental protein expression	Testosterone is decreased in men with wasting
	Stimulation of growth hormone release	
	Antiglucocorticoid effects	
Growth hormone	↑protein synthesis	Growth hormone resistance has been observed in wasting, resulting in decreased IGF-1 production
	↑collagen synthesis	
	Stimulation of release of IGF-1	
Insulin-like growth factor-1	↑protein synthesis	IGF-1 is decreased in wasting
	Stimulation of replication and differentiation of muscle precursor cells	Increased degradation of binding proteins in wasting leads to decreased IGF-1 activity
Catabolic agents Tumour necrosis factor Î±	Stimulation of protein degradation	TNF-Î± levels are elevated in wasting
	Alteration of hormone receptor sensitivity	
	Decrease in anabolic hormone levels	
	Indirect stimulation of cortisol release	
	↑in resting energy expenditure	
Cortisol	Inhibition of protein synthesis	Elevated cortisol levels are common in persons with wasting
	↑protein degradation	
	↑proteolytic enzymes	

IGF, insulin-like growth factor; TNF, tumour necrosis factor.
From Dudgeon *et al.* (2006).

7.7   Nutritional requirements

7.7.1   Energy requirements

The optimum daily energy and protein intake to prevent HIV-associated weight loss is uncertain. A World Health Organization (WHO) working group recommended an intake above 10% of expected energy for asymptomatic HIV infection (Hsu *et al.*, 2005). However, in ESPEN guidelines for HIV and infectious disease it was concluded that there is no evidence that the energy requirement in HIV infection is any different from other patient groups as studies of total energy expenditure have not demonstrated hypermetabolism. Such studies, however, were not designed to evaluate the requirements for energy intake, although they did demonstrate the importance of adequate energy intake (Ockenga *et al.*, 2006). However, there is better agreement between the two reports in that

- during the recovery phase after opportunistic infections nutritional requirements may be increased by 20 to 50% in both children and adults (Hsu *et al.*, 2005; Ockenga *et al.*, 2006)
- additionally, the anabolic phase after initiation of ART is likely to increase energy requirements (Mangili *et al.*, 2006; Ockenga *et al.*, 2006).

7.7.2   Protein requirements

While the WHO review found no evidence to increase the proportion of protein in the diet beyond the recommended 12–15%, according to ESPEN guidelines for nutritional care in HIV and infectious diseases the target for protein intake should be 1.2 g/kg bw/day in stable phases of the disease, while it may be increased to 1.5 g/kg bw/day during acute illness. Albeit no controlled trials have addressed this question and dose response has not been studied systematically, studies of nitrogen balance using stable isotopes have demonstrated positive nitrogen balance in symptomatic HIV patients with a protein intake between 1.2 and 1.8 g/day (Ockenga *et al.*, 2006). See Appendix 8. Additionally, it may be difficult for people on low incomes to afford a high intake of protein. There is debate about how well metabolism responds to feeding in HIV/AIDS, and if increased amino acid and protein levels are utilised adequately when infection is not well managed. It is also thought that clinical status can deteriorate if hyper-alimentation is given in the presence of sepsis and body composition analysis showed that weight gain in HIV-positive patients treated with total parenteral nutrition was predominantly fat (Hsu *et al.*, 2005).

It should be noted that PLHIV often have pre-existing protein-energy malnutrition (PEM), resulting from inadequate intake or poor utilisation of food. This type of deficiency is not just caused by lack of protein in the diet but lack of total kilocalories from food. Therefore, foods must be balanced to contain adequate protein as well as energy. The increase in energy required by PLHIV, described above, can also be met by eating more protein. Despite some research showing improvements in body cell mass (muscle stores (Schwenk, 1999)) and total body weight (Charlin, 2002; Tabi, 2006) with increased protein intake, further research is required to determine whether PLHIV have additional protein needs compared to people living without HIV.

As there are shortcomings in knowledge and individuals in this patient group present with a very wide range of disease pathologies and nutritional complications, in the clinical setting in the UK prediction equations and factors are commonly used to estimate energy and protein requirements in this and other patient groups (see Appendices 5 and 7). The UK National Institute for Health and Clinical Excellence recommend estimating energy requirements on a per kilogram body weight basis (NICE, 2006, Appendix 6). This less precise method may be appropriate for some unstressed patients who do not present in a malnourished state (Woodham, 2007). The best indication for whether the patient is receiving adequate energy for weight gain or maintenance is provided by nutrition monitoring. If there is no change in weight then energy should be increased and the underlying cause of weight loss should be treated.

7.8 Nutritional management

The role of nutrition support in HIV infection has been poorly investigated, so there is a paucity of evidence to demonstrate improved clinical outcomes through dietary interventions (Ockenga et al., 2006).

Dietary support may improve clinical outcomes in individuals with HIV infection by reducing the incidence of HIV-associated complications and attenuating progression of HIV disease, thereby improving quality of life and ultimately reducing disease-related mortality (Mahlungulu et al., 2007).

In this Cochrane review, Mahlungulu et al. investigated whether macronutrient interventions for reducing morbidity and mortality in people with HIV, such as a balanced diet or high-protein, high-carbohydrate, or high-fat diets given orally, influence morbidity and mortality in adults and children living with HIV infection. The review was based on eight small trials (with a total of 486 participants) conducted in high-income countries. The selection criteria was based on randomised controlled trials evaluating the effectiveness of macronutrient interventions compared with no nutritional supplements or placebo in the management of adults and children infected with HIV. Overall, macronutrient supplementation (with or without nutritional counselling) significantly improved energy intake (5 trials; $n = 254$) and protein intake (3 trials; $n = 128$) compared with no nutritional supplementation or placebo. There was no evidence of an effect on body weight (8 trials; $n = 423$), fat mass (6 trials; $n = 305$), fat-free mass (5 trials; $n = 311$) or CD4 count (6 trials; $n = 271$) (Mahlungulu et al., 2007).

However, these reviewers found no evidence that such supplementation translates into reductions in disease progression or HIV-related complications, such as opportunistic infections or death. The authors concluded that given the current evidence base, which is limited to a few small trials in high-income countries, no firm conclusions can be drawn about the effects of macronutrient supplementation on morbidity and mortality in people living with HIV (Mahlungulu et al., 2007). These findings were supported by a more recent review of macronutrient supplementation for malnourished adults with HIV infection. Of the few studies that analysed HIV progression most had relatively short follow-up periods (e.g. 3–6 months). Only 1 of the 9 randomised controlled trials included in the study reported an improvement in CD4 T-cell count with supplementation (Koethe et al., 2009).

All randomised controlled trials of enteral nutrition in HIV-infected patients have been conducted in populations with normal or only mildly impaired nutritional status. Positive outcome of nutritional intervention in patients with advanced AIDS wasting has been described in several non-controlled observation trials (Ockenga *et al.*, 2006).

7.8.1 Management of weight-stable individuals and those newly diagnosed with HIV

The optimum time to commence nutrition intervention is soon after an HIV-positive diagnosis. For many people this will be early in the course of the disease but others may be diagnosed at an advanced stage when there may already be considerable depletion of nutrient reserves.

For asymptomatic weight-stable individuals, general nutrition advice aims to:

- achieve an ideal body weight
- prevent nutrient deficiencies
- optimise nutritional stores.

Baseline nutritional assessment should include a diet history in combination with measurement of:

- height
- weight
- body mass index (BMI)
- CD4
- viral load
- blood glucose
- blood lipids.

Full anthropometric assessment is advised prior to starting ART, (Pribram and Lanigan, 2007) (see Chapter 8 'Nutritional Screening and Assessment').

Dietary advice should promote a regular, balanced intake of all nutrients in line with current recommendations (Department of Health, 1991).

Nutritional supplementation

Patients should be encouraged to meet daily nutritional requirements from food. Nutritional supplementation, such as oral sip feeds, may be required for relatively weight-stable individuals during episodes of acute illness, increased requirements and limited oral intake due to symptoms or the effects of medication (Pribram and Lanigan, 2007).

7.8.2 Management of patients with decreased/impaired nutritional status

Aims of nutritional interventions in the presence of decreased nutritional status include:

- improve nutritional status and meet daily requirements of all nutrients
- preserve or increase fat-free mass
- achieve and maintain an ideal body weight
- decrease functional impairment from undernutrition (muscular fatigue, bedridden state and work incapacity)
- improve immune function
- limit disease-specific complications
- improve tolerance to antiretroviral treatment
- provide symptomatic relief and alleviate gastrointestinal symptoms of HIV illness (nausea, diarrhoea and bloating) and
- improve quality of life and survival (Ockenga *et al.*, 2006;Mahlungulu *et al.*, 2007).

Nutritional assessment

Assessment of nutritional status is crucial in the management of patients with weight loss and wasting. This is to:

- establish severity of decreased nutritional status
- help determine degree of fat mass and lean body mass that is repleted with nutritional support and
- help differentiate between weight loss, wasting and lipodystrophy or altered fat metabolism (see Chapters 4 and 8 for further information on Nutritional Screening and Assessment in children and adults).

In addition to standard nutritional assessment, the following actions and investigations should be considered:

- Search for an opportunistic infection or other complications of disease or therapy.
- Determine testosterone concentration.
- Determine LH/FSH, thyroid function.
- Look for signs of lipodystrophy (loss of subcutaneous fat, triceps skinfold thickness and waist/hip ratio).
- Exclude diabetes mellitus.
- If nausea/vomiting: is this an adverse drug reaction?
- Exclude malassimilation/malabsorption.
- If abdominal pain or dysphagia: suspect candida oesophagitis, and perform upper GI endoscopy or therapeutic trial with fluconazole.
- Start nutritional support while awaiting results of the diagnostic tests.
- Distinguish between predominant muscle mass depletion (wasting) and peripheral fat loss (lipoatrophy) by changes in body shape and muscular function. Wasting and lipoatrophy may be combined in patients failing on long-term antiretroviral treatment (see Chapter 8 'Nutritional Screening and Assessment').

In case of weight loss, despite sufficient ART, special consideration has to be given to:

- depression
- anorexia

- self-neglect
- food security
- dry mouth and lack of saliva caused by medication (e.g. antiviral therapy)
- dental problems
- addictions (e.g. drugs and alcohol) (Ockenga *et al.*, 2006).

How to introduce nutritional interventions for patients with weight loss and wasting

If patients are failing to meet their nutritional needs, a stepwise approach to nutritional support should be adopted for patients without dysphagia:

- Initially, the adequacy and quality of dietary intake should be assessed and the degree of malabsorption and/or hypermetabolism (dependent on stage of HIV) taken into account.
- Nutrition counselling should be used to improve oral food intake (Grinspoon and Mulligan, 2003).
- Oral sip feeds for malnourished individuals or Ready-to-use Therapeutic Food (RUTF) for children in developing countries may be needed in combination with advice about nourishing foods and food fortification strategies
- If a patient still fails to achieve an adequate oral intake, enteral tube feeding should be considered. If support is likely to be required in the short term, for example to aid repletion after an opportunistic infection, nasogastric feeding is usually the route of choice, although this may be difficult if the patient has nausea and vomiting or severe *Candida* overgrowth of the oesophagus. This route is also useful to assess response to feeding prior to the insertion of a gastrostomy or post-pyloric feeding.
- For long-term artificial nutritional support, a percutaneous endoscopic gastrostomy (PEG) should be considered.
- Parenteral nutrition is indicated in cases where it is not possible to feed via the gastrointestinal tract.
- Institution of nutritional support should be preceded by a search for a potential reason for undernutrition (Ockenga *et al.*, 2006).

There is a lack of controlled intervention trials supporting the use of tube feeding over normal food. No controlled studies comparing normal food and EN in patients with AIDS wasting have been published (Ockenga *et al.*, 2006). Some open randomised trials compare different types of nutritional support. Choice of the mode of nutritional support is therefore based on expert opinion only (Ockenga *et al.*, 2006).

Nutritional counselling and oral nutritional supplements (ONS)

- Nutritional counselling with ONS, or counselling alone, have been shown to be equally efficient at the beginning of nutritional support and/or for preserving nutritional status.
- In settings where qualified nutritional counselling cannot be provided, ONS may be indicated in addition to normal food but this should be limited in time.
- ONS may increase total energy intake by about 20% for limited periods.

- They should be prescribed, where available, as part of a structured nutritional counselling process. The effect should be evaluated at least every 2 to 3 months.
- Patients should be advised to use ONS between meals and avoid interfering with oral intake at mealtimes.
- No data are available regarding the optimal duration of the nutritional counselling or ONS before escalating to more invasive nutritional strategies. This has to be decided individually according to the clinical situation (Ockenga *et al.*, 2006).

Tube feeding (TF)

Tube feeding is indicated in patients with dysphagia and where it has not been possible to meet daily nutritional requirements by nutritional counselling and ONS. For those unable to swallow, a nasogastric (NG) tube is often required for life-saving administration of medicine as well as nutrition. All clinical studies of tube feeding in such patients have documented some weight gain, but this was shown to be fat rather than muscle in cases where body composition was measured. However, study participants were mostly bedridden and inactive and nutritional support is unlikely to restore muscle in the absence of physical activity (Ockenga *et al.*, 2006).

Enteral support is usually used as a supplementary rather than total source of nutrition. If oral intake during the day is insufficient due to causes that cannot be influenced (e.g. lack of saliva or neurological causes), then nocturnal TF may be used to increase nutrient intake. Particularly at home this is a very comfortable way of combining oral (social) feeding with an optimised intake (Ockenga *et al.*, 2006).

What type of enteral formulae should be used?

Generally, no advantage for any specific formula has been shown. Most patients, even those with diarrhoea, tolerate a standard low-lactose feed. Standard formulae should therefore be used, although in patients with diarrhoea and severe undernutrition, MCT-containing formulae are advantageous. For some patients with severe gastrointestinal complications and/or malabsorption states, elemental or semi-elemental feeds may be best tolerated. Soluble fibre-enriched feeds may be useful in mild-to-moderate diarrhoea.

Conflicting results have been obtained from studies investigating the impact of immune-modulating formulae. They are not therefore recommended (Ockenga *et al.*, 2006).

Parenteral Nutrition

In patients with diarrhoea and severe malabsorption, a controlled trial over 3 months of peptide-based ONS versus parenteral nutrition (PN) showed similar efficacy, but PN was more expensive. Patients on PN achieved higher energy intake and gained more weight but this was almost entirely due to gain in fat mass. EN has a positive impact on stool frequency and consistency and those receiving EN had a better quality of life and greater physical activity.

Only one small multi-centre prospective controlled trial of PN versus nutritional counselling was conducted in severely immunocompromised and malnourished patients (N = 31) with severe digestive disease, but free of opportunistic infections. The results were an increase of 7 kg in LBM in 2 months of treatment in the treated group with an increase in survival and quality of life, while at the same time the control group continued to lose weight.

As patients with advanced disease often present with very low weights and rapid rates of recent weight loss, there is a high risk of refeeding syndrome in this population group. Further information about clinical management of this condition can be found in Nutritional Support for Adults (NICE, 2006).

Ethical considerations have rightly prevented the conduct of large powerful controlled studies of nutritional intervention which include an untreated control group in severely malnourished patients with AIDS, as most experts agreed on the need to give nutritional support in the presence of significant malnutrition. This has led to a lack of unequivocal evidence for its efficacy (Ockenga et al., 2006).

The composition of the diet and most effective route of administration is dependent on the nutritional status, presenting symptoms and stage of disease of the patient. The multifactorial nature of AIDS can produce a different combination of symptoms in each individual. Any nutritional interventions should be acceptable to the patient and form part of an agreed care plan (Pribram and Lanigan, 2007).

A summary of ESPEN statements on HIV and nutritional therapy (Ockenga et al., 2006) can be found in Appendix 8. Full guidelines of nutritional support in adults, including management of those at risk of refeeding syndrome and nutritional management of seriously ill patients can be found in NICE, 2006.

7.9 Non-nutritional treatments for HIV-related muscle wasting

Numerous treatments for HIV/AIDS muscle wasting have been proposed and studied. In addition to nutritional interventions, these treatments include resistance exercise training (see Chapter 14 'Exercise and Physical Activity and Long-Term Management of HIV'), hormone therapy and cytokine treatments (Table 7.2). Resistance exercise training is a more easily accessible method of promoting lean body mass than some of the pharmacological treatments, and it holds promise in counteracting the process of HIV wasting, as it has been successfully used to increase lean tissue mass in healthy and clinical populations (Dudgeon et al., 2006).

7.9.1 Pharmacological interventions to treat weight loss and wasting

Drug treatment and EN may complement each other (Ockenga et al., 2006). Many of the studies investigating pharmacological interventions of weight loss and wasting were carried out in the early years of the pandemic, before the advent of effective treatment and in many of these studies pharmacological interventions were investigated in combination with exercise, so it is sometimes difficult to separate the effects of the two types on interventions. Results and side effects of some of these interventions are summarized in Table 7.2.

Appetite stimulants

Appetite may be increased by treatment with high doses of megestrol acetate and this is associated with weight gain, although, in men, the weight gained was shown

Table 7.2 Effects of various therapies on body composition and muscular strength in HIV-infected persons with wasting.

Therapy	Treatment duration (weeks)	Weight	LTM	FM	BCM	Muscular strength	Side effects
Total parenteral nutrition	4–42	↑	NC	↑	↑	—	None reported
l-glutamine	12	↑	—	NC	↑	—	None reported
Testosterone/ nandrolone decanoate		↑	↑	—	↑	↑	Acne, gynaecomastia, breast tenderness, testicular shrinkage
Growth hormone/IGF-1 fasting	1–24	↑	↑	—	—	NC	Jaw pain, myalgia, arthralgia, oedema, hyperglycaemia, diarrhoea, headaches
TNF-Î± blockers interference	2–12	↑	—	—	—	—	Potential innate immune system
Resistance exercise	8	↑	↑	—	—	↑	None reported
Resistance exercise and testosterone	8–16	↑	↑	NC	—	↑	See testosterone side effects

LTM, lean tissue mass; FM, fat mass; BCM, body cell mass; ↑, increase following therapy; NC, no change following therapy; —, not measured; IGF, insulin-like growth factor; TNF, tumour necrosis factor.
From Dudgeon *et al.*, 2006.

to consist almost entirely of fat mass (56; 57). In a randomised clinical trial of 40 participants with a BMI of 21 or more, a mean weight gain of 2.8 kg over the course of 2 months was found in the group that received megestrol acetate, compared with a 2.5-kg mean weight gain in the group that received the anabolic steroid, oxandrolone. LBM increased 39% with megestrol acetate and 56% with oxandrolone. Both were effective in increasing weight in participants with HIV-associated weight loss and resulted in a significant increase in LBM (Mangili *et al.*, 2006).

Whilst cannabinoids may improve perceived appetite, they do not impact weight to the same extent. The use of these drugs is limited by high cost and adverse reactions (Ockenga *et al.*, 2006).

Anabolic steroids

Anabolic steroids include testosterone and its derivatives. Testosterone has been demonstrated to increase muscle mass and LBM in testosterone-deficient but otherwise healthy men (Johns *et al.*, 2005).

Testosterone
HIV-positive patients with testosterone deficiency should receive testosterone substitution to restore muscle mass. It is currently not licensed for use in HIV wasting in Europe. In a recent meta-analysis eight trials of testosterone therapy met the inclusion criteria and 417 randomised patients were included. Overall, the incidence of adverse effects was similar in both groups. Testosterone therapy was shown in this

review to increase LBM more than placebo. These studies, however, were limited by small numbers and heterogeneity of the population, which potentially introduced bias into the methods and results. There is a concern about the adverse metabolic effects of long-term testosterone administration and long-term follow-up for these patients is needed (Ockenga *et al.*, 2006).

The efficacy of anabolic drug treatment in populations with access to modern drugs needs to be reassessed in future studies, as almost all controlled studies were conducted before the introduction of effective ART (Ockenga *et al.*, 2006). Nandrolone decanoate (ND) is a testosterone analogue. The rationale for using ND in treating HIV/AIDS wasting is that it has high androgenic/anabolic activity accompanied by fewer androgenic side effects than testosterone.

Shevitz *et al.* (2005) showed that nutritional treatment alone was as effective in improving body composition as oxandrolone and strength training combined in 50 participants with HIV-associated wasting. Strength training was associated with the highest improvement in quality of life and had the lowest intervention cost (Mangili *et al.*, 2006).

In a Cochrane Review of anabolic steroids for the treatment of weight loss in HIV-infected individuals, including 13 randomised clinical trials in the primary analysis, results suggested that anabolic steroids increased both LBM and body weight. However, results were not consistent among individual trials, the average increase was small and may not be clinically relevant. Other limitations included small sample sizes, short duration of treatment and of follow-up, heterogeneity in terms of the study populations, the anabolic interventions and concomitant therapies. The authors concluded that while results suggest that anabolic steroids may be useful in the treatment of weight loss in HIV-infected individuals, because of limitations, treatment recommendations cannot be made. Further information is required regarding the long-term benefit and adverse effects of anabolic steroid use, the specific populations for which anabolic steroid therapy may be most beneficial, and the optimal regime. In addition, the correlation of improvement in LBM with more clinically relevant endpoints, such as physical functioning and survival, needs to be determined (Johns *et al.*, 2005).

Growth hormone

Moderate gain in body weight and fat-free mass has been achieved by recombinant human growth hormone (rhGH) at high cost (Ockenga *et al.*, 2006). The literature for recombinant human growth hormone is extensive and shows clear effects on nitrogen retention and improved physical functioning and quality of life, but the side effects and the cost implications are substantial (Hsu *et al.*, 2005). Many of these results were attained before the availability of effective treatment, so the outcomes must be viewed cautiously given the influences of ART on fat distribution and skeletal muscle function (Dudgeon *et al.*, 2006).

Insulin-like growth factor-1

Studies have shown that IGF-1 is not as effective as growth hormone at increasing nitrogen retention and subjects frequently experience hypoglycaemic effects along with myalgia, gynaecomastia and headaches (Dudgeon *et al.*, 2006).

Cytokine treatments

Research has shown that pro-inflammatory cytokines (specifically TNF-α) can induce catabolic pathways in skeletal muscle and suppress the expression and function of the anabolic hormone IGF-1 (Spate and Schulze, 2004). Additionally, TNF-α has been shown to be elevated in patients with AIDS and AIDS-related weight loss Thus, cytokine therapies may be beneficial in combating muscle wasting in HIV-infected individuals (Dudgeon *et al.*, 2006).

7.10   Micronutrients

Micronutrient deficiencies, commonly observed with advanced HIV disease, have been associated with higher risks of HIV disease progression and mortality (Scrimshaw and SanGiovanni, 1997; Cunningham-Rundles *et al.*, 2005). Micronutrients including Vitamins A, C, E, B6 and B12, riboflavin, zinc, copper and selenium are essential for maintaining proper immunologic function (Drain *et al.*, 2007). Observational studies have shown low or deficient serum concentrations of several micronutrients, including thiamine, selenium, zinc and vitamins A, B-3, B-6, B-12, C, D and E to be individually associated with either low CD4 cell counts, advanced HIV-related diseases, faster disease progression or HIV-related mortality among HIV-positive persons not receiving ART. Micronutrient concentrations have been shown to be lower among patients with HIV wasting syndrome (Drain *et al.*, 2007).

7.10.1   Aetiology of deficiencies

Vitamin and mineral deficiencies are caused by a similar combination of mechanisms as weight loss and wasting (decreased food intake, gastrointestinal malabsorption and increased metabolic demand). Nutritional and metabolic disturbances such as elevated cytokines may contribute to the chronic oxidative stress observed in HIV-positive persons, leading to HIV disease progression through impairment of immune function, enhancement of HIV replication, or both (Drain *et al.*, 2007). These disturbances can also lead to altered acute phase response proteins in response to acute or chronic inflammation, namely decreased albumin and elevated C-reactive protein concentrations which have been shown to be associated with low serum concentrations of several micronutrients in HIV-negative persons (Mayland *et al.*, 2004; Ghayour-Mobarhan *et al.*, 2005) and with low serum concentrations of vitamin A and selenium in HIV-positive persons not receiving ART. Furthermore, both serum albumin and C-reactive protein are independent predictors of mortality in HIV-positive persons not receiving ART (Melchior *et al.*, 1999; Feldman *et al.*, 2003). These studies suggest that micronutrient deficiencies that persist after initiation of ART could be due to an inflammatory response (Drain *et al.*, 2007).

7.10.2   Evidence of beneficial effects

Mixed beneficial effects on immunologic status, plasma viral load and clinical outcomes have been shown by micronutrient intervention studies in HIV-infected persons receiving ART. However, intervention studies have been few in number and have individually had major limitations, most commonly a small sample size and a short intervention period. The largest and longest randomised trial conducted found that daily selenium supplementation for 2 years decreased hospital admissions in HIV-positive users of injection drugs, but less than 50% were receiving ART (Drain *et al.*, 2007).

Cellular and clinical benefits of micronutrient interventions have been shown mainly in the era before the advent of successful antiretroviral treatment. Benefits have been shown for vitamins C and E, including results of randomized placebo-controlled trials, in which a daily supplement of vitamins C and E for 3 months reduced oxidative stress (Drain *et al.*, 2007). A daily multivitamin supplement for 48 weeks reduced mortality in subjects with baseline CD4 counts <100 cells/μL (Jiamton *et al.*, 2003) and a single large dose of vitamin A to neonates improved survival at 6 weeks in those who were HIV-positive by polymerase chain reaction (Humphrey *et al.*, 2006). In a randomized placebo-controlled trial in HIV-infected pregnant women, a daily multivitamin resulted in significant reductions in clinical HIV disease progression, improvements in CD4 and CD8 counts and HIV viral loads, and a reduction in HIV-related mortality (Fawzi *et al.*, 1998; Fawzi *et al.*, 2004).

7.10.3   Anaemia

Anaemia is more common and more severe with advanced HIV disease progression (Belperio and Rhew, 2004) and studies disagree on whether this is principally due to iron deficiency anaemia or to anaemia of chronic disease (Drain *et al.*, 2007). Several longitudinal studies have reported either a significant increase in haemoglobin concentration or a significant decrease in clinical anaemia 1 year after HIV-positive persons began ART. In a multivariate analysis in which BMI, opportunistic infections and sex were adjusted for, mean haemoglobin concentrations increased significantly by 0.223 g/L per month in HIV-positive persons receiving ART. In another multivariate analysis, adjusted for CD4 cell count, plasma viral load and anaemia treatments, ART was strongly associated with not becoming anaemic during the follow-up period (Drain *et al.*, 2007).

Although HIV-associated anaemia is caused by several factors, results of various trials have found beneficial effects of epoetin-alfa on anaemia. Benefits include improved haemoglobin concentrations and reduced frequency and number of blood transfusions, and improved quality of life both for those taking and not taking zidovudine (AZT) (Drain *et al.*, 2007). Finally, an HIV Working Group recently endorsed initiating weekly epoetin-alfa therapy if correctable causes of anaemia have been ruled out and the haemoglobin concentration is <13 g/dL in men and <12 g/dL in women (Volberding *et al.*, 2004; Drain *et al.*, 2007).

Although conclusive evidence is lacking, some data suggest that increased iron intake may be detrimental in HIV infection (Friis, 2005).

7.10.4   Possible detrimental effects of micronutrient supplementation

Potential negative effects of vitamin and mineral supplementation in HIV infection have been shown:

- Iron can enhance the production of reactive iron species and cause more oxidative stress, which could activate NF-κB and increase viral transcription; increasing iron concentrations could propagate HIV replication despite HAART.
- Greater zinc intakes from foods and supplements have been associated with faster HIV disease progression and mortality in a clear dose-response relation, in asymptomatic HIV-positive men (Drain et al., 2007).
- Maternal vitamin A and β-carotene supplements have been shown to significantly increase risk of mother-to-child transmission of HIV in randomised trials and can increase mortality in some children born to mothers HIV while positive benefits and conflicting results have been shown in other studies (Friis, 2005; Drain et al., 2007).
- Other randomised trials have shown that supplementation with vitamin A and with a multivitamin containing selenium can cause increased viral shedding in the female genital tract (Drain et al., 2007).

Additionally, micronutrient supplements may have adverse effects on cellular mechanisms in HIV-positive persons.

Micronutrient interventions have also been shown to alter the bioavailability, metabolism and pharmacokinetics of certain HIV medications:

- A daily vitamin C supplement (1000 g) for 7days reduced the peak blood concentrations of indinavir by 20% ($P = 0.04$) and the area under the curve by 14% ($P = 0.05$) in 7 HIV-negative healthy volunteers.
- Calcium supplements have been shown to increase serum concentrations of nelfinavir and its metabolite (M8) in 15 HIV-positive persons receiving ART.
- In a small randomised trial of HIV-positive persons experiencing chronic diarrhoea or wasting, 7days of glutamine or alanyl-glutamine improved clinical outcomes, but increased HIV drug concentrations by 45% compared with the control group ($P = 0.02$).
- St John's Wort and garlic supplements, both popular herbal treatments, have also been shown to significantly reduce plasma concentrations of indinavir and saquinavir, respectively. These studies raise concerns about the possibility of micronutrient and herbal supplementation leading to increased toxicity (Drain et al., 2007). For further information, see University of Liverpool website on HIV drug interactions http://www.hiv-druginteractions.org/.

In conclusion, although in some cases micronutrient supplements have been shown to provide some benefit in HIV-infected persons not receiving ART, results have been mixed and little evidence is available to support or refute the benefits of providing micronutrient supplements to HIV-positive persons receiving HAART (Drain et al., 2007). Benefits shown to date include reduced diarrhoeal morbidity and mortality and all-cause mortality in children younger than 5 years of age and post-natal mother-to-child HIV transmission (Friis, 2005). Due to widespread vitamin A deficiency in populations greatly affected by HIV, there is an urgent need to clarify whether adverse effects shown are due to the form or dose given or the presence of a factor that adversely modifies its effect so that global commitment to combat vitamin A deficiency may be continued without the risk of increasing mother-to-child HIV transmission (Friis, 2005).

Authors of a Cochrane review on micronutrients in adults and children with HIV found no conclusive evidence to show that micronutrient supplementation effectively reduces morbidity and mortality among HIV-infected adults, but there is evidence of benefit of vitamin A supplementation in children (Irlam *et al.*, 2005). They suggested it is reasonable to support the current WHO recommendations to promote and support adequate dietary intake of micronutrients at RDA levels wherever possible and the long-term clinical benefits, adverse effects and optimal formulation of micronutrient supplements require further investigation. It is hoped that this could result in affordable and feasible interventions to help improve micronutrient intake and status which could contribute to a reduction in the magnitude and impact of the global HIV epidemic (Friis, 2005).

In the UK, micronutrient supplementation is indicated and may be beneficial in the presence of symptoms such as malabsorption, increased requirements and inadequate oral intake if the individual is unable to meet daily nutritional requirements from food and fluid alone (BMA, 2008). Referral to a dietitian is advised for nutritional assessment, counselling and support, if required, for example if these conditions continue over a prolonged period. It is also advisable, during dietary intake assessment, to ask about use of vitamin and mineral supplements. Consumption of high doses of vitamins and minerals should be discouraged.

7.11 Conclusions

Weight loss in adults and weight loss and growth failure in children are common in HIV even in the era of ART, and this is associated with increased morbidity and mortality. Nutritional requirements are increased particularly in the convalescent catch-up period after an episode of opportunistic infection in both children and adults. The energy deficit in patients with HIV infection results from a combination of reduced dietary intake, malabsorption, increased energy expenditure and abnormal utilization of substrates. Reduction in nutrient intake is the predominant factor causing weight loss in patients with HIV infection.

Deficiency of protein stores and abnormal protein metabolism occur in HIV. Management of this condition includes nutritional interventions in the form of counselling, oral nutritional support, and artificial nutritional support such as enteral tube feeding and parenteral nutrition, if required. Nutritional status can be improved by physical exercise regimens and, in a limited number of cases, by adding appetite stimulant or anabolic agents such as anabolic steroids, hormone therapy and cytokine treatment. Micronutrient status has also been shown to be impaired in HIV infection and although some benefits have been shown in various types of studies, data is conflicting.

New agricultural and social welfare policies are necessary to address deficiencies of household food security among individuals with HIV/infection and families affected by HIV/AIDS. The short- and long-term benefits in terms of immune status, disease progression, physical function, and decreased morbidity and mortality resulting from nutritional interventions have not been proven. There is a strong need for further well-designed trials and research into nutritional interventions for the maintenance and improvement of nutritional status in HIV/AIDS, including at the start of ART (Hsu *et al.*, 2005; Koethe *et al.*, 2009).

Acknowledgements

This Chapter was reviewed by:

Louise Houtzager, BSc, MSc (Nutrition and Dietetics), Accredited Practising Dietitian (APD), Honorary Associate Lecturer in the School of Molecular and Microbial Biosciences, University of Sydney, Australia. Manager, Nutrition Development Division, Albion Street Centre, Sydney, Australia.

References

Arpadi SM, Cuff PA, Kotler DP *et al.* Growth velocity, fat-free mass and energy intake are inversely related to viral load in HIV-infected children. *J Nutr* 2000; **130**(10):2498–502.

Belperio PS, Rhew DC. Prevalence and outcomes of anemia in individuals with human immunodeficiency virus: a systematic review of the literature. *Am J Med* 2004; **116**(Suppl):27S–43S.

British Medical Association/Royal Pharmaceutical Society of Great Britain, BNF 56 - September 2008. Published jointly by the British Medical Association and the Royal Pharmaceutical Society.

Centers for Disease Control and Prevention. Revised classification system for HIV infection and expanded surveillance case definition for AIDS among adolescents and adults. *MMWR Recomm Rep* 1992 Dec 18; **41**(RR-17):1–19. Available online at www.cdc.gov/mmwr/preview/mmwrhtml/00018871.htm.

Chang E, Sekhar R, Patel S, Balasubramanyam A. Dysregulated *Energy Expenditure* in HIV-infected patients: a mechanistic review. *Clin Infect Dis* 2007; **44**:1509–17.

Charlin V, Carrasco F, Sepulveda C, Torres M, Kehr J. Nutritional supplementation according to energy and protein requirements in malnourished HIV-infected patients. *Arch Latinoam Nutr* 2002; **52**(3):267–73.

Cunningham-Rundles S, McNeeley DF, Moon A. Mechanism of nutrient modulation of the immune response. *J Allergy Clin Immunol* 2005; **115**:1119–28.

Department of Health (DH). *Dietary Reference Values for Food Energy and Nutrients for the United Kingdom.* Report on Health and Social Subjects 41. London: HMSO, 1991.

Drain PK, Kupka R, Mugusi F, Fawzi WW. Micronutrients in HIV-positive persons receiving highly active antiretroviral therapy. *Am J Clin Nutr* 2007; **85**(2):333–45.

Dudgeon WD, Phillips KD, Carson JA, Brewer RB, Durstine JL, Hand GA. Counteracting muscle wasting in HIV-infected individuals. *HIV Med* 2006; **7**(5):299–310.

Fawzi WW, Msamanga GI, Spiegelman D *et al.* Randomized trial of effects of vitamin supplements on pregnancy outcomes and T cell counts in HIV-1-infected women in Tanzania. *Lancet* 1998; **351**:1477–82.

Fawzi WW, Msamanga GI, Spiegelman D *et al.* A randomized trial of multivitamin supplements and HIV disease progression and mortality. *N Engl J Med* 2004; **351**:23–32.

Feldman JG, Gange SJ, Bacchetti P *et al.* Serum albumin is a powerful predictor of survival among HIV-1-infected women. *J Acquir Immune Defic Syndr* 2003; **33**:66–73.

Friis H. *Micronutrients and HIV Infection: A Review of Current Evidence, Consultation on Nutrition and HIV/AIDS in Africa: Evidence, Lessons and Recommendations for Action.* Durban, South Africa: Department of Nutrition for Health and Development, World Health Organization, 2005.

Ghayour-Mobarhan M, Taylor A, New SA, Lamb DJ, Ferns GA. Determinants of serum copper, zinc, and selenium in healthy subjects. *Ann Clin Biochem* 2005; **42**:364–75.

Grinspoon S, Mulligan K, Department of Health and Human Services Working Group on the Prevention and Treatment of Wasting and Weight Loss. Weight loss and wasting in patients infected with human immunodeficiency virus. *Clin Infect Dis* 2003; **36**(Suppl 2):S69–S78.

Grunfeld C, Kotler DP. The wasting syndrome and nutritional support in AIDS. *Semin Gastrointest Dis* 1991; **2**(1):25–36.

Hsu JW-C, Pencharz PB, Macallan D, Tomkins A. *Macronutrients and HIV/AIDS: A Review of Current Evidence, Consultation on Nutrition and HIV/AIDS in Africa: Evidence, Lessons and*

Recommendations for Action. Durban, South Africa: Department of Nutrition for Health and Development World Health Organization, 2005.

Humphrey JH, Iliff PJ, Marinda ET *et al*. Effects of a single large dose of vitamin A, given during the postpartum period to HIV-positive women and their infants, on child HIV infection, HIV-free survival, and mortality. *J Infect Dis* 2006; **193**:860–71.

Irlam JH, Visser ME, Rollins N, Siegfried N. Micronutrient supplementation in children and adults with HIV infection. *Cochrane Database Syst Rev* 2005; Issue 4. Art. No.: CD003650. DOI: 10.1002/14651858.CD003650.pub2.

Jiamton S, Pepin J, Suttent R, *et al*. A randomized trial of the impact of multiple micronutrient supplementation on mortality among HIV-infected individuals living in Bangkok. *AIDS* 2003; **17**:2461–9.

Johns K, Beddall MJ, Corrin RC. Anabolic steroids for the treatment of weight loss in HIV-infected individuals. *Cochrane Database Syst Rev* 2005; Issue 4. Art. No.: CD005483. DOI: 10.1002/14651858.CD005483.

Koethe JR, Chi BH, Megazzini KM, Heimburger DC, Stringer JS. Macronutrient supplementation for malnourished HIV-infected adults: a review of the evidence in resource-adequate and resource-constrained setting. *Clin Infect Dis* 2009; **49**:787–98.

Kosmiski LA, Kuritzkes DR, Lichtenstein KA *et al*. Fat distribution and metabolic changes are strongly correlated and energy expenditure is increased in the HIV lipodystrophy syndrome. *AIDS* 2001; **15**:1993–2000.

Kotler DP, Tierney AR, Want J, Pierson RN. Magnitude of body-cell-mass depletion and the timing of death from wasting in AIDS. *Am J Clin Nutr* 1989; **50**(3):444–7.

Macallan DC. Wasting in HIV infection and AIDS. *J Nutr* 1999; **129**(1 Suppl):238S–42.

Macallan DC, Noble C, Baldwin C *et al*. Energy expenditure and wasting in human immunodeficiency virus infection. *N Engl J Med* 1995; **333**(2):83–8.

Mahlungulu S, Grobler LA, Visser ME, Volmink J. Nutritional interventions for reducing morbidity and mortality in people with HIV. *Cochrane Database Syst Rev* 2007; Issue 3. Art. No.: CD004536. DOI: 10.1002/14651858.CD004536.pub2. This version first published online: July 18, 2007. Date of last substantive update: May 22, 2007.

Mangili A, Murman DH, Zampini AM, Wanke CA. Nutrition and HIV infection: review of weight loss and wasting in the era of highly active antiretroviral therapy from the nutrition for healthy living cohort. *Clin Infect Dis* 2006; **42**:836–42.

Mayland C, Allen KR, Degg TJ, Bennet M. Micronutrient concentrations in patients with malignant disease: effect of the inflammatory response. *Ann Clin Biochem* 2004; **41**:138–41.

Melchior JC, Niyongabo T, Henzel D *et al*. Malnutrition and wasting, immunodepression, and chronic inflammation as independent predictors of survival in HIV-infected patients. *Nutrition* 1999; **15**:865–9.

NICE (National Institute for Health and Clinical Excellence). *Nutritional Support in Adults: Oral Nutrition Support, Enteral Tube Feeding and Parenteral Nutrition*. Clinical Guideline 32. London: National Institute for Clinical Excellence, 2006.

Ockenga J, Grimble R, Jonkers-Schuitema C *et al*. ESPEN guidelines on enteral nutrition: wasting in HIV and other chronic infectious diseases. *Clin Nutr* 2006; **25**:319–29.

Pribram V, Lanigan J, Nutrition and HIV. In: Thomas B, Bishop J, eds. *Manual of Dietetic Practice*. 4th ed., Oxford: Blackwell Publishing, 2007.

Quach LA, Wanke CA, Schmid CH, *et al*. Drug use and other risk factors related to lower body mass index among HIV-infected individuals. *Drug Alcohol Depend* 2008 May 1; **95**(1–2): 30–6.

Reiter G. *Tufts*. The HIV Wasting Syndrome. Published in AIDS Clinical Care November 1, 1996. http://aids-clinical-care.jwatch.org/cgi/content/full/1996/1101/1. 2005. Accessed on May 3, 2010.

Schwenk A, Steuck H, Kremer G. Oral supplements as adjunctive treatment to nutritional counseling in malnourished HIV-infected patients: randomized controlled trial. *Clin Nutr* 1999; **18**(6):371–4.

Scrimshaw NS, SanGiovanni JP. Synergism of nutrition, infection, and immunity: an overview. *Am J Clin Nutr* 1997; **66**(Suppl):464S–77.

Shevitz AH, Wilson IB, McDermott AY *et al*. A comparison of the clinical and cost-effectiveness of 3 intervention strategies for AIDS wasting. *J Acquir Immune Defic Syndr* 2005; **38**: 399–406.

Spate U, Schulze PC. Proinflammatory cytokines and skeletal muscle. *Curr Opin Clin Nutr Metab Care* 2004; **7**:265–9.

Tabi M, Vogel R. Nutritional counselling: an intervention for HIV-positive patients. *J Adv Nurs* 2006; **54**(6):676–82.

Volberding PA, Levine AM, Dietrich D *et al*. Anemia in HIV infection: clinical impact and evidence-based management strategies. *Clin Infect Dis* 2004; **38**:1454–63.

Williams SB, Bartsch G, Muurahaienen N, Collins G, Raghavan SS, Wheeler D. Protein intake is positively associated with body cell mass in weight-stable HIV-infected men. *J Nutr* 2003; **133**:1143–6.

Woodham S. In: Thomas B, Bishop J, eds. *Estimating Nutritional Requirements, Manual of Dietetic Practice*. 4th ed., Oxford: Blackwell Publishing, 2007.

8 Nutritional Screening and Assessment

Sarah Woodman, Michelle Sutcliffe and Amy McDonald

Key Points

- Nutritional screening and assessment are fundamental aspects of the care of individuals living with HIV.
- Nutritional screening is a quick process using a simple tool to recognise undernutrition and overnutrition and to identify individuals who require more in-depth nutritional assessment.
- Comprehensive nutritional assessment using anthropometric, biochemical, clinical and dietary parameters will provide a more in-depth assessment of nutritional status.
- Nutritional assessment must be ongoing so that trends for an individual can be identified over time and compared to a baseline.
- During nutritional assessment, consideration must be made to the physical changes in HIV, e.g. lipodystrophy and changes in lean and fat tissues.

8.1 Overview

The impact of HIV infection and associated complications on overall nutritional status have been identified since the early stages of the pandemic. Poor nutritional status is known to have a detrimental effect on immune system development and function, while declining immune function can impact negatively on nutritional status and compound the problem of malnutrition for people living with HIV (PLHIV). It is important that nutritional screening and assessment form part of routine care for PLHIV in order to detect changes in nutritional status at an early stage, as nutritional status is strongly predictive of survival and functional status during the course of HIV infection and nutritional interventions can help maintain and improve health outcomes (Knox *et al.*, 2003; Family Health International, 2007).

At an individual level, a broad range of factors may contribute to declining health and nutritional status for PLHIV. Factors that determine nutritional status in PLHIV can be categorised as:

Psychosocial: e.g. household income, food availability, personal beliefs and social and cultural issues.

or

Biological: e.g. metabolic factors and nutrient requirements, chronic infections and illnesses, gastrointestinal complications and antiretroviral treatment (ART).

Causes and effects of changes in nutritional status and special considerations for particular groups are covered in other chapters. Broadly speaking, alterations in nutritional status and body composition in PLHIV are linked to undernutrition, overnutrition or the effects of treatment and infection, including HIV itself.

8.1.1   Undernutrition

Weight loss is associated with adverse outcomes in HIV. Poor nutritional status, and particularly the loss of metabolically active lean tissue, has been associated with increased mortality and faster disease progression (Kotler *et al.*, 1989; Wheeler *et al.*, 1998).

While serial weight measurements have been used to identify wasting syndrome in PLHIV, studies have shown that measurement of body weight alone failed to identify dramatic losses in body cell mass leading to death because of relative increases in body water with disease progression. Measurements of body compartments are, therefore, crucial in identifying persons with HIV who are at risk for serious consequences of malnutrition (Knox *et al.*, 2003). Serum albumin levels have also been shown to predict survival in HIV, and micronutrients including serum vitamin A, vitamin B_{12}, selenium and zinc have been associated with progression of HIV infection (Knox *et al.*, 2003).

8.1.2   Disease and treatment related alterations in body composition and metabolism

A diverse range of adverse effects associated with HIV and ART are known. Fat redistribution (often referred to as lipodystrophy) and metabolic abnormalities have been a major concern for PLHIV, particularly since the advent of effective ART, and these morphological changes have been linked to combination antiretroviral treatment. To date, there is no universally accepted definition (see, Further Reading).

The main features of fat redistribution are:

Lipoatrophy characterised by:

- loss of subcutaneous fat from the cheeks (buccal fat pads)
- subcutaneous tissue is depleted from the arms, shoulders, thighs and buttocks (peripheral wasting), with prominence of the superficial veins in these sites.

Lipohypertrophy or fat accumulation. Presentation includes:

- Fat accumulation around the shoulders (dorsocervical fat pad, sometimes referred to as "buffalo hump") (see Chapter 10 'The Nutritional Management of Complications Associated with HIV and Antiretroviral Therapy').
- Central adiposity caused by an increase in central visceral fat. This may be difficult to distinguish from central fat gain through general obesity.
- Breast hypertrophy (Roblee and Olson, 2008).

Metabolic changes that may occur (to varying degrees) include raised levels of total and LDL cholesterol, altered HDL cholesterol level, and abnormalities in glucose and insulin levels (Grinspoon, 2005).

These features may present in isolation or in combination.

Wide variation exists in the literature regarding the prevalence of HIV lipodystrophy. Various studies show the prevalence rate of this syndrome is 2–60% in all patients who are HIV positive; a 2007 meta-analysis found a prevalence rate of 14–40% in HIV-positive patients on ART. In untreated patients with HIV infection, a 4% prevalence rate is reported. The incidence of associated new-onset hypercholesterolemia, hypertriglyceridemia, and hyperglycemia is 24, 19 and 5%, respectively. International rates of HIV-associated lipodystrophy vary according to country. A prospective cohort study in England demonstrated a 17% prevalence rate after an 18-month follow-up. Variations in the reported prevalence rates are related to a variety of factors, including age, genetics, HIV medications and case definition (Roblee and Olson, 2008).

Baseline and serial measurements of limbs and truncal regions are useful in order to monitor the presence of fat redistribution and to plan intervention strategies (Knox et al., 2003) (see Appendix 9), while full lipid profile and blood glucose levels should be monitored routinely (see Sections 8.4.2 and 8.4.3).

8.1.3   Overnutrition

Studies have shown a high prevalence of overweight, obesity and poor quality of diet among PLHIV (Kruzich et al., 2004; Amorosa et al., 2005; Hendricks et al., 2006). This could be due to a number of factors including cultural differences in perceptions of ideal body weight, social economic status, income and ability to purchase and access a wide range of foods including fruits and vegetables, lifestyle issues, mobility and food habits. Studies have also shown accelerated arteriosclerosis and increased incidence of myocardial infarction associated with HIV infection (Friis-Moller et al., 2003; Bergersen, 2006; see Chapter 10, 'The Nutritional Management of Complications Associated with HIV and Antiretroviral Therapy'). In a wider context, rapid economic development along with an increased urbanisation over the last decade has brought about considerable changes in diets and lifestyles of people all over the world, e.g. increased consumption of energy-dense diets high in fat, particularly saturated fat. These patterns are combined with a decline in energy expenditure that is associated with a sedentary lifestyle (WHO/FAO, 2003). The resulting overnutrition can have adverse effects on health outcomes, particularly related to cardiovascular disease risk and the development of co-morbidity.

Clinicians need to employ skills in nutritional screening and assessment to aid in the identification of lipodystrophy and cardiovascular risk by undertaking baseline and serial measurements and histories.

8.2   Nutritional screening in the clinical setting

Nutritional screening is an important component of care for individuals living with HIV. It is a quick, easy and non-specific method used to identify those who are at risk of undernutrition. Early identification of individuals at nutritional risk is vital to ensure timely and effective nutritional intervention as the presence of malnutrition may increase an individual's susceptibility to infection, which can impair strength and functional ability and adversely affect the outcome in people with HIV (Kotler et al., 1989; Ott et al., 1993; Süttmann et al., 1995).

Nutritional screening is distinct from nutritional assessment which is discussed later in this chapter.

As the numbers of people successfully treated for HIV continues to grow, patient population groups are likely to increase in size. It is not feasible for all individuals with HIV to receive an in-depth nutritional assessment. Additionally, this may not be necessary for all PLHIV, particularly if HIV is diagnosed at an early stage and treatment is initiated preventing the development of nutritional complications.

Nutritional screening will identify which individuals require a more in-depth assessment and further intervention. It may form part of a wider screening program used by HIV teams, which may include other risks, e.g. cardiovascular disease risk (see Chapter 11).

Screening should be the responsibility of the whole multidisciplinary team, and can be undertaken by any suitably trained health care professional. It should be undertaken routinely and at regular intervals, in both inpatient and outpatient settings (see Chapter 11, 'Community Interventions in Resource-Limited Settings'). Minimum measurements that should be included in nutritional screening in the clinical setting are:

Measurements	Height
	Weight
	Body mass index (kg/m^2)
	Waist circumference
History	
	Weight history since developing HIV
	Current and previous lifestyle history including exercise, smoking, intake of alcohol, recreational drugs, stimulants and sleep patterns
	Presence of symptoms and conditions that may affect nutritional status such as infections, diarrhoea, nausea, vomiting and loss of appetite

8.2.1 Screening tools

There are a variety of different screening tools available, but it is important to ensure that whichever tool is chosen meets the following criteria:

- easy to use
- universal
- reliable and repeatable
- valid
- evidence based
- acceptable to patients and health care providers
- triggers further assessment and intervention where appropriate.

The nutritional screening tool used should also identify current nutritional status, any recent changes and predict the likelihood of future changes.

Although there are several tools available, the Malnutrition Universal Screening Tool, used in the UK, incorporates all of these elements, and will be discussed in more detail below.

MUST

The Malnutrition Universal Screening Tool (MUST) was developed by the British Association of Parenteral and Enteral Nutrition (BAPEN) and is supported by many professional bodies, including the British Dietetic Association and Royal College of Physicians. It is recommended for use by the National Institute for Health and Clinical Excellence (NICE, 2006).

MUST is an evidence-based tool (Elia, 2003), and is designed to identify those who are at risk of over- and undernutrition. It has been developed for use with all adults (both ill and healthy), in a variety of different settings (including in-patient, out-patient and public health settings). Although it can be applied to all types of patient groups (Stratton *et al.*, 2004), it has not been specifically validated for use in the HIV-positive population.

MUST requires height and weight to calculate body mass index (BMI) and changes in weight. Where height cannot be measured, reported height, ulna length or knee height can be used (see Section 8.3.1). If it is not possible to measure weight, use mid-upper arm circumference (MUAC) to estimate BMI, using the following reference tool:

- if MUAC <23.5 cm, BMI <20 kg/m^2 (underweight)
- if MUAC >32 cm, BMI >30 kg/m^2 (obese)

(See Section 8.3.2 for instruction on measuring MUAC.)

If recent weight loss cannot be calculated, use self-reported weight loss or changes in MUAC (5% reduction in MUAC suggests a weight loss of 5%). If neither BMI nor weight change can be calculated, use professional judgement to obtain a clinical impression of the individuals overall weight, i.e. very thin or overweight (see Section 8.3 for more details).

8.2.2   Frequency of screening

Full nutritional screening should be part of routine clinical care and should happen at first contact. The future frequency of screening should reflect the ongoing health of the individual. For some individuals, screening annually will suffice, whereas for acutely unwell individuals who are hospitalised, weekly screening may be more appropriate.

8.3   Nutritional assessment

While nutritional screening is a broad assessment that can be used to identify PLHIV in need of nutritional therapy, nutritional assessment involves a detailed investigation of individual nutritional status by a dietitian or trained health professional (FHI, 2007). Initial assessment provides a baseline against which future assessments can be compared, allowing the development of individualised dietary plans where necessary. Detailed below is the ABCD model of nutritional assessment in HIV. This involves anthropometric, biochemical, clinical and dietary assessment of the patient. The practicalities, benefits and limitations of each method will be discussed.

8.3.1 Anthropometric assessment

Anthropometry is the external measurement of body composition and plays a vital role in assessing nutritional status. It can involve simple techniques and basic equipment such as a tape measure or more sophisticated techniques with more complex tools such as DEXA (dual energy X-ray absorptiometry) scanners.

Anthropometric measurements can be used to assess lean body mass (LBM), fat mass and body water. Untreated HIV infection may lead to alterations in fat mass and fat-free mass (lipodystrpohy). In such cases anthropometric measurements may have limited value detecting total body fat but remain useful for detecting regional changes (Knox et al., 2003).

In order to fully interpret the anthropometric measurements, the clinician must be aware of the effect that HIV disease and treatment has on the body. Studies assessing the validity of these measurements among PLHIV have shown mixed results (Batterham et al., 1999; Schwenk et al., 2001).

Typically, in clinical practice, anthropometric measurements will include:

- body weight (and changes in body weight)
- height (including surrogate measures)
- measurements of adiposity (including BMI, waist circumference and skinfold thicknesses)
- measurements of muscle mass (including mid-arm muscle circumference)
- estimates of body composition (including bioelectrical impedance techniques).

The most critical baseline measurements to obtain are height and weight, and although simplistic, are also the most precise (Ulijaszek and Kerr, 1999).

Body weight

Change in body weight, or weight loss may indicate an early change in nutritional status or nutritional compromise. Taken regularly, it is a useful tool to monitor nutritional status, particularly in resource-limited settings. However, weight should never be used in isolation as a measure of nutritional assessment in PLHIV, as dramatic losses in cell mass can be masked by relative increases in body water (Knox et al., 2003).

Body weight should be measured under standardised conditions. Where possible, weight should be recorded using the same scales and at the same time of day. Individuals should be asked to remove shoes, heavy jewellery and clothing, and to empty pockets.

Five percent or greater weight loss in 3 months in patients with HIV may indicate the need for nutrition support (Ockenga et al., 2006). Percentage weight change is calculated by the following formula:

$$\text{Weight Change}\,(\%) = \frac{[\text{Usual Weight (kg)} - \text{Actual Weight (kg)}]}{\text{Usual Weight (kg)}}100$$

The following points should be considered when interpreting the significance of weight change in HIV infection:

- Body weight measures only whole body composition and is not sensitive to change in fluid status secondary to ascites or oedema. In HIV-associated weight loss, loss of metabolically active lean tissue may be accompanied by an increase in total body water, therefore masking malnutrition.

- Body weight in those with lipodystrophy may increase, decrease or remain unchanged, dependent on the relative decrease in subcutaneous adipose fat to increase in visceral adipose fat. For this reason, body weight or change in body weight is not a good marker for lipodystrophy.

When weight cannot be measured

When weight cannot be measured, or there is limited access to accurate weighing scales, weight can be ascertained from surrogate measures:

- Self-reported usual weight – although the overweight are likely to underestimate, and the underweight are likely to overestimate (Rowland, 1990; Roberts, 1995).
- Educated guess by health professionals, relatives or carers – first-degree relatives can frequently estimate weight to within 3–5% of measured weight (Reed and Price, 1998).
- Other measurements which have a linear relationship with weight change can be recorded, e.g. MUAC.

Height

Height can be measured using a portable or fixed stadiometer (height measuring instrument). Subjects should be instructed to stand with feet flat and heels almost together against the wall or stadiometer. Legs should be straight, arms at their side, shoulders relaxed and the individual should be looking straight ahead. The head plate is lowered until it rests gently on the subject's head and the measurement is taken to the nearest centimetre (Gibson, 1990; NHANES, 2002) (Figure 8.1).

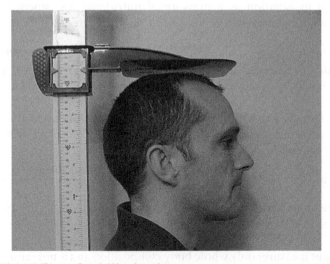

Figure 8.1 'Height' (Photo: Sarah Woodman).

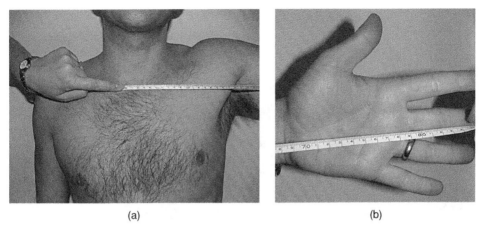

(a)   (b)

Figure 8.2   (a) Sternal notch and (b) finger (Photo: Sarah Woodman).

When height cannot be measured
In the absence of a stadiometer, or for individuals who are unable to stand for a measurement, several surrogate markers for height have been shown to be useful:

- Self-reported heights: this is the superior measure of height when height cannot be measured (BAPEN, 2003). However, people are not always aware of the reduction in height with age, and can overestimate their height by approximately 2 cm (although this is unlikely to affect BMI category) (Rowland, 1990; Spencer *et al.*, 2002).
- Knee height: using callipers or a tape measure, measure the distance from the top of the knee to the heel, with the leg at right angles. Equations to calculate height are available in Appendix 10.1.
- **Demispan:** using a tape measure, measure the distance between the centre of the sternal notch and in between the bases of the ring and middle fingers with arm outstretched horizontally (see Figure 8.2). Equations to calculate height are available in Appendix 10.2.
- **Ulna length:** using a tape measure, measure the distance between the central part of the styloid process and the centre of the bony prominence (olecranon) at the elbow, with the arm bent diagonally across the chest. (Figure 8.3). Estimates of height from ulna length measurements are shown in Appendix 10.3 (Elia, 2003)

Measurements of adiposity

Body mass index (BMI)
Body mass index is calculated with the formula:

$$\text{BMI} = \frac{\text{Weight (kg)}}{[\text{Height (m)} \times \text{Height (m)}]}$$

The resultant figure is then compared with accepted population norms, independent of age or sex, and an assessment of nutritional status is made. Calculation of BMI relies on an accurate measurement of weight and height as described above. BMI

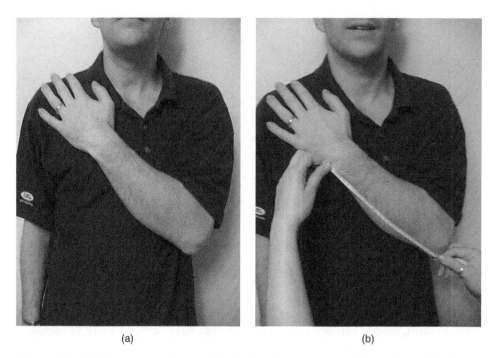

(a)   (b)

Figure 8.3   (a) Ulna length position and (b) ulna length measurement (Photo: Sarah Woodman).

cut-offs were largely developed for public health purposes using free-living Caucasian adults. However, WHO have expanded to include other populations which are outlined in Table 8.1.

As an indirect measure of body fatness, the BMI classification does not take into account differences in size, proportion and muscularity between different ethnicities, ages and genders (Prentice *et al.*, 2001; Movsesyan *et al.*, 2003). Despite such limitations of BMI classification in relation to risk among different population groups, an increasing BMI beyond ideal range represents an increasing health risk and needs to be addressed.

Although BMI measures have widespread application, it should be used with caution in people with altered fluid balance, high muscle mass or high visceral fat.

Table 8.1   BMI reference ranges.

Classification	Caucasian	Asian, Caribbean, African and Aboriginal	Polynesians
Underweight	<18.5		
Normal range	18.5–24.99	18.5–23	
Overweight	>25.00	23–26	26–32
Obese	>30.00	26–30	>32
Morbidly obese	>40.00	>30	

From Report of a WHO consultation on obesity, Geneva, 1997. With permission from WHO.

Table 8.2 Waist circumference reference ranges.

	Increased risk	Substantial risk
Caucasian men	>94 cm	>102 cm
Caucasian women	>80 cm	>88 cm
Asian men	No data	>90 cm
Asian women	No data	>80 cm

WHO 1998. With permission from WHO.

Waist circumference

Waist circumference is a measure of central adiposity. The waist circumference requires limited equipment, is minimally invasive and highly reproducible if a standard site is used (Wang *et al.*, 2003). Serial measurements can track changes in central adiposity. Abdominal fat is an independent predictor of health risk for those with a healthy BMI. It can be a better indicator of health than BMI in older people and those from black and minority ethnic groups (Lean *et al.*, 2005).

Waist circumference is measured with a tape measure at the end of expiration. Subjects should be standing, the tape parallel to the ground. The tape should be snug but should not compress the skin. The measurement is taken halfway between the lowest rib and hip bone (which is usually in line with the individual's umbilicus).

Waist measurements as a health risk predictor are summarised in Table 8.2.

In individuals with HIV, an increasing waist circumference cannot distinguish between generalised adiposity and increased visceral adipose tissue. Moreover, a loss of subcutaneous fat can go hand in hand with an accumulation of visceral fat, making the waist circumference less reliable.

Skinfold thickness

Skinfold assessment estimates adiposity by measuring, with calipers, the layer of subcutaneous fat under the skin. Measurements should be taken by a trained observer, in triplicate, and recorded to the nearest millimetre while the observer continues to hold the skinfold (Gibson, 1990).

To increase the accuracy of the readings, skinfold measurements should be taken at a number of sites, generally the triceps, biceps, subscapular and ileac crest.

Durnin and Wormcrsley (1974) validated a predictive formula to estimate a person's total body fat percentage from the sum of skinfold thicknesses from these four anatomical sites. The measurement of skinfold thickness at each of these sites is described in Table 8.3.

Reproducibility and reliability of skinfold measurements relies heavily on observer skill and there is a large inter-observer variability seen with these measurements (Gibson, 1990). Small changes in body fat (<0.5 kg) cannot be detected by skinfold thickness which can limit the value as a short-term monitoring tool (Heynsfield and Caspar, 1987). Predictive equations make assumptions about body density, which may differ amongst different genders, ethnic groups, ages and individual variation. The relationship between subcutaneous fat and total body fat remains fairly constant but there may be variations in individuals and between individuals at different points in time, as with increasing age a greater proportion of body fat is deposited internally rather than subcutaneously.

Table 8.3 Description of skinfold thickness technique.

Anatomical site	Technique
Triceps* (see Figure 8.4a)	Measured on the non-dominant arm, whilst hanging freely at the side at the midpoint arm between the acromial and olecranon processes.
Subscapular (see Figure 8.4b)	With the patient standing, grasp the fold of skin diagonally 1–2 cm below the point of the shoulder blade and 1–2 cm towards the arm.
Biceps (see Figure 8.4c)	With the patient standing, take the measurement on the anterior surface of the arm over the belly of the bicep at the mid point of the arm
Suprailiac (see Figure 8.4d)	A diagonal pinch just above the front forward protrusion of the iliac crest

*The tricep skinfold (TSF) thickness is used in estimating the mid-arm muscle circumference.

People of African-Caribbean origin tend to have a greater proportion of visceral and upper body fat deposition than Caucasians (Zillikens and Conway, 1990). Also, Asian adults have more upper body subcutaneous fat and a higher body fat to BMI ratio than Caucasian adults, which is more pronounced in women (Wang, 1994).

8.3.2 Measurements of muscle mass

Mid-arm muscle circumference (MAMC)

In order to estimate the MAMC the observer needs to measure the mid-upper arm circumference (MUAC). Mid-upper arm circumference is an indirect measure of both adipose and lean tissue. It is measured using a flexible non-stretch tape, at the midpoint arm between the acromial and olecranon processes To prevent an inaccurate measurement it is important that the arm hangs loosely beside the body and the bicep is not flexed (NHANES, 2002).The midpoint of the arm is found with the arm bent at right angles across the front of the body, see Figure 8.5.

MUAC is simple and minimally invasive. As upper arms are rarely affected by oedema it has the advantage of being less affected in oedematous individuals than other anthropometric measurements. A single MUAC measurement in the non-HIV population can be used to make an estimate of nutritional status using published age-dependent guidelines (see Appendices 11 and 12) (Bishop et al., 1981). These reference tables are not validated specifically for use with individuals currently living with HIV, so should be referred to with some caution and clinical judgement. As with all anthropometric measurements, a baseline measurement should be taken at the earliest opportunity against which subsequent readings can be compared.

When measuring the MUAC, keep a record of which arm the measurement was taken on so that subsequent measures can be repeated on the same arm.

Estimating the mid-arm muscle circumference (MAMC) uses MUAC and the triceps skinfold thickness (TSF) employing the formula below:

$$\text{MAMC (cm)} = \text{MUAC (cm)} - [\text{TSF (mm)} \times 0.314].$$

Figures for interpreting the MAMC are found in Appendix 12.

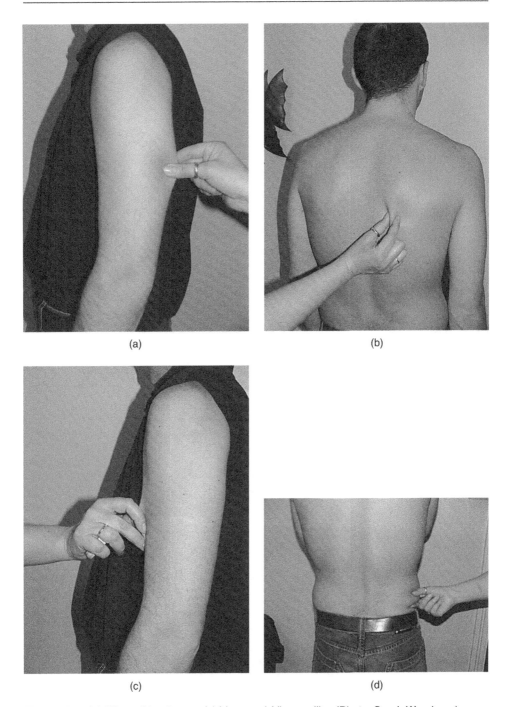

Figure 8.4 (a) Tricep, (b) subscap, (c) bicep and (d) suprailiac (Photo: Sarah Woodman).

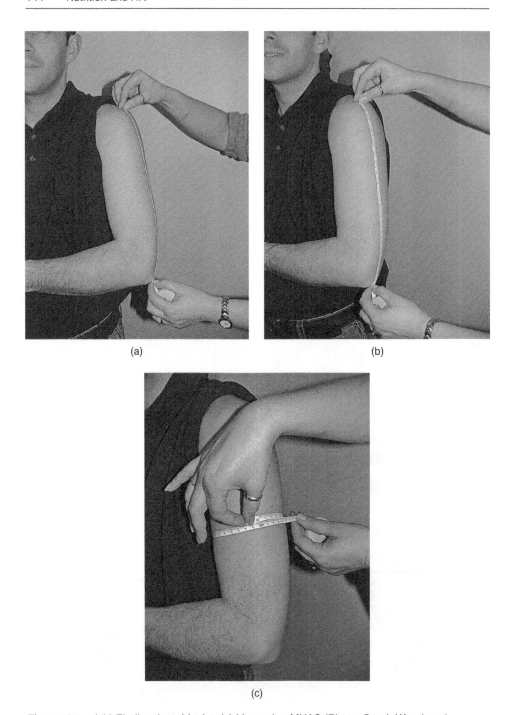

Figure 8.5   (ab) Finding the midpoint. (c) Measuring MUAC (Photo: Sarah Woodman).

8.3.3   Estimates of body composition

Other more sophisticated techniques are available to distinguish between lean and fat mass. They are principally research tools; however, some centres are able to use these techniques in routine clinical care.

Dual energy X-ray absorptiometry

Dual energy X-ray absorptiometry (DEXA) is a whole body scan using x-ray radiation measuring body fat, fat-free mass and bone density. Compared with other methods of anthropometric assessments previously described, DEXA is costly and time-consuming. It can be used to measure limb fat in HIV-associated lipoatrophy, but is unable to distinguish visceral and subcutaneous fat and so cannot accurately predict the presence of visceral abdominal obesity. It should be noted that DEXA machines of different manufacture are not necessarily consistent.

Bioelectrical impedance analysis

Bioelectrical impedance analysis (BIA) is a quick, non-invasive, portable and relatively cheap method to assess body composition that can be utilized in a variety of settings. There is very limited intra- and inter-observer error. BIA assesses body composition by measuring the impedance or resistance to an electrical signal as it travels through the body. Body fat slows conduction of an electric current because it contains minimal amounts of water. Due to its high water content (assumed 73%) lean tissue allows an electrical current to pass much more easily. The variations in bioelectrical impedance allow an estimate of lean body mass to be made. Fat mass is then predicted by subtraction of lean body mass from total body mass assuming a constant hydration. Accurate weight and height measurements are needed.

Many factors can influence the accuracy of impedance measurements. Standardised conditions should therefore be employed according to the type of measuring device used. Some require the individual to lie supine on a non-conductive surface with limbs abducted slightly, others are based on stand-on scales which just require removal of footwear. For all BIA measurements, individuals should avoid alcohol and vigorous exercise for 24 hours before testing. The individual should ideally be fasted, but not dehydrated and should have voided before the measurement. The skin surface at the sites of electrode placement should be cleaned with alcohol and electrodes should be accurately placed with reference to anatomical markers (Gibson, 1990; Kyle et al., 2003).

BIA only measures whole body fat and lean body mass. Consequently, it cannot detect abnormalities of fat redistribution and so may be inaccurate in individuals with lipodystrophy (Knox et al., 2003).

8.3.4   Summary

No single anthropometric measurement of body composition can be accurate and precise. Where possible several measures, employing different anthropometric measurements should be taken and compared over time to a baseline. When using these measurements with HIV-positive individuals, caution should be used, as there is limited validated information specifically for this population group.

8.4 Biochemical assessment

Biochemical markers can provide further insight into the individuals' nutritional status. They can help guide subsequent nutritional education and treatment.

The following markers can be used to assess nutritional status in the HIV population, although different centres will have their own guidelines for the frequency of these measurements. The more common reference ranges are in Appendix 13.

8.4.1 Serum albumin

Historically, low serum albumin has been used as a marker for malnutrition. However, serum albumin alone is an insensitive and non-specific marker of nutritional status (Anderson and Wochos, 1982). Albumin can be affected by a number of factors, including age, hydration, infection and zinc deficiency. Low serum albumin in the presence of acute inflammation and an increased C-reactive protein is more likely to indicate inflammation than malnutrition. A serum albumin level of less than 35 g/l, along with a history of prolonged inadequate nutritional intake and other physical signs of malnutrition indicates severe malnutrition (Scott *et al.*, 1998). In order to identify trends, a baseline measure should be taken, which can then be compared with future results.

In HIV, low serum albumin remains a marker of mortality (Feldman *et al.*, 2003; Shah *et al.*, 2007). Shah *et al.* (2007) found that low levels of albumin and haemoglobin were strong independent prognostic factors for risk of AIDS and death, regardless of gender.

8.4.2 Lipid profile

Untreated HIV is associated with a decrease in total, HDL and LDL cholesterol (Riddler *et al.*, 2003). Some antiretroviral treatments may have adverse effects on lipid levels, leading to an increase in triglycerides, total and LDL cholesterol levels (Stein, 2007; Bergensen, 2006).

A full lipid profile that includes total cholesterol, HDL cholesterol and triglycerides should be taken. LDL cholesterol can be calculated from the other values. A fasted sample should be requested in those with an elevated triglyceride level greater than 1.7 mmol/L on random sampling. Different centres are likely to use slightly different reference ranges for their biochemical results. (See Chapter 10, 'The Nutritional Management of Complications Associated with HIV and Antiretroviral Therapy'.)

8.4.3 Glucose

In the HIV population, the prevalence of diabetes is estimated at between 8 and 10% and results from decompensated insulin resistance (Carr, 2003). The incidence of diabetes may increase in this population group, as insulin resistance and abnormal glucose homeostasis have been shown to occur in an additional 15–45% (Carr, 2003). Measurement of random blood glucose should therefore be performed routinely.

Diagnostic criteria for diabetes are defined as:

> The presence of classical diabetes symptoms plus either a random venous plasma glucose concentration >11.1 mmol/L or fasting venous plasma glucose concentration >7.0 mmol/L or >11.1 mmol/L as part of an oral glucose tolerance test (OGTT) (WHO, 1999).

8.4.4   Ferritin

A number of haematological parameters can be used to assess iron deficiency. Serum ferritin reflects iron stores and the level will fall prior to any change in haemoglobin levels. There is a high prevalence of anaemia in the HIV population resulting from nutritional deficiencies and impaired red blood cell production, consumption or destruction.

8.4.5   Folate

Folic acid deficiency is generally caused by either dietary deficiency or malabsorption. Suboptimal folate status predisposes to megaloblastic anaemia (enlarged red blood cells) and cardiovascular disease. A low folate level along with a low vitamin B12 indicates true vitamin B12 deficiency (Remacha et al., 2003).

8.4.6   Vitamin B12

Vitamin B12 deficiency affects the production of red blood cells in the bone marrow. In HIV-infected patients, vitamin B12 deficiency may result from dietary deficiency or malabsorption. Low concentrations of vitamin B12 and red blood cell folate have been found in 20 and 10% of HIV-infected patients respectively (Ramesha et al., 1999).

8.4.7   Vitamin D

A high incidence of osteopenia and osteoporosis has been observed in individuals infected with HIV (Mondy et al., 2005). Vitamin D enhances absorption of calcium and phosphate from the gut, modifies serum calcium concentration, both directly and through PTH and promotes skeletal mineralisation (Munns et al., 2006).

When individuals with darker skin migrate to an area of lower UVB activity, the potential for vitamin D deficiency is high (Hollis, 2005). Chronic liver and kidney disease as well as drugs such as rifampacin and isonaizid, used for the treatment of tuberculosis, a common infection seen in HIV, can affect the body's ability to synthesise or can increase degradation of vitamins (Munns et al., 2006; see also Chapter 10).

An increase in alkaline phosphatase is a non-specific marker of vitamin D deficiency.

8.4.8   Testosterone

In the era of ART, approximately 20% of males with HIV-associated weight loss have been found to have low levels of testosterone (Rietschel *et al.*, 2000). This is a useful biochemical test, especially in those who present with weight loss. (See Chapter 7 'Decreased Nutritional Status and Nutritional Interventions for People Living with HIV'.)

8.4.9   Immunological assessment: CD4 and viral load

A decreased CD4 count is a surrogate marker for immunocompromise and may be associated with an increased nutritional risk. CD4 count should be monitored regularly in patients.

An increased viral load is associated with an increase in resting energy expenditure (Batterham *et al.*, 2003), although this is not a uniform finding. (See Chapter 1: 'Introduction to Human Immunodeficiency Virus' and Chapter 7 'Decreased Nutritional Status and Nutritional Interventions for People Living with HIV'.)

8.5   Clinical assessment

Chronic illness can have a marked effect on an individual's nutritional status. As part of a nutritional assessment, it is important to consider symptoms, medical history and other medical conditions. These may all carry a direct or indirect impact on the nutritional status of the individual. Clinical signs can often be non-specific markers of nutritional status.

Clinical parameters which may have nutritional implications include:

- physical appearance (including weight change)
- physical symptoms (including gastrointestinal symptoms, dehydration, functional capacity and lipodystrophy)
- co-morbid conditions
- increased nutritional requirements
- appetite.

8.5.1   Physical appearance

Loss of subcutaneous fat or lean tissue may be highlighted by low body weight, loose-fitting clothing or jewellery and ill-fitting dentures. Loss of hair and a pale complexion can also indicate poor nutritional status. Skin becomes more fragile and may be prone to pressure ulcers, and suffer from poor wound healing. This can also indicate impaired immunity. Dryness of skin, decreased turgor and breakdown can indicate both poor nutritional status and dehydration.

Weight change

Unintentional, rapid weight loss is likely to be associated with loss of lean body mass in the general population (Gibson, 1990) (see Section 8.1). Patients who have oedema or ascites should be carefully monitored using anthropometric techniques, such as

MAMC and skinfold thickness (as described earlier in this chapter), as their fluid status may mask loss of lean body mass. Obese patients should also be monitored, as rapid weight change can indicate poor nutritional intake and loss of LBM (see Chapter 7 'Decreased Nutritional Status and Nutritional Interventions for People Living with HIV').

8.5.2   Physical symptoms

Dehydration

Decreased skin turgor, dry mucous membranes, confusion and sunken eyes can indicate a poor hydration status.

Gastrointestinal symptoms

Gastrointestinal symptoms may be due to a direct consequence of an opportunistic infection such as oesphageal candidiasis, or may be due to adverse effects of medication (see Chapter 1 'Introduction to Human Immunodeficiency Virus'). Anything that impairs an individual's ability to eat, swallow, digest and absorb food, if prolonged, is likely to compromise nutritional status.

Functional capacity

A decrease in functional capacity can cause lethargy and muscle weakness. This can impair an individual's ability to buy and prepare food resulting in poor nutritional intake. Lethargy, apathy and impaired concentration are also indicators of poor nutritional status.

Lipodystrophy/fat redistribution

During routine clinical appointments, clinicians should be observant for alterations which may indicate presence of HIV-associated fat redistribution such as changes in weight, increased abdominal girth, breast hypertrophy, thinning of legs, arms, face and/or buttocks, dorsocervical fat pad, and metabolic abnormalities such as dyslipidaemia and irregularities in blood glucose levels (see Sections 8.1.2 and 8.3.1, Chapter 11). Clinical assessment may identify overt signs of lipodystrophy. Self-reported clinical signs or physician-noted signs have been used successfully to identify the presence of lipodystrophy (Schwenk, 2002). Although a subjective assessment introduces the possibility of bias, the patient perception of body-shape changes remains important. For some individuals lipodystrophy may be stigmatising and of great concern, for others it may be an accepted side effect of treatment. Routine clinical monitoring of full lipid profile and blood glucose is essential (see Sections 8.4.2. and 8.4.3). Body composition assessment such as anthropometry measurements should be available and offered to the patient and this should include baseline measurements before commencement of ART (see Appendix 9).

8.5.3 Co-morbid conditions

Other diseases, in addition to HIV, may have a bearing on nutritional requirements and the development of a nutritional care plan (see Chapters 18–22).

Assessment of an individual's cardiovascular risk and screening for metabolic syndrome should form an integral part of a nutritional screening. (For a more detailed discussion, see Chapter 10, 'The Nutritional Management of Complications Associated with HIV and Antiretroviral Therapy'.)

The DAD trial (Data on Adverse Events of Anti-HIV Drugs), a multi-national population study, showed a 26% relative increase in the rate of myocardial infarction per year of exposure to antiretroviral therapy (ART), during the first 4–6 years of use (Friis-Moller et al., 2003). Unsurprisingly traditional risk factors such as smoking, male gender and increasing age of patients in this population contributed to the increased risk of CVD.

This increasing morbidity and mortality through cardiovascular complications has the potential to become a significant factor among successfully treated individuals with HIV, due to the increasing age of this population group. The British HIV Association (BHIVA) guidelines state: 'Evaluation of CVD risk could begin with a nonfasting lipid profile including total cholesterol (TC) and high density lipoprotein (HDL), and (TC:HDL ratio). The lipid profile should be repeated within 3–6 months of HAART initiation, and then annually. In view of the potential for HIV to increase cardiovascular risk, patients naïve to HAART or off HAART should also have cardiovascular risk assessment and appropriate advice or management'. See Chapter 10, 'The Nutritional Management of Complications Associated with HIV and Antiretroviral Therapy' for further information (Gazzard, 2008).

8.5.4 Increased nutritional requirements

Factors that may increase nutritional requirements include diarrhoea, pyrexia, untreated infection and untreated HIV.

8.5.5 Appetite

Altered taste sensation and poor appetite will predispose an individual to malnutrition.

8.6 Dietary and lifestyle assessment

A dietary assessment should be completed as part of the overall nutritional assessment. Poor micronutrient and macronutrient intake can have adverse effects on general health and immune function. There are several methods available to assess an individual's dietary intake, each of which has its limitations. It is therefore important to use whichever tool is most appropriate for the information required. Some tools will provide *actual* intake (e.g. recorded intake), and others *usual* intake (e.g. food frequency questionnaires and 24-hour recall). Dietary assessment is only as accurate as the information provided by the individual. Some individuals will under- or over-report intake or modify their diet for the period they are recording to what they perceive the health professional wishes to hear. Dietary assessment should take place regularly (e.g. at each consultation or more frequently if there are specific concerns).

8.6.1   Common methods of assessing dietary intake

Diet history

A diet history, in which the individual is asked to report their usual dietary patterns and intake, is a useful and commonly employed tool. It relies on good patient recall and needs to be conducted by a skilled interviewer, typically, a Registered Dietitian. A diet history would be taken as part of a consultation and typically comprise a recall of intake during the previous 24 hours, open questions to assess usual intake and asking about frequency of consumption of certain foods as a cross-reference. Depth of questioning is limited to time available to conduct the diet history. Particular questions may be asked to probe further if there are other specific health concerns or if the individual is following a restricted diet.

The dietitian can make a crude analysis of the individual's diet based on the diet history to formulate relevant dietary advice. A diet history can highlight the need for a more detailed, recorded food intake to assess actual intake, e.g. a food diary.

Food diaries

Individuals can be asked to complete a recorded food intake prior to a consultation to record actual intake of food and drink to provide a more detailed insight into meal pattern, food choices and overall dietary balance. In order to get a representative view of oral intake, the food diary should be kept over at least three days (including one weekend day) but, generally, the longer the duration of the diary, the greater the accuracy.

Food diaries can be weighed, i.e. the individual measures precisely everything consumed, or unweighed, i.e. described in household measures, e.g. spoonfuls and slices.

Maintaining a food diary requires organisation, cooperation and for the individual to have skills in literacy. Further questioning can take place during the consultation and more information gained as necessary, e.g. about portion sizes or cooking methods.

Computer analysis

There are computer packages available that will allow a skilled practitioner to input data gained from a detailed dietary assessment in order to attain a more accurate breakdown about an individual's dietary intake. Due to the time taken to gain, input and analyse the data, it is not realistic, in many centres, for everyone to have such a full analysis. It is a useful tool, however, in certain individuals for whom the nutritional assessment process has caused concern.

8.6.2   Food and water safety

For individuals who are severely immunocompromised, special consideration should be given during the dietary assessment to foods and food preparation practices that present a high risk of causing food poisoning, such as consumption of unpasteurised dairy products, raw and undercooked meat and seafood or failure to store foods at the correct temperature (see Chapter 17 'Food and Water Safety').

8.6.3   Alcohol

The type, amount and frequency of alcohol consumed should be recorded during the dietary assessment. Individuals who consume very high intakes of alcohol are at risk of an unbalanced diet and may require micronutrient supplementation. Although alcohol does not interfere with the absorption of ART, it may exacerbate some of the side effects of medication.

8.6.4   Social and environmental factors

Social and environmental factors can affect the ability of an individual to buy, prepare and consume food and will influence the type of food selected and eaten. Such factors include:

- household finances
- ability and knowledge to buy, prepare and cook food
- food storage and preparation facilities
- ethnic or cultural background
- mental health
- social isolation
- alcoholism
- mood, e.g. apathy or lethargy.

8.6.5   Use of complementary therapies, herbs and vitamins

The use of herbal supplements and other complementary therapies is widespread amongst individuals with HIV. Individuals should be encouraged to discuss openly the use of supplements and herbal remedies, as they have the potential to interact with ART medication (see Chapter 16 'Complementary and Alternative Therapy').

8.6.6   Exercise

Exercise in HIV can increase weight, lean body mass, strength and functional performance (Bhasin et al., 2000; Lucrecia et al., 2006). Performing regular exercise has been shown to improve general fitness, decrease visceral adipose tissue, abdominal fat, cholesterol and triglyceride and increase HDL levels (Thoni et al., 2002; also see Chapter 14 'Exercise and Physical Activity and Long-Term Management of HIV').

The amount, duration and frequency of exercise being undertaken should be assessed and documented. This may take the form of structured exercise, e.g. at the gym, or in leading a generally active lifestyle, e.g. a physically active job. In assessing nutritional requirements the amount of regular activity undertaken needs to be considered (see Chapter 14, 'Exercise and Physical Activity and Long-Term Management of HIV').

8.7 Conclusion

Nutritional care remains an important element of care for individuals living with HIV and screening and assessment of nutritional status are fundamental elements of the overall ongoing assessment of health for individuals with HIV. Nutritional assessment should be based on information gained from a variety of sources including anthropometric, biochemical, clinical and dietary assessments. Ongoing nutritional screening and assessment will identify trends for an individual and highlight the need for timely and effective nutritional intervention.

Acknowledgements

The authors would like to thank Robert Cramb, Consultant Chemical Pathologist, University Hospital Birmingham NHS Foundation Trust and Mohsen Shahmanesh, Consultant GU Medicine, Heart of Birmingham Teaching PCT Trust.

Further reading

Carr A, Emery S, Law M, Puls R, Lundgren JD, Powderly WG. HIV Lipodystrophy Case Definition Study Group. An objective case definition of lipodystrophy in HIV-infected adults: a case-control study. *The Lancet* 2003; **361**(9359):726–735. doi: 10.1016/S0140–6736(03) 12656–6.

The Fat Redistribution and Metabolic Change in HIV Infection (FRAM) Study Team. Fat distribution in women with HIV infection. *J Acquir Immune Defic Syndr* 2006; **42**(5):562–71.

References

Amorosa V *et al.* A tale of two epidemics. The intersection between obesity and HIV infection in Philadelphia. *J Acquir Immune Defic Syndr* 2005; **39**(5):557–61.

Anderson CF, Wochos DN. The utility of serum albumin values in the nutritional assessment of patients. *Mayo Clin Proc* 1982; **57**:181–4.

BAPEN. *Malnutrition Universal Screening Tool: 'MUST'.* British Association for Parenteral and Enteral Nutrition, Redditch, 2003.

Batterham MJ, Garsia R, Greenop P. Clinical assessment of HIV-associated lipodystrophy syndrome: bioelectrical impedance analysis, anthropometry and clinical scores. *J Am Diet Assoc* September 1999; **99**(9):1109–11.

Batterham MJ, Morgan-Jones J, Greenop P *et al.* Calculating energy requirements for men with HIV/AIDS in the era of highly active antiretroviral therapy. *EJCN* 2003; **57**(2):209–17.

Bhasin S, Storer TW, Javanbakht M et al. "Testosterone replacement and resistance exercise in HIV- infected men with weight loss and low testosterone levels". *JAMA* 2000; **283**(6):763–70.

Bergersen BM. Cardiovascular risk in patients with HIV infection: impact of antiretroviral therapy. *Drugs* 2006; **66**(15):1971–87.

Bishop CW, Bowen PE, Ritchey SJ. Norms for nutritional assessment of American adults by upper arm anthropometry. *Am J Clin Nutr* 1981; **34**:2530–39.

Chumlea WC, Guo S. Equations for predicting stature in white and black elderly individuals. *J Gerontol* 1992; **47**(6):M197–M203.

Chumlea WC, Guo SS, Steinbaugh ML. Prediction of stature from knee height for black and white adults and children with application to mobility –impaired or handicapped persons. *J Am Diet Assoc* 1994; **94**:1388–91.

Chumlea W, Roche AF, Steinbaugh ML. Estimating stature from knee height for persons 60–90 year of age. *J Am Geriatr Soc* 1985; **33**:116–20.

Durnin JVGA, Womcrsley J. Body fat assessed from total body density and its estimation from skinfold thickness, measurements on 481 men and women aged from 16 to 72 years. *Br J Nutr* 1974; **32**:77–97. Available at http://journals.cambridge.org/download.php?file= %2FBJN%2FBJN32_01%2FS0007114574000614a.pdf&code=8494f4a6db65b004e5fb4dfe7 e2a40f0. Accessed on October 23, 2009.

Elia M. (Chairman & Editor). Screening for Malnutrition: a multidisciplinary responsibility. *Development and Use of the Malnutrition Universal Screening Tool (MUST) for Adults.* Redditch: BAPEN, 2003.

Family Health International. *A Practical Guide for Technical Staff and Clinicians,* 2007. Available at http://www.fhi.org/NR/rdonlyres/ee664prpqnshwqhfx3u2×75bzfl6d6jtngph365xsfyqzbhvw 762qy6zoe2zeo3y3xems66lkn746j/HIVNutritionFoodPracticalGuideHV.pdf.

Feldman JG, Gange SJ, Bacchetti P, *et al.* Serum albumin is a powerful predictor of survival among HIV-1-infected women. *J Acquir Immune Defic Syndr* 2003; **33**:66–73.

Friis-Moller N, Weber R, Reiss P *et al.* Cardiovascular disease risk factors in HIV patients - association with antiretroviral therapy. *AIDS* 2003; **17**(8):1179–93.

Gazzard BG. BHIVA Treatment Guidelines Writing Group. British HIV Association guidelines for the treatment of HIV-1-infected adults with antiretroviral therapy 2008. *HIV Med* 2008; **9**(8):563–608.

Gibson RS. *Principles of Nutritional Assessment.* New York: Oxford University Press, 1990.

Grinspoon SK. Metabolic syndrome and cardiovascular disease in patients with human immunodeficiency virus. *Am J Med* 2005; **118**(Suppl 2):23S–28S.

Hendricks KM, Willis K, Houser R, Jones CY. Obesity in HIV-infection: dietary correlates. *J Am Coll Nutr* 2006; **25**(4):321–31.

Heynsfield SB, Casper K. Anthropometric assessment of the adult hospital. *J Parenter Enteral Nutr* 1987; **11**:36S–41S.

Hollis BW. Circulating 25-hydroxyvitamin D levels indicative of vitamin D sufficiency: implications for establishing a new effective dietary intake recommendation for vitamin D. *J Nutr* 2005; **135**(2):317–22.

Knox TA, Zafonte-Sanders M, Fields-Gardner C, Moen K, Johansen D, Paton N. Assessment of nutritional status, body composition, and human immunodeficiency virus–associated morphologic changes. *Clin Infect Dis* 2003; **36**:S63–S68, Chicago.

Kotler D, Tierney A, Wang J, Pierson R. Magnitude of body-cell mass depletion and the timing of death from wasting in AIDS. *Am J Clin Nutr* 1989; **50**:444–7.

Kruzich L, Marquis G, Wilson C, Stephensen C. HIV-infected US youth are at high risk of obesity and poor diet quality: a challenge for improving short- and long-term health outcomes. *J Am Diet Assoc* 2004; **104**(10):1554–60.

Kyle UG, Genton L, Hans D, Pichard C. Validation of a bioelectrical impedance analysis equation to predict appendicular skeletal muscle mass (ASMM). *Clin Nutr* 2003; **22**:537–43.

Lean MEJ, Hans TS, Morrison CE. Waist circumference as a measure for indicating need for weight management. *British Medical Journal* 1995; **311**:158–61.

Lundgren JD, Battegay M, Behrens De Wit GS *et al.* EACS *(European AIDS Clinical Society), Guidelines on the Prevention an Management of Metabolic Diseases in HIV,* 2007. Revised on 2008. Available at http://www.eacs.eu/guide/index.htm.

Mondy K, Powderly W, Claxton S, *et al.* Alendronate, vitamin D, and calcium for the treatment of osteopenia/osteoporosis associated with HIV infection. *J Acquir Immune Defic Syndr* 2005; **38**:426–31.

Movsesyan L, Tankó LB, Larsen PJ, Christiansen C, Svendsen OL. Variations in percentage of body fat within different BMI groups in young, middle-aged and old women. *Clin Physiol Funct Imaging* 2003; **23**(3):130–33.

Munns C, Zacharin MR, Rodda CP, Batch JA, Morley R *et al.* Prevention and treatment of infant and childhood vitamin D deficiency in Australia and New Zealand: a consensus statement. *MJA* 2006; **185**:268–72. Available at http://www.mja.com.au/public/issues/185_05_040906/mun10153_fm.html. Accessed on 15 May 2010.

National Health and Nutrition Examination Survey (NHANES). National Center for Health Statistics (NCHS). U.S. Department of Health and Human Services, Centers for Disease Control and Prevention. Hyattsville, MD, 2002.

National Institute for Health and Clinical Excellence (NICE). Nutrition support in adults: oral nutritional support, enteral tube feeding and parenteral nutrition. *Clin Guide* **32**. London: NICE, 2006.

Ockenga J, Grimble R, Jonkers-Schuitema C *et al.* ESPEN guidelines on enteral nutrition: wasting in HIV and other chronic infectious diseases. *Clin Nutr* 2006; **25**:319–29.

Ott M, Lambke B, Fischer H *et al.* Early changes of body composition in human immunodeficiency virus-infected patients: tetrapolar body impedance analysis indicates significant malnutrition. *Am J Clin Nutr* 1993; **57**:15–19.

Prentice AM, Jebb SA. Beyond body mass index. *Obes Rev* 2001; **2**(3):141–7.

Reed DR, Price RA. Estimates of the heights and weights of family members: accuracy of informant reports International. *J Obes Relat Disord* 1998; **22**:827–35.

Remacha AF, Cadafalch J. Cobalamin deficiency in patients infected with the human immunodeficiency virus. *Semin Hematol* 1999; **36**:75–87.

Remacha AF, Cadafalch J, Sarda P, Barcelo M, Fuster M. Vitamin B-12 metabolism in HIV-infected patients in the age of highly active antiretroviral therapy: role of homocysteine in assessing vitamin B-12 status. *Am J Clin Nutr* 2003; **77**:420–24.

Riddler S, Smit E, Cole S *et al.* Impact of HIV infection and HAART on serum lipids in men. *JAMA* 2003; **289**(22):2978–82.

Rietschel P, Corcoran C, Stanley T, *et al.* Prevalence of hypogonadism among men with weight loss related to human immunodeficiency virus infection who were receiving highly active antiretroviral therapy. *Clin Infect Dis* 2000; **31**(5):1240–44.

Roberts RJ. Can self reported data accurately describe the prevalence of overweight? *Public Health* 1995; **109**:275–84.

Roblee DT, Olson JM. Lipdystrophy, HIV. emedicine from WebMD, updated December 2008. Available at http://emedicine.medscape.com/article/1082199-print.

Rowland ML. Self reported weight and height. *Am J Clin Nutr* 1990; **52**:1125–33.

Shah S, Smith CJ, Lampe F *et al.* Haemoglobin and albumin as markers of HIV disease progression in the highly active antiretroviral therapy era: relationships with gender. *HIV Med* 2007; **8**:38–45. DOI: 10.1111/j.1468-1293.2007.00434.x

Stein JH. Cardiovascular risks of antiretroviral therapy. *N Engl J Med* 2007; **356**:1773–5.

Süttmann U, Ockenga J, Selberg O, Hoogestraat L, Deicher H, Müller MJ. Incidence and prognostic value of malnutrition and wasting in human immunodeficiency virus-infected patients. *J Acquir Immune Defic Syndr Hum Retrovirol* 1995; **8**:239–46.

Schwenk A. Methods of assessing body shape and composition in HIV-associated lipodystrophy. *Curr Opin Infect Dis* 2002; **15**/1(9–16) 0951-7375.

Schwenk A, Breuer P, Kremer G, Ward L. Clinical assessment of HIV-associated lipodystrophy syndrome: bioelectrical impedance analysis, anthropometry and clinical scores. *Clin Nutr* 2001.

Scott A, Skerratt S, Adam S. *Nutrition for the Critical Ill: A Practical Handbook.* London: Arnold, 1998.

Spencer EA, Appleby PN, Davey GK, Key TJ. Validity of self reported height and weight in 4808 Epic-Oxford participants. *Public Health Nutr* 2002; **5**:561–5.

Stratton RJ, Hackston A, Longmore D et al. Malnutrition in hospital out patients and in patients: prevalence, concurrent validity and ease of use of the Malnutrition Universal Screening Tool (MUST) for adults. *Br J Nutr* 2004; **92**:799–808.

Terry L, Sprinz E, Stein R, Medeiros NB, Oliveira J, Ribeiro JP. Exercise training in HIV-1-infected individuals with dyslipidemia and lipodystrophy. *Med Sci Sports Exerc* 2006; **38**(3):411–17. doi: 10.1249/01.mss.0000191347.73848.80.

Thoni GJ, Fedou C, Brun JF et al. "Reduction of fat accumulation and lipid disorders by individualized light aerobic training in human immunodeficiency virus infected patients with lipodystrophy and/or dyslipidemia". *Diabetes Metab* 2002; **28**(5):397–404.

Todorvic V, Micklewright A (eds). *A Pocket Guide to Clinical Nutrition.* 3rd ed., Parenteral and Enteral Nutrition Group (PENG) of the British Dietetic Association. PEN Group Publications, 2005.

Ulijaszek SJ, Kerr DA. Anthropometric measurement error and the assessment of nutritional status. *Br J Nutr* 1999; **82**:165–77.

Wang Z, Hoy WE. Waist circumference, body mass index, hip circumference and waist-to-hip ratio as predictors of cardiovascular disease in Aboriginal people. *Eur J Clin Nutr* 2004; **58**(6):888–93.

Wheeler DA, Gilbert CL, Launer CA et al. Weight loss as a predictor of survival and disease progression in HIV infection. *J Acquir Immune Defic Syndr Hum Retrovirol* 1998; **18**:80–85.

WHO/FAO. Diet, nutrition and the prevention of chronic diseases: report of a joint WHO/FAO expert consultation, Geneva, 28 January – 1 February 2002. World Health Organization 2003.

World Health Organization (WHO) *Definition, Diagnosis, and Classification of Diabetes Mellitus and Its Complications*. Geneva: WHO, 1999.

Zillikens MC, Conway JM. Anthropometry in blacks: applicability of generalized skinfold equations and differences in fat patterning between blacks and whites. *Am J Clin Nutr* 1990; **52**:45–51.

Zhu S, Heymsfield S, Totoshima H, Wang Z, Pietobelli A, Heshka S. Race-ethnicity-specific waist circumference cutoffs for identifying cardiovascular risk factors. *American Journal of Clinical Nutrition* 2005; **81**:409–15.

9 Symptom Control and Management

Louise Houtzager and Tim Barnes

Key Points

- Symptoms of HIV infection or related illnesses contribute to both primary and secondary malnutrition in people living with HIV (PLHIV).
- Dietary symptom control strategies can help improve nutritional status prior to taking ART and also reduce side effects whilst taking medications.
- This chapter covers the potential causes, control and management of the following symptoms: diarrhoea, poor appetite, mouth pain, swallowing difficulties, taste changes, nausea and vomiting, and fatigue.
- Patients with risk of nutritional deficiencies should be referred to a dietitian.
- Nutrition screening is a procedure to assist health care providers to determine which patients require a dietetic referral.
- Individual dietary counselling and monitoring of PLHIV with symptoms is required to ensure they meet their specific nutritional requirements with appropriate, acceptable and affordable foods.

9.1 Symptoms experienced by people living with HIV

Symptoms of HIV infection or related illnesses contribute to both primary and secondary malnutrition in people living with HIV (PLHIV). Symptoms may impact on nutritional status by reducing the desire to eat, changing the types of foods consumed, reducing the amount of food eaten and by affecting the absorption and utilisation of nutrients.

Most patients in Clinical Stage 1 HIV infection (asymptomatic/early infection) do not experience symptoms that require dietary modification. In Clinical Stage 2 and 3 (mild and moderate symptomatic stages) and Clinical Stage 4 (late-stage infection/AIDS), however, dietary modifications may be necessary to help control symptoms and maintain nutritional status.

Energy requirements in symptomatic patients with tuberculosis, chronic lung disease and persistent diarrhoea increase by 25–30% in adults (WHO, 2008a). Nutrition interventions can assist PLHIV to meet these increased needs whilst they are undergoing medical management, and improve their response to treatments.

Where possible, PLHIV should be referred to, or be reviewed by, medical practitioners for investigation of all symptoms. While good nutrition cannot cure HIV, it is essential to maintain the immune system and help achieve optimal quality of life. Antiretroviral therapy (ART) and nutrition interventions are both required for management of symptomatic HIV infection. Dietary symptom control strategies can help improve nutritional status prior to taking ART and also reduce side effects whilst taking medications. Symptoms experienced by PLHIV in the UK are discussed in Box 9.1.

Box 9.1   Symptoms experienced by PLHIV in the United Kingdom

In a national survey of PLHIV in the UK, 42% of all respondents had experienced problems with their appetite or ability to eat and drink in the previous 12 months ($n = 756$). Of these respondents, 663 had appetite problems and 220 had physical problems with eating or drinking. Reported problems included:

- nausea and/or vomiting
- diarrhoea, digestion and stomach problems
- mouth and throat problems
- taste changes
- lack of energy to cook and
- depression.

Source: Weatherburn *et al.* (2002).

9.2   Referring patients to a dietitian for symptom control and management

Patients at high nutritional risk should be seen by a dietitian within 1 week of identification and those at moderate risk within 1 month.

High-risk patients include patients with more than 5% unintentional weight loss within 4 weeks in conjunction with one of the symptoms below:

1. chronic oral candidiasis
2. oesophageal candidiasis
3. dental problems
4. swallowing difficulty (dysphagia)
5. chronic nausea or vomiting
6. acute or chronic diarrhoea
7. underweight (i.e. BMI < 18.5).

Moderate-risk patients include those experiencing one of the above symptoms with less than 5% weight loss.

Nutritional screening is a procedure to assist health care providers to determine which patients require a dietetic referral. This can be done using a screening tool which can be administered by a health professional or by the patient. Nutrition screening allows early intervention and better health outcomes for PLHIV.

An example of a self-administered symptom screening tool is shown in Table 9.1. Nutritional screening and assessment is described in detail in Chapters 4 and 8.

Table 9.1 Example of a self-administered symptom screening tool*

	I have not had this symptom	I had this symptom and...			
		It has not disturbed me	It has disturbed me a little	It has disturbed me	It has disturbed me a lot
1. Fatigue or less energy than usual	☐ (0)	☐ (1)	☐ (2)	☐ (3)	☐ (4)
2. Nausea or vomiting	☐ (0)	☐ (1)	☐ (2)	☐ (3)	☐ (4)
3. Diarrhoea or loose bowel movements ('the runs')	☐ (0)	☐ (1)	☐ (2)	☐ (3)	☐ (4)
4. Bloating, pain or wind in your abdomen	☐ (0)	☐ (1)	☐ (2)	☐ (3)	☐ (4)

*Clients tick the relevant box if they have experienced these symptoms in the last 4 weeks. For each item a score of 1 or more indicates the need for dietitian referral. A score of 3 or 4 indicates urgent referral is required, in addition to medical review.
Source: National Institute of Allergy and Infectious Diseases (NIAID).

9.3 Goals of dietary symptom management strategies

The goals of dietary management for the control of all HIV-related symptoms are to:

- prevent malnutrition
- improve the health and nutritional status of PLHIV, thereby slowing the progression of the disease
- improve quality of life.

Dietary management of HIV-related symptoms can impact on the outcome of care, support and treatment of PLHIV by:

- reducing the severity of symptoms and improving absorption and utilisation of nutrients
- reducing pain during and after eating
- helping to increase food (nutrient) consumption
- preventing dehydration during diarrhoea and fever and
- improving response to medical treatment.

9.4 Symptom control and management of diarrhoea

Diarrhoea is the passage of three or more loose or liquid stools per day, or more frequently than is normal for the individual (WHO, 2008b). Diarrhoea can also be defined as stool weight greater than 200 grams per day. Usual stool weight in healthy individuals is 100–200 grams per day. Many people consider any increased stool fluidity to be diarrhoea, regardless of the number of stools passed. Conversely, others who ingest fibre and pass multiple 'bulkier' (more formed) stools daily may not consider themselves to have diarrhoea.

Diarrhoea is one of the most common symptoms experienced by PLHIV.

9.4.1 Assessing diarrhoea

'Mild', 'moderate', 'severe', 'acute' or 'chronic' are gradings or terms used to describe diarrhoea. In the assessment of diarrhoea, clinicians need to consider the impact that any change of stool consistency or frequency may have on an individual. For some people, more than three motions per day may be considered 'mild to moderate' diarrhoea while others may consider this 'severe', depending on the type of bowel motion. Very urgent, watery bowel motions causing pain and/or cramping may be considered severe.

Acute diarrhoea

Acute diarrhoea usually lasts for less than 14 days (Post, 2006) and, depending on severity, may have little impact on nutritional status.

Chronic diarrhoea

Chronic diarrhoea has many definitions including 'loose stools occurring three days per week'; or 'two or more loose watery stools per day for at least 30 days'. Many PLHIV have had chronic diarrhoea for several years and often do not report this symptom when seeing their doctor, as it has become 'normal' to have recurrent loose bowel motions. As weight loss and nutrient deficiencies often occur in PLHIV with chronic diarrhoea, clinicians and dietitians should routinely ask PLHIV about stool volume, consistency and frequency, together with gauging the impact these are having on the patient.

The volume and frequency of diarrhoea will vary depending on the affected part(s) of the intestines. In diseases of the small intestine, stools are usually voluminous and watery or fatty. In colonic (large intestine) disease, stools are frequent, sometimes small in volume, and possibly accompanied by blood, mucus, pus and abdominal cramping or discomfort (WHO, 2006).

9.4.2 Causes of diarrhoea in PLHIV

Parasites, bacteria and viruses may account for up to 80% of diarrhoea experienced by PLHIV. Medications, including ART, may also cause or exacerbate diarrhoea in this population. The causes of diarrhoea will vary depending on an individual's immune status. Common causes at different CD4 counts are described below.

CD4 counts below 100 cells/μL

Cryptosporidiosis is a disease that causes typically large-volume watery diarrhoea, and can be life-threatening in individuals who are severely immune suppressed. It is a common cause of disease in both the developed and the developing world. A 'Cochrane review' of trials found insufficient evidence to establish whether any drug is able to effectively eliminate the organism amongst symptomatic individuals (Abubakar *et al.*, 2007).

Microsporidiosis typically causes fever, pain, watery stools with or without malabsorption and wasting. However, microsporidiosis may respond to antimicrobial therapy. In developed countries, before ART was widely available, severe malnutrition and dehydration were causes of death in PLHIV with cryptosporidiosis.

CD4 count below 50 cells/μL

The incidences of **Cytomegalovirus** (CMV) and **Mycobacterium avium complex** (MAC) have significantly reduced in response to the increased availability of ART. Fever, watery diarrhoea with or without blood and wasting is the usual presentation with these diseases. Effective treatment options are available, though in the absence of immune restoration PLHIV are likely to remain on long-term secondary prophylaxis to minimize the risk of recurrent disease.

At any CD4 count

Campylobacter jejuni, *Salmonella spp* and *Shigella sonnei* infections are common causes of diarrhoea worldwide, though they are more common in HIV infection, particularly at lower CD4 counts. Effective treatments are available but prevention is important to help maintain nutritional status (see Chapter 17, 'Food and Water Safety').

Giardiasis *(G. lamblia = intestinalis)* causes up to 5% of acute diarrhoeal illness in PLHIV. Symptoms include bloating, cramping and watery stools and the response to antimicrobial treatment is not dependent on HIV status.

'HIV enteropathy' is changes in the intestinal mucosa as a direct effect of HIV. Stools are classically of smaller volume, variable in frequency and associated with milder degrees of weight loss. Diagnosis is by exclusion of pathogenic causes of diarrhoea (Kotler *et al.*, 1984).

Other less common causes of diarrhoea in PLHIV include: Clostridium difficile cyclospora, isospora, adenovirus, herpes simplex virus, rotavirus Entamoeba hisotlytica, Kaposi's sarcoma and lymphoma.

9.4.3   Control and management of diarrhoea

Diarrhoea is a symptom. When possible, the underlying cause of diarrhoea should be identified and treated. In some instances symptomatic treatment alone may be adequate or all that is available but in most cases investigation is preferable to determine the cause prior to medical intervention. Symptom control strategies include dietary modification, fluid and electrolyte replacement and antidiarrhoeals. These are usually necessary in addition to further medical interventions, particularly in cases of moderate-to-severe diarrhoea in PLHIV.

Medications to help control diarrhoea

With or without treatment of the underlying cause of diarrhoea, several common symptomatic treatment options are widely available, including use of antidiarrhoeals such as:

- loperamide 2–4 mg tds or qds (preferably given 30 minutes before meals or after lose motions, not exceeding 16 mg daily)
- diphenoxylate 2.5–5 mg (tablets or liquid) tds or qds
- codeine phosphate 15–30 mg bd or tds.

Note: Antidiarrhoeals can be used to reduce symptoms of frequent or watery diarrhoea when there are no signs of systemic toxicity. These agents should not be used in cases of bloody diarrhoea of unknown cause.

Fluid replacement

Fluid and electrolyte replacement are essential particularly in severe diarrhoea. PLHIV should be counselled on adequate fluid and electrolyte replacement.

When electrolytes are low, e.g. in sodium and potassium deficiency, oral rehydration solution (ORS) is the preferred fluid for replacement. Extra potassium can also be obtained from eating high potassium foods such as ripe bananas (1–2 per day), which are usually well tolerated.

Parenteral fluids delivered by intravenous infusion (IV crystalloids) may be administered when patients present with severe dehydration in either inpatient or outpatient settings. For example, 500 ml of IV fluid with appropriate added electrolytes (usually sodium and potassium) could be administered over a 1–2-hour period.

Box 9.2   Fluid replacement guide for PLHIV

- Drink as much fluid as possible to replace lost fluid. Aim for more than 2 litres per day.
  - These fluids should include clean or boiled water, ORS such as gastrolyte, rice water, diluted tea, weak or diluted fruit juice (1/4 juice to 3/4 water) or diluted sports drinks.
- If PLHIV do not have ORS they can replace with one of the solutions below:
  - **Sugar and salt solution**: mix 1/2 teaspoon of table salt and 8 teaspoons of sugar into 1 litre of boiled water.
  - **Cereal solution**: add 1/2 teaspoon of table salt and 8 teaspoons of rice flour or maize flour to 1 litre of water. Boil for 5–7 minutes until the solution looks like thin porridge. Allow the solution to cool before drinking.

* Take a glass of one of these solutions every time you vomit or pass stool.

Dietary modifications to control and manage diarrhoea

The response to dietary modifications in PLHIV will depend on the cause of diarrhoea and compliance with the prescribed diet.

Management strategies will also differ depending on the part of the intestine affected. In disease of the small intestine, malabsorption is common and a low fat, low lactose diet may be recommended. In severe cases, an elemental diet, or with very severe diarrhoea, TPN may be indicated. In disease of the large intestine, not associated with opportunistic infections, soluble fibre supplementation may be beneficial in improving stool consistency (Anastasi *et al.*, 2006).

Scientific evidence for the effectiveness of dietary interventions is limited. One clinical trial of symptom management in HIV-related diarrhoea using normal foods (i.e. non-supplemental) showed a significant reduction in stool frequency and consistency. The intervention diet included 50% reduction in intake of fat, lactose and insoluble fibre, 50% increase in soluble fibre and the elimination of caffeine. These dietary modifications resulted in a 28% reduction in stool frequency in the treatment group compared to 15% in the control group. Stool consistency improved 20% in the treatment group vs. 8% in the control group (Anastasi *et al.*, 2006).

In practice, dietitians find that a reduction in chilli and spicy foods, fruit juice, alcohol and sugar-free gums, in addition to altering the fat, fibre and caffeine components of the diet, may be effective in reducing urgency and frequency of diarrhoea. Restricting lactose usually depends on the severity of diarrhoea as lactose may be tolerated in PLHIV with mild diarrhoea. Gluten should only be restricted in those with coeliac disease and wheat products restricted only in those with known intolerance. Vitamin and mineral supplement use should be assessed and adjusted; for example, a single dose of more than 1 g of vitamin C may cause bloating and diarrhoea.

In patients with mild-to-moderate diarrhoea, soluble fibre supplements may be useful. Psyllium or methylcellulose compounds provide beneficial bulking. Although usually prescribed for constipation, bulking agents given in small doses decrease the fluidity of liquid stools. Up to one tablespoon twice daily may be well tolerated.

If diarrhoea does not improve with dietary change, antidiarrhoeal agents as discussed above should be trialled.

A dietitian should be consulted for an individualised approach to managing patients' diarrhoea, especially when other symptoms are present. Box 9.3 outlines some dietary modifications for controlling diarrhoea. This diet should not be followed for more than 7 days without review by a dietitian. When severe diarrhoea persists for more than 2 days in PLHIV, medical review is required.

The goals of dietary management of diarrhoea include:

- maintenance of normal electrolyte balance
- prevention of dehydration
- reduction in frequency of bowel motions
- improvement in consistency of stools
- maintenance of weight and nutritional status.

Box 9.3   Dietary modifications for management of diarrhoea in PLHIV

Drink at least 8–10 glasses of fluid per day
Choose water, diluted juice, weak cordial, herbal teas and diluted sports drinks.

Limit selected drinks, especially those containing caffeine (coffee, strong tea, cola and 'energy' drinks), alcohol, carbonated drinks and undiluted fruit juices as they can make diarrhoea worse and increase dehydration.

Avoid foods that are high in fibre (particularly insoluble fibre from seeds and grains)
- Limit your intake of fresh fruits and vegetables, especially broccoli, cabbage, cauliflower, beans and fruits with skin.
- Avoid high-fibre and grainy breads, wholemeal rice and pasta.
- Avoid high-fibre breakfast cereals and choose low-fibre alternatives such as cornflakes and rice bubbles.

- Avoid dried beans, peas and pulses (e.g. baked beans, lentils and red kidney beans).
- Avoid dried fruit, nuts and seeds.
- However, in mild-to-moderate diarrhoea, soluble fibre may be included. Oats or porridge for breakfast or snacking and psyllium husks (1 teaspoon to 1 tablespoon) added to cereal are easy, economical options.

Eat foods high in potassium
Severe diarrhoea can result in a loss of potassium from the body. To replace this loss, choose foods high in potassium such as bananas, potatoes and fruit juices daily. Remember that fruit juices should be diluted (i.e. 1/4 juice, 3/4 water).

Reduce high fat foods
Limit pastries, pies, deep fried and takeaway foods, cream and fatty meats as they can make diarrhoea worse and induce nausea.

Avoid spicy food, particularly foods containing chilli

Minimise lactose (the sugar in milk)
Especially in more severe cases of diarrhoea when malabsorption is more common, the lactose in milk can make diarrhoea worse. Lactose-free or low-lactose milks or soya milk are good alternatives. Yoghurt and hard cheese have little or no lactose, so should not have to be excluded.

Avoid large doses of fructose
Limit fruit to 2–3 serves per day and dilute juices (<1/4 juice, 3/4 water)

Eat plenty of 'helpful' foods
The following foods can help make your stools firmer and control your diarrhoea:

- Boiled potato
- Plain white bread or toast
- Boiled white rice or pasta
- Banana
- Stewed apple (skin removed)

Try to eat small, frequent meals 5 or 6 times per day to help maintain weight.

Try to include one to two serves of lean meat, chicken, fish or eggs daily
Protein foods have little effect on diarrhoea and are an important part of the diet. Choose lean options.

Take good care of personal hygiene
When you have diarrhoea it is even more important to be careful about hygiene, including washing hands before food preparation and eating meals and after going to the toilet.

If you are taking a nutritional supplement, check with your Doctor or Dietitian that it will not make your diarrhoea worse.

9.5   Symptom control and management of loss of appetite

Loss of appetite leading to reduced intake of food (and nutrients) is one of the main factors contributing to weight loss in PLHIV. Poor appetite may occur for many reasons including psychological problems (e.g. depression, anxiety and stress), metabolic changes, infections affecting the gastrointestinal tract, other illnesses, fever and adverse effects of medications.

Explaining the importance of eating regularly to PLHIV can assist in motivating them to change their eating habits. PLHIV should be counselled that even if they do not feel hungry it is important to eat to prevent malnutrition. Malnutrition shortens the time frame between initial HIV infection and advanced disease and increases the risk of opportunistic infections. Box 9.4 explains strategies to help PLHIV maintain nutritional status when appetite is poor.

9.6   Mouth pain, taste changes and swallowing difficulties

Oral health conditions affect 90% of PLHIV at some time during the course of their disease (Sifri et al., 1998).

9.6.1   Painful mouth, dysphagia and taste changes

Oral lesions may be associated with a variety of infectious, neoplastic or inflammatory conditions.

Oral candidiasis occurs frequently in PLHIV and usually presents as white or yellow plaques on the roof of the mouth, tongue and inside cheeks. Candida colonisation increases with age, smoking and the use of antibiotics. The incidence and severity of oral candidiasis increases as the CD4 count decreases. Oropharyngeal candidiasis is more common in patients with CD4 counts less than 200 cells/µl.

Common causes of oral and pharyngeal ulceration include herpes simplex virus (HSV), CMV and aphthous (inflammatory) ulcers. Neoplasms such as Kaposi's sarcoma and lymphoma may also result in ulcerating mass lesions.

Mouth infections including candidiasis can alter taste and reduce appetite.

Oesophageal candidiasis is the most common cause of oesophageal symptoms in PLHIV, chiefly dysphagia (difficulty swallowing) and odynophagia (painful swallowing).

Painful lesions in the mouth, throat and oesophagus contribute significantly to the reduction in food and liquid intake in PLHIV and warrant aggressive investigation and management where possible.

Treatment of candidiasis in PLHIV includes topical antifungal agents where oral disease is mild (e.g. Nystatin emulsion, Miconazole gel or Amphotricin lozenges), and systemic antifungal treatment with Fluconazole or Itraconazole for more severe disease. In prolonged severe cases resistance to available agents may occur and here the most effective strategy is to induce immune recovery with ART. Specific antiviral agents are available for HSV and CMV.

Dietary modifications

There are no particular foods which affect recovery from candidiasis or ulceration, although ulcerated lesions are usually more sensitive to salty, spicy and acidic foods.

Box 9.4   To help maintain weight when appetite is poor

Eat frequent meals and snacks

- Aim to eat at regular times to avoid missing meals. Skipping meals can further reduce appetite, exacerbating weight loss and poor health.
- Six small meals per day might be easier to manage than three large meals.
- Serve only small portions. Large servings of food can be off-putting.
- Eat when you are hungry, even if at odd times (e.g. eat toast at two in the morning if that's what you feel like).

Keep nutritious food at hand for frequent snacking

- It is easier to eat when food is available and ready to be eaten. For example, keep food in your bag, in front of the TV, in the car and at work.
- Good choices include cheese and biscuits, dried fruit and nuts, muesli bars, fruit yoghurt, fruit smoothies, raisin toast and bread with peanut butter.

Avoid foods and drinks that are low in energy

- Avoid diet soft drinks, tea, coffee and water, especially before and during meals, as they can fill you up and further reduce your appetite.
- Choose nourishing drinks such as milk, fruit juice, soya milk, soups or nutritional supplements (if advised by your dietitian).

Other tips:

- Try to eat meals before drinking. This will enable more to be eaten without overloading the stomach.
- **Exercise** can also increase appetite. Try engaging in light exercise or stretching about 30 minutes before eating.
- Try to make meal times as enjoyable as possible. For example, eat with friends or family, eat in pleasant surroundings, use candles or listen to music to make the atmosphere as pleasant as possible.
- Relaxation techniques or talking with a counsellor may help to reduce stress, anxiety and depression, all of which could be contributing to reduced appetite.
- Limit substances that reduce appetite such as tobacco, caffeine and recreational drugs such as amphetamines.
- Avoid cooking smells. Avoid the kitchen when food is being prepared. Cooking smells can reduce appetite and increase nausea.

Eating a healthy diet is important for good health, though is often difficult with altered taste, mouth soreness or painful swallowing.

The goals of dietary management for mouth pain, taste changes, chewing and swallowing difficulties include:

- to assist patients in maintaining a safe and comfortable food intake
- to prevent development of further oral health problems and
- to maintain nutritional status and prevent weight loss.

Table 9.2 describes recommended dietary interventions for patients with sore mouth, painful swallowing and taste changes.

Table 9.2 Dietary interventions for PLHIV with sore mouth, painful swallowing and/or taste changes.

Symptom	Recommended nutrition management for PLHIV
Sore mouth	• Choose foods that are soft and smooth such as eggs, boneless fish, canned fruit, soups, pasta dishes, custard, puddings and yoghurt • Blend, mince and chop food finely to reduce chewing time • Cook meat and vegetables until very tender and noodles and pasta until soft • Avoid hot foods – allow cooling to a comfortable temperature (for not more than 30 minutes before being eaten) • Avoid acidic, spicy and salty foods • Have nutritious 'wet' dishes such as hearty soups and casseroles or add sauces, gravies or custard to foods to make them moist but not sticky • Biscuits, bread and other dry foods can be made softer by dipping them in liquids such as milk and soups • Drink plenty of cool fluids, especially with meals to help moisten the food • Try using a straw for drinks

Difficult or painful swallowing	• A blended or pureed meal may be required
	  – blend each item of food with a little fluid to keep it moist
	  – blend each item of food separately to make it more appetising
	• Maintain an upright posture whilst eating
	• Avoid mashed potatoes, cooked rice and peanut butter, which will often stick in your throat. Boiled, cubed potato, mashed potato with added pumpkin and margarine or noodles may be easier to swallow
	• See a dietitian to check whether you need extra nutritional supplements to maintain your health
	• Assessment of swallowing by speech pathology is recommended if aspiration is suspected

Taste changes	• Keep your mouth clean • Rinse your mouth before you eat to clean the palate • Use marinades to alter taste of meats if meat tastes unusual to you • Add sugar or honey to foods you find too salty or acidic • Add salt, lemon juice, vinegar or coffee powder to foods you find too sweet • Use flavour and smell enhancers to help food taste less bland, e.g. bacon, cheese, ham, onion, salt, pepper, herbs, packet soup mixes, garlic, sauces, pickles and chutneys. Smell food before you taste it • Try adding gravies and sauces to meals, as moist foods may have a stronger flavour than dry foods • Use plastic cutlery and try not to drink out of metallic containers if food tastes metallic • Vary the texture (e.g. smooth, crunchy or rough), colour, and temperature of foods you eat to enjoy the way food feels and looks • Try a straw for liquids: an easy way to bypass your tastebuds

Note: A dietitian can provide further individualised advice, recipes and nutritional supplement prescriptions if required.

When oral intake is inadequate for mechanical or biological reasons, enteral feeding should be considered in addition to a textured modified/liquid diet, or in some instances, as the main source of nutrition.

9.6.2 Dry mouth and dental problems

Xerostomia

Xerostomia (decreased saliva flow) is common in PLHIV, whether or not they are taking ART. A dry mouth is a side effect of many other medications as well as recreational drugs including amphetamines, heroin and cocaine.

Assessing xerostomia

Positive responses to the following questions can be reliable indicators of decreased salivary flow (Edgar and O'Mullane, 1996):

- Do you sip liquids to help in swallowing dry foods?
- Does your mouth feel dry when eating a meal?
- Do you have difficulties swallowing?

Reduced saliva flow cannot only affect eating but results in food accumulation in the mouth which promotes tooth decay and periodontal diseases. Dietary management strategies to increase salivary flow and reduce the effects of dry mouth are described in Box 9.5.

Box 9.5 Management of xerostomia (dry mouth)

- Regularly suck on ice (made from water, no added sugar)
- Chew sugar-free gum or sugar-free sweets to stimulate saliva flow
- Carry a water bottle and sip water throughout the day
- Rinse mouth with an alcohol-free mouthwash or sodium bicarbonate solution daily
- Limit alcohol and caffeine drinks as they dry the mouth
- Try artificial saliva products containing carboxymethylcellulose, glycoproteins, glycerine, enzymes and fluoride.

Periodontal disease and gingivitis

Periodontal disease and **gingivitis** occur more often in PLHIV than the general community. Gingivitis occurs less frequently in patients on ART. Necrotising ulcerative gingivitis and necrotising ulcerative periodontitis are severe forms of gum disease occurring more often in advanced HIV infection in patients not taking ART. Both periodontitis and gingivitis can cause pain and thus lead to reduced food intake.

Referral to a periodontist is recommended. Treatment may include antibiotics such as metronidazole, amoxicillin or tetracyclines. **Dietary strategies** to maintain intake with a painful mouth are described in Table 9.2.

Periodontal disease and diabetes: periodontal disease increases when diabetes is poorly controlled. PLHIV with diabetes should receive dietary advice for their diabetes in addition to regular medical review to optimise their diabetes management.

Smoking has been associated with dental caries, periodontal diseases, oral mucosal lesions and oral cancer. Smoking, alcohol and other drug use should be discussed with PLHIV and referrals made to assist clients with cessation or reduction as appropriate.

Dental decay

Dental decay is strongly linked to the consistency and frequency of sugar consumption. When PLHIV are trying to gain weight, dietary strategies should take into consideration impacts on oral and dental health. Box 9.6 provides practical dietary tips to prevent dental decay.

Box 9.6   Practical dietary and oral hygiene tips for preventing dental decay and erosion

- Use sugar substitutes for hot and cold drinks
- Always rinse your mouth after the consumption of sugary and sticky foods such as biscuits, toffee, potato chips and raisins
- Eat sweets only with main meals
- Use decaffeinated products
- Drink 'diet' cordials instead of soft drinks, other sugary drinks or carbonated drinks
- When taken, acidic and sugary drinks should only be consumed with meals, preferably using a straw to reduce the contact time with teeth.
- Frequently drink or sip water
- Chew sugar-free gum or suck on sugar-free lozenges
- Eat dairy foods at least 3 times per day to help protect teeth
- Remove food that sticks or lodges between teeth
- Floss then brush teeth at least 2 times a day.

Dental erosions can occur from not only frequent vomiting or reflux but externally through diet with consumption of acidic foods and drinks such as regular and sugar-free soft drinks and fruit juices.

Box 9.7 lists recommended dietary modifications when chewing is difficult due to dental problems.

Note: PLHIV with dental decay who are underweight should be advised to snack on unflavoured milk, unsweetened yoghurt and cheese rather than sugary foods to assist with weight gain. If nutritional supplements are prescribed PLHIV should be advised to drink them in one go rather than sip on them and to rinse their mouth with water after taking supplements.

Referrals

Poor oral health is commonly associated with compromised nutritional status. As explained in chapter one, maintaining nutritional status is particularly important for PLHIV.

Box 9.7   Recommended dietary modifications when chewing is difficult

- To reduce chewing time and pressure, blend, mince and finely chop firm foods and increase the balance of soft or moist foods. Examples include stews, casseroles, soups, pasta, baked beans, creamed corn, savoury mince, etc.
  - Soften cereal with warm milk
  - Cook meat until very tender
  - Cook vegetables until tender and serve with sauce
  - Add extra water to rice or noodles for a soft sticky texture
- Avoid rough, dry and crunchy foods, especially foods such as crackers, crisps, nuts and hard toast.
- Remove crusts from bread
- Cut food into small pieces
- If you need to gain weight, eat at least 5–6 times per day
  - Include nutritious drinks like milkshakes and soups instead of tea and coffee
- Include healthy high-fat foods like avocado, olive oil and nut spreads.

Dentists, periodontists, dietitians and other health care workers should be screening PLHIV for oral health problems, providing education and initiating referrals to each other as part of comprehensive client care.

9.7 Reflux (heartburn)

Pain and discomfort associated with indigestion is caused by stomach acid entering the oesophagus (reflux). Even when symptoms are mild or intermittent, extensive ulceration and inflammation may result. Painful swallowing is likely to adversely affect food and liquid intake. Refluxing into the mouth is associated with dental damage.

Reflux may be caused by some ART and other medications, laxity in the valve between the oesophagus and stomach or may be a sign of a more serious underlying problem. Medical investigation is recommended. Table 9.3 describes some symptom management strategies for reducing reflux.

Table 9.3   Recommended nutritional management for reflux.

	Recommended nutritional management for PLHIV
Reflux (heartburn)	<ul><li>Avoid large meals, eat six small meals/snacks per day</li><li>Avoid lying down during and within 30 minutes following eating</li><li>Take a short break (e.g. 30 minutes) after eating before drinking fluids and drink only small amounts with your meals</li><li>Take time to enjoy your meals – eat slowly and chew thoroughly</li><li>Avoid tight or restrictive clothing as these can cause pressure on the stomach</li><li>Get support to lose weight if you are overweight – research shows reflux decreases with weight loss in people who are overweight</li><li>Limit the following if they worsen your reflux: chocolate, caffeine, alcohol, fatty foods, citrus fruits and juices</li><li>Get support to stop smoking. Smoking increases the incidence and severity of heartburn by relaxing the valve between the oesophagus and stomach</li></ul>

9.8 Symptom control and management of nausea and vomiting

Nausea and vomiting present in PLHIV for many reasons including anxiety, medication side effects, food poisoning, infections and even hunger.

Severe vomiting can lead to dehydration, so it is important to frequently drink small amount of fluids. Anti-nausea medications prescribed by your doctor should preferably be taken 30 minutes prior to a meal.

9.8.1 Goals of dietary management for nausea and vomiting

- Minimise nausea and vomiting to improve quality of life and normalise daily activities and routine.
- Avoid dehydration and electrolyte imbalances.
- Maintain nutritional status and weight.

Box 9.8 provides examples of management strategies for the control of nausea and vomiting.

9.9 Symptom control and management of fatigue

Fatigue and tiredness occur often in PLHIV. There are many causes of fatigue including:

- HIV infection raising energy expenditure in the body's response to HIV
- anaemia due to factors discussed below
- psychological problems including depression, sleeping difficulties and stress
- low levels of testosterone
- weight loss with lean muscle mass loss
- decreased food intake or poor absorption of foods leading to micronutrient deficiencies.

Fatigue can affect nutritional status by reducing physical activity and energy for activities of daily living including buying food, cooking meals and even eating.

PLHIV should be referred for medical investigation for the cause of the fatigue and treatment if required.

Box 9.9 describes some strategies for managing fatigue and maintaining nutritional status during periods of fatigue.

9.9.1 Fatigue related to anaemia

Anaemia is a condition where the blood is unable to carry adequate oxygen to tissues due to a low level of haemoglobin found in red blood cells. Oxygen is a

Box 9.8   Strategies to control and manage nausea and vomiting

Before you eat

- Rinse your mouth to clean the palate.
- Consider using relaxation techniques which may alleviate nausea related to anxiety.
- Try to make meal times as enjoyable as possible, e.g. eat with friends or family, eat in pleasant surroundings, use a table cloth or put on music.
- Consider taking an anti-emetic 30 minutes prior to your meal.

When to eat

- Eat your largest meal of the day when you feel best. This is often at breakfast.
- Do not skip meals as an empty stomach will often increase nausea. At least have a small snack.

What to eat

- Six small meals per day may be easier to manage than three large meals.
- Eat and drink slowly, chewing food well.
- After a sleep eat some plain, salty crackers or thin crisp bread before activity.
- Cool foods are often more appealing. Try sandwiches, salads and cold milk pudding.
- Avoid strong food odours such as cabbage and coffee.
- If possible, avoid the kitchen when food is being prepared. Sit in a well ventilated room or outside where food smells are not confined to small spaces.
- Try not to over-rely on your favourite foods during times of nausea. This will help stop you from developing a dislike for these foods. Keeping variety in your food choices is important.
- Avoid greasy or fatty foods such as fried food, pastries, pies, sausage rolls, sausages and cream.
- Small quantities of salty foods such as crackers or soup, or sour/tart foods such as lemon or citrus foods, may help reduce nausea.
- If you cannot manage solid foods try liquids, e.g. low fat milk drinks, cordial, clear soup, jelly, diluted juices, flavoured ice blocks and fruit beverage-based nutritional supplements (on recommendation from your dietitian).

After you eat

- Rest after meals, but avoid lying flat. Use pillows to keep your head and shoulders slightly raised if you lie down and avoid sitting where you are curved strongly forward putting pressure on your stomach.

Vomiting

- Maintaining fluid balance is very important and liquids such as flat dry ginger ale, lemonade or glucose drinks are usually well tolerated. (See Box 9.2 for recipe for oral rehydration solution (ORS).)

- As vomiting settles, try drinking clear broth or nibbling on salty biscuits or toast (without butter).

As soon as you are able, gradually increase your intake of food. Continue to avoid high fat foods until well recovered.

Box 9.9   Nutritional strategies for managing fatigue

- Eat regular meals and snacks.
    Include low glycaemic index (low GI) foods in meals and snacks. These may give more sustained energy throughout the day. These foods include grainy breads, oats, sweet potato, pasta, fruit and yoghurt.
- Stock and eat easy-to-prepare canned or frozen foods, cooked cereals and pastas with ready-to-eat sauce, for example.
- Cook large quantities on days you feel good and freeze individual portion sizes in small containers that can be thawed and reheated at a later date.
- Add left-over meat, poultry, canned fish or eggs to ready-to-eat soup.
- Make home-made shakes with regular or soya milk, fruit and frozen yogurt.
- Decrease your consumption of coffee – it may actually add to the problem of fatigue.
- Sign up with community food and assistance programs (if available) to help you shop, cook and clean up.
- Include at least 30 minutes of daily exercise, e.g. walking. Exercise may help to increase energy levels.

See a dietitian to find out if you need to increase any specific foods or require nutritional supplements

---

basic requirement for cell function. Anaemia is a common problem for PLHIV and contributes to fatigue and malaise as well as increasing the risk of HIV disease progression.

There are a number of different causes of anaemia in PLHIV including:

- deficiency in iron, B12 or folate from inadequate intake or malabsorption
- chronic illnesses such as TB and malaria
- HIV medications, particularly Zidovudine
- increased iron needs, e.g. pregnancy
- HIV infection per se
- blood loss.

Box 9.10 describes recommended dietary guidelines for PLHIV with iron deficiency anaemia.

Box 9.10   Strategies for the dietary management of iron deficiency anaemia

- Eat iron-rich foods containing haem iron such as red meat, i.e. beef, lamb, poultry and fish at least 3–4 times per week (if these foods are normally consumed in the diet).
- Eat iron-rich foods containing non-haem iron such as pulses (e.g. red kidney beans, soya beans), tofu, tempeh, dark green leafy vegetables (e.g. spinach), nuts and seeds (e.g. sesame seeds and cashew nuts), eggs and iron-fortified cereals. Non-haem iron should be eaten with a food or drink rich in vitamin C to enhance absorption.

The best way to prevent anaemia is by eating a wide variety of nutritious food. The iron absorption is influenced by the body's stores of iron. It is not just the amount of iron in your diet that counts, but the amount that the body can absorb.

You may need iron supplements. Discuss with your doctor or other health care workers before taking them.

Ways to improve your iron absorption:

1. Hot drinks like tea, coffee and cocoa contain substances that reduce the absorption of iron from your food. Drink these beverages only about one hour after meals or between meals (SNDRI, 2010).
2. Eat haem iron sources (e.g. meat) with non-haem iron sources (e.g. vegetables, pulses or tofu) as this increases the absorption of non-haem iron by the body. For example, try putting a small amount of meat into your cooked beans.
3. Eat vitamin-C-rich foods. They can increase the absorption of non-haem iron by up to 4 times. For example combine non-meat meals with high vitamin C foods including orange, lemon, berries, canned pineapple, fruit juice broccoli, peppers, tomato and cabbage. For example, drink a glass of orange juice with your meals, cook your spinach or red kidney beans with tomatoes or add chilies to your tofu/tempeh.

9.10   Conclusion

There is no one diet for people living with HIV. Individual dietary counselling and monitoring of PLHIV with symptoms is required to ensure they meet their specific nutritional requirements with appropriate, acceptable and affordable foods.

Nutritional interventions should be provided concurrently with medical management as part of routine care for symptomatic PLHIV.

Acknowledgements

Robert Cherry, Clinical Nurse Specialist and Tim Errington, HIV information line, both from the Albion St Centre, Sydney, Australia, and Antionette Ackerie HIV Dietitian, Royal Prince Alfred Hospital, Sydney Australia for their review of and technical advice for this chapter. Thanks to the Dietitians Association of Australia's

HIV interest group for sharing their knowledge and expertise in patient management over the last 12 years.

References

Abubakar I, Aliyu SH, Arumugam C, Hunter PR, Usman NK. Prevention and treatment of cryptosporidiosis in immunocompromised patients. *Cochrane Database Syst Rev* 2007; CD004932.

Anastasi JK, Capili B, Kim AG, McMahon D, Heitkemper MM. Symptom management of HIV-related diarrhea by using normal foods: A randomized controlled clinical trial. *J Assoc Nurses AIDS Care*, 2006; **17**:47–57.

Edgar WM, O'Mullane DM. *Saliva and Oral Health*, 2nd edn. London: British Dental Association, 1996.

Kotler DP, Gaetz HP, Lange M, Klein EB, Holt PR. Enteropathy associated with teh acquired immunodeficiency syndrome. *Ann Inernt Med* 1984; **101**:421–8.

Post J. Gastrointestinal manifestations, approach to gastrointestinal symptoms. *HIV Management in Australia, A Guide to Clinical Care*. Sydney: Australasian Society for HIV medicine, Inc, ASHM 06, 2006: 175–78.

Sifri R, Diaz VA, Gordan L *et al*. Oral health care issues in HIV disease: developing a Core curriculum for primary care physicians. *J Am Board Fam Pract* 1998; **11**: 434–44.

SNDRI (Scottish Nutrition and Diet Resources Initiative), Iron-Deficiency Anaemia, What You Eat Can Help, Glasgow, 2010. available at: http://www.gcal.ac.uk/sndri/pdf/Iron_deficiencyanaemia.pdf- 51.8KB – Glasgow Caledonian University. Accessed 01/3/10.

Weatherburn P, Anderson W, Reid D, Henderson, L. What do you need? Findings from a national survey of people living with HIV. London: Sigma Research, 2002.

WHO. Antiretroviral therapy for HIV infection in adults and adolescents in resource-limited settings: towards universal access recommendations for a public health approach. Rev. Geneva: WHO, 2006.

WHO. Regional consultation on Nutrition and HIV/AIDS, Evidence, lessons and recommendations for action in South East Asia, October 2007 New Delhi: World Health Organisation, 2008a.

WHO: World Health Organization. Diarrhoea, Geneva, WHO 2008b. Available at: http://www.who.int/topics/diarrhoea/en/ (last accessed 28 May 2008).

10 The Nutritional Management of Complications Associated with HIV and Antiretroviral Therapy

Alastair Duncan and Karen Klassen

Key Points

- HIV infection itself and antiretroviral therapy (ART) can lead to a variety of metabolic disturbances that may increase risk for development of diabetes, coronary heart disease and bone fracture.
- A higher prevalence of reduced bone mineral density, vitamin D deficiency, impaired glucose tolerance and cardiovascular risk has been reported in HIV-positive people than in HIV-uninfected individuals.
- All HIV-positive people should be monitored for signs of development of metabolic side effects and assessed for risk of developing coronary heart disease and bone demineralisation.
- A small number of research trials have demonstrated that individualised dietary and lifestyle interventions can have a positive effect on dyslipidaemias, impaired glucose tolerance, diabetes and lipohypertrophy.
- The impact of many years' duration of both HIV infection and antiretroviral treatment on human metabolism will gradually become evident. Research must continue to look at both prevention and treatment.

10.1 Introduction

Antiretroviral use has seen a dramatic fall in HIV-related mortality, resulting in a population living and gradually ageing with chronic but controlled HIV infection. As a result, people with HIV are now experiencing an increased rate of diseases associated with normal life expectancy, including diabetes, cancer, osteoporosis and heart disease (Palella *et al.*, 2006). These diseases may also be associated with antiretroviral therapy itself, in part driven by metabolic side effects.

Metabolic complications have been observed as a side effect of even the earliest types of ART. These complications include dyslipidaemias, altered glucose metabolism, bone demineralisation, altered body fat metabolism characterised by changes in body composition and lactic acidaemia. The majority of antiretroviral medicines used to treat HIV interfere with viral genetic material. Many human metabolic processes are operationally similar to those of HIV, and so it is unfortunate

Table 10.1 Metabolic complications associated with ART.

Complication	Description
Dyslipidaemia	• Hypertriglyceridaemia • Raised total or low density lipoprotein (LDL) cholesterol • Suppressed high density lipoprotein (HDL) cholesterol • These may occur in isolation or in combination, leading to increased coronary heart disease risk
Altered glucose metabolism	• Central fat accumulation increases risk of impaired glucose tolerance • Insulin resistance leading to impaired glucose tolerance and raised serum glucose; may result in development of diabetes

Fat redistribution, known as lipodystrophy	• Reduced levels of subcutaneous fat in one or several sites (*lipoatrophy*):
	  o Face (temporal, intra-orbital, buccal and/or malar fat pads)
	  o Abdomen
	  o Buttocks (gluteal fat pads)
	  o Arms and/or legs (characterised by prominent vasculature)
	• Increased deposition of fat in one or several sites (*lipohypertrophy*):
	  o Neck
	  o Between the shoulders (dorsocervical fat pad)
	  o Breasts (in both men and women)
	  o Visceral fat within the abdomen
	• These changes may be isolated or combined, and usually not associated with loss of muscle tissue

Altered bone mineralization	• Altered vitamin D metabolism and deficiency • Reduced bone mineral density, osteopaenia, osteoporosis and increased fracture risk
Non-alcoholic hepatic steatosis	• Deposition of fat within the liver, secondary to insulin resistance and central adiposity
Peripheral neuropathy	• Nerve damage in the peripheral areas of the limbs, leading to discomfort, pain, reduced mobility and reduced quality of life
Lactic acidosis	• Mitochondrial toxicity, where ARTs disrupt mitochondrial ribonucleic acid metabolism, leading to increased serum lactic acid levels • Asymptomatic hyperlactataemia may be common, but symptomatic and potentially life-threatening lactic acidosis is rare when ARTs closely associated can be avoided

but not altogether surprising that ART can be associated with the side effects described in Table 10.1. One or more of these side effects may be experienced in combination.

There remains an absence of robust evidence for treatment of many of these ART side effects; treatment plans for these complications in HIV infection are partially developed from the medical guidelines for general populations (British HIV Association, 2008), with nutritional management being an important factor.

10.2 Aetiology of metabolic side effects

Prior to the advent of combination ART, certain metabolic abnormalities had been observed in association with HIV infection, including diminished 1,25-

dihydroxyvitamin D_3 levels (Aukrust *et al.*, 1994), raised triglyceride levels (Grunfeld *et al.*, 1991), and increased rates of heart disease. Around half of those presenting with AIDS showed signs of cardiac abnormalities (Fong *et al.*, 1993); this high rate has been attributed to a combination of factors including HIV and opportunistic infections, accelerated atherosclerosis, cocaine use and malnutrition.

During 1997, case reports emerged detailing unusual metabolic occurrences, such as death caused by massively raised triglyceride levels leading to acute pancreatitis, and accumulation of large quantities of abdominal visceral fat (Capaldini, 1997). This central fat accumulation appeared to be associated with the protease inhibitor (PI) Indinavir, widely used at the time. Patients became increasingly unhappy with their physical appearance, with some choosing to stop taking ART. These factors led to detailed investigations of the syndrome, which became known as lipodystrophy.

An understanding of the mechanisms by which ART causes metabolic side effects remains elusive. These side effects may become evident after months or years of treatment, and may occur in isolation or in combination as part of a wider syndrome. Aetiology theories can be grouped into two general categories: interactions between HIV and the host genotype, for example cytokine-mediated changes resulting from chronic viral infection followed by immune reconstitution, and ART-specific side effects such as mitochondrial toxicity. A review article by Stankov and Behrens (2007) provides further reading.

10.3   Prevalence of metabolic side effects

The prevalence of ART-related metabolic side effects varies, depending on treatment used. Where possible, particular agents associated with a side effect are used less, bringing about reduced prevalence of the side effect. For example, the prevalence of fat redistribution has declined over the last 10 years due to reduced use of certain PIs such as Indinavir, and nucleoside reverse transcriptase inhibitors (NRTIs) including d4T. In practice, physicians tailor the combination of agents used on an individual basis. In less well-resourced regions, choice of ART is limited, and so a much higher prevalence of metabolic side effects is seen (Mutimura *et al.*, 2007).

Since the advent of effective ART in 1998, the rate of HIV-positive people in the United States dying as a result of cardiovascular-related disease has increased from 20 to 26% (Sackoff *et al.*, 2006); in addition the incidence of both coronary heart disease (CHD) and myocardial infarction (MI) in HIV-positive Americans is double that of HIV-negative comparison groups (Triant *et al.*, 2007).

There is conflicting data around the prevalence of the metabolic syndrome in HIV. Jacobson *et al.* (2006) report comparable rates for both HIV-positive patients on ART and HIV-negative comparison populations presenting with a combination of abnormal lipids, hypertension and central obesity. However, in the large Women's Interagency HIV Study, Sobieszczyk *et al.* (2008) show a 33% prevalence rate amongst HIV-positive women compared with 22% in HIV-negative controls. This increase is largely due to dyslipidaemias.

10.4   Assessment of metabolic parameters and cardiovascular disease risk

10.4.1   Background

Given the increased risk for CVD in HIV, regular assessment should be a routine component of care (Wierzbicki *et al.*, 2008). CVD risk should be assessed:

- annually in all HIV-infected adults
- before the initiation of ART
- two to four months after any change in antiretroviral treatment.

Factors contributing to increased CVD risk in people living with HIV not seen in the general population (Hadigan *et al.*, 2001b) include:

- changes in body composition, e.g. loss of subcutaneous fat and/or accumulation of visceral fat
- inflammation whether by direct effects of the virus
- renal impairment: more common in HIV, and can contribute to CVD through microalbuminaemia and sodium retention potentiating hypertension
- direct effects of specific antiretrovirals
- higher incidence of traditional risk factors, including smoking, dyslipidaemia, insulin resistance and impaired glucose tolerance (Friis-Moller *et al.*, 2003).

Box 10.1   CVD risk factors for consideration in annual assessments.

- History of established atherosclerotic CVD
- History of CVD risk estimates
- Diabetes mellitus (type 1 or 2)
- Hypertension
- Family history of premature coronary heart disease
- Weight, height, BMI
- Waist circumference
- Smoking status
- Ethnicity
- Age
- Gender
- Diet
- Physical activity
- Fasting lipid profile (Total, HDL and LDL cholesterol and triglycerides)
- Fasting glucose (HbA1C in those with existing diabetes)
- Steroid use

Adapted from NCEP, 2002, British Cardiac Society, 2005.

HIV-infected patients with lipodystrophy share many characteristics with the metabolic syndrome. It is uncertain, however, whether the risk factor thresholds characterising the metabolic syndrome in general populations, using guidelines such as those from the International Diabetes Federation (IDF, 2006) or National Cholesterol Education program, are applicable in HIV.

10.4.2   Calculating cardiovascular risk

All patients with established atherosclerotic disease or diabetes are considered at high risk for cardiovascular disease – calculation is not required. Accurate prediction of CVD risk depends on assessing a range of interrelated factors. There are a number of tools available for calculation of cardiovascular risk. The validity of any risk calculator in determining long-term cardiovascular risk among younger patients with HIV has not been determined. Most risk calculators use data biased towards Caucasian ethnic origin. The most commonly used calculators are based on the Framingham equation, which uses data derived from a predominately Caucasian North American population. Health professionals should choose the most appropriate tool based on the population or individual they are assessing.

The Joint European Societies recommend the use of the SCORE system, which estimates the 10-year risk of a fatal coronary event as opposed to any cardiovascular event (http://www.benecol.net/healthcareprofessionals.asp?viewID=2374).

Alternatively in the UK, there are cardiovascular risk prediction charts from the Joint British Societies/British National Formulary based on the Framingham (1991) algorithm (http://cvrisk.mvm.ed.ac.uk/calculator/bnf.htm).

In the UK the QRISK2 algorithm has been developed from Primary Care databases and includes family history, deprivation and ethnicity as risk factors. Although postcode data can be entered, this has not yet been validated. It could be argued that this is the most appropriate tool to use for calculating CVD risk in the British HIV-positive population (http://qr2.dyndns.org) (Figure 10.1).

10.5   Management of dyslipidaemias

10.5.1   Introduction

HIV infection, ART and traditional risk factors (including obesity, smoking and lifestyle) all contribute to the prevalence of dyslipidaemia. In addition, anabolic steroids used to treat HIV wasting may be atherogenic: studies have shown that they lower HDL levels (Grunfeld et al., 2006).

In the largest survey of dyslipidaemia in HIV, the Data Collection on Adverse Events of Anti-HIV Drugs (D:A:D) study, dyslipidaemia rates were reported as in Table 10.2 (Friis-Moller et al., 2003).

The management of dyslipidaemias in HIV follows guidelines for the general population. Modification of diet, exercise and smoking cessation are first-line treatments. However, modification of ART and lipid-lowering medication can also be considered.

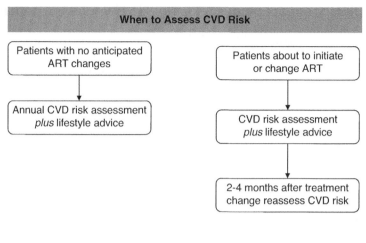

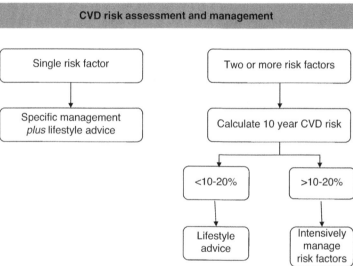

Figure 10.1   Clinical algorithm for investigation and management of CVD risk in HIV (Adapted from Wierzbicki *et al.*, 2008).

Table 10.2   Dyslipidaemia rates from the D:A:D study.

	Raised total cholesterol (%)	Suppressed HDL (%)	Raised triglycerides (%)
ART including a PI	27	27	40
NNRTI but no PI	23	19	32
NRTIs only	10	25	23
ART naive	8	26	15

10.5.2   Dietary impact on dyslipidaemia in HIV-infected patients

The impact of dietary saturated fat and cholesterol intake on serum lipid levels, well known in the general population, has not been particularly well-studied in HIV. In observational studies, Joy *et al.* (2007) looked at the relationship between dietary composition and lipid levels in HIV-infected adults with metabolic abnormalities. They found that higher dietary saturated fat intakes were related to higher serum triglyceride levels, but not to total- or LDL-cholesterol. Hadigan *et al.* (2001a) showed that those with a lower dietary fibre and higher saturated fat intake had higher insulin levels. In addition, alcohol intake was positively associated with increased LDL and decreased HDL.

In a 12-month controlled trial conducted in Brazil, Lazzaretti *et al.* (2007) randomised 90 patients commencing ART to either an intervention of three-monthly personal appointments with a dietitian or to a control group given standard non-individualised diet advice. After one year, the control group had seen an increase in triglycerides of 18%, total cholesterol (26%) and LDL (25%), with no change in HDL. The intervention group experienced statistically significant changes in total cholesterol (increased 5%), triglycerides (decreased 25%) and LDL (decreased 5%), with no change in HDL.

There is weak evidence to suggest that a low fat, high fibre and low glycaemic index (GI)-diet with exercise will decrease BMI, waist circumference and improve lipid profiles and blood pressure (Roubenoff *et al.*, 2002; Fitch *et al.*, 2006). Other small intervention studies have shown that only those compliant with diet experienced statistically significant changes in their lipid levels (Moyle *et al.*, 2001; Barrios *et al.*, 2002). As in HIV-uninfected adults, dietary intervention often failed to normalize lipid levels, suggesting that additional interventions may be required. Billing and Hunt (2008) describe a dietary advice approach in routine care for dyslipidaemia in an HIV clinic in the UK. Outside of the research setting, they report difficulties with adherence to diet, with only 20% of clients attending for follow-up.

10.5.3   Considerations for lipid-lowering medications in HIV-infection

Depending on antiretroviral therapy, some lipid-lowering agents may interact with ART metabolism at the level of CYP3A4 (Dube *et al.*, 2003). Pravastatin (no CYP metabolism) and fluvastatin (CYP2C9) are least likely to interact with protease inhibitors. Atorvastatin (CYP3A4/3A6) can be used with caution and usually in lower doses than is normally prescribed. Simvastatin and lovastatin are contraindicated in patients taking PIs. With non-nucleoside reverse transcriptase inhibitors (NNRTIs), higher doses of statins may be needed as the two drugs are competing for the same metabolic pathway. Rosuvastatin may be metabolised by CYP2C19 and should be used with caution as blood levels can increase with ritonavir. The European Aids Clinical Society (Lundgren *et al.*, 2008) recommends that statins should be first-line treatment for both isolated raised LDL and for elevated LDL and triglycerides in combination. Fibrates are recommended for severe hypertriglyceridaemia (>10 mmol/L) and for isolated low HDL.

10.5.4   Omega-3 fatty acids

In the general population, omega-3 fatty acids are known to significantly lower triglyceride levels. A Cochrane review of omega-3 supplements in people with Type 2 Diabetes found that triglyceride levels were significantly lowered in those taking supplements (Hartweg *et al.*, 2008). Omega-3 fatty acids have also been shown to reduce blood triglyceride levels in HIV-infected adults (Wohl *et al.*, 2005; De Truchis *et al.*, 2007). Doses should start at 2 grams per day and increased to 4 grams and up to 12 grams per day as needed (BNF, 2009). Caution may be warranted in patients at risk of bleeding, those receiving warfarin, or those with high levels of LDL. Also of note, cod liver oil contains a smaller dose of omega-3s and high amounts of vitamin A, potentially toxic if combined with other vitamin supplements. Vitamin A doses over 1500 mcg (5000 IU) per day may be associated with an increased risk of developing osteoporosis (Weber and Raederstorff, 2000).

10.5.5   Lifestyle modifications: smoking, exercise and diet

Reducing saturated fat intake and other dietary interventions to improve diet quality is known to improve serum lipids in the general population, and has been associated with reduced mortality in patients with coronary artery disease (Please see Box 10.2 Dietary advice for improving dyslipidaemia). A Cochrane review revealed that dietary advice was effective in significantly reducing total cholesterol and LDL levels (Brunner *et al.*, 2007). Data from cohort studies in non-HIV populations suggests that small changes made early in life can lead to substantial long-term reductions in CVD (Law *et al.*, 1994).

A thorough dietary assessment is necessary to help individualise advice given. Weight reduction for overweight or obese patients will enhance total cholesterol, LDL and triglyceride lowering, and also improve other health outcomes (Patalay *et al.*, 2005).

10.5.6   Smoking

Cigarette smoking is the most important modifiable cardiovascular risk factor for HIV-infected patients. In the D:A:D study (Friis-Moller *et al.*, 2003), approximately 50% of participants were current or former cigarette smokers; smoking conferred a greater than twofold increased risk of myocardial infarction. Cessation of smoking is more likely to reduce cardiovascular risk than either the choice of ART or the use of any lipid-lowering therapy. Knowledge of local smoking cessation services and use of online resources is important for all clinicians (www.smokefree.nhs.uk).

10.5.7   Exercise

Physical activity favourably modifies several risk factors: it has been reported to lower LDL and triglyceride levels, raise HDL, improve insulin sensitivity and lower blood pressure in the general population, however, there are conflicting results from studies specifically investigating the effect of an exercise intervention on improving dyslipidaemia in HIV-infected adults (Fitch *et al.*, 2006).

Box 10.2 Dietary advice for improving dyslipidaemia.

Saturated fatty acids

- Reducing saturated fat, whilst maintaining or increasing intakes of unsaturated fat, can help to reduce total and LDL cholesterol.
- UK guidelines on primary prevention of CVD suggest that higher risk individuals should consume less than 30% of total energy from fat, less than 10% of total energy from saturated fat and to consume less than 300 mg/day of dietary cholesterol (NICE, 2008).
- Dietary impact on LDL should be seen 6 weeks after the implementation of the low saturated fatty acid diet.

Plant stanols/sterols

- Some data show that plant-derived stanol/sterol esters at dosages of 2 g/day (the amount present in the commercially available yogurt drink products) lower LDL levels by 6–15% with little or no change in HDL cholesterol or triglyceride levels (SIGN, 2007). Their mode of action is different to statins and so they can be used as an adjunct therapy.
- The long-term safety of plant stanol/sterols is unknown.

Omega-3 fatty acids

- For those at risk of developing CVD, regular intake of fish (2 servings of fish per week, one of which should be oily) and other sources of omega-3 fatty acids are recommended (British Cardiac Society, 2005, NICE, 2008).
- For secondary prevention, those who have had an MI should consume at least 7 grams of omega-3 fatty acids per week from 2 to 4 portions of oily fish per week. For those unable to achieve this amount from their diet, 1 gram daily of an omega-3 fatty acid supplement is recommended (NICE, 2008).

When encouraging fish intake the health professional should consider environmental issues such as sustainability and the potential for toxic contamination (the (UK) Marine Conservation Society website www.fishonline.org provides further information).

Salt

- Evidence suggests that high blood pressure can be reduced or prevented by consuming less salt (NCEP, 2002). British Cardiac Society (2005) guidelines recommend that those at risk of developing CVD limit their intake of salt to 100 mmol/L day (the equivalent of 6 g of sodium chloride or 2.4 g of sodium daily).

Fibre/complex carbohydrates

- Soluble fibre (e.g. oats, guar, pectin, and psyllium) can help decrease total and LDL cholesterol. Increasing intake can be therapeutically beneficial (NCEP, 2002)
- Low glycaemic index (GI) diets have been found to lower triglyceride levels, and have beneficial effects on insulin sensitivity (Zivkovic et al., 2007). In addition, a Mediterranean-style diet consisting of 50–60% carbohydrates and high in soluble fibre is more effective at reducing features of the metabolic syndrome, primarily dyslipidaemia (Esposito et al., 2004).

Others

- Jenkins *et al.* (2003) investigated a combination of lipid-lowering foods – 'The Portfolio Diet'. This included low saturated fat intakes, almonds, soy products, plant sterols, high soluble fibre and high vegetable protein sources. All of these components individually have been shown in previous studies to have a modest effect on serum lipids. Compliance was poor overall; those who adhered to the diet achieved significant lowering of LDL by 20%.
- Patients with dyslipidaemia may consider alternative therapies and nutritional or herbal supplements. Some herbs and high doses of nutrients may interact with ART or stimulate HIV itself. For example, garlic is commonly promoted as a 'heart healthy' supplement, however, capsules containing a garlic concentrate have been shown to interact with the PI saquinavir and should be avoided. There is no indication that routine use of garlic in cooking poses a problem (Piscitelli *et al.*, 2002) (more information about interactions between HIV medication and complementary and alternative therapies can be found in Chapter 16).

Alcohol

- Heavy drinking increases CVD risk and has been associated with impaired fasting glucose/diabetes mellitus, hypertriglyceridaemia, abdominal obesity, and high blood pressure (Fan *et al.*, 2008). Moderate alcohol intake may reduce CVD risk mediated by a beneficial effect on HDL. Patients should be advised to follow advice for the general population and to limit alcohol consumption to 3–4 units per day for men and 2–3 units per day for women, with two alcohol-free days per week, and to avoid binge drinking (NICE, 2008).

Encouraging increased physical activity is appropriate for all individuals as this will help to achieve optimal lean body mass (LBM) and may improve lipid profiles. NICE (2008) recommends that people at high risk of developing CVD should be advised to take 30 minutes of physical activity at least 5 days a week. Dietitians and other health professionals can be instrumental in providing exercise advice and referring to hospital and community exercise programmes.

10.6   Management of impaired glucose metabolism

10.6.1   Aetiology

Most researchers agree that impaired glucose metabolism secondary to ART use is multifactorial in aetiology, however, there remains no clear explanation for the mechanism of action as results conflict between in vitro studies and clinical data (Blumer *et al.*, 2008). One compelling theory is that accumulation of adipose tissue within both muscle tissue and the liver lead to reduced insulin sensitivity.

Development of both impaired glucose tolerance and diabetes occurs with antiretroviral use, particularly AZT, d4T (both NRTIs), and the PIs. The risk increases with duration of ART, and with onset of accumulation of both visceral and subcutaneous abdominal fat. Haugaard *et al.* (2005) demonstrated that in those patients receiving ART who developed clinically overt signs of lipohypertrophy or lipoatrophy also showed disturbances in glucose metabolism, including insulin resistance at the level of hepatic glucose production, peripheral glucose utilisation and lipolysis.

10.6.2 Prevalence

The prevalence of both impaired glucose tolerance and diabetes increases with ART use. In patients prescribed PIs, 61% presented with peripheral insulin resistance; PI use resulted in a threefold increased risk of developing diabetes compared with HIV-negative controls (Justman et al., 2003). There was no increased risk associated with PI-sparing regimens. In another cohort study diabetes occurred in 7% of patients with fat atrophy or fat accumulation, a rate 14 times higher than in healthy, matched controls (Brown et al., 2005). In the D:A:D study, de Wit et al. (2008) showed that duration of treatment with ART increases risk of developing diabetes. They also showed that the NRTIs AZT and d4T confer an independent risk for developing both insulin resistance and diabetes.

10.6.3 Monitoring and treatment

HIV patients should be routinely monitored for signs of impaired glucose metabolism. Fasting glucose should be assessed prior to commencing ART. A follow-up measurement should be repeated 3–6 months after starting treatment (British HIV Association, 2008). The International Diabetes Federation (2008) suggests that patients with fasting plasma glucose levels 5.6 mmol/L or above should be offered an oral glucose tolerance test.

Treatment of impaired glucose metabolism in HIV should mirror that of the general population (British HIV Association, 2008), shown in Figure 10.2, and targets for diabetes management in HIV should be derived from targets for those with Type 2 diabetes, shown in Table 10.3.

Dietary and lifestyle advice for management of impaired glucose metabolism in HIV can be found in section 10.11 of this chapter. In addition, the UK national guidelines for specific dietary management for impaired glucose metabolism (NICE, 2008) include:

1. Individualised and ongoing nutritional advice taking into account the individual's needs, culture and beliefs, being sensitive to their willingness to change and the effects on their quality of life.
2. Encourage high-fibre, low-glycaemic-index sources of carbohydrate in the diet, such as fruit, vegetables, wholegrains and pulses; include low-fat dairy products and oily fish; and control the intake of foods containing saturated and trans fatty acids.
3. Integrate dietary advice with a personalised diabetes management plan, including other aspects of lifestyle modification, such as increasing physical activity and losing weight.
4. Advise individuals that limited substitution of sucrose-containing foods for other carbohydrates in the meal plan is allowable, but that care should be taken to avoid excess energy intake.
5. Discourage the use of foods marketed specifically for people with diabetes, as these tend to be high in saturated fat or sorbitol.

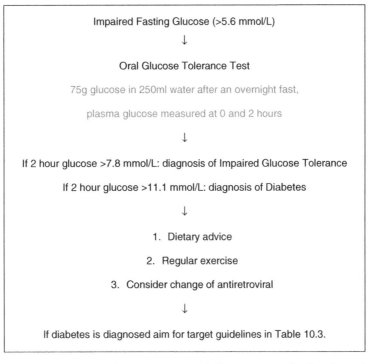

Figure 10.2 Treatment of impaired glucose metabolism as a result of antiretroviral therapy (Adapted from BHIVA, 2008).

There are other dietary considerations for insulin resistance specific to HIV. Agh-dassi *et al.* (2008) have demonstrated the benefit of chromium supplementation in patients on ART with proven insulin resistance. In a small randomised placebo-controlled trial, 400 μg of chromium nicotinate daily for 16 weeks significantly reduced insulin levels, triglycerides and trunk fat mass without affecting serum glucose.

Regarding the use of diabetic medicines in HIV-positive people receiving ART, recommendations are to follow general guidelines for the management of diabetes, however, there are certain caveats. The biguanide Metformin should be used with caution where signs of lipoatrophy are apparent, where its use may exacerbate

Table 10.3 Targets for diabetes management.

Parameter		Goal
Glycaemic control	Glycosylated Haemoglobin (HbA1C), %	<7.0
	Pre-prandial capillary plasma glucose (mmol/L)	5.0–7.0
	Peak postprandial capillary plasma glucose (mmol/L)	<10.0
	Blood pressure, mm Hg	<130/80
Lipids	Total cholesterol (mmol/L)	<4.0
	LDL cholesterol (mmol/L)	<2.0
	Triglycerides (mmol/L)	<1.70

Adapted from International Diabetes Federation (2008) and NICE (2008).

peripheral fat loss (Kohli *et al.*, 2007). Glitazones should be used with caution in patients with dyslipidaemias as they may increase LDL levels (Hadigan *et al.*, 2007). The British HIV Association (2008) urge caution with the use of the following oral hypoglycaemic agents given the lack of evidence for their use in those receiving ART: the sulfonylureas gliclazide and glipizide, glinides, exenatide and alpha-glucosidase inhibitors. Also recommended is the use of aspirin in all those with diabetes (British Cardiac Society, 2005).

10.7   Management of altered fat distribution

10.7.1   Aetiology

Although there are several theoretical mechanisms, the aetiology of body-shape changes secondary to ART use remains controversial. PIs and NRTIs are known to have different effects on fat mass. This can be shown by observing changes in body composition when patients cease using PIs or NRTIs, instead switching to alternative therapy. Where lipoatrophy has already occurred, cessation of PI use does not lead to fat mass recovery, whereas replacing d4T (stavudine) or AZT with an alternative NRTI, such as abacavir (ziagen), will enable fat mass to recover (Carr *et al.*, 2002).

Although theories regarding aetiology remain controversial, a fuller understanding of the body-shape changes themselves has developed. For example, the Fat Redistribution and Metabolic Change in HIV study (Bacchetti *et al.*, 2005) showed that in lipoatrophy there is less peripheral and central subcutaneous fat along with less visceral fat. Previously, it was thought that peripheral lipoatrophy was usually associated with central fat accumulation. Lean body mass is preserved with both lipoatrophy and lipohypertrophy, allowing a clear distinction between fat redistribution and wasting. It can be more difficult to distinguish between development of lipohypertrophy and normal weight gain, and this is later discussed in the case study in Box 10.3, as well as being illustrated in Picture 10.3. Leptin deficiency may also exacerbate lipohypertrophy (Mulligan *et al.*, 2009). Risk factors for developing fat redistribution are described in Table 10.4 (see Figures 10.3 and 10.4).

Wasting of subcutaneous fat in the legs often leads to more prominent vasculature and musculature (Figure 10.4).

Table 10.4   Risk factors for developing fat redistribution (lipodystrophy).

Increased risk of lipoatrophy	Increased risk of lipohypertrophy
Male gender	Female gender
Use of d4T, AZT or unboosted PI	Use of PIs
Duration of antiretroviral treatment	Duration of antiretroviral treatment
Low body weight	Overweight
Ethnicity – Caucasian highest risk, Black and East Asian lowest risk	Increasing age
Low CD4 prior to initiation of antiretrovirals (less than 200)	
Increasing age	

Adapted from Kotler *et al.* (1999).

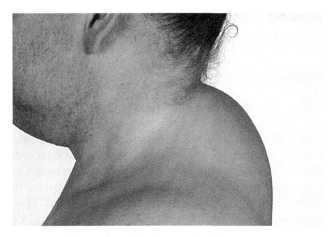

Figure 10.3 Deposition of fat in the neck: dorsocervical fat pad.

10.7.2 Prevalence

The prevalence of antiretroviral-associated body-shape changes is difficult to quantify, as no unifying classification of the syndrome has been agreed. Various studies have reported the prevalence to be between 10 and 83%. For example, Miller *et al.* (2003) showed that the prevalence of fat redistribution in an Australian cohort receiving antiretroviral therapy of 1348 patients was 53%. Antiretrovirals more closely associated with fat redistribution such as d4T, ddI and Indinavir are being used less frequently in developed regions and so incidence is rapidly reducing; compared to an increasing prevalence in Africa where choice of antiretroviral agent is more limited

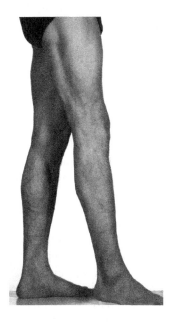

Figure 10.4 Lipoatrophy.

by price: Mutimura *et al.* (2007) describe a fat redistribution prevalence of 70% in those receiving antiretrovirals in Rwanda.

10.7.3   Monitoring

Monitoring for signs of fat redistribution should be carried out routinely. The British HIV Association guidelines (2008) suggest sequential measurements using manual anthropometry should be taken, including annual waist measurements. Ideally, a range of skinfold and circumference measurements should be recorded at the initiation of ART, along with height and weight. These measurements can be repeated annually or more frequently if changes in body shape are suspected or observed.

Magnetic resonance imaging (MRI), computed tomography (CT) and dual-energy X-ray absorptiometry (DEXA) can provide good quality data regarding body composition, however, their use is largely confined to research secondary to cost (The British HIV Association, 2008). DEXA scanning has been widely used in this context and provides a detailed breakdown of fat and lean tissue by body compartment, with a margin of error of less than 5%. There are no standard reference values for patient comparison. The abdomen is analysed as a whole, however, and so the data is unable to distinguish between subcutaneous and visceral fat. Fatty infiltration of muscle and liver tissue may also be missed. MRI and CT scans can provide an accurate measure of both subcutaneous and visceral abdominal fat, but are prohibitively expensive for routine clinical use.

10.7.4   Treatment

Where clinicians are able to employ an informed management of the use of various antiretroviral agents in combination with each other, lipoatrophy is at best slowly reversible (Carr *et al.*, 2002; Martin *et al.*, 2004; Tebas *et al.*, 2007). The British HIV Association (2008) therefore recommends avoiding causative agents such as d4T or to switch away from them. With facial lipoatrophy, inert fillers such as polylactic acid have a well-documented and greatly beneficial effect (Moyle *et al.*, 2006).

Box 10.3   Case study: obesity or lipohypertrophy?

- A 43-year-old Caucasian male was 1.80m tall, with a reported usual weight of 82 kg. However, he attended his GP as he was worried about weight loss, where he weighed 69 kg. He was diagnosed with HIV, with a CD4 count of 131.
- At the HIV clinic he agreed with his physician to commence antiretroviral therapy. Standard practice at his HIV clinic included baseline measurement of body shape by the dietitian using skinfold caliper and tape measure. These measurements were repeated at 6-month intervals.
- At month 12, the patient became anxious that he was developing antiretroviral-related lipohypertrophy. He reported that none of his trousers would fit any more. On examination, his physician agreed that he had an accumulation of central fat. His anthropometry was as follows:

	Usual weight	Baseline	Month 6	Month 12	Month 18
Weight, kg	82	69.0	75.2	84.7	83.4
BMI, kg/m^2	25	21.3	23.2	26.1	25.7
Mid-arm circumference, cm (population centiles)		28.2 (<5th)	29.4 (10th)	33.6 (50th)	35.1 (75th)
Triceps skinfold, mm (population centiles)		7.9 (15th)	7.8 (15th)	9.0 (15–25th)	9.2 (15–25th)
Waist, cm		98.8	107.1	112.5	106.5
Suprailiac skinfold, mm (population centiles)		12.3 (5–10th)	12.7 (10th)	11.9 (5th)	12.7 (10th)
Hips, cm (population centiles)		97.1 (20–50th)	102.0 (50–75th)	101.3 (50–75th)	104.6 (75th)
Mid-thigh circumference, cm (population centiles)		48.3 (15–25th)	52.9 (50–75th)	53.5 (50–75th)	55.0 (75th)
Mid-thigh skinfold, mm		16.8	18.2	17.5	17.6

Discussion:
At month 12 the patient had gained significant amounts of weight since commencing antiretrovirals, commonly seen with a return to health. There was some evidence of increase in LBM: arm and thigh circumferences had increased without substantial increase in skinfold measurements. The waist size had increased dramatically, without an increase in suprailiac skinfold, and only a modest increase in hips.

This data suggests that antiretroviral-associated lipohypertrophy may be implicated as a cause of increased waist size as opposed to obesity. During normal weight gain, both subcutaneous and visceral fat are deposited in the abdomen. Added to this, appendicular fat gain was minimal, in this case, while mid-thigh and mid-arm circumference increased substantially, indicating increased muscle mass. Thus, with regular repeat simple anthropometric measurements it is possible to track changes in body composition in this patient group, without the need for expensive, time-consuming scanning techniques which may involve exposure to radiation.

The patient was motivated to adopt a lifestyle approach to treating his body-shape changes. He attended the gym 3 times per week, with a balance of cardiovascular and resistance exercises. His month 18 anthropometry reflects a decrease in visceral fat: his waist has reduced without a loss in suprailiac skinfold size. In addition, increasing hips, and arm and thigh circumferences indicate increasing LBM.

Various strategies to reduce visceral fat (e.g. thiazolidinedione, metformin, recombinant human growth hormone and testosterone) have been evaluated with limited effect (Pirmohamed, 2009). Growth hormone analogues, and tesamorelin, a growth hormone-releasing hormone analogue, have shown promise, however, these therapies are expensive, require parenteral administration, and the unknown long-term effects on cardiovascular risk will limit their use until more evidence is available (British HIV Association, 2008; Pirmohamed, 2009). In a pilot study, Mulligan et al. (2009) suggest that patients with a deficiency of leptin – a hormone produced by

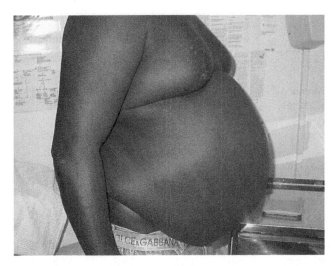

Figure 10.5 Deposition of truncal fat. It is often difficult to distinguish between normal-pattern central obesity and HIV-related deposition of visceral fat. This is discussed in Box 10.3.

fat cells – will benefit from replacement injections. Improvements included a decrease in visceral fat with no change in peripheral fat, in addition to a reduction in LDL, and increases in HDL and insulin sensitivity. Larger and longer, well-designed, placebo-controlled, clinical trials of recombinant human leptin for the treatment of HIV-associated lipoatrophy and metabolic syndrome are required.

Liposuction of regional subcutaneous fat accumulation has been used, but there is often reaccumulation. Surgical removal of visceral fat in the abdomen is contraindicated. For 'buffalo hump', excisional lipectomy may be an alternative that is associated with a smaller risk of reaccumulation. Nutritional interventions (diets low in saturated fats and high in fibre) either alone or in combination with exercise training may also be beneficial if adhered to over the long term (Pirmohamed, 2009).

Diet and exercise are considered to be of primary importance in the treatment of lipohypertrophy (British HIV Association, 2008; Lundgren *et al.*, 2008), however, the role of diet in prevention of both lipohypertrophy and lipoatrophy remains controversial. Saint-Marc *et al.* (1999) showed that reduced energy intake was not responsible for HIV-related lipoatrophy. Batterham *et al.* (2000) investigated dietary intake and body composition. No correlation was found between saturated or total fat and those with fat redistribution. Jones *et al.* (2006) found no correlation between dietary intake of any specific vitamin or mineral or combination of micronutrients and fat redistribution. However, some evidence indicates that increased dietary fibre may aid prevention of development of lipohypertrophy. In an American case-controlled study, Hendricks *et al.* (2003) found that HIV-positive patients without fat deposition had statistically significant higher intakes of both soluble and insoluble fibre, as well as greater protein and energy intakes. Dong *et al.* (2006) found no association between dietary glycaemic index and onset of fat deposition, but again observed a reduced rate of fat deposition with higher fibre intakes. These studies also observed that resistance exercise and non-smoking were protective in terms of lipohypertrophy.

Cho *et al.* (2006) found that 74% of their HOPS cohort reporting fat redistribution was using complementary and alternative medicines to help treat body-shape changes. In terms of perceived positive impact on their body-shape changes, 44% of study participants felt that exercise had helped, vitamins/minerals had helped 35%, and diet 32%. However, there is no evidence that vitamins, minerals, herbs or other dietary supplements can have a positive impact on fat redistribution (Liu *et al.*, 2005).

10.8   Altered bone metabolism

10.8.1   Aetiology

Several antiretrovirals have been implicated in altering bone mineral and vitamin D metabolism at a cellular level (Cozzolino *et al.*, 2003; Pan *et al.*, 2006). In addition, HIV infection and disease severity may contribute to altered bone turnover and formation (Aukrust *et al.*, 1999). Several biological mechanisms support a direct effect of HIV itself on bone metabolism, such as increased cytokine production which may stimulate osteoclast activity and/or inhibit osteoblast function (Aukrust *et al.*, 1999). In addition, HIV infection is associated with an increased metabolic rate, with its associated weight loss and muscle wasting prior to antiretroviral treatment. Low body weight is a known risk factor for decreased bone mineral density (BMD) in both the general population (Kanis *et al.*, 2007) and in HIV-infected individuals (Bolland *et al.*, 2007).

Vitamin D deficiency is a possible factor contributing to decreased BMD. Several studies have shown that 1,25-dihydroxyvitamin D_3 ($1,25(OH)_2D_3$) is decreased in HIV-infected patients with advanced disease (Aukrust *et al.*, 1994). In addition, some classes of ART such as PIs, NNRTIs and NtRTIs, may interact with vitamin D metabolism (Cozzolino *et al.*, 2003; Gyllensten *et al.*, 2006). In particular, Efavirenz (an NNRTI) has been signifcantly associated with an increased prevalence of vitamin D deficiency in several cohort studies. Tenofovir (a nucleotide reverse transcriptase inhibitor) may impact on renal vitamin D metabolism as several studies have shown an association with tenofovir and increased parathyroid hormone (PTH) and alkaline phosphatase (ALP). (Mallon 2010). This area needs further research to explore the possible mechanisms affecting vitamin D metabolism. ART has also been implicated in the pathogenesis of bone metabolism. The relationship between other metabolic complications such as fat redistribution and bone disorders is controversial, as several studies have produced conflicting findings (Huang *et al.*, 2001).

10.8.2   Prevalence

A recent meta-analysis of studies evaluating BMD in HIV-infected patients estimated the current prevalence of osteoporosis and reduced BMD to be 15 and 67% respectively (Brown and Qaqish, 2006). Triant *et al.* (2008) observed that fracture prevalence is significantly higher amongst HIV-positive African-American and Caucasian females and Caucasian males compared to HIV-negative subjects. Several studies in the UK have reported that prevalence of vitamin D deficiency (<50 nmol/L) amongst HIV-infected individuals in the UK ranges from 57%–84% (Klassen *et al.*, 2008;Rosenvinge *et al.*, 2008). It is still unclear if vitamin D deficiency is more common in HIV-infected patients compared to uninfected controls. However, there appears to be a number of HIV-related factors, such as antiretroviral therapy, that may be contributing to the incidence of vitamin D deficiency.

10.8.3   Fracture risk

Bone is a changing tissue constantly undergoing remodelling: formation by osteoblasts produces bone mass while resorption by osteoclasts reduces bone mass. Reduced bone formation or increased bone resorption will consequently result in diminished BMD, increasing the risk of fracture. BMD is most often measured by DEXA including sites most vulnerable to fracture, such as the spine, hip, distal forearm and proximal humerus. Osteoporosis is diagnosed when the DEXA t-score is greater than 2.5 standard deviations below the mean in a young female population (Anonymous, 1993). The less severe osteopaenia is defined as a bone mass that has a DEXA *t*-score of less than 1 standard deviation. Further descriptions of the diagnosis of osteoporosis and osteopaenia is available in other texts (Kanis *et al.*, 2007).

Box 10.4   Potential risk factors contributing to bone loss.

- Longer duration of HIV infection
- Cigarette smoking
- Steroid exposure
- Rheumatoid arthritis
- Family history of hip fracture or osteoporosis
- History of broken bones
- Consumption of >16 g alcohol (2 units in the UK) per day
- Post-menopausal women
- Increased age
- Vitamin D deficiency
- Other nutritional deficiencies (chronic poor dietary calcium intake)
- Caucasian, Asian and Latin ethnicity
- Low sex hormones
  - ◦ Androgen deficiency (low testosterone levels)
  - ◦ Low oestrogen levels
  - ◦ Amenorrhoea
- History of anorexia nervosa or underweight
- Loss of height
- Hyperthyroidism
- Hyperparathyroidism
- Renal insufficiency
- Certain medication, e.g. anticonvulsants
- Opiate use

To calculate a 10-year fracture risk, the FRAX tool developed by WHO (Kanis *et al.*, 2007) can be accessed at: http://www.shef.ac.uk/FRAX

10.8.4   Nutritional management of those at risk for bone disease

Diet is an important factor in forming and maintaining healthy bones. To date, no completed randomised controlled study has investigated the role of diet in treating or preventing decreased bone mineral density associated with HIV infection. Current best practice, therefore, is to base dietary advice on nutritional strategies for bone health in the general population.

The role of the dietitian is to help identify those at risk of bone disease through nutrition assessment and to provide nutritional advice and further refer these patients for a DEXA scan where appropriate. A thorough weight history should be obtained, including lowest weight as an adult, in addition to the appropriate anthropometric measurements to assess muscle mass. Using a validated food frequency questionnaire to assess dietary intake may be useful in assessing the adequacy of nutrient intake related to bone health.

Vitamin D

Calcium and vitamin D are essential nutrients for bone health. The skeleton acts as a metabolic reservoir of calcium and phosphate, the movement of which is regulated by vitamin D. Vitamin D was discovered as an essential nutrient for absorbing calcium and phosphate from the intestine and promoting normal bone formation and mineralization. Vitamin D status is best evaluated by measuring serum 25(OH)D [25-hydroxyvitamin D] as it is the main circulating form of vitamin D. Expert opinion suggests that the optimal serum level of 25(OH)D is at least 75 nmol/L (Holick, 2007) for optimal intestinal calcium absorption and maximal parathyroid hormone suppression. Severe vitamin D deficiency impairs bone mineralisation causing rickets in children and osteomalacia in adults. Vitamin D deficiency decreases calcium absorption which stimulates production of PTH, causing secondary hyperparathyoroidism, which in turn increases absorption, bone mobilisation and renal concentration of calcium and increased excretion of phosphate resulting in hypophosphatemia. Symptoms of vitamin D deficiency can include muscle aches, muscle weakness and bone pain.

In the UK there is no vitamin D synthesis from the sun during the winter months and those of African and Asian descent are at a higher risk of deficiency due to increased pigmentation reducing vitamin D production in the skin (Cosman et al., 2007). In addition, some patients avoid sun exposure due to photosensitivity or are covered due to cultural or religious reasons. Recommending an increased exposure to the sun for those infected with HIV should be done with caution as one large study found an increased risk of skin cancer in this patient group (Crum-Cianflone et al., 2007). Few clinical trials of vitamin D supplementation have been done in HIV-infected individuals. A pilot study supplemented vitamin D-deficient patients with 2000 IU cholecalciferol daily (van den Bout-van den Beukel, 2008b). This amount appeared to be sufficient to increase 25(OH)D to optimal levels, decrease parathyroid hormone (PTH) and increase $1,25(OH_2)D_3$, However, after another 24 weeks of supplementation with half this dose, only $25(OH)D_3$ levels remained significantly different from baseline, while the other parameter levels returned to baseline, suggesting a dose-response effect.

Vitamin D deficiency and supplementation in HIV is not yet well understood, therefore, careful monitoring while supplementing those with vitamin D deficiency is essential in order to provide adequate supplementation and optimal care.

Dietary Vitamin D is consumed through eating oily fish, fortified cereals, margarines, eggs and liver. Those found to have deficient or insufficient levels of 25(OH)D, will need pharmacological supplementation with ergocalciferol or cholecalciferol. Those with established vitamin D deficiency may need ongoing supplementation with a low dose of vitamin D in order to maintain their serum levels. There currently is no Reference Nutrient Intake (RNI) for vitamin D in the UK for children and adults of less than 65 years. For men and women over the age of 65 the RNI is 10 µg/d.

Box 10.5   Risk factors for vitamin D deficiency.

- African or South Asian ethnicity
- Elderly
- Housebound and indoor living
- Malabsorption
- Alcohol abuse
- Renal or liver impairment
- P450 enzyme inducing drugs (e.g. rifampicin, phenytoin)
- Limited exposure to sunlight or excessive use of sunblocks
- Limited or no dietary intake
- Low serum phosphate
- Obesity

Calcium

Vitamin D status, intestinal transit time and mucosal mass are the best established factors affecting calcium absorption. Evaluating each patient's calcium intake and identifying those with low calcium intake, especially long-term, and providing dietary advice will decrease the risk for osteoporosis. There is no functional marker for calcium status as serum calcium is closely regulated. Calcium requirements vary depending on the age, gender and menopausal status of the individual. Most people should be able to meet their needs for calcium through a well-balanced diet, however, some individuals may not. In these cases supplements should be considered. The RNI for adults is 700 mg daily, however, for those at risk of osteoporosis, the National Osteoporosis Society recommends consuming 1200 mg/day.

Phosphorus

When dietary phosphorus is low or when phosphorus is not adequately absorbed from the intestine, urinary phosphorus concentrations fall and serve as good indicators of altered phosphorus regulation. The result is enhanced resorption from bone. Urinary phosphorus losses can be measured using a 24-hour urine collection or by using a urinary fluid phosphate measurement to calculate the fractional phosphate excretion percentage. Intestinal phosphate absorption is increased by vitamin D while renal tubular absorption is inhibited by PTH and phosphatonins, most importantly of those being fibroblast growth factor 23 (FGF-23).

In contrast, excessive intakes of phosphorus when combined with low calcium may have harmful effects on bone metabolism. An increase in serum phosphorus concentration arising from a high dietary phosphorus intake stimulates PTH secretion and FGF-23 levels (Burnett *et al.*, 2006), both of which suppress $1,25(OH)_2D$ production and intestinal calcium absorption. Increased phosphorus reduces calcium lost through the urine, counteracting the adverse effects on calcium absorption and bone metabolism in healthy adults. For these reasons monitoring the ratio of dietary phosphorus to calcium is more important for bone health than phosphorus alone.

The RNI for phosphorus is 550 mg/day for adults, with almost all UK adults exceeding this. The main food sources of phosphorus in the UK are meat, cereals and dairy products.

Protein

It has been hypothesised that excess dietary protein can result in increased urinary calcium excretion creating a negative calcium balance in the blood, resulting in loss of calcium from the bones. This has not been scientifically proven. There is stronger evidence to support low protein intakes leading to increased bone loss (Bonjour, 2005). A risk factor for bone disease in HIV infection is low body weight; for those who are undernourished, maintaining an optimal protein intake to encourage an ideal weight is advisable.

Alkali and potassium

A number of studies have demonstrated a link between high potassium intake and an improvement in calcium balance and reduction of bone resorption. A diet rich in fruit and vegetables as well as increasing potassium intake may also result in a more alkaline environment, which has been shown to reduce urinary calcium excretion and improve bone health (Prynne *et al.*, 2006). The current RNI for potassium in adults is 3500 mg/day. The Dietary Approaches to Stop Hypertension (DASH) diet is a low-sodium, calcium-rich diet that emphasizes fruit, vegetables and low-fat dairy products. It has been shown to lower blood pressure and, more recently (Lin *et al.*, 2003), significantly reduce bone turnover in adults. The DASH diet recommends 4700 mg of potassium daily, however, any increase in fruit and vegetables would be beneficial to patients to reduce both their cardiovascular and osteoporosis risk.

Vitamin K

Vitamin K is required for the production of osteocalcin. Observational data suggests low serum vitamin K concentrations are associated with an increased risk for osteoporotic fractures. However, in a long-term observational study in girls, higher vitamin K status did not improve bone mineral content (Kalkwarf *et al.*, 2004). There currently is no RNI for vitamin K in the UK.

Vitamin A

Vitamin A is essential for bone health, yet excessive intakes of vitamin A, usually achieved by taking supplements, have been associated with lower bone mineral density and higher fracture risk. Experts at the Linus Pauling Institute (2007) recommend a multivitamin/multimineral supplement that provides no more than 2,500 IU (750 mcg/day) to avoid the potential detrimental effects on bone health.

Other nutrients

Bone metabolism may also be improved by a number of other nutrients, including zinc, fluoride, magnesium, vitamin C, B vitamins, omega-3 fatty acids, phytoestrogens and non-digestible oligosaccharides. In contrast, factors that may be potentially harmful to bone health are excess alcohol, caffeine, sodium, fluoride, phosphorus, and omega-6 polyunsaturated fatty acids (Cashman, 2007).

10.8.5   Bisphosphonates

There have been a number of studies evaluating the use of bisphosphonates for the treatment of osteoporosis in HIV. The majority of these studies have included supplementation with calcium (usually 1000 mg of calcium carbonate) and vitamin D (400 IU) in both the treatment (alendronate) and control (placebo) arms (Mondy *et al.*, 2005; McComsey *et al.*, 2007). The improvements in BMD seen with calcium and vitamin D alone were similar in these trials to those seen in other osteoporosis trials, but significantly lower than those treated with bisphosphonates in addition to calcium and vitamin D. However, bisphosphonates are not routinely used in younger people (under 65 years old) as their long-term safety is still unknown; diet and lifestyle interventions remain important for patients who develop osteoporosis at a young age.

10.8.6   Conclusion

Nutrition plays a crucial role in maintaining healthy bones as a variety of nutrients are necessary for the optimization of bone metabolism. A thorough evaluation of individual nutritional intake is advised in order to ensure micro- and macronutrient adequacy. In cases where there is dietary insufficiency, an appropriate micronutrient supplement is advisable.

Box 10.6   Bone health case study.

- Mr M, a 44-year-old Pakistani man, diagnosed with HIV 6 years before, was referred to see the dietitian because he was worried that he had gained 10 kg in the past year, had slightly high cholesterol and also complained of constipation
- Anthropometry: weight 76.1 kg, BMI 24.8 and waist circumference 92.0 cm. He reported he had lost weight when he was diagnosed with HIV infection and had a BMI of 19.6 at that time.
- Biochemistry: Phosphate 1.04 mmol/l (normal); corrected calcium 2.36 mmol/l (normal); alkaline phosphatase 116 u/l (normal) vitamin D deficiency (<15 nmol/L) with a raised parathyroid hormone level of 13.2 pmol/L
- Diet history: longstanding calcium deficiency as he only had 2 teaspoons of milk in his tea each day. Otherwise, he consumed little saturated fat and ate 2 portions of vegetables and 1 portion of fruit each day. He did not smoke and drank 1–2 units of alcohol per week. No exercise and he was rather reclusive.
- Medical history: chronic back pain, sensory polyneuropathy secondary to previous ddI use, and depression. Antiretrovirals: tenofovir, abacavir, lamivudine, atazanavir, ritonavir Previous antidepressant and antacid use.
- Assessment: His risk factors for poor bone health are: history of low BMI, vitamin D deficiency, poor long-standing dietary calcium intake, lack of exercise and history of antacid use
- Due to these risk factors, his BMD was measured. Using DEXA, t-scores less than 1.0 indicate osteopaenia, and less than −2.5 indicate osteoporosis

- The t-scores from the DEXA scan were:
  - R femur: −1.7, L femur: −1.3
  - Lumbar spine 2–4: -3.0
- From these results we can see that the patient has osteoporosis of his lumbar spine, and osteopaenia of femur
- Plan: He was given 7.5 mg of ergocalciferol intramuscularly and was commenced on calcium with vitamin D supplements equivalent to 1200 mg calcium and 800 IU cholecalciferol daily
- Dietary advice given was to improve his lifestyle factors relating to bone health and high cholesterol and constipation, considering his mental health. He was therefore advised to increase his fruit and vegetable intake, especially legumes and nuts, drink more water and to increase his physical activity, especially weight-bearing exercise.

10.9 Management of lactic acidaemia

It is thought that hepatic steatosis, often associated with the NRTIs, d4T and AZT used together in combination, results in the liver becoming unable to clear lactic acid, followed by an inevitable systemic accumulation. Asymptomatic hyperlactataemia may be relatively common amongst those receiving ART, occurring in up to 39% of patients. Symptomatic lactic acidosis is rare, however, presenting in only 0.4% of a developed countries cohort (John *et al.*, 2001).

In recent years, increased use of NRTIs in developing countries has seen an increased incidence of symptomatic lactic acidosis. For example in Botswana, Wester *et al.* (2007) describe an incidence of over 2%. Women with a BMI greater than 25 are at highest risk of developing fatal lactic acidosis, and this is thought to correlate with increased deposition of fat within the liver.

Symptomatic raised serum lactic acid as a result of ART is a potentially life-threatening condition requiring immediate withdrawal of ART and any other possible contributory agents (British HIV Association, 2008). Patients should receive fluid resuscitation and remain under close observation.

Claims are made for the role of nutritional therapies in the treatment of lactic acidosis, however there is a lack of an evidence base for efficacy. Riboflavin (vitamin B2), thiamine (vitamin B1) and L-carnitine have all been proposed as treatments for hyperlactataemia (Falcó *et al.*, 2002). Although the evidence remains inconclusive, in Falcó's small study only 4 of 18 people with lactic acidosis died after treatment with riboflavin or thiamine, significantly fewer than expected. It has also been suggested that vitamins C and E, and coenzyme Q may protect against damage to the mitochondria, although this remains unproven. Further research is needed regarding dosing and efficacy of these nutritional therapies. Given their relative low cost, potential for some benefit and low risk for harm, an argument can be made for ongoing treatment without a more substantial evidence base.

10.10 Peripheral neuropathy

Peripheral neuropathy (PN) can be caused by HIV itself directly damaging nerve tissue. An association between PN and use of the NRTIs, ddI, d4T and to a lesser extent

3TC (lamivudine) has also been demonstrated (Hulgan *et al.*, 2005). It is thought that mitochondrial toxicity from these antiretrovirals contributes to development of neuropathic damage.

The prevalence of PN has decreased since the introduction of effective ART. In a study published by Lichtenstein *et al.* (2005), 147 out of 509 participants developed PN; 73% of those with PN were receiving either d4T or ddI as part of their ART. As treatment continues, however, the prevalence of PN declines, associated with an improving immune system.

There is no definitive treatment for PN, and so management relies heavily on symptom relief through pain control. Nicholas *et al.* (2007) describe a wide range of self-care strategies adopted by the majority of people experiencing PN, including exercise, medication and complementary therapies.

In terms of nutrition, it is known that vitamin B_{12} deficiency can lead to neuropathy. Researchers have explored the possibility that nutritional therapies might prevent or treat HIV or antiretroviral related PN. It should be noted, however, that high doses of vitamin B_6 can itself cause neuropathy. In a Cochrane review Ang *et al.* (2008) concluded that there is insufficient evidence that B vitamins are helpful or harmful in the treatment of peripheral neuropathies. In summary, there is little evidence for a beneficial role for nutritional therapies, with treatment relying on symptom relief.

10.11   Routine assessment, dietary and lifestyle management of metabolic complications

All patients prescribed ART should be routinely assessed for metabolic side effects as part of their Standard of Care. Assessment should be completed on initiation of ART, and then annually or more frequently if clinically indicated. Methods for assessment are described in Chapter 8, 'Nutritional Screening and Assessment'.

Patients experiencing metabolic side effects as a result of ART should follow a healthy balanced diet, and be encouraged to adopt healthier lifestyle strategies. These are summarised in Box 10.7. Further guidance on healthy eating and exercise in HIV can be found in the relevant chapters in this book.

Diet and lifestyle modification should be individualised and carefully monitored. Many of the studies described in this chapter discuss the difficulties involved in ensuring compliance to dietary change. Motivation is key; this has been shown to be best achieved through regular three-monthly appointments with a specialist dietitian (Thompson *et al.*, 2003).

Ideally, the number of individual appointments each patient is invited to attend should be kept to a minimum. This will ensure minimal disruption to the patients' routine, and reduce non-attendance rates in clinics. To this end, many HIV clinics in the UK provide special sessions where, in a single appointment, patients experiencing metabolic side effects can be given advice regarding all aspects of lifestyle modification from the appropriate clinicians and health professionals. These might include an HIV or lipid physician, pharmacist, dietitian, physiotherapist, nurse, or psychologist.

Box 10.7   Diet and lifestyle modification for treatment of metabolic side effects of ART.

Diet

- Energy intake should be modified in order to achieve an ideal body weight
- An adequate protein intake should be achieved
- Saturated fats should be limited
- Monounsaturated and polyunsaturated fats should be encouraged
- Dietary omega-3 fatty acids should be encouraged
- Lower glycaemic load carbohydrates should be encouraged, and sugary foods should be avoided
- The daily diet should provide adequate soluble fibre
- Fruits and vegetables should be encouraged
- Low-fat dairy products are an excellent source of calcium
- Salt should be limited

Exercise

- A balance of both regular cardiovascular and regular resistance exercise should be encouraged
- A target of 30 minutes, 5 times per week is achievable

Smoking

- Smoking cessation should be strongly encouraged

Alcohol

- Limit alcohol consumption to 3–4 units per day for men and 2–3 units per day for women
- Avoid binge drinking

Special care must be taken regarding body composition during treatment of metabolic side effects. Prior to the introduction of ART, studies demonstrated that preservation of LBM and fat mass conferred protection in terms of increased survival through maintenance of immune function (Guenter *et al.*, 1993). Clearly higher levels of fat mass can be a risk factor for increased risk of cardiovascular disease. In addition, lower levels of LBM are a risk factor for reduced bone mineral density. With these factors in mind, diet and exercise advice should be individualised to ensure preservation of LBM, with a goal to achieve ideal fat levels.

10.12 Summary

- HIV infection itself and antiretroviral therapy can both lead to a variety of metabolic disturbances that may increase patients' risk of developing diabetes, coronary heart disease and bone fracture. The effect of individual antiretrovirals on metabolism is summarised in Table10.5. Interventions may have specific effects on metabolism; these are summarised in Table 10.6.

Table 10.5 Effect of individual antiretrovirals on metabolism.

Drug	Effect on lipid levels and cardiovascular risk	Effect on changes in body habitus	Effect on glucose metabolism	Effect on bone metabolism	References
Protease inhibitors					
Atazanavir	No change, but may ↑HDL	No change	No change in insulin sensitivity	May be associated with reduced BMD	Brown and Qaqish (2006); Duvivier et al. (2009)
Amprenavir / Fosamprenavir	↑ total, LDL and HDL cholesterols, and ↑TG	Some ↑ risk of VAT	No change in insulin sensitivity	Unknown	Guffanti et al. (2007)
Darunavir	Neutral	Not known	Not known	Did not increase bone turnover ex vivo	Moyle (2007)
Kaletra	↑ total, LDL and HDL cholesterols, and ↑TG	Some ↑ risk of VAT	↑insulin resistance	Not known	Moyle (2007); Eckhardt and Glesby (2008)
Indinavir	↑ total, LDL cholesterols, and ↑TG. No effect on HDL	↑ risk of dorsocervical fat pat and VAT	↑insulin resistance	Did not increase bone turnover ex vivo	Eckhardt and Glesby (2008)
Nelfinavir	↑ total, LDL and HDL cholesterols. No effect TG	↑ risk of VAT	↑insulin resistance	Possible increase in bone turnover and alteration in vitamin D metabolism	Cozzolino et al. (2003); Mallon (2007); Eckhardt and Glesby (2008)
Ritonavir	↑cholesterol and TG	↑ risk of dorsocervical fat pat, Some ↑ risk of VAT	↑insulin resistance	Possible increase in bone turnover and alteration in vitamin D metabolism	Cozzolino et al. (2003); Eckhardt and Glesby (2008)
Tipranavir	↑cholesterol and TG	Some ↑ risk of VAT	Not known	Possible increase in bone turnover and alteration in vitamin D metabolism	Cozzolino et al. (2003); Mallon (2007); Moyle (2007)
Saquinavir	No change or slight ↑cholesterol and TG	↑ risk of dorsocervical fat pat, ↑ risk of VAT	↑insulin resistance	Not known	Eckhardt and Glesby (2008)
				Not known	Mallon (2007); Moyle (2007); Eckhardt and Glesby (2008)

	Lipids	Fat distribution	Insulin	Bone/other	References
NRTIs					
ddI	Generally unknown, possible risk of ↑MI	Probable ↑ risk of lipoatrophy when administered with stavudine; ↑ risk of dorsocervical fat pat	↑insulin resistance	Not known	Mallon (2007); Moyle (2007); Eckhardt and Glesby (2008)
d4T	↑total cholesterol and TG, especially in patients with lipoatrophy	↑ risk of lipoatrophy; ↑ risk of dorsocervical fat pat	↑ insulin resistance	Not known	Mallon (2007); Moyle (2007); Eckhardt and Glesby (2008)
AZT	Generally unknown	↑ risk of lipoatrophy; ↑ risk of dorsocervical fat pat	↑ insulin resistance	Not known	Mallon (2007), Moyle (2007); Eckhardt and Glesby (2008);
Tenofovir	No change	No change	No change	Possible increased secondary hyperparathyroidism and decreased BMD	Gallant et al. (2004); Moyle (2007); Eckhardt and Glesby (2008)
NNRTIs					
Efavirenz	↑ total and HDL cholesterols, and ↑TG	No change	No change	CYP3A4 inducer: potential for affecting vitamin D metabolism	Gyllensten et al. (2006); Moyle (2007); Eckhardt and Glesby (2008)
Nevirapine	↑ total and HDL cholesterols, and ↑TG	No change	Not known	Not known	Moyle (2007); Eckhardt and Glesby (2008)
Entry inhibitors					
Enfuvirtide	No change	Not known	No change	Not known	Moyle (2007); Eckhardt and Glesby (2008)

Abbreviations: ↑ = may effect an increase; HDL = high density lipoprotein cholesterol; NNRTI = non-nucleoside reverse transcriptase inhibitor; NRTI = nucleoside/tide reverse transcriptase inhibitor; PI = protease inhibitor; TG = triglycerides, VAT = visceral adipose tissue.

Table 10.6 Interventions and their effect on metabolic changes.

Intervention	Lipo-atrophy	Lipo-hypertrophy	Dyslipidaemia	Low HDL	Insulin resistance	Comment	References
ART switch							
d4T or AZT switch to ABC or TDF	Improves	No effect	May improve	No effect	No effect	May take 5–10 years to return to 'normal' body shape	Carr et al. (2002), Martin et al. (2004)
PI to Nevirapine or ABC	No effect	May improve	Improves: ↑HDL, ↓TG	No effect	Can improve if no lipoatrophy	May reduce VAT	Calza et al. (2005)
d4T or AZT to Kaletra	Improves	Improves	Worsens	Unknown	Unknown		Tebas et al. (2007)
PI to Atazanavir	Unknown	↓Waist size	↓Total and LDL cholesterols, and ↓TG	No effect	Improves		Moyle (2007), Mallolas et al. (2009)
Other interventions							
Diet	No effect	Fibre may prevent and improve	Improves	Improves	Improves	See body of chapter	
Exercise	No effect	Improves	Improves	Improves	Improves		Lindegaard et al. (2008)
Fibrates	No effect	No effect	↓TG, small ↓ in total and LDL cholesterols	Improves	No effect	May be less effective than in HIV negative adults	Badiou et al. (2004), Normen et al. (2007)
Statins	No effect, or may improve	No effect	Total and LDL-cholesterols fall by up to 25%	Improves	No effect	Seek advice on interactions between statins and ART	Lundgren et al. (2008), Mallon (2007)
Metformin	May worsen and lead to ↓weight	Improves	May ↓TG	No effect	Improves	Theoretical risk of lactic acidosis	Sutinen (2005), Lundgren et al. (2008)

Effect on:

						References
Thiazo-lidinediones	No effect	No effect	$\uparrow$TG and LDL	No effect	Improves	Possible reduction in blood pressure	Sutinen (2005), Hadigan et al. (2007), Lundgren et al. (2008)
Human Recombinant Growth Hormone	May worsen at higher doses	Improves	No effect on TG, improves total and LDL cholesterols	May improve	May worsen	Maintenance therapy required to sustain effect on intra-abdominal fat	Sutinen (2005)
Growth hormone-releasing hormone	May improve	Improves	May improve	No effect	No effect		Sutinen (2005)
Ezetimibe	Not known	Not known	$\downarrow$LDL	Not known	Not known		Lundgren et al. (2008)
Nicotinic Acid	Not known	Not known	$\downarrow$TG	Not known	Not known		Lundgren et al. (2008)
Omega-3 (Fish) Oil	Not known	Not known	$\downarrow$TG	May improve	Not known		De Truchis et al. (2007)
Anabolic steroids	May worsen	No effect	Worsens	Worsens	Worsens	Increases lean body mass	Sutinen (2005)
Testosterone	May worsen	$\downarrow$VAT	No effect	May worsen	No effect	Increases lean body mass	Schambelan (2002)

Abbreviations: $\uparrow$ = may effect an increase; $\downarrow$ = may effect a decrease; ABC = abacavir; ART = antiretroviral therapy; HDL = high-density lipoprotein cholesterol; LDL = low-density lipoprotein cholesterol; NNRTI = non-nucleoside reverse transcriptase inhibitor; NRTI = nucleoside reverse transcriptase inhibitor; PI = protease inhibitor; TDF = tenofovir; TG = triglycerides; VAT = visceral adipose tissue.

- Monitoring for signs of development of metabolic problems and annual assessment of physical, biochemical and dietary factors are indicated.
- Diet and lifestyle modification, such as high fibre and exercise, have an important role in both prevention and treatment of antiretroviral-related side effects.
- Individualised advice should be offered by specialist health professionals, for example Registered Dietitians with specialist HIV knowledge. Regular appointments have been shown to have the best outcomes.
- Future research should focus on lifestyle interventions for both the prevention and treatment of coronary heart disease and bone demineralisation.

Acknowledgements

This chapter was reviewed by:

Alan Lee, CDE CDN CFT RD, Nutrition Consultant, North General Hospital Center, Greyston Health Services, TOUCH Inc., Congers, Asian & Pacific Islander Coalition On HIV/AIDS, all New York, USA.

Alison Mead, BSc PGDip AdDip RD, Specialist Dietitian and MSc Coordinator, Cardiovascular Medicine, NHLI and Nutrition and Dietetic Department, Imperial College and Imperial Healthcare NHS Trust

Barry Peters, MBBS MRCP UK DFFP MD Elected FRCP, Reader & Hon Consultant Physician in HIV Medicine, Department of Infectious Diseases, Guy's & St Thomas Hospital NHS Foundation Trust

Michelle Phillpot, Bsc (Hons) AdDip RD, Specialist Dietitian, Nutrition & Dietetics Department, Imperial Healthcare NHS Trust

Clare Stradling, BSc MSc RD, Specialist Dietitian, Birmingham Heartlands HIV Service, Heart of England NHS Foundation Trust

Anthony S Wierzbicki, DPhil DM FRCPath FAHA, Consultant in Metabolic Medicine & Chemical Pathology, Guy's & St Thomas Hospital NHS Foundation Trust

References

Aghdassi E, Salit I, Mohammed S et al. Chromium supplementation decreases insulin resistance and trunk fat. 2008. Conference on Retroviruses and Opportunistic Infections 2008, abstract 936.

Ang C, Alviar M, Dans A et al. Vitamin B for treating peripheral neuropathy. Cochrane Database Syst Rev 2008; Issue 3.

Anonymous. Consensus development conference: diagnosis, prophylaxis and treatment of osteoporosis. Am J Med 1993; 94:646–50.

Aukrust P, Haug C, Ueland T et al. Decreased bone formative and enhanced resorptive markers in human immunodeficiency virus infection: indication of normalization of the bone-remodelling process during HAART. J Clin Endocrinol Metab 1999; 84:145–50.

Aukrust P, Liabakk N-B, Muller F et al. Serum levels of tumor necrosis factor (TNF)a and soluble TNF receptors in human immunodeficiency virus type 1 infection – correlations to clinical, immunologic, and virologic parameters. J Infect Dis 1994; 169:420–4.

Bacchetti P, Gripshover B, Grunfeld C et al. Fat distribution in men with HIV. J Acqu Immune Defic Syndr 2005; 40(2):121–31.

Badiou S, De Boever CM, Dupuy A et al. Fenofibrate improves the atherogenic lipid profile and enhances LDL resistance to oxidation in HIV-positive adults. Atherosclerosis 2004; 172: 273–9.

Barrios A, Blanco F, Garcia-Benayas T *et al.* Effect of dietary intervention on highly active antiretroviral therapy-related dyslipidaemia. *AIDS* 2002; 16:2079–81.

Batterham M, Garsia R, Greenop P. Dietary intake, serum lipids, insulin resistance and body
composition in the era of HAART. *AIDS* 2000; 14(12):1839–43.

Billing N, Hunt C. A study of dietary advice and care provided to HIV positive patients referred for lipid lowering: as part of a service improvement initiative. *J Hum Nutr Diet* 2008;
21(4):380–380.

Blumer R, van Vonderen M, Sutinen J *et al.* Zidovudine / lamivudine contributes to insulin resistance
within 3 months of starting combination antiretroviral therapy. *AIDS* 2008; 22:227–36.

Bolland MJ, Grey AB, Gamble GD, Reid IR. Low body weight mediates the relationship between
HIV infection and low bone mineral density: a meta-analysis. *J Clin Endocrinol Metab* 2007;
92:4522–8.

Bonjour J. Dietary protein: an essential nutrient for bone health. *J Am Coll Nutr* 2005; 24(Suppl
6):526S.

British Cardiac Society. JBS 2: Joint British Societies' guidelines on prevention of cardiovascular
disease in clinical practice. *Heart* 2005; 91(Suppl 5): v1–52.

British HIV Association. Treatment of HIV-infected adults with antiretroviral therapy. *HIV Med*
2008; 9:563–608.

British National Formulary No. 57. BMJ Publishing Group Limited, March 2009.

Brown T, Cole S, Li X. Antiretroviral therapy and the prevalence and incidence of diabetes mellitus
in the Multicenter AIDS Cohort Study. *Arch Intern Med* 2005; 165:1179–84.

Brown T, Qaqish R. Antiretroviral therapy and the prevalence of osteopenia and osteoporosis: a
meta-analytic review. *AIDS* 2006; 20:2165–74.

Brunner E, Rees K, Ward K *et al.* Dietary advice for reducing cardiovascular risk. *Cochrane
Database Syst Rev* 2007, Issue 4. Art. No.: CD002128.

Burnett S, Gunawardene S, Bringhurst F *et al.* Regulation of C-terminal and intact FGF-23 by
dietary phosphate in men and women. *J Bone Miner Res* 2006; 21:1187–96.

Calza L, Manfredi R, Colangeli V *et al.* Substitution of nevirapine or efavirenz for protease inhibitor
versus lipid-lowering therapy for the management of dyslipidaemia. *AIDS* 2005; 19: 1051–8.

Capaldini L. Protease inhibitors' metabolic side effects: cholesterol, triglycerides, blood sugar, and
'Crix belly.' *AIDS Treat News* 1997; 15(277):1–4.

Carr A, Workman C, Smith D *et al.* Mitochondrial Toxicity (MITOX) Study Group; Abacavir
substitution for nucleoside analogs in patients with HIV lipoatrophy: a randomized trial. *J Am
Med Assoc* 2002; 288(2):207–15.

Cashman, KD. Diet, nutrition, and bone health. *J Nutr* 2007; 137:2507S–12S.

Cho M, Ye X, Dobs A, Cofrancesco J. Prevalence of complementary and alternative medicine
use among HIV patients for perceived lipodystrophy. *J Altern Complement Med* 2006;
12/5(475–82):1075–5535.

Cosman F, Nieves J, Dempster D, Lindsay R. Vitamin D economy in blacks. *J Bone Miner Res*
2007; 22(S2):V34–8.

Cozzolino M, Vidal M, Arcidiacono M *et al.* HIV-protease inhibitors impair vitamin D bioactivation
to 1,25-dihydroxyvitamin D. *AIDS* 2003; 17:513–20.

Crum-Cianflone N, Marconi V, Weintrob A *et al.* Increased incidence of skin cancers among
HIV-infected persons. Fourth IAS Conference on HIV Treatment, Pathogenesis and Prevention,
Sydney, abstract MoPeB086, 2007.

De Truchis P, Kirstetter M, Perier A *et al.* Reduction in triglyceride level with n-3 polyunsaturated
fatty acids in HIV-infected patients taking potent antiretroviral therapy. *J Acqu Immune Defic
Syndr* 2007; 44:278–85.

de Wit S, Sabin C, Weber R *et al.* Incidence and risk factors for new-onset diabetes in HIV-infected
patients: The D:A:D Study. *Diabetes Care* 2008; 31(6):1224–29.

Dong K, Wanke C, Tang A *et al.* Dietary glycemic index of human immunodeficiency virus-positive
men with and without fat deposition. *J Am Diet Assoc* 2006; 106(5):728–32.

Dube M, Stein J, Aberg J *et al.* Guidelines for the evaluation and management of dyslipidemia
in human immunodeficiency virus (HIV)-infected adults receiving antiretroviral therapy. *Clin
Infect Dis* 2003; 37:613–27.

Duvivier C, Kolta S, Assoumou L *et al.* Greater decrease in bone mineral density with protease
inhibitor regimens compared with nonnucleoside reverse transcriptase inhibitor regimens in
HIV-1 infected naive patients. *AIDS* 2009; 23:817–24.

Eckhardt B, Glesby M. Antiretroviral therapy and cardiovascular risk: are some medications cardioprotective? *Curr Opin HIV AIDS* 2008; **3**:226–33.

Esposito K, Marfella R, Ciotola M *et al*. Effect of a Mediterranean style diet on endothelial dysfunction and markers of vascular inflammation in the metabolic syndrome: a randomized trial. *J Am Med Assoc* 2004; **292**:1440–6.

Falcó V, Rodriguez D, Ribera E. Severe nucleoside-associated lactic acidosis in human immunodeficiency virus-infected patients: report of 12 cases and review of the literature. *Clin Infect Dis* 2002; **34**:838–46.

Fan A, Russell M, Naimi T *et al*. Patterns of alcohol consumption and the metabolic syndrome. *J Clin Endocrinol Metab* Rapid Electronic Publication first published as doi:10.1210/jc.2007–2788, 2008.

Fitch K, Anderson E, Hubbard J *et al*. Effects of a lifestyle modification program in HIV-infected patients with the metabolic syndrome. *AIDS* 2006; **20**(14):1843–50.

Fong I, Howard R, Elzawi A *et al*. Cardiac involvement in HIV infected patients. *J Acquir Immune Defic Syndr* 1993; **6**:380–85.

Friis-Moller N, Weber R, Reiss P *et al*. Cardiovascular disease risk factors in HIV patients – association with antiretroviral therapy. *AIDS* 2003; **17**(8):1179–93.

Gallant J, Staszewski S, Pozniak A *et al*. Efficacy and safety of tenofovir DF vs stavudine in combination therapy in antiretroviral-naive patients: a 3-year randomized trial. *JAMA* 2004; **292**:191–201.

Grunfeld C, Kotler DP, Dobs A *et al*. Oxandrolone in the treatment of HIV-associated weight loss in men: a randomized, double-blind, placebo-controlled study. *J Acquir Immune Defic Syndr* 2006; **41**:304–14.

Grunfeld C, Kotler D, Shigenaga J *et al*. Circulating interferon alpha levels and hypertriglyceridemia in the acquired immunodeficiency syndrome. *Am J Med* 1991; **90**:154–62.

Guenter P, Muurahainen N, Simons G *et al*. Relationships among nutritional status, disease progression, and survival in HIV Infection. *J Acquir Immune Defic Syndr* 1993; **6**:1130–38.

Guffanti M, Caumo A, Galli L *et al*. Switching to unboosted atazanavir improves glucose tolerance in highly pretreated HIV-1 infected subjects. *Eur J Endocrinol* 2007; **156**:503–9.

Gyllensten K, Josephson F, Lidman K, Saaf M. Severe vitamin D deficiency diagnosed after introduction of antiretroviral therapy including efavirenz in a patient living at latitude 59-N. *AIDS* 2006; **20**:1906–1907.

Hadigan C, Jeste S, Anderson E *et al*. Modifiable dietary habits and their relation to metabolic abnormalities in men and women with HIV infection and fat redistribution. *Clin Infect Dis* 2001a; **33**(5):710–17.

Hadigan C, Mazza S, Crum D, Grinspoon S Rosiglitazone increases small dense low-density lipoprotein concentration and decreases high-density lipoprotein particle size in HIV-infected patients. *AIDS* 2007; **21**:2543–6.

Hadigan C, Meigs J, Corcoran C *et al*. Metabolic abnormalities and cardiovascular disease risk factors in adults with HIV infection and lipodystrophy. *Clin Infect Dis* 2001b; **32**:130–9.

Hartweg J, Perera R, Montori V *et al*. Omega-3 polyunsaturated fatty acids (PUFA) for type 2 diabetes mellitus. *Cochrane Database Syst Rev* 2008; Issue 1. Art. No.: CD003205. DOI:10.1002/14651858.CD003205.pub2.

Haugaard S, Andersen O, Dela F *et al*. Defective glucose and lipid metabolism in HIV-infected patients with lipodystrophy involve liver, muscle tissue and pancreatic beta-cells. *Eur J Endocrinol* 2005; **152**:103–12.

Hendricks K, Dong K, Tang A *et al*. High-fiber diet in HIV-positive men is associated with lower risk of developing fat deposition. *Am J Clin Nutr* 2003; **78**(4):790–5.

Holick M. Vitamin D deficiency. *N Engl J Med* 2007; **357**:266–81.

Huang J, Rietschel P, Hadigan C *et al*. Increased abdominal visceral fat is associated with reduced bone density in HV-infected men with lipodystrophy. *AIDS* 2001; **15**:975–82.

Hulgan T, Haas D, Haines J *et al*. Mitochondrial haplogroups and peripheral neuropathy during antiretroviral therapy: An adult AIDS clinical trials group study. *AIDS* 2005; **19**:1341–49.

International Diabetes Federation. The IDF consensus worldwide definition of the Metabolic Syndrome. 2006. Accessed at http://www.idf.org/webdata/docs/IDF_Meta_def_final.pdf on July 20, 2008.

International Diabetes Federation (IDF) guidelines. (2008) http://www.idf.org/home/index.cfm?node=1457.

Jacobson D, Tang A, Spiegelman D *et al.* Incidence of metabolic syndrome in a cohort of HIV-infected adults and prevalence relative to the US population. *J Acquir Immune Defic Syndr* 2006; **43**(4):458–66.

Jenkins D, Kendall C, Marchie A *et al.* Effects of a dietary portfolio of cholesterol-lowering foods vs lovastatin on serum lipids and CRP. *JAMA* 2003; **290**:502–10.

John M, Moore C, James I *et al.* Chronic hyperlactatemia in HIV-infected patients taking antiretroviral therapy. *AIDS* 2001; **15**(6):717–23.

Jones C, Tang A, Forrester J *et al.* Micronutrient levels and HIV disease status in HIV-infected patients on HAART in the nutrition for healthy living cohort. *J Acquir Immune Defic Syndr* 2006; **43**(4):475–82.

Joy T, Keogh H, Hadigan C *et al.* Dietary fat intake and relationship to serum lipid levels in HIV-infected patients with metabolic abnormalities in the HAART era. *AIDS* 2007; **21**(12):1591–600.

Justman J, Benning L, Danoff A *et al.* Protease inhibitor use and the incidence of diabetes mellitus in a large cohort of HIV-infected women. *J Acquir Immune Defic Syndr* 2003; **32**:298–302.

Kalkwarf H, Khoury J, Bean J, Elliot J. Vitamin K, bone turnover, and bone mass in girls. *Am J Clin Nutr* 2004; **80**:1075–80.

Kanis J, Burlet N, Cooper C *et al.* European guidance for the diagnosis and management of osteoporosis in postmenopausal women. *Osteoporos Int* 2007; **19**:399–428.

Kohli R, Shevitz A, Gorbach S, Wanke C. A randomized placebo controlled trial of metformin for the treatment of HIV lipodystrophy. *HIV Med* 2007; **8**:420–26.

Kotler D, Thea D, Heo M *et al.* Relative influences of sex, race, environment, and HIV infection on body composition in adults. *Am J Clin Nutr* 1999; **69**:432–39.

Klassen K, Winston A, Portsmouth S. Risk factors for hypovitaminosis D in HIV positive individuals. In: *Abstracts of the 14th annual conference of the British HIV Association; Belfast 2008.* HIV Medicine 9: Abstract P95A, 2008.

Law M, Wald N, Thompson S. By how much and how quickly does reduction in serum cholesterol concentration lower risk of ischaemic heart disease? *Br Med J* 1994; **308**:367–72.

Lazzaretti R, Pinto-Ribeiro J, Kuhmmer R *et al.* Dietary intervention when starting HAART prevents the increase in lipids independently of drug regimen: a randomized trial. 4th IAS Conference on HIV Pathogenesis, Treatment, and Prevention. Sydney. Abstract WEAB303. 2007.

Lichtenstein K, Armon C, Baron A *et al.* Modification of the incidence of drug associated symmetrical peripheral neuropathy by host and disease factors in the HIV outpatient study cohort. *Clin Infect Dis* 2005; **40**:148–157.

Lin P, Ginty F, Appel L *et al.* The DASH diet and sodium reduction improve markers of bone turnover and calcium metabolism in adults. *J Nutr* 2003; **133**:3130–6.

Lindegaard B, Hansen T, Hvid T *et al.* The effect of strength and endurance training on insulin sensitivity and fat distribution in HIV-infected patients with lipodystrophy. *J Clin Endocrinol Metab* 2008; **93**(10):3860–69.

Linus Pauling Institute. Vitamin A and bone health. 2007. Accessed at http://lpi.oregonstate.edu/infocenter/vitamins/vitaminA/.

Liu J, Mannheimer E, Yang M. Herbal medicines for treating HIV infections and AIDS. *Cochrane Database Syst Rev* 2005; **20**(3): CD003937.

Lundgren J, Battegay M, Behrens G *et al.* European AIDS Clinical Society (EACS) guidelines on the prevention and management of metabolic diseases in HIV. *HIV Med* 2008; **9**(2):72–81.

Mallolas J, Podzamczer D, Milinkovic A *et al.* Efficacy and safety of switching from boosted lopinavir to boosted atazanavir in patients with virological suppression receiving a LPV/r-containing HAART: the ATAZIP study. *J Acquir Immune Defic Syndr* 2009; **51**:29–36.

Mallon PW. HIV and bone mineral density. *Curr Opin Infect Dis* 2010; **23**:1–8.

Mallon PW. Pathogenesis of lipodystrophy and lipid abnormalities in patients taking antiretroviral therapy. *AIDS Rev* 2007; **9**:3–15.

Martin A, Smith D, Carr A *et al.* Reversibility of lipoatrophy in HIV-infected patients 2 years after switching from a thymidine analogue to abacavir. *AIDS* (2004) 30; **18**(7):1029–36.

McComsey G, Kendall M, Tebas P *et al.* Alendronate with calcium and vitamin D supplementation is safe and effective for the treatment of decreased bone mineral density in HIV. *AIDS* 2007; **21**:2473–82.

Miller J, Carr A, Emery S *et al.* HIV lipodystrophy: prevalence, severity and correlates of risk in Australia. *HIV Med* 2003; **4**(3):293–301.

Mondy K, Powderly W, Claxton S *et al.* Alendronate, vitamin D, and calcium for the treatment of osteopenia/osteoporosis associated with HIV infection. *J Acquir Immune Defic Syndr* 2005; 38:426–31.

Moyle G. Metabolic issues associated with protease inhibitors. *J Acquir Immune Defic Syndr* 2007; 45:S19–26.

Moyle G, Brown S, Lysakova L, Barton S. Long-term safety and efficacy of poly-L-lactic acid in the treatment of HIV-related facial lipoatrophy. *HIV Med* 2006; 7(3):181–5.

Moyle G, Lloyd M, Reynolds B *et al.* Dietary advice with or without pravastatin for the management of hypercholesterolaemia associated with protease inhibitor therapy. *AIDS* 2001; 15:1503–8.

Mulligan K, Khatami H, Schwarz J *et al.* The effects of recombinant human leptin on visceral fat, dyslipidemia, and insulin resistance in patients with HIV-associated lipoatrophy and hypoleptinemia. *J Clin Endocrinol Metab* 2009; 94(4):1137–44.

Mutimura E, Stewart A, Rheeder P, Crowther N. Metabolic Function and the Prevalence of Lipodystrophy in a Population of HIV-Infected African Subjects Receiving HAART. *J Acqu Immune Defic Syndr* 2007; 46(4):451–5.

National Cholesterol Education Program. NIH Publication No. 02–5215. Third Report of the NCEP Expert Panel on Detection, Evaluation, and Treatment of High Blood Cholesterol in Adults: Final Report. 2002.

NICE Guidelines on Diabetes Management. 2008. http://www.nice.org.uk/Guidance/CG66/NiceGuidance/doc/English.

Nicholas K, Kemppainen J, Canaval G *et al.* Symptom management and self-care for peripheral neuropathy in HIV/AIDS. *AIDS Care* 2007; 19(2):179–89.

Normen L, Yip B, Montaner J *et al.* Use of metabolic drugs and fish oil in HIV-positive patients with metabolic complications and associations with dyslipidaemia and treatment targets. *HIV Med* 2007; 8:346–56.

Palella F, Baker R, Moorman A *et al.* Mortality in the highly active antiretroviral therapy era: changing causes of death and disease in the HIV outpatient study. *J Acquir Immune Defic Syndr* 2006; 43(1):27–34.

Pan G, Yang Z, Ballinger S, McDonald J. Pathogenesis of osteopenia/osteoporosis induced by highly active anti-retroviral therapy for AIDS. *Ann N Y Acad Sci* 2006; 1068:297–308.

Patalay M, Lofgren I, Freake H *et al.* The lowering of plasma lipids following a weight reduction program is related to increased expression of the LDL receptor and lipoprotein lipase. *J Nutr* 2005; 135:735–9.

Pirmohamed M. Clinical management of HIV-Associated Lipodystrophy. *Curr Opin Lipid* 2009; 20(4):309–14

Piscitelli S, Burstein A, Welden N *et al.* The effect of garlic supplements on the pharmacokinetics of saquinavir. *Clin Infect Dis* 2002; 34:234–8.

Prynne C, Mishra G, O'Connell M *et al.* Fruit and vegetable intakes and bone mineral status: a cross-sectional study in 5 age and sex cohorts. *Am J Clin Nutr* 2006; 83:1420–8.

Rosenvinge M, Gedela K, Wilkinson A *et al.* Unexpectedly high rates of vitamin D deficiency in an inner-city London HIV clinic. *HIV Med* 2008; 9(Suppl 1): Oral abstract O15.

Roubenoff R, Schmitz H, Bairos L *et al.* Reduction of abdominal obesity in lipodystrophy associated with human immunodeficiency virus infection by means of diet and exercise. *Clin Infect Dis* 2002; 34:390–3.

Sackoff J, Hanna D, Pfeiffer M, Torian L. Causes of death among persons with AIDS in the era of HAART. *Ann Intern Med* 2006; 145:397–406.

Saint-Marc T, Partisani M, Poizot-Martin I *et al.* A syndrome of peripheral fat wasting (lipodystrophy) in patients receiving long-term nucleoside analogue therapy. *AIDS* 1999; 13(13): 1659–67.

Schambelan M, Benson C, Carr A *et al.* Management of metabolic complications associated with antiretroviral therapy for HIV-1 infection. *J Acquir Immune Defic Syndrs* 2002; 31:257–75.

SIGN (Scottish Intercollegiate Guidelines Network). Risk estimation and the prevention of cardiovascular disease: National clinical guidelines. 2007. Available at www.sign.ac.uk. Accessed on July 26, 2009.

Sobieszczyk M, Hoover D, Anastos K *et al.* Prevalence and predictors of metabolic syndrome among HIV-infected and HIV-uninfected women in the Women's Interagency HIV Study. *J Acquir Immune Defic Syndr* 2008; 48(3):272–80.

Stankov M, Behrens G. HIV-therapy associated lipodystrophy: experimental and clinical evidence for the pathogenesis and treatment. *Endocr, Metab Immune Disord* 2007; **7**(4):237–49.

Sutinen J. Interventions for managing antiretroviral therapy-associated lipoatrophy. *Curr Opin Infect Dis* 2005; **18**(1):25–33.

Tebas P, Zhang J, Yarasheski K *et al.* Switching to a protease inhibitor-containing, nucleoside-sparing regimen (lopinavir/ritonavir plus efavirenz) increases limb fat but raises serum lipid levels. *J Acquir Immune Defic Syndr* 2007; **45**(2):193–200.

Thompson RL, Summerbell CD, Hooper L *et al.* Dietary advice given by a dietitian versus other health professional or self-help resources to reduce blood cholesterol. *Cochrane Database Syst Rev* 2003; Issue 3. Art. No.: CD001366. DOI:10.1002/14651858.CD001366.

Triant V, Lee H, Hadigan C, Grinspoon S. Increased acute myocardial infarction rates and cardiovascular risk factors among patients with human immunodeficiency virus disease. *J Clin Endocrinol Metab* 2007; **92**:2506–2512.

Triant V, Brown T, Lee H, Grinspoon S. Fracture prevalence among human immunodeficiency virus (HIV)-infected versus non-HIV-infected patients in a large U.S. healthcare system. *J Clin Endocrinol Metab* 2008; **93**:3499–3504.

Van Den Bout-Van Den Beukel C, Fievez L, Michels M *et al.* Vitamin D deficiency among HIV type 1-infected individuals in the Netherlands: effects of antiretroviral therapy. *AIDS Res Hum Retroviruses* 2008a; **24**(11):1375–82.

Van Den Bout-van den Beukel C, Van Den Bos M, Oyen W *et al.* The effect of cholecalciferol supplementation on vitamin D levels and insulin sensitivity is dose related in vitamin D-deficient HIV-1-infected patients. *HIV Med* 2008b; **9**(9):771–9.

Weber P, Raederstorff D. Triglyceride-lowering effect of omega-3 LC-polyunsaturated fatty acids – a review. *Nutr Metab Cardiovasc Dis* 2000; **10**:28–37.

Wester W, Okezie O, Thomas A *et al.* Higher-than-expected rates of lactic acidosis among highly active antiretroviral therapy-treated women in Botswana. *J Acquir Immune Defic Syndr* 2007; **46**(3):318–22.

Wierzbicki A, Purdon S, Hardman T *et al.* Clinical aspects of the management of HIV lipodystrophy. *Br J Diabetes Vasc Dis* 2008; **8**:113–9.

Wohl D, Tien H, Busby M *et al.* Randomized study of the safety and efficacy of fish oil (omega-3 fatty acid) supplementation with dietary and exercise counseling for the treatment of antiretroviral therapy-associated hypertriglyceridemia. *Clin Infect Dis* 2005; **41**:1498–504.

Zivkovic A, German J, Sanyal A. Comparative review of diets for the metabolic syndrome: implications for non-alcoholic fatty liver disease. *Am J Clin Nutr* 2007; **86**:285.

Further resources

Cardiovascular risk calculators (British Cardiac Society, 2005): Framingham CVD risk calculator: http://hp2010.nhlbihin.net/atpiii/calculator.asp.

Joint European Societies calculator: http://www.benecol.net/healthcareprofessionals.asp?viewID=2374.

Joint British Societies/British National Formulary based on the Framingham (1991) algorithm: http://cvrisk.mvm.ed.ac.uk/calculator/bnf.htm.

QRISK2 can be accessed at: http://qr2.dyndns.org.

Target lipid levels depend on the cardiovascular risk of the individual (including age, sex, cigarette smoking, systolic blood pressure, lipid ratios, and family history of premature CHD: www.nhlbi.nih.gov/guidelines/cholesterol/atglance.

Resources to help with smoking cessation can be accessed at: www.smokefree.nhs.uk.

Resources regarding safe consumption of fish can be accessed at: www.fishonline.org.

11 Community Interventions in Resource-Limited Settings

Claire de Menezes and Kate Ogden

Key Points

- Many resource-limited settings affected by HIV are high on the global hunger index as well as the poverty index.
- Early identification of HIV to establish healthy living and good dietary habits is an essential part of a positive living strategy in resource-limited settings, as risk of mortality is significantly increased if individuals are malnourished when starting ART.
- A holistic approach needs to be taken, integrating nutrition care with health and psychological care, access to safe water (sufficient for drinking and hygiene needs), and providing sustainable food access that meets all the requirements of a balanced diet enriched with essential micronutrients.
- Nutrition counselling and education should form a part of any HIV intervention and any programme to treat or prevent malnutrition in order to provide individuals, households and communities with the information they need to optimise nutritional intake.
- Treatment of severe acute malnutrition (SAM) has been well researched and standard international guidelines are in place for both inpatient and community-based care.
- Empowering communities and moving the emphasis of responsibility back to the communities themselves can provide support to help implement interventions in a sustainable manner, incorporating both nutrition and HIV responses.

11.1 Introduction

It is often difficult for people living with HIV (PLHIV) to achieve and maintain their recommended nutritional intake; even for those fortunate enough to have full access to an optimal diet, financial resources and social safety nets. How then can nutrition recommendations for PLHIV be put into practice in resource-limited settings? These are the very settings most affected by the phenomenal impact of HIV and yet those in which malnutrition and poverty are commonplace and seasonal hunger is the norm. This chapter is about community nutritional interventions that can be applied in resource-limited settings affected by HIV and some of the social and financial constraints which make nutrition and HIV a challenging priority requiring maximum input and political support.

11.1.1 Background

Nutrition has been slow to be recognised as an essential part of HIV and AIDS care in resource-limited settings, with the emphasis having been very much focused on gaining access to antiretroviral therapy (ART). In 2003, WHO established a technical advisory group on nutrition and HIV and this was followed with key initiatives such as the Durban technical consultation of 2005 (WHO, 2005), which called to strengthen political commitment for the inclusion of nutrition into HIV policy and the 59th World Health Assembly (WHO, 2006), which called to incorporate HIV and AIDS into nutrition policies. In 2006, the World Bank released a strategic paper: 'Repositioning Nutrition as Central to Development', and publicly stated that without addressing malnutrition, there will be no eradication of poverty (World Bank, 2006). This strategy has strong implications for the HIV agenda with its well-defined links to both malnutrition and poverty. Undoubtedly, political will and international awareness are now increasing and nutrition is slowly being recognised as an integral part of HIV care alongside ART but many practical issues remain unresolved. Where combined nutrition and HIV programmes are emerging, they are linked very much to the provision of ART. This is predominantly based on the need to ensure adequate nutrition when taking therapy at the same time as managing ART-related side effects to help increase adherence to therapy. Whilst there is still a paucity of evidence to support the view that being in optimal nutritional health will delay the onset of AIDS and the need for ART, the plausibility of the argument stands and it has been shown that if individuals are malnourished when starting ART, the risk of mortality is significantly increased (Obimbo et al., 2004; Zachariah et al., 2006; Cross Continents Collaboration for Kids, 2008). It is therefore justifiable to look at ways to implement nutrition interventions in HIV-affected communities before individuals have completed the process of diagnosis, referral and commencement of ART, in addition to those interventions aimed at increasing adherence to ART.

11.2   HIV and nutrition in resource-limited settings

Due to the social nature of HIV and environments most conducive for successful transmission of the virus, the impact of the disease is predominantly felt by the most vulnerable groups of society. This is particularly true for those in under-resourced countries who bear the brunt of the public health impact of HIV. The regions of Eastern and Southern Africa continue to be the most affected with an estimated 17.4 million people living with HIV, 1.4 million of which are children. The next most affected regions are West and Central Africa, South Asia, East Asia and Latin America respectively. Approximately 12 million children have been orphaned by AIDS worldwide and have been left without their usual social care and protection leaving them vulnerable to the risk of malnutrition and further exposure to HIV (UNAIDS, 2006).

Access to ART has improved significantly on the global scale but remains limited in resource-poor settings, partly because of the vast amount of resources needed to support ART services, including human resources and supplies related to monitoring and management of therapy, which are all additional to the cost of the drugs them-selves. Without ART and in contexts where malnutrition and communicable disease are commonplace, there is little to stop deterioration in immune response. Inevitably, HIV infected individuals are faced with the vicious cycle of increased frequency of infections, worsening nutrition status (macro- and micronutrient deficiencies), de-creased physical capacity, reduced income and inadequate food access, leading to further increase of infections as the cycle continues.

Identifying those who are HIV positive in order that they can be more pro-active regarding their nutritional health is a key issue for tackling HIV-related nutrition problems in resource-limited settings. Early identification of HIV to establish healthy living and good dietary habits whilst the immune system is still robust is an essential part of a positive living approach (FAO, 2002). Unfortunately, it remains the case that the majority of those infected with HIV in resource-poor settings are unaware of their diagnosis until deteriorating health and serious infections take hold. Even then, stigmatisation and lack of community information, particularly in rural settings, remain key obstacles in encouraging people to come forward for HIV testing. However, over the last decade the stigma associated with HIV testing has gradually decreased with raised awareness of the pandemic. In addition to individual health-seeking behaviour, vast improvements to services are needed as effective HIV testing facilities and reliable surveillance systems are lacking in many resource-limited settings – factors which contribute to the numbers of undiagnosed individuals. Every opportunity should be taken to introduce easy access to HIV testing in as many community settings as possible and nutrition programmes in an HIV context provide a perfect setting as many affected by undernutrition are also likely to be vulnerable to the risks of HIV exposure and transmission. Opt-out approaches to HIV testing rather than individuals being asked to opt in are certainly encouraged for nutrition programming.

Many resource-limited settings affected by HIV are also high on the global hunger index as well as the poverty index. For example, sub-Saharan Africa hosts 64% of those living globally with HIV; 47% of those living below the poverty line (UNIDO, 2005) and nearly one-third of the world's underweight children (Black et al., 2008). Globally, malnutrition contributes to approximately 60% of deaths in the under-fives in developing countries (Black et al., 2003), and in settings where malnutrition and HIV are commonplace, the proportion of children being admitted for the treatment of severe malnutrition who are testing HIV positive is alarmingly high, as is the related mortality (Kessler et al., 2000; Amadi et al., 2001). This illustrates the clear need to address nutrition in HIV-affected communities before the manifestation of severe malnutrition and to address the combination of the three factors (malnutrition, HIV and poverty) in order to prevent the already vulnerable from suffering the double burden of poverty or seasonal related hunger plus malnutrition related to HIV.

When the causal factors of malnutrition are considered (Figure 11.1), it is clear how HIV is able to exacerbate many of the potential causes and, in turn, how the potential causes of malnutrition themselves are exacerbated by HIV. The causal framework of malnutrition forms the basis of a wider analysis and will be developed in the livelihoods and food access section. The three pillars of HIV care are often referred to as prevention, care (treatment and support) and mitigation. Nutrition plays an important role in each of these pillars. By maintaining good nutrition status in those infected with HIV and ensuring they have sufficient access to nutrition to maintain a healthy diet and lifestyle, significant health gains can be made. The frequent question in resource-limited settings, often in the face of both hunger and poverty, is how to address the root causes of malnutrition and at the same time provide the additional nutritional needs recommended for those infected with HIV. There is little point in providing extra energy when baseline nutritional needs are not met, or providing food when households lack other essential resources for survival, as the food assistance is then likely to be sold or exchanged for other goods or essential medical care. A holistic approach needs to be taken, integrating nutrition care with health and psychological care, access to safe water (sufficient for drinking and hygiene needs), and providing sustainable food access that meets all the requirements of a balanced diet enriched with essential micronutrients.

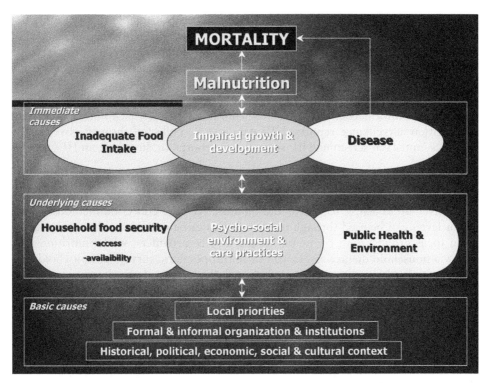

Figure 11.1 Conceptual framework of malnutrition. Adapted from UNICEF, Strategy for Improved Nutrition of Children and Women in Developing Countries. UNICEF Policy Review. New York, UNICEF. 1990.

A broad framework for integrated nutrition and HIV activities should consider (FANTA, 2007):

- Assessment of the community including nutrition status of the targeted population and dietary availability looking at macronutrients and micronutrients
- Community sensitisation around nutrition and HIV, nutrition education and nutrition counselling
- Targeted food supplementation programmes
- Livelihood support and ensuring food access
- Community mobilisation for support of PLHIV
- Integrated links between nutrition, health and hygiene services covering HIV and health care, counselling, psychosocial support, access to safe water and sanitation to enable safe food storage and preparation.

11.3   Assessment of needs and capacities

As with any intervention, the decision on what is required starts with an assessment. The assessment aims to understand the impact of HIV on communities and how this affects the nutritional situation of the community population. The needs of the communities and households within them can then be defined as well as their capacity to address these needs. There are various tools available to thoroughly assess elements within the causal framework related to nutrition in the context of HIV. There are tools to assess community and urban settings, infant feeding practices and how traditional and cultural factors may affect diet and intra-household distribution of food at household and individual level (FHI, 2003; FAO, 2006; FANTA, WFP, 2007). Prevalence and type of malnutrition are important baseline indicators and this information can be gained from health clinics, past nutrition surveys or nutrition surveillance reports. HIV data can be collected through government statistics (antenatal screening/HIV surveillance reports) or directly from HIV service providers.

Aspects such as local food availability, food access (including an evaluation of economic opportunities) and the health environment need to be understood to ensure the holistic approach. Qualitative and quantitative data collection methods at different levels can be used through interviews and questionnaires, either individually or in focus groups, with communities and service providers, whilst nutrition surveys via household dietary assessment or anthropometric surveys at household and community levels can be conducted. Although these methods are commonly used in developmental settings there are many additional challenges of undertaking assessments in the HIV context with regard to achieving a clear and representative picture of the situation. For example, the impact of HIV may not yet be clearly evident in its entirety (potential future impacts need to be considered); the complications of stigma may hinder a true assessment of the situation and the multiple factors, which affect households and communities affected by HIV, may indeed be complicated to disentangle in order for priorities to be set.

Given that both HIV and hunger disproportionately affect women, gender must form an integral part of the initial assessment (Guijt and Kaul Shah, 2001). Similarly, the voices of other marginalized community groups, often those most in need (elderly, female, and child-headed households, and those with lower social standing within the community), must be heard and their opinions included (Case Study 11.1). All aspects affecting nutrition (Figure 11.1) must be considered in the assessment to identify the integrated services that may be required to improve the nutritional situation.

Case Study 11.1   Involving all sectors of the community in assessment.

Ensuring the voice of marginalized community groups: John – Kitwe, Zambia

At just 19 years old, John is the head of his household. His father died when he was 16, and his mother died 18 months later and he is now responsible for 10 family members. Although John would like to have a voice in planning and managing future community projects, decision making within communities in Kitwe district is often in the hands of the influential, higher earning males. John does not attend community meetings because he does not feel his opinion would be considered or valued; although he is the head of his household, he is young and considered uneducated and inexperienced. Without his elder family members to consult for guidance, he has no one with which to discuss community or family matters.

From Organ, 2007, with permission from Action contre la Faim (ACF-UK).

11.3.1   Setting objectives

Once the assessment and the subsequent analyses are complete, the objectives of the nutrition intervention should be defined. Different objectives will drive different approaches for specifying targeting criteria and the type of nutrition intervention chosen. They will also help to determine the duration of the intervention. Box 11.1 gives some examples of potential objectives.

Box 11.1   Potential objectives for community nutrition interventions

- To protect and improve nutritional status of HIV-infected individuals
- To treat acute malnutrition in those infected with HIV
- To provide nutritional care from the point of HIV diagnosis and throughout HIV care
- To provide nutrition to promote and improve adherence to medical treatment
- To address maternal nutrition in HIV-infected mothers to improve birth outcomes and promote HIV-free survival in children
- To promote growth and development in infants and young children born to HIV-infected mothers
- To improve food diversity and access to food in HIV-affected communities

---

In the case that the assessment report results in recommendations for direct food assistance, existing and potential channels of food distribution would need to be further assessed. Where the recommendation is made to implement more general approaches to improve food security, the feasibility, capacities and resources available locally have to be reviewed both at the community and household levels. Sustainability of the interventions is a key issue, especially as the very nature of the HIV context implies long-term needs and thus long-term solutions. The principle of DO NO HARM must always be applied. Food assistance programming should be seen as a short-term solution to improve food security and more sustainable options should be sought to promote positive coping strategies for the longer term. Any food assistance programming must be targeted appropriately to only those in need in order to avoid negative consequences.

11.4   Targeting

The targeting of nutrition programmes in HIV contexts in resource-limited settings has been controversial. Targeting can be done at different levels: regional (for large actors such as the World Food Programme (WFP)), community, household or individual. Targeting should be an output of the needs assessment and be refined according to defined objectives. For example, if the objective is to improve food security, then inclusion criteria for the programme should be based on indicators of food insecurity; if the objective is to improve nutrition or health status, then criteria should be linked to nutrition or health indicators. Despite knowing that there are recommendations for those living with HIV to consume more energy, how can people with HIV be considered more in need of nutritional support above others who are not known to be infected but nevertheless have a suboptimal diet due to poverty or environmental factors? In line with this school of thought, many nutritional programmes target beneficiaries using vulnerability criteria, but can the vulnerability of two households really be compared when one is facing a time bomb of extra impact that, once exploded, will be hard to reverse? At present there is no answer to this question and, in most cases, resources dictate that only those meeting certain vulnerability criteria (for which there are no agreed international standards for use in the HIV context), will receive assistance from programmes intended to reduce the negative impact of HIV on nutrition, regardless of individual HIV status.

There are few documented projects that target HIV status alone. Indeed, direct targeting of those infected with HIV, without additional evidence of vulnerability which is visible to the community, can create issues (although it may also bring enhanced benefits to infected individuals in advance of visible signs of malnutrition or vulnerability). In societies where infected persons are viewed as promiscuous or somehow to blame for their condition, the negative consequences of singling out HIV-infected people for assistance may outweigh any benefits of the nutrition intervention by leading to increased social disharmony. Alternatively, encouraging people to know their HIV status in order to benefit from interventions that can enhance their lives can help to challenge stigma as communities become more aware and more open about HIV and the numbers affected. Use of proxy indicators to avoid the necessity to know HIV status can be useful but also has the potential to increase stigma as all the 'chronically sick' or all those who lose a main income-earning member of the household may become labelled as HIV positive. Proxy indicators can also be open to manipulation. Examples include reports of single-parent households registering their children as orphans and households with working males earning away from home, registering as female or elderly headed when there is an elder woman residing in the house, in order to benefit from assistance. In rural areas it may be a long-standing tradition (and one that is well managed at the household level) that the 'workers' travel elsewhere for income which they send home; it does not therefore necessarily follow that all female- or elderly headed households are affected by HIV as proxy indicators would have us believe. Field-level verification should always complement the first-level selection of beneficiaries.

Different target groups for nutrition interventions may include:

- Communities with high HIV prevalence
- HIV-infected individuals targeted through HIV services
- Households living with HIV and AIDS (accessing home-based care or other services)
- Orphans and child-headed households
- Households hosting orphans or the chronically sick
- Elderly headed households
- HIV-positive pregnant women
- Infants and young children of HIV-positive mothers.

Some examples of targeting criteria that have been used in the field are given in Table 11.1.

11.5 Nutrition counselling and education

Nutrition counselling and education should form a part of any HIV intervention and any programme to treat or prevent malnutrition in order to provide individuals, households and communities with the information they need to optimise nutritional

Table 11.1 Examples of targeting criteria used.

Type of programme	Criteria used	Comments noted
Food supplementation for positive patients starting ART 6 month duration (extended to 12 months in special circumstances) AMPATH, Kenya (Byron *et al.*, 2006)	At least one of the following: – Insufficient access to food to support patient recovery; – Body Mass Index (BMI) below 19; – Household income less than 3,000 Kenyan shillings. per month; – CD4 count less than 200	Targeted to HIV-infected individuals only Beneficiaries may go to collection points further afield to avoid stigma (in this case it was related to the food supplement packaging which was adorned with HIV education messages)
Supplementary Feeding using proxy indicators (Monitors to review eligibility criteria with beneficiaries) WFP, Malawi	Food security indicators – at least 3 of the following: – Limited access to land; – No major common livestock; – No formal wages; – <3 months stock from harvest time; – Caring for chronically ill family members; – Caring for orphans; – Child/Female/elderly headed households; – Any households caring for more than two orphans who have lost both parents.	Indirectly reaching HIV affected households HIV prevalence may factor in the targeting of geographical zones
Supplementary feeding with agricultural inputs Action Against Hunger, Malawi (2003–2004)	Community identification of vulnerable households Representative community committee set up to identify the vulnerable in the community based on family size, orphans, assets, access to land etc	System was open to community 'favouritism' and not all vulnerable were identified as they did not have community representation. A perception of 'unfairness' was reported by nearly 15% of the community
Supplementary feeding for HIV affected households by proxy indicators Concern, Malawi	Orphan/female/elderly headed households Chronically ill Surviving on only one meal per day	Triangulated approach to cross check selection using HIV services and other NGOs.
MOH/Action Against Hunger, Malawi (Action Against Hunger, 2007)	HIV positive people starting ART Adults BMI <17.5 Pregnant and lactating women MUAC <22 cm Children weight/height <80% or MUAC <12 cm	Little impact noted on anthropometric nutrition status indicating earlier nutrition intervention is required for the maximum benefit Positive impact on improvement in physical strength and ability to return to casual labour
Organic Farm and supplementary feeding for OVCs CINDI, Zambia	Presence of OVC in household Elderly/Child/Female headed households	

intake. It can be delivered on an individual level or on a group or community level and can be linked to a multitude of services. These can include community nutrition interventions, nutrition surveys, vaccination campaigns, clinics (HIV-related or 'mother and child health related'), home-based care (HBC) and any community groups offering health education including schools, traditional birth attendants (TBAs), community health workers, women's groups, youth groups, water projects, as well as agricultural projects and community gardens. Nutrition counselling and education should centre around the knowledge of a healthy balanced diet and ways in which to achieve optimal nutrition through looking at local and affordable foods, helping the community to value the nutritional importance of local produce and to make informed choices with the financial means they have available. Nutrition education does not only cover the nutritional values of food available but also the appropriate storage, handling and preparation of food. Done effectively, this can help to reduce the risk of contamination, optimise use of fuel resources and reduce wastage. Infant and young child feeding forms an essential part of any nutrition education (see Chapter 3.4).

When looking at nutrition tools – counselling cards, posters, booklets and other IEC[1] materials, the importance of standardisation and translation must always be considered. To get effective messages across on a wide scale, consistency is essential and materials must be accessible, easy to use and understandable for all. Coordination between service groups, governmental groups such as ministries of health, education and agriculture, and community based organisations (CBOs)/non-government organisations (NGOs) can only strengthen the messages and their impact (Box 11.2). Training for those delivering nutrition education should help ensure consistency and effective use of materials. The Living Well manual (FAO, WHO, 2002) provides an excellent and handy guide to use for comprehensive nutrition education with communities affected by HIV.

Box 11.2   Using nutrition education in home-based care (HBC)

HOSPAZ, an umbrella organisation for HBC in Zimbabwe, provides training for HBC volunteers with a mandate to provide effective standards for HBC. Volunteers from multiple organisations are given training and issued with a set of counselling cards, with simple pictorial and written messages, to use within the households they support. The cards cover food hygiene and medical issues with important nutrition messages, including how to use nutrition to cope with symptoms of illness and the side effects of medications, and the importance of safe water. The information cards and training the volunteers receive are based on Ministry of Health nutrition guidelines but made simple and accessible for all.

Community groups can be used in the first instance to help devise what foods are affordable and acceptable for people to eat. They can further be used as a method of service delivery, with demonstration cooking and communal eating as an integral part of the nutrition education. HIV education and forums for discussion

---

[1] IEC materials are health education tools that cover Information, Education and Communication. Websites with examples of IEC materials on HIV and nutrition include www.fantaproject.org and www.aed.org.

can be integrated around the food and nutrition focus. There are often traditional or cultural factors that may block community acceptance to certain foods and available products. The reasons for this can be explored with community groups to see if available products of nutritional value could be accepted into the diet and utilised.

Nutrition gardens in the form of community or school gardens offer a great setting for nutrition education. Youth clubs where children learn about cultivation and nutrition can help replace the channels of information that have been lost where households have lost their capacity for home cultivation. Demonstration gardens can also be used as illustrated in Box 11.3.

Box 11.3   The linkage trust, Zimbabwe

The Linkage trust in Makoni, Zimbabwe is an organisation offering nutrition education and counselling to those affected by HIV. Using demonstration gardens and community workers, they offer labour and resource saving techniques for gardening such as drip kits and 'fertility trenches' to encourage families to grow nutritious food and produce that can be used for personal consumption and income-generating activities. Their emphasis is on education for the use of common herbs and products that can be used for control of illness-related symptoms and small-scale agriculture to enable self-sustainability.

11.6   Targeted food supplementation programmes

Targeted food supplementations usually involve a nutrition supplement that is delivered either through a health care channel, or community channels such as community support groups, religious groups or home-based care. With the exception of severe malnutrition and therapeutic feeding, nutrition supplements are precisely that – a supplement to be taken in addition to the normal diet. They are not meant to provide the full energy requirement and there is no standard ration used for HIV nutrition programmes. Nutrition supplements of various types can be used, depending on local resources and context. At the planning stage of the intervention it is best to see what is locally available to meet the additional nutritional requirements needed. Assessment will show whether there is enough food available and if the target group/community would benefit from nutrition education on how to increase and improve their intake, or whether there are certain missing elements in the diet such as essential macronutrients and micronutrients. Typical examples of this are households who can only afford the staple food and do not get a balanced diet, and those for whom meat or fish are classed as a luxury and thus only affordable on limited occasions. When checking for micronutrient deficiencies, sources of commonly deficient micronutrients such as vitamin A, vitamin C, iron, zinc, riboflavin and iodine should be confirmed. Where the staple diet is maize or sorghum, it is important to check for additional sources of niacin (pulses, nuts or dried fish). If the staple is polished rice, additional sources of thiamine (such as pulses, nuts or eggs) should be checked. In emergency settings following poor harvests, severe weather, conflict or other natural disasters, full support of macro- and micronutrients may be required. In these instances especially, it is worth providing an increased ration above that has been calculated for individual needs, as intra-household sharing will be commonplace. Guidelines for rations in emergency settings can be found in the Sphere Handbook (The Sphere Project, 2004).

Importing of specialised supplementary foods may be a good solution in the short term if there is an immediate shortage of locally available products and if they are deemed acceptable by the community involved. However for the purpose of sustainability, which will undoubtedly be needed in the HIV context, it is better to look at local solutions already available and potential solutions such as generating local agricultural or small businesses to provide for community programmes (Valid International, 2006). Some supplementary foods have been marketed especially for the HIV-infected population and are widely advertised in certain countries as 'miracle' cures. Care should be taken when considering use of these products for several reasons. There are no 'special' dietary needs recommended for those infected with HIV other than to increase the overall amount of energy intake depending on clinical status. This should be increased in the normal proportional balance of carbohydrate, protein and fats, and micronutrients should not exceed the recommended daily intakes as given for the general population. Additionally, some of these products have been so widely marketed for 'HIV use' that there is an element of stigma attached that could backfire on a well-intended nutrition intervention. Therefore, it is important to research the product carefully:

- Check the nutritional component is well balanced and suitable for the supplementation intended (by proportion of daily intake)
- Confirm neutral packaging
- Ensure that the product is affordable
- Finally, consider if the ingredients of the 'specialised' supplement are not cheaper to buy, or produce locally.

Just as it is important to define the type of nutrition intervention and approach, it is also important to define the aim of use of the nutrition supplement. If the aim is to treat acute malnutrition, the supplement needs to be proven in terms of quality and effectiveness. Similarly, when treating acute malnutrition in the community, the supplement should be clearly intended for the individual so that sharing is less likely within the household and there must be regular provision with no break in supply. In areas where there is general hardship, a family ration of the staple diet can be provided alongside the individual supplementary ration to try and prevent sharing. If community services such as HBC are involved in the distribution of food supplements to support households affected by HIV, it is imperative that volunteers are able to recognise the signs of acute malnutrition in order to refer for detailed assessment and specialised nutrition supplements if any member of the household becomes malnourished. When community-based treatment of acute malnutrition is ongoing in the community, the beneficiaries must be monitored regularly in terms of weight, height and/or MUAC in order to confirm response to treatment, to refer for medical treatment if necessary and ultimately to be appropriately discharged from a specialised programme back to more generalised household nutrition support. Indeed, all types of food supplementation should be seen as part of a process which includes preventative approaches to strengthen household food security wherever possible.

In an ideal setting, to ensure practicality in terms of intake, rations intended for those with HIV should:

- meet the nutritional value required
- be easy to eat/palatable

- be fortified with micronutrients (not exceeding RDA[2])
- include processed cereals for minimum cooking and preparation
- be easily digestible and
- not be too large a quantity for ingestion, as it must be perceived as a supplement only.

If the ration is for a small child, the food supplement must be suitable in quantity and consistency for the age range. Similarly, for a sick adult, it cannot be expected for the individual to consume large quantities of difficult to digest supplement on top of their normal diet. The supplement must be both palatable and nutrient-dense so as not to result in large quantities either for dietary intake or for the logistics of delivery or collection. When planning the ration, it is worth looking at the market value. Is the ration more likely to be sold for its worth rather than used by the individual for the intended use? If using valuable commodities such as oil and sugar in a ration, it is often worth premixing the ration to decrease the selling off of certain components. This, however, will reduce the shelf life of the ration and also limit the use of the ration (i.e. no oil for cooking if the oil is premixed into a porridge preparation). Monitoring household consumption by checking remaining levels of rations during community visits will help to determine appropriate use and necessary duration of interventions.

11.6.1   Different types of targeted food supplementation programmes

There are many different channels for providing targeted food supplements, linked to various types of services. It is, however, important to remember that distributing food through a clinic or other service systems, such as HBC, will inevitably overlook individuals that are either unaware of their HIV status, or have not yet tapped into services. This does not necessarily reflect that they don't have the need for support but can be a result of stigma, pride or simply due to lack of awareness of the services and support available. Care should be taken to reach out to men, and women who do not have young children, two particular groups who are less likely to be routinely accessing health services. Channels for targeted food supplements that may be considered in an HIV context are set out in (Table 11.2).

11.7   Support of HIV-positive pregnant women

All women in pregnancy automatically require increased energy to meet the needs of both themselves and their unborn child. Without this increase, there is a risk that the child will not receive all the essential nutrients required for health and development in the womb. By providing the mother with increased energy, the unborn baby can feed off the mother without any detrimental effect on maternal health and nutritional status (see Chapter 3, 'Malnutrition, Infant Feeding, Maternal and Child Health').

In women infected with HIV there is an increased risk of delivering small full-term babies and premature babies (Arpadi, 2005; Black *et al.*, 2008). With the added risk of malnutrition in resource-limited settings, there is a higher risk of adverse birth outcomes highlighting the increased importance of adequate nutrition during pregnancy for mothers with HIV. Essentially, women have to be diagnosed before

---

[2] Recommended daily allowance.

Table 11.2 Different forms of food distribution.

Targeted nutrition intervention	Prevention	Care (Treatment and support)	Mitigation
Supplementary Feeding (Community based outposts; schools; community based organisations (CBO); HBC; HIV services (eat in or take home); MCH clinics	Food insecure Infant and young child feeding (IYCF) support Pregnant and lactating women support	Treatment of low BMI, MUAC, or weight for height (moderate acute malnutrition) Losing weight Complement to treatment for infection /TB etc Palliative care	Family ration for vulnerable households School feeding in high HIV-prevalent communities
Therapeutic Feeding		Treatment of severe acute malnutrition	
Food as an incentive	Participation in PMTCT Attendance to awareness and sensitisation campaigns Food for training (agricultural or livelihood strategies/HBC nutrition training)	Improve adherence to ART/TB treatment Improve adherence to PMTCT follow up (treatment for infants)	Food for education Food for work (can be used as incentive for HBC volunteers)

Adapted from (FANTA, WFP, 2007).

they can be targeted for such nutrition interventions. Prevention of mother-to-child transmission (PMTCT) programmes are becoming more widespread in resource-limited settings but uptake remains disappointingly low, reaching approximately only 10% of HIV-infected women (Mbori-Ngacha, 2006). Reasons for this are believed to be a combination of factors including individual health-seeking behaviour, quality of services offered and issues around health infrastructures. Community intervention needs to look at sensitisation and mobilisation of TBAs and other key matriarchal community figures to maximise the role they can play in increasing uptake and understanding of PMTCT. Male support groups can also be used as a method of educating the men around the importance of knowing HIV diagnosis in pregnancy, the importance of good nutrition in pregnancy and the importance of choosing appropriate infant feeding for their babies.

If PMTCT approaches are limited to clinical health care settings in environments where on average only 47% of pregnant women deliver in health care facilities or with a skilled health care attendant (WHO, 2006), it is unlikely they will achieve the coverage needed to make an impact on mother-to-child transmission in high HIV-prevalent areas. If TBAs and matriarchal community figures can be mobilised to help women access HIV counselling and testing, complementary nutrition supplements can then be linked in through the channels of diagnosis such as community antenatal services and community-based primary health care clinics. This integrated approach can offer several benefits to mother and child health through encouragement by incentive of nutrition supplementation to attend general antenatal and post-natal checks as well as PMTCT services.

Information about nutritional requirements during pregnancy is provided in Chapter 3. Energy and micronutrients that are not sufficiently available in the diet can be provided through fortification of the intended nutrition supplement, or micronutrient supplements can be used (WHO, WFP, UNICEF, 2006). If there is severe maternal iron deficiency in pregnancy (<7 g/dl Hb), the infant will have a higher risk of prematurity, associated low haemoglobin, and a higher risk of morbidity and mortality (Mocroft et al., 1999; Clark et al., 2002). Given the association between HIV and iron deficiency, it is important to be aware of maternal iron deficiency early in the pregnancy. Simple field techniques are available for checking haemoglobin and can be integrated into community surveys, and primary health care obstetric services, especially if the initial assessment shows a lack of iron-rich food sources available. Care must be taken however regarding the administration of iron supplements in HIV-positive pregnant women as anaemia may be due to chronic infection rather than iron deficiency. Women can be advised on optimal diet and recommended doses of supplements given if necessary, but repeated courses for treatment of non-responding haemoglobin levels must be avoided as this can potentially increase the risk of mother-to-child HIV transmission (Prentice et al., 2008).

11.8   Breastfeeding and infant feeding support

As with support for pregnant women, community interventions need to look at sensitisation and mobilisation of TBAs and key matriarchal community figures to maximise the role they can play for breastfeeding and infant feeding support (see Chapter 3). Breastfeeding advice traditionally comes from elder women in many cultures (to be clarified as part of the assessment) and they may form as an essential target group as the pregnant women themselves. By supporting early initiation of breastfeeding and early solutions to breastfeeding problems (such as engorgement and mastitis) in the home environment, rates of exclusive breastfeeding can be improved to help reduce the risk of HIV transmission. Peer education from other new mothers is also an effective mode of support.

As with support of pregnant women, the additional maternal nutrition requirements for lactating women (see Chapter 3, 'Malnutrition, Infant Feeding, Maternal and Child Health') are recommended regardless of HIV status. However, with the additional associated risk of malnutrition for mother (Papathakis et al., 2006; Taha et al., 2006) and baby (Kessler et al., 2001) infected with HIV, the pertinence of nutrition interventions at this stage is highlighted. Even if a mother is malnourished, the quantity of her milk is unlikely to be affected, but the milk may contain fewer vitamins and fat for the baby and, additionally, the baby may take what he/she needs at the expense of the mother's own nutrient stores. This is particularly true for iron and both mother and baby should be monitored accordingly, given the common association between HIV and anaemia.

Nutrition supplements are ideally linked to community network interventions that are also providing breastfeeding and post-natal support. Mother and child health (MCH) clinics are often a good location for setting up HIV counselling, nutrition education and supplementary feeding. Mothers can come and be weighed with their babies and receive advice and treatment from health care workers and peer support from other mothers.

In community settings, or even work areas, breastfeeding corners can be set up from simple resources to provide a calm and relaxing protected environment for mothers to take a break and breastfeed their babies. Support groups can be set up in

easy to access community settings at a time of day that is suitable for women to con-
gregate. Nutrition and infant feeding education can be provided whilst mothers share
experiences. Men can also be included if culturally acceptable, or have separate partner support groups. Male involvement can assist the breastfeeding process through
support and encouragement for women to breastfeed, perhaps through reduction of
some duties that can be shared or by understanding of the optimal conditions or
environment needed in the home setting to breastfeed.

Of course, not all mothers with HIV will be breastfeeding, although this is the
more common likelihood in resource-limited settings (WHO 2009). For those who
are counselled and make an informed choice to use breast milk alternatives (see
Chapter 3), it is essential that any community intervention that is assisting with
formula milk must adhere to the International Code of Marketing of Breast-Milk
Substitutes (WHO, 1981).

Nutritional support of breastfeeding women should ideally be provided for
the maximum of 6 months of exclusive breastfeeding accompanied by nutritional education. One of the limitations of the PMTCT programmes to date has been their lack
of follow-up. If PMTCT services are moved out into the community and integrated
with existing community networks, then it is hoped that improved follow-up will
progress. Follow-up would include continued support for infant feeding choice, management of breast conditions and feeding problems, nutrition support to mother and
growth monitoring of the baby, all in a community setting. Well before the baby is 6
months of age, sources of appropriate complementary foods need to be explored and
discussed with the mother in preparation for weaning. Again peer support from other
mothers and key matriarchal community figures are invaluable and will just need
occasional input from a health or nutrition worker for support and training updates.

One of the common obstacles that arise when setting up community support
networks is the issue of incentives. Offering financial incentives to 'volunteers' can
have the potential effect of encouraging the less genuinely motivated community
members to come forward and hence reduce the sustainability of a programme. The
ideal is to encourage those who are already unofficially active in the maternal and
child health arena, such as TBAs, experienced mothers and elder matriarchs in the
community, to set up an official system of support. In return, technical training can be
given as incentive and even some sort of qualification such as certification for 'breast
feeding counsellor' or certificate in nutrition. There are excellent training modules
available from WHO that can be used precisely for such interventions (WHO, 1993;
WHO, 2000; WHO, 2003; WHO, 2006).

At the beginning of a project it may be that experienced workers work alongside
the community volunteers to provide 'on the job' training. This period should be
limited in duration to prevent barriers between paid and non-paid members of a
network.

Infant and young child feeding practices, as seen in Box 11.4, often have their basis
in food insecurity either as a result of lack of availability of appropriate food or lack
of access to it. Recent work, although not specific to HIV, has shown that inability
to afford nutritious diets results in a substantial shortfall in a household's ability to
feed their children. Recommendations point to improved cash-based social protection
interventions to alleviate this shortfall. Whilst this work was not specifically related
to HIV settings, it illustrates the added pressure to provide appropriate infant and
young child feeding when all the exacerbating factors of HIV are taken into account
and again reiterates the need for a holistic approach (Chastre et al., 2007).

Box 11.4   ACF-International, Burundi 2007.

After more than 10 years of political, economic and social crisis Burundi has exceptionally high levels of poverty and HIV prevalence is estimated between 3 and 11% (rural/urban). Prevention programmes are being encouraged to prevent worsening of the situation.

In the province of Ruyigi, Action Contre la Faim (ACF) conducted a 'Knowledge, Attitudes and Practices' (KAP) survey via questionnaires and focus group discussions to assess infant feeding practices within the population. It showed that breastfeeding rates were high but inappropriate foods were commonly introduced at a premature stage introducing risk of diarrhoeal disease and increasing the risk of HIV transmission by mixed feeding. The assessment revealed how even though some nutrient-rich foods were available, they were not consumed due to cultural taboos and dietary restrictions. Food insecurity was the main reason for inappropriate infant and young child feeding with undernourished mothers experiencing a lack of belief in their ability to produce enough breast milk and poor availability of complementary foods for weaning.

A programme was designed to address these issues through increasing community awareness of the benefits of exclusive breastfeeding and appropriate infant feeding practices in the HIV context, and to provide psychological support to enhance breastfeeding practices among HIV-positive women. The project was designed to complement an existing PMTCT program run by the Italian NGO, LVIA. The main objective is to reduce vertical transmission of HIV and consequently HIV-related malnutrition.

11.9   Support for other vulnerable groups

Supplementary feeding can be provided using many different approaches. There are programmes that are aimed at treatment of acute moderate malnutrition, which will target only those within certain nutrition parameters and those who will target any other vulnerable group such as HIV-infected individuals, pregnant and lactating women, those attending particular medical clinics such as TB, PMTCT or ART, or households affected by HIV or other chronic illness through avenues such as home-based care. A range of the supplements that may be used in supplementary feeding is given in Table 11.3.

Programmes with strict nutrition parameters in resource-limited settings are usually intended for individuals with clinically diagnosed acute malnutrition and follow the guidelines commonly implemented during times of emergency or seasonal hunger gaps. They are often in conjunction with other nutrition interventions such as general food distributions and population-wide micronutrient supplementation (WHO, 1999). The type of nutrition supplements used will vary depending on the context and type of programme. If the programme is implemented for the treatment of moderate malnutrition, regardless of HIV status, the ration will meet a specific nutrition standard and usually be fortified with micronutrients. Standard methods of monitoring and evaluating programmes should be followed and once beneficiaries have reached the target weight gain they will be discharged.

Table 11.3 Supplementary feeding products.

Food supplements available	Forms
Ready to Use Food	Commercial or locally produced RUTF or RUSF (ready to use Therapeutic or Supplementary food)
Fortified cereals	CSB/UNIMIX/SP450
Fortified Biscuits	BP5/high energy biscuits
Fortified drinks	HEPS (high energy protein and soya drink)
Locally available foods	Cereal, oil, sugar, dried milk, pulses, eggs, fruit and vegetables
Breast milk substitutes	MUST adhere to the international breastfeeding code

With other forms of supplementary feeding, such as those often used as an adjunct to HIV programmes, there may be less stringent admission criteria and beneficiaries may be recruited on vulnerability or medical grounds rather than anthropometric criteria. In these cases the discharge standards may become unclear and could potentially affect the sustainability of the programme if there is insufficient capacity for increasing numbers. Examples of eligibility criteria that may be used are shown earlier in this chapter in Table 11.1. Box 11.5 below, gives an example of a community form of supplementary feeding.

The nutrition supplements used in these instances will probably depend on resources available. In many home-based care programmes any commonly eaten and available foods may be distributed as a support ration without real emphasis on the nutritional value. This is not because the nutritional value is not considered important, but if the ideal foods are not available, giving any extra commodities to a household in need will give some extra nutrition or alternatively extra commodities to exchange or sell for income. The income can then be used to purchase fresh produce or other essentials.

Once again an adequate analysis of household food intake and sources of food is essential to determine the most appropriate programming. It may be that a cash-based intervention improving direct access to available foodstuffs is more effective at improving food diversity for households and is cheaper to implement (Creti and Jaspers, 2006; Action contre la Faim, 2007).

Box 11.5 Community-based supplementary feeding of orphans and vulnerable children.

From 2004 to 2006 Children in Distress (CINDI) in Kitwe, Zambia, working in one of the highest HIV-prevalent areas in the Copperbelt region, supported 28 'nutrition centres' in the township. Caregivers volunteered use of their homes (the 'nutrition centres') on a rotational basis to cook for up to 50 children 4 days a week in the community. Nshima and porridge was provided by CINDI and the volunteers all worked for free. The programme enabled a low-cost opportunity to feed many vulnerable children with accompanying health and nutrition education.

Another form of community-based supplementary feeding is school feeding, often provided by WFP. Communities with high HIV prevalence can benefit from school feeding to ensure vulnerable children receive at least one meal per day. The food provided can also act as an incentive for school attendance and improve concentration whilst receiving education.

Table 11.4 Examples of diversity of SFP rations.

Type of programme	Target group	Ration
Church group, Zimbabwe	HIV infected individuals and affected HIV households	Individual food baskets of 10 kg CSB plus a household basket of 10 kg mealie-meal/600 ml oil/2 kg pulse
HBC group, Harare	HIV infected individuals	CSB, oil, beans and Epap*
CINDI, Kitwe	OVCs	Pre-mix of ground kapenta, mealie-meal and salt plus milk and eggs (farm partnership)
PMTCT programme, Zimbabwe	HIV positive pregnant women	Food basket to feed family of 5 (monthly per person: cereal 8 kg/pulse 1.5/oil 0.5 kg/CSB 1.5)
HBC, Ndola, Zambia	HIV infected individuals	HEPS high energy protein soya (drink of mealie-meal, soya and DSM)
ACF Malawi	Those starting ART with moderate malnutrition	CSB and oil

*Epap is a commercial food supplement marketed in southern Africa for those with HIV.

In summary, there is no right or wrong when it comes to supplementary feeding for HIV support. The degrees of impact, however, will vary tremendously in accordance with the rations used, the frequency with which they are given and whether or not they are accompanied by nutrition counselling and education. Many HIV programmes simply include nutrition as a popular addition to an intervention without necessary concern for the actual nutritional impact. Table 11.4 gives an illustration of the variety of approaches that have been observed in the field, usually dictated by the availability (or lack) of funding and resources.

There is a large move by some NGOs towards the distribution of ready-to-use therapeutic food (RUTF) – available as a commercial brand (Nutriset, Feeding Children, France, 2006) but can also be locally made from raw ingredients in HIV programmes as a nutrition supplement to support those on ART, those on TB medication or even those who have had recent acute illness. Whilst the recipients unarguably benefit from weight gain, there is no evidence as yet that this is suitable use of the product and until then, care should be taken that detrimental effects do not result from giving a specialised nutrient-dense product intended for therapeutic feeding to those who do not have the same physical constitution of severe acute malnutrition. This applies particularly to those starting ART who may potentially suffer other initial side effects of therapy. If those who are attending HIV treatment clinics do meet the criteria for severe acute malnutrition, then they should be treated accordingly (Valid International, 2006).

11.10   Treatment of severe acute malnutrition in HIV context

Severe acute malnutrition (SAM) is classified as weight for height <70% of the median or less than −3z-scores compared to the reference population, and/or presence of bilateral oedema. Treatment of SAM has been well researched and standard international guidelines are in place for both inpatient and community-based care (Valid International, 2006). Treatment of severe acute malnutrition should ideally include access to HIV counselling and testing as well as nutrition counselling and education. There are no alterations to the nutritional treatment that should be given to a child with SAM and HIV but there should be extra care in the management of persistent diarrhoea to avoid the risk of fluid overload and effective antibiotic use in bacteraemia may move away from standard antibiotic regimes recommended in international guidelines. Research by Action Against Hunger in Malawi suggests that whilst full recovery can be achieved, the duration of treatment may be longer with slower weight gain and resources should be planned accordingly. Hunger and HIV, Action Against Hunger, Hunger Watch Publication 2007.

11.11   Micronutrient supplementation programmes

In most resource-limited settings, micronutrient supplementation programmes are commonplace. Common micronutrient deficiencies in these settings include vitamins A, B3, and vitamin C; thiamine, riboflavin, iodine and iron deficiency anaemia. Micronutrient interventions can be linked to immunisation campaigns or any nutrition or health intervention, making them extremely cost-effective and simple with regard to logistics (WHO, WFP & UNICEF, 2006). They provide a valuable, low-cost enhancement to nutrition status in contexts where locally available diet is often insufficient to meet essential micronutrient requirements. This is true, of course, for any micronutrient-deficient population but there may be added benefit in HIV contexts where even asymptomatic HIV may impair micronutrient status. Common micronutrient deficiencies independently associated with both HIV and malnutrition include iron, selenium, zinc and vitamins A, C and E (Golden and Golden, 1986; Waterlow, 1992; Mofenson, 2003) and assessment of local dietary availability of these micronutrients should be included in initial assessments. With advanced HIV disease, micronutrient deficiencies are more likely to occur due to increased utilisation and loss of nutrients often associated with infection. Micronutrient intake can be increased with fortified nutrition supplements or multiple micronutrient supplementation in the form of tablets or specialised food supplements.[3] Optimum dosage for HIV-affected individuals is not yet known and caution should be used when considering the multi-micronutrients available and the normal RDA should not be exceeded (Friis, 2006). Due to the interaction between certain micronutrients such as vitamin C and iron, or zinc and copper, where increase or decrease in one can affect the utilisation or levels of another, it is necessary to consider the complete picture of available micronutrients for intake.

11.12   Livelihood support and ensuring access to food

The impact of the HIV pandemic on already vulnerable households is well documented and wide-reaching (Harvey, 2004; Gillespie and Kadlyala, 2005; The World Bank, 2007) and a detailed account of the subject is outside the scope of this chapter. The aim here is to summarise the main points of community livelihood programming.

HIV-affected households face a greater risk of experiencing a reduction in their household food and nutrition security as a result of numerous interlinking factors (Figure 11.1). Households are in an extremely difficult position, with clear risks to

---

[3] An illustration of the variety of micronutrient supplements available can be browsed at: http://www.micronutrient.org.

health when trying to maintain adequate and appropriate food within the household, when sick members have increased dietary needs at the same time that providers may have reduced capacity to provide for those needs.

During the assessment of the context, answers to numerous questions must be sought before solutions can be defined. Some of the priority questions are listed below:

- How is food access sustained when the main breadwinner is ill and the labour capacity in the household is reduced due to sickness?
- As more time is given to care of the sick by healthy members, what economic opportunities are available to the households and by which means can they supplement their income?
- What proportion of income is channelled into purchase of medical expenses, water, hygiene and funeral costs at the expense of food (in societies where food purchase usually takes a high proportion of total income)?
- Are children taken out of school to assist in the daily struggle to ensure that the basic needs for the family are met; what is the potential future impact of this reduction in education?
- How has the proportion of own-production as a total of food sources changed when land cannot be cultivated because of lack of time; what are the labour and input constraints?
- Can markets be reached when constraints include lack of transport means, sickness or necessity to stay at home to care for the sick?
- What other coping strategies do households have to resort to in order to survive?
- Are productive assets being sold?
- What impact does caring have on the carer and the rest of the household when the carer becomes sick, weakened or desperate from putting all his/her energy into caring?

In resource-limited settings, vulnerable households often struggle to ensure a minimum of two meals per day and it is often difficult to consider whether daily food intake is nutritionally balanced and appropriate for sick individuals. The picture is bleak but it is the reality for millions of households living with HIV in resource-limited settings as illustrated below by case study 11.2 in a country heavily affected by HIV.

Case Study 11.2   Case study, Zimbabwe.

Action Contre la Faim (ACF), Zimbabwe September – December 2007:

In a survey undertaken by ACF in Zvishavane, a zone with the highest HIV prevalence in Zimbabwe, more than 90% of households interviewed devoted their entire income to staple food purchase. A combination of factors contributed to this rise [compared to the previous period], (i) an increase in food prices, (ii) diminishing food reserves and (iii) increased reliance on the market for food. Market analysis showed a critical decrease of cereal availability. There was a shortage of basic commodities on the formal market as most goods like maize grain, cooking oil and sugar could only be found in the informal market or close to bigger cities (which people used despite the high cost of transport). All prices had skyrocketed [during the 3 month period preceding the survey]. As the hunger gap went deeper, households significantly increased the use of consumption coping strategies: limiting the portion size at meal times, reducing the number of meals, and taking days without eating. In addition, the 2007–2008 cropping season was compromised, as households were unable to access enough agricultural inputs to fulfil their cultivation plans.

Source: ACF Zimbabwe Food Security Surveillance Bulletin #3

Interventions to address population needs should be integrated to reflect the numerous causes and interlinking factors. All factors must be addressed. For example: addressing ART without improved nutrition; nutrition education without means to ensure access to good nutrition; diversification of production without labour capacity or storage means will have limited impact. All such links must be considered to enable effective interventions.

Where direct food shortage occurs at the local level, such as in the case study above, there will clearly be certain households or individuals for whom there is no other immediate solution except support with food assistance delivered from external sources and community interventions. In this case there may also be a need for additional supplements for HIV-infected people in order to meet their needs for macronutrients and micronutrients. Food assistance for HIV-infected individuals may have the objective to maintain or delay decline in nutritional status as well as giving households opportunities to maintain a balanced diet to avoid adverse consequences as a result of a decline in food availability.

As with all nutrition interventions, the aim at the outset would be to replace food assistance with actions which allow a sustainable supply of adequate food for vulnerable or affected households. This could be in the form of activities which can generate income for the household, monetary assistance via food vouchers or direct cash transfers. Any activity-based food security intervention is likely to require external support in the initial stages to ensure that households have the necessary inputs and training to set up the activity (Box 11.6).

Box 11.6 Community gardens.

Zimbabwe January 2007.

Gardens set up by an international NGO in Zimbabwe (Medicins du Monde – MDM) were established following a direct request from the community to further support those community members receiving ART from the same NGO. At the same time as providing a diversified source of food and generating income from the sale of their produce, the HIV-affected community members benefiting from the garden project, received psycho-social support and were a source of mutual assistance being proactive in breaking down stigma against themselves and being seen as valued members of the community.

Source – author's (KO) discussion with MDM medical project team and garden committee members during a field visit January 2007.

In resource-limited settings with high prevalence of HIV, the resilience of the community as well as the household is likely to be reduced. Traditional practices such as sharing and other support mechanisms may become weakened or break down simply due to limited means and lack of resources. Analyses should focus on vulnerabilities and capacities of communities to support their members and to advocate for better services with authorities and governments. Interventions should aim to build on and strengthen community cohesion and should involve community members from the analytical and project identification phases.

In Box 11.1 it was suggested that a potential objective for community nutrition interventions is to improve food diversity and access to food. Programmes to improve the availability and access to diverse foods whilst at the same time reducing labour requirements for reasons stated earlier in this section, require an innovative approach. It is only thorough assessment and analysis of the specific context and needs of individuals which will define the appropriate project type – there are no carbon-copy solutions. Vegetable production as a solution to increased food diversity needs land, water and knowledge. Does this exist in the community under assessment or is it something that can be improved through the project? Tapping into local knowledge, foods and practices is extremely important not only to capitalise on and develop the transmission of information but also for the dignity and empowerment of the community to work to develop their future. Food production support (which can include seeds, irrigation systems and training) and advice and help for post-harvest processing and sale should all be addressed in this kind of project. Cooking methods with support for optimum use of fuel should be addressed either through training or physical inputs such as fuel-efficient stoves.

Evidence of the impact of such projects, however, is not conclusive and certainly differs from household to household and from community to community.

Box 11.7 illustrates vegetable production support on Zimbabwe. There was, however, some conflict relating to communal gardens due to imbalance of power, too much bureaucracy and limited control over produce. These are aspects which are not insurmountable and could work very well in other contexts or communities but necessitate the total implication and participation of the community as well as a clear understanding between community members on roles and rights in all aspects of the project. Nevertheless, those plots which were individually cultivated but within a protected communal plot met with success in terms of community cohesion, sharing and exchange of resources and shared learning – ever more important in a context where resources are limited and learning passed on from generation to generation is drastically diminished. In the case study in question it was, nevertheless, the individual gardens which proved the most popular for their flexibility, their privacy, their management and their capacity to empower the owner.

Key lessons to learn from these experiences are that in order to reach the objective of improving food diversity and nutritional intake there is no one method that is the most appropriate and much will depend on the context, on communities and on individual households. Whilst taking more time to define and to put in place, tailor-made solutions will optimise the impact and thus make a greater contribution to improved nutritional situation of HIV-infected individuals and affected households.

Box 11.7   Vegetable production using drip kits.

Zimbabwe 2006–2007.

A vegetable production project targeting vulnerable households, including those with chronically ill members using drip irrigation kits to overcome the lack of water, was implemented in Zimbabwe. The aims were to diversify food available, to improve micronutrient intake, to reduce labour requirements, to provide income from sale of vegetables and to provide a vehicle for training on nutritional practices.

Indeed, impact evaluation showed a diversification for households receiving distributed seed. For able households with a low dependency ratio, there was an increase in productivity with time freed up to spend on other activities such as attending to a chronically ill person. For less able households or those with a high dependency ratio, the drip irrigation system increased the workload in terms of time and labour required to fill the water tank. Whilst the project period was short (11 months) there was evidence that households were harvesting in the hunger gap providing a much-needed food source during this critical period. However, the real increase in food availability was seasonal and thus increased meal diversity and frequency was not seen over the whole year. There was some income generated from sale of vegetables and a positive effect was that power dynamics shifted in favour of women. An unexpected but also positive outcome was that households adopted environmentally friendly cropping strategies including use of plants as pesticide which further freed up valuable financial resources and benefited the environment.

From the Programme Evaluation Report ECHO Zimbabwe with permission from Action contre la Faim (ACF-France).

11.13   Community mobilisation to support people living with HIV

Community-based safety nets and support systems have been effective for decades in preventing those hit by trauma in the community from slipping into destitution. This is however now under threat as the scale of HIV has increased the burden of responsibility with fewer earners and higher dependency ratios, but essentially the practices remain intact and with support, particularly of resources and organisational capacity, these safety nets can continue.

As already outlined, community interventions can be implemented through various channels of delivery: religious groups; women's groups; traditional healers and leaders; community workplaces or common meeting places; home-based care groups or community health posts. Community participation in the planning stages of the intervention can help improve the impact of nutrition programming through improved uptake of more appropriate services, improved coverage and acceptance of the programme and potentially will help reduce opportunity costs at the outset. Frequent opportunity costs cited by beneficiaries of nutrition programmes include transport expenses and time spent away from the homestead or from income-earning opportunities. Direct cash transfers can help to alleviate such aspects and provide capital for longer term sustainable actions. Also, by involving community members,

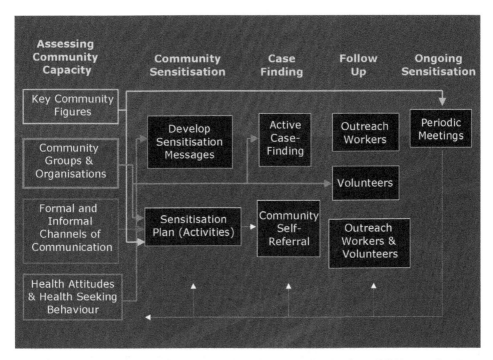

Figure 11.2 Elements of community mobilisation. With permission from Valid International.

community ownership will be encouraged and in the long term this should ease the process of withdrawing external support, enabling long-term nutrition support. Community participation in the planning and implementation stages can also help ensure that activities will not increase stigma in any way and will not adversely discriminate against those who are not directly affected by HIV but may require similar nutritional assistance.

Every context will be different but aspects of community participation will include:

- Assessing community capacity
- Liaison with key community figures
- Community sensitisation for the aims of the nutrition/HIV programme, including who it is intended for
- Case finding for beneficiaries
- Identifying and planning approaches for follow-up systems and continual nutrition sensitisation.

Figure 11.2 illustrates the different elements of community mobilisation.

Participatory communication strategies and participatory tools have been shown to be effective instruments for involving the community and aiding development of programmes that the community will both value and benefit from (ELDIS, 2009).Sustainable programmes can be developed by linking community dialogue with methods of action and support, with a clear exit strategy for the external support from the beginning. Whatever the size of the community intervention, it is important to develop continuing support, with agreed guidelines and policies in order to leave clear directions to enable the programme to continue. These can be devised with the community in the participatory process. As stated earlier, it is vital not only to include key community members but also representatives of the minority groups within the community to ensure interventions are accessible and beneficial to all those in need. The community can be strengthened through capacity building, not only through training on technical issues, such as nutrition and HIV, but also around practical issues on how to run and maintain an effective programme including storage and provision of resources, financial and legal issues (Box 11.8). Advocacy issues are key for both HIV and nutrition and all vulnerable groups must be given a voice in the community.

Box 11.8 Empowering communities: Children in Distress (CINDI), Kitwe 2006–2010.

In partnership with Action Against Hunger UK, (CINDI) in Kitwe, Zambia planned a 3-year project to support 11 rural communities to form their own community-based organisations (CBO) to support families affected by HIV. Training was given on the formation (legal and financial) of a CBO so that registration could be attained and committee members were trained on the activities that they would help initiate with affected households. Income-generating activities such as hydroponic gardening, basket weaving, rabbit and poultry rearing were initiated and committee members were also trained in HIV counselling to encourage community members to go forward for testing. The project has been successful and received further funding for a one year extension.

When planning an exit strategy, (something which should be started at the inception of the programme), there must be identified service providers who will be responsible for the continuation of the intervention. All education and counselling materials must be agreed and provided, essential nutrition equipment supplied and provisions made for repair or replacement and guidelines must be in place. Ideally, some aspect of the intervention will be income generating with a reliable/trained financial committee in place to provide revolving funds for the maintenance of the intervention.

11.14 Monitoring

Whatever intervention is carried out and wherever it takes place, a key aspect in the project's cycle is monitoring. This applies to following up anthropometric indicators for individuals, monitoring the use of food rations at household level, harvests and changes in income as a result of project interventions and monitoring changes in food security and nutritional indicators at community level. The importance and value of selecting key indicators and having a baseline against which to measure them cannot be emphasised enough. At the project identification phase monitoring indicators should be defined and adapted throughout the project term to take into account new and developing situations. This helps to ensure quality interventions that can adapt to contextual or other changes and that can be documented to help in learning lessons for further project improvement. As national and international organisations are still learning in HIV contexts, monitoring takes on an even greater importance.

11.15   Other issues

11.15.1   Integrated links

As mentioned in the assessment phase, it is important to address other factors that impact on nutrition status within the community. Food assistance alone will rarely solve the intricate problem of HIV-related malnutrition. Communication between community-based and non-governmental organisations to build an integrated response looking at livelihood support and food access, access to sufficient safe water, infant feeding practices and essential health care must be ongoing. Simple health care interventions such as impregnated bed nets against malaria and health education can accompany any nutrition response.

11.15.2   Social protection in the context of HIV (as a part of integrated community interventions)

Although not directly nutrition linked, the integrated approach to assist communities to improve their overall nutrition should include aspects of support for social protection in the HIV setting. Links with organisations that advocate against early marriage, child labour and sexual exploitation are invaluable in helping to slow the transmission rates of HIV and protect nutrition status in the long term. Likewise, simple acts such as birth registration in countries where less than half of newborn babies are registered (UNICEF, 2006) can have an impact on social safety nets and help create protective environments for children to grow and develop. Only with effective social safety nets, and ongoing sufficient food and safe water, can the cycle of HIV, poor nutrition, poor school performance and poor economic opportunities be broken.

11.15.3   Funding issues

Funding for nutrition projects in resource-limited settings have generally appeared to be on the downward trend with nutrition funding streams getting soaked up into major humanitarian crises such as Darfur. The Lancet series on maternal and child undernutrition (January 2008) may help reverse trends or at least have some impact towards improving availability of funds for nutrition interventions. However, nutrition through HIV funding appears to be more forthcoming and should be utilised to the maximum. One of the problems, as seen earlier, remains that whilst arguments are plausible for the benefits of nutrition in delaying the onset for expensive ART therapies, the clear-cut scientific evidence has not yet been presented and until this stage should arrive, funding will be limited to nutrition interventions that target those 'seen' to be in need, such as those who are already malnourished or those starting on ART. Commitment is needed to coordinate and strengthen funding for nutrition to scale up and integrate effective responses. Comprehensive community-based interventions can offer potential for sustainable approaches. They can act as a channel for nutrition assistance and incentive to encourage HIV testing, access to HIV services and appropriate infant and young child feeding and care practices. As the World Bank have stated, improving nutrition increases productivity and economic growth and the returns from programmes improving nutrition far outweigh their costs (World Bank, 2006). This will surely reap additional benefits when applied in HIV contexts.

11.16 Conclusion

Without the practical and technical resources required to support and enable national policies and guidelines, widespread, effective HIV linked nutrition programmes have yet to materialise in most resource-limited settings. Whilst progress has been made and many countries now have a national plan of action for nutrition and HIV, the challenge remains to implement those plans and either free up the resources required to make them happen or enable communities to deliver interventions through strengthening their resilience and capacity. Ensuring good nutrition status in the face of HIV is not just about provision of food but about integrated approaches to encourage healthy and productive communities. Empowering communities and moving the emphasis of responsibility back to the communities themselves can provide support to help implement interventions in a sustainable manner, incorporating both nutrition and HIV responses.

As a final reminder, resource-limited settings are not just in developing countries, but also exist at household level in many developed world settings where HIV affects many people with unstable immigration and poor socio-economic status. In these settings the main message remains to work with the families and individuals to find their own affordable and acceptable solutions for optimal nutrition. There will always be a way: the challenge is to find the right mode of delivery.

References

Action Against Hunger. *Hunger and HIV; From Crisis to Integrated Care*. London: Action Against Hunger, 2007.

Action contre la Faim. *Implementing Cash-Based Interventions: A Guideline for Aid Workers*. Paris: Action contre la Faim, 2007.

Amadi B, Kelly P, Mwiya M, Mulwazi E, Sianongo S. Intestinal and systemic infection, HIV and mortality in Zambian children with persistent diarrhoea and malnutrition. *J Pediatr Gastroenterol* 2001; **32**:550–4.

Arpadi SM. *Growth Failure in HIV-Infected Children. Consultation on Nutrition and HIV/AIDS in Africa: Evidence, Lessons and Recommendations for Action*. Durban: WHO Geneva, 2005.

Black RE, Allen LH, Bhutta ZA et al. Maternal and child undernutrition: global and regional exposures and health consequences. *Lancet* 2008 Jan 19; **371**(9608):243–60 Review.

Black RE, Morris SS, Bryce J. Where and why are 10 million children dying every year? *Lancet* 2003; **361**(9376):2226–33.

Black RE et al. 2008.

Byron E, Gillespie S, Nangami M. *Integrating Nutrition Security with Treatment of People Living with HIV: Lessons Being Learned in Kenya*. Washington: IFPRI, 2006.

Chastre C, Duffield A, Kindness H, LaJeune S, Taylor A. *The Minimum Cost of a Healthy Diet. Findings from Piloting a New Methodology in Four Study Locations*. London: Save_UK, 2007.

Clark TD, Mmiro F, Ndugwa C et al. Risk factors and cumulative incidence of anaemia among human immunodeficiency virus-infected children in Uganda. *Annals of Tropical Paediatrics* 2002 Mar; **22**(1):11–7.

Cross Continents Collaboration for Kids (3Cs4kids). Markers for predicting mortality in untreated HIV-infected children in resource-limited settings: a meta-analysis. *AIDS* 2008 Jan 2; **22**(1):97–105.

ELDIS. Livlihoods Connect, Institute of Development (IDS). Available at:www.livelihoods.org/info/pcdl/self/self_instruction_materials18.html. 2009.

FANTA/Academy for education development (AED), UNICEF, WHO. *Nutrition Care and Support for People Living with HIV/AIDS in Eastern and Southern Africa: Progress, Experience and Lessons.* Washington: FANTA Project, 2007.

FANTA, WFP. *Food Assistance Programming in the Context of HIV.* FANTA project Washington Chapter 3. 2007.

FANTA, WFP. *Food Assistance Programming in the context of HIV.* FANTA project Washington, Chapter 4.4 p. 80, 2007.

FAO. *HIV/AIDS: A Guide For Nutritional Care and Support,* 2nd edn, Food and Nutrition Technical Assistance Project, Academy for Educational Development, Washington DC, 2004.

FAO. *Improving Nutrition Programmes ; an Assessment Tool for Action.* Rome, 2006.

FAO. *Improving Nutrition Programmes: an Assessment Tool for Action. Users' Training Manual.* FAO, Rome, 2004.FAO, WHO.

FHI. *Baseline Assessment Tools for Prevention of Mother to Child Transmission of HIV.* Family Health International, Elizabeth Glaser Paediatric AIDS Foundation, Arlington, VA., 2003.

Friis H. *Micronutrients and HIV Infection; a Review of Current Evidence.* (http://www.who.int/nutrition/topics/Paper%20Number%202%20-%20Micronutrients.pdf). 2006.

Gillespie S, Kadlyala S. *HIV/AIDS and Food and Nutrition Security. From Evidence to Action.* Food Policy Review 7. Washington, D.C: International Food Policy Research Institute, 2005.

Golden M, Golden B. Zinc deficiency and oedema. *Paediatrics* 1986 Jan; 77(1):132–3.

Guijt I, Kaul Shah M. eds. *The Myth of Community-Gender Issues in Participatory Development.* London, 2001.

Harvey P. *HIV/AIDS and Humanitarian Action.* Humanitarian Policy Group Research Report 16. London: Overseas Development Institute, 2004.

Kessler L, Daley H, Malenga G, Graham S. The impact of the human immunodeficiency virus type 1 on the management of severe malnutrition in Malawi. *Ann Trop Paediatr* 2000; 20(1): 50–6.

Kessler L, Daley H, Malenga G, Graham SM. The impact of HIV infection on the clinical presentation of severe malnutrition in children at Queen Elizabeth Central Hospital. *Malawi Med J* 2001; 13(3):30–3.

Mbori-Ngacha D. *The 2006 HIV/AIDS Implementers Meeting of the President's Emergency Plan for AIDS Relief.* Durban, South Africa: Keynote Address, 2006.

Mocroft A, Kirk O, Barton SE *et al.* Anaemia is an independent predictive marker for clinical prognosis in HIV-infected patients from across Europe. Euro SIDA study group. *AIDS* 1999 May; 13(8):943–50.

Mofenson LM. Paediatric HIV infection in developed and developing countries: epidemiology and natural history In: Shearer WT, Hanson IC, eds. *Medical Management of AIDS in Children.* USA: Saunders, 2003.

Nutriset, Feeding Children, France. Available at: www.nutriset.fr. 2006.

Obimbo EM, Mbori-Ngacha DA, Ochieng JO *et al.* Predictors of early mortality in a cohort of human immunodeficiency virus type-1 infected African children. *Paediatr Infect Dis J* 2004 Jun; 23(6):536–43.

Creti, P. Jaspers S. (eds.) *Cash Transfer Programming in Emergencies.* Oxford: Oxfam Skills & Practice Series, Oxfam GB, 2006..

Papathakis PC, Van Loan MD, Rollins NC *et al.* Body composition changes during lactation in HIV-infected and HIV-uninfected South African women. *J Acquir Immune Defic Syndr* 2006; 43(4):467–74.

Prentice AM, Gershwin ME, Schaible UE *et al.* New challenges of studying nutrition-disease interactions in the developing world. *J Clin Invest* 2008; 118(4):1322–9 names in full.

Taha TE, Kumwenda NI, Hoover DR *et al.* The impact of breastfeeding on the health of HIV-positive mothers and their children in sub-Saharan Africa. *Bull World Health Org* 2006; 84(7), 546–554.

The Sphere Project. *Humanitarian Charter and Minimum Standards in Disaster response.* Sphere, Geneva http://www.sphereproject.org/index.php?option=content&task=view&id=27&Itemid =84. 2004.

The World Bank. *HIV/AIDS, Nutrition and Food Security: What Can We Do? A Synthesis of International Guidance.* Washington, DC: The World Bank, 2007.

UNAIDS. *Report on the Global AIDS Epidemic.* Geneva, 2006.

UNICEF. *State of the Worlds Children.* New York: UNICEF, 2006.

UNIDO. *United Nations Industrial Development Report 2005. Capacity Building for Catching Up. Historical, Empirical and Policy Dimensions.* Vienna, 2005.

Valid International. *Community-Based Therapeutic Care (CTC): A Field Manual*, 1st edn. Oxford: Valid International. Chapter 11, 2006.

Valid International. *Community Mobilisation. Community-Based Therapeutic Care (CTC)- a Field Manual*, 1st edn. Oxford: Valid International. Chapter 5, 2006.

Waterlow JC. *Protein Energy Malnutrition*, 2nd edn. England: Edward Arnold, 1992; revised re-print 2006.

WHO. *The International Code of Marketing of Breast-Milk Substitutes.* Geneva: WHO, 1981.

WHO. *Breastfeeding Counselling: A Training Course.* Geneva: WHO, 1993.

WHO. *Management of Severe Malnutrition: a Manual for Physicians and Other Senior Health Workers.* Geneva: WHO, 1999.

WHO. *HIV and Infant Feeding Counselling: A Training Course.* Geneva: WHO, 2000.

WHO. *Nutritional Care and Support for People Living with HIV/AIDS: A Short Counselling Course.* Geneva: WHO, 2003.

WHO. *Infant and Young Child Feeding Counselling: An Integrated Course.* Geneva: WHO, 2006.

WHO. Online reproductive Health indicators database. http://www.who.int/reproductivehealth/en/ accessed 11/5/2010. 2006.

WHO (World Health Organization), HIV and infant feeding, Revised Principles and Recommendations, RAPID ADVICE, Geneva, Switzerland, November 2009. Available at: http://www.who.int/hiv/pub/paediatric/advice/en/index.html. (Accessed 4 January 2010).

WHO, WFP, UNICEF. *Joint Statement on Preventing and Controlling Micronutrient Deficiencies, in Populations Affected by an Emergency.* Geneva: WHO, 2006.

WHO, WFP & UNICEF. Preventing and controlling micronutrient deficiencies in populations affected by an emergency. Multiple vitamin and mineral supplements for pregnant and lactating women and for children aged 6–59 months. Joint statement of the World Health Organisation, the World Food programme and the United Nations Children's Fund. 2006.

World Bank. *Repositioning Nutrition as Central to Development: A Strategy for Large-Scale Action.* Washington: World Bank, 2006.

Zachariah R Fitzgerald M Massaquoi M *et al.* Risk factors for high early mortality in patients on antiretroviral treatment in a rural district of Malawi. *AIDS* 2006 Nov 28; 20(18):2355–60.

Section 4
HEALTHY LIVING AND LONG-TERM MANAGEMENT

12 Medications, Adherence and Interactions with Food

Angela Bailey

Key Points

- Antiretroviral therapy (ART) is highly effective at preventing HIV-related morbidity and mortality.
- ART should be started if : symptomatic; CD4 < 200; CD4 < 350 but >200 and ready to start; may be indicated if CD4 > 350 and significant co-morbidities/older age.
- ART drugs have interactions with commonly used medications – check if you are not sure. There are also interactions with food and some ART.
- ART only works if you take it – adherence support is key.
- Choice of regimen should be guided by up to date local guidelines.
- ART is also used in prevention of HIV-PMTCT (Prevention of Mother-to-Child Transmission), PEP (Post-Exposure Prohyslaxis) and may be used for other strategies in future.

12.1 HIV medications – background

Effective anti-HIV medications ('antiretrovirals') have transformed HIV infection from a progressive, terminal illness to a chronic, manageable disease (Mocroft *et al.*, 1998; May *et al.*, 2007). This chapter aims to discuss the classes of drug used and their mechanisms of action; how regimens are chosen and constructed; adverse effects of these medications; drug–drug and drug–food interactions; and the importance of adherence in treating HIV.

12.1.1 Some terminology

There are a number of terms in use for describing HIV therapy, such as 'Highly Active Antiretroviral Therapy' (HAART) and 'Combination Antiretroviral Therapy' (cART). The only combinations now in general use are those shown to be highly active and therefore in this book we use the term ART (antiretroviral therapy).

12.1.2 How do antiretroviral drugs work?

There are six different classes (including two classes blocking HIV entry) of drugs working at different stages of the HIV life cycle (see Figure 12.1). The currently available drugs are listed in Table 12.1 by class, including those in the later stages of clinical trials.

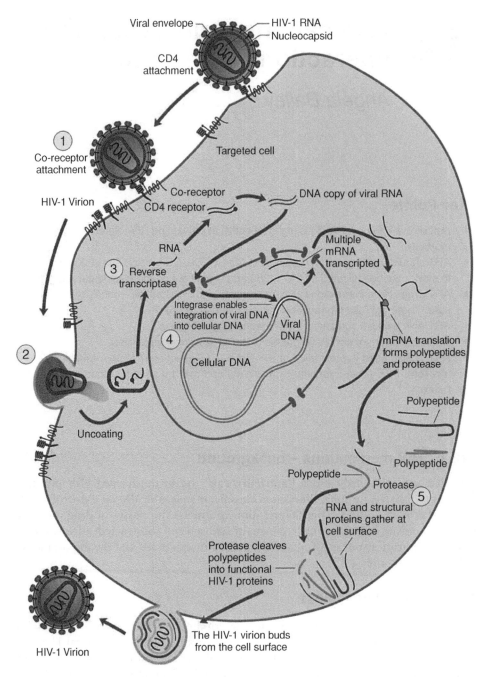

Figure 12.1   The lifecycle of HIV and mechanism of action of antiretroviral drugs. From Leake, 2007.

Table 12.1   Currently available antiretroviral drugs by class.[*]

NRTI	NNRTI	Protease inhibitors	Entry inhibitors	Integrase inhibitors
Abacavir[a]	Efavirenz[b]	Atazanavir	Enfuvirtide	Raltegravir
Didanosine	Etravirine	Darunavir	Maraviroc	(Elvitegravir)[c]
Emtricitabine[b,d]	Nevirapine	Fosamprenavir	(Vicriviroc)[c]	
Lamivudine[a,e]	(Rilpivirine)[c]	Indinavir		
Stavudine		Lopinavir[f]		
Tenofovir[b,d]		Nelfinavir		
Zidovudine[e]		Ritonavir[f]		
		Saquinavir		
		Tipranavir		

[*]This table refers to the UK. In resource limited settings, generic versions of some drugs, mainly stavudine, zidovudine, lamivudine, nevirapine, efavirenz, and various fixed-dose combinations of these are available at much lower prices than the proprietary brands, and are the mainstay of the World Health Organization push to roll out antiretroviral treatment globally (World Health Organisation, 2006).
[a]Co-formulated as Kivexa®
[b]Co-formulated as Atripla®
[c]Unlicensed medications shown in brackets.
[d]Co-formulated as Truvada®
[e]Co-formulated as Combivir®
[f]Co-formulated as Kaletra®

Their mechanisms of action are as follows, illustrated in the HIV life cycle (Figure 12.1).

1.   Entry inhibitors – currently available drugs bind to CCR5 receptors on immune cells, blocking their use as a co-receptor for cell entry by HIV. There are investigational agents which block the other co-receptor for HIV entry, the CXCR-4 receptor but these remain far from clinical practice. The CCR5 inhibitors are the only antiretroviral drug class targeting a human receptor, which has led to concerns about safety but those currently available have had a good safety profile in clinical trials (Landovitz *et al.*, 2008; MacArthur and Novak, 2008).
2.   Fusion inhibitors block gp41, a viral surface protein, preventing the conformational change necessary to allow fusion of viral and cell membranes, thereby preventing entry of viral nuclear material into the cell (Cervia and Smith, 2003).
3.   Two classes of drug act on the viral reverse transcriptase enzyme which converts viral RNA into the DNA copies needed to integrate into the host cell DNA and make new viruses:
       Nucleoside reverse transcriptase inhibitors (NRTIs) and closely related nucleotide reverse transcriptase inhibitors (NtRTIs) are nucleic acid analogues and work by terminating the DNA chain as reverse transcriptase copies viral RNA into DNA. They also have an effect on some human DNA processing enzymes, particularly mitochondrial DNA (Leake Date and Fisher, 2007).
       Non-nucleoside reverse transcriptase inhibitors (NNRTIs) bind tightly to and block the reverse transcriptase enzyme (Leake Date and Fisher, 2007).
4.   Integrase inhibitors block the integrase enzyme which incorporates viral copy DNA into the cellular DNA (Jegede *et al.*, 2008).
5.   Protease inhibitors (PIs) bind to the viral protease blocking cleavage of the viral amino acid chain to its constituent proteins. The can be pharmacologically 'boosted' by giving a small dose of one PI, ritonavir, a potent inhibitor of the

liver enzyme which breaks down these drugs, alongside other PIs to improve levels and half-life in the body. This improves potency and allows more flexible dosing (Leake Date and Fisher, 2007).

12.1.3 Combining antiretrovirals in ART regimens

In the early days of HIV therapy it rapidly became clear that monotherapy and dual therapy have limited effect due to the development of viral resistance. HIV mutates rapidly and therefore is able to evolve resistance to drugs and combinations of drugs which don't (almost) completely suppress viral replication.

The breakthrough came when three drugs from two classes (initially 2 NRTIs and a PI) were combined suppressing viral replication sufficiently to prevent evolution of resistance, allowing recovery of the immune system and long-term healthy survival in the patient. (Hammer *et al.*, 1997). The current convention is still to use three drugs – 2 NRTIs plus an NNRTI or a boosted PI. International guidelines concur on this approach and the specific drug recommendations are summarised in Table 12.2. It is essential to consult the geographically appropriate website for the most current recommendations, as they are updated frequently in light of emerging evidence.

The initial goals of ART were to prevent HIV-related mortality and morbidity. This is now achievable (Murphy *et al.*, 2001) and developments are aimed towards improving tolerability, reducing long-term side effects and providing convenience in administration. We will now discuss in more detail considerations for selecting ART drugs and regimens and the reasons behind current recommendations.

12.1.4 Choosing an ART regimen in antiretroviral naïve patients

A number of factors need to be considered when selecting a regimen.

Efficacy/potency

It is important to use only combinations of medications that are proven in clinical trials as not all regimens are the same. For example, tenofovir + didanosine + efavirenz was tried and discarded due to such high virological failure rates that a study was stopped at 12 weeks (Maitland *et al.*, 2005). Some previously used combinations are regarded as insufficiently potent, for example combinations of 3 NRTIs alone, and unboosted protease inhibitors, since they performed less well than comparators (Walmsley *et al.*, 2002; Gulick *et al.*, 2004).

Efficacy: Boosted PI or NNRTI?
Regimens based on boosted PIs and those based on NNRTIs are known to be potent. There is data comparing the two classes directly from several studies. Firstly, the ACTG5142 study, where patients were randomised to Lopinavir/ritonavir with 2NRTIs, Efavirenz with 2NRTI or Lopinavir/ritonavir plus Efavirenz (sparing the NRTI class). The efavirenz/NRTI arm in this study performed better than the Lopinavir/ritonavir/NRTI arm, with a higher proportion of patients remaining virologically suppressed at 96 weeks. The ACTG 5202 study compared efavirenz with atazanavir/ritonavir, with a second randomisation to abacavir/lamivudine or tenofovir/emtricitabine. The PI arm was non-inferior to efavirenz with both backbones and independent of viral load at baseline. Finally, the ARTEN study compared

Table 12.2 Summary of most recent guidelines for treatment of HIV-infected adults.

Guidelines	Summary of preference	NRTIs	NNRTIs	PIs
BHIVA (Gazzard, 2008) 2008 preferred www.bhiva.org	2NRTIs + efavirenz	Tenofovir + emtricitabine Or Abacavir + lamivudine	Efavirenz	
BHIVA 2008 alternative		Didanosine + lamivudine or emtricitabine Zidovudine + lamivudine		Lopinavir/rit Fosamprenavir/rit Atazanavir/rit Saquinavir/rit
DHHS (Panel on Antiretroviral Guidelines for Adult and Adolescents, 2008) 2008 preferred www.aidsinfo.nih.gov	2NRTIs + NNRTI or boosted PI	Tenofovir + emtricitabine	Efavirenz	Atazanavir/rit Darunavir/rit od Fosamprenavir/rit bd Lopinavir/rit od or bd
DHHS 2008 alternative		Abacavir + lamivudine Didanosine + lamivudine or emtricitabine Zidovudine + lamivudine	Nevirapine	Atazanavir unboosted od Fosamprenavir/rit od or unboosted bd Saquinavir/rit bd
EACS (Clumeck et al., 2008) 2008 preferred http://www.europeanaidsclinicalsociety.org/	2NRTIs + NNRTI or boosted PI	Tenofovir + emtricitabine Or Abacavir + lamivudine	Efavirenz or Nevirapine	Fosamprenavir/rit od or bd Lopinavir/rit od or bd Saquinavir/rit od or bd Atazanavir/rit
EACS 2008 Alternative		Zidovudine + lamivudine Didanosine + lamivudine or emtricitabine		Darunavir/rit od
WHO (2006) 2006 preferred http://www.who.int/hiv/pub/arv/adult/en/index.html	2NRTIs + NNRTI	Zidovudine or tenofovir plus lamivudine or emtricitabine	Efavirenz or nevirapine	For second-line use only
WHO 2006 alternative		Stavudine* or abacavir plus lamivudine or emtricitabine		

*2009 guidelines from WHO recommend phasing out stavudine from national ART programmes, although this may take some time to implement as the alternatives are more expensive.

atazanavir/ritonavir with nevirapine, both with tenofovir/emtricitabine and demonstrated non-inferiority for nevirapine alongside good tolerability (Daar *et al.* 2010, Soriano V *et al.*, 2009). Direct randomised comparisons of other boosted PIs with efavirenz or nevirapine, are so far unavailable.

Efficacy: Which NNRTI?
Within the NNRTI class, a head-to-head trial (2NN) comparing nevirapine and efavirenz, was performed to compare efficacy and while the nevirapine arm did not meet criteria for non-inferiority to efavirenz, the efavirenz arm was not statistically superior (van Leth *et al.*, 2004). There is cohort data suggesting that efavirenz might be more potent (Phillips *et al.*, 2001; Bannister *et al.*, 2008) and in the light of the ACTG5142 study (see the above paragraph) and the toxicity outcomes of 2NN (to be discussed shortly), most guidelines recommend efavirenz with nevirapine used as an alternative for some patient groups.

Efficacy: Which boosted PI?
Within the boosted PI class, there is recent data in naïve patients showing that darunavir/ritonavir once daily is superior to lopinavir/ritonavir (mixed population of once and twice daily dosing)(Ortiz *et al.*, 2008). Other studies have shown non-inferiority of atazanavir/ritonavir (once daily)(Molina *et al.*, 2008), fosamprenavir/ritonavir (twice daily)(Eron *et al.*, 2006) and saquinavir/ritonavir (twice daily) (Walmsley *et al.*, 2009) to lopinavir/ritonavir (dosed twice daily). Comparisons of other PIs with darunavir are not yet available.

Efficacy: Which NRTIs?
Moving on to NRTIs, tenofovir + emtricitabine combination has demonstrated superiority (Arribas *et al.*, 2007) and abacavir + lamivudine has demonstrated non-inferiority (DeJesus *et al.*, 2004) to the previous gold standard of zidovudine + lamivudine in randomised trials. However, there is some concern about the potency of abacavir + lamivudine in patients with baseline viral loads above 100 000 copies/ml. ACTG5202 is a double-blind, randomised controlled trial with a two-way randomisation, first to abacavir + lamivudine or tenofovir + emtricitabine and then to efavirenz or boosted atazanavir (Sax *et al.*, 2008). Participants were stratified by baseline viral load and the high viral load arm was unblinded early due to a planned review of data indicating that those on abacavir + lamivudine in the high viral load stratum were less likely to suppress to undetectable. The low viral load stratum remained blinded and the study was ongoing at the time of going to press. Previous trials using once daily abacavir + lamivudine have not shown this finding (Pappa *et al.*, 2008; Smith *et al.*, 2008) but this large trial must be taken seriously while further data and other comparative studies are awaited.

There was a concern over the efficacy of tenofovir + lamivudine or emtricitabine when used with nevirapine (but not with efavirenz or boosted PIs). Two small studies, one each using lamivudine and emtricitabine, have shown unacceptably high rates of early virological failure (Lapadula *et al.*, 2008; Rey *et al.*, 2009). A larger randomised study, the ARTEN study, showed acceptable efficacy and tolerability of tenofovir + emtricitabine with nevirapine, providing reassurance that this combination works well (Soriano V *et al.*, 2009).

Other NRTI combinations which have shown acceptable efficacy include didanosine + lamivudine (Berenguer *et al.*, 2008) or emtricitabine (Molina *et al.*, 2007) and stavudine + lamivudine (Squires *et al.*, 2000).

Efficacy: Newer agents

Raltegravir has been evaluated in treatment-naïve individuals and been shown to be non-inferior to efavirenz when combined with tenofovir + emtricitabine (Markowitz *et al.*, 2007).

Maraviroc was compared to efavirenz in this group in combination with zidovudine + lamivudine in the MERIT study, and failed to demonstrate non-inferiority (Saag *et al.*, 2007). However, in a reanalysis of the MERIT data after excluding patients with CXCR4 tropic virus at baseline on a newer, more sensitive assay for tropism than that available when MERIT was undertaken, the criteria for non-inferiority are met (Saag *et al.*, 2008). This reanalysis is post hoc and not truly randomised but is interesting and may lead to a revisiting of the role of this drug in naïve patients.

Rilpivirine, a second-generation NNRTI, has shown promising efficacy and tolerability in a 96-week follow-up of a phase IIB study compared to efavirenz. Phase III studies were in progress with data expected to be available in a few years at the time of going to press.

Etravirine, a second-generation NNRTI currently licensed in treatment-experienced patients, has not been investigated in treatment-naïve patients in phase III studies and is unlikely to be in the near future. Similarly, tipranavir, a second-generation PI, is not characterised in this population.

12.1.5   Toxicity and tolerability

Both long and short-term toxicities are important in selecting drugs. Some side effects such as nausea or tiredness are common in the early stages of taking a regimen, and can be managed symptomatically or expectantly. However, if such symptoms persist they may impact on adherence and, consequently, long-term success of the treatment (Chesney *et al.*, 2000; Bartlett, 2002).

The improved life expectancy with ART, with patients expected to survive for decades if treated, has led to a renewed focus on identifying, avoiding and preventing long-term toxicity.

Toxicity: PI or NNRTI?

In ACTG 5142 (comparing lopinavir/ritonavir + 2NRTIs, efavirenz + 2NRTIs and lopinavir/ritonavir + efavirenz), there was no difference in treatment limiting adverse events across the three arms (Riddler *et al.*, 2008). However, there are differences in side effect profiles associated with efavirenz and lopinavir/ritonavir, with efavirenz causing rashes and central nervous system symptoms such as vivid dreams and dizziness, whereas lopinavir/ritonavir more frequently causes diarrhoea. In the metabolic sub-study of this trial, the NRTI sparing regimen caused a significantly greater increase in lipids than the other two arms. The PI class is associated with lipid abnormalities, gastrointestinal disturbance and lipodystrophy, whereas the NNRTI class is more associated with rash and has fewer metabolic toxicities. The D:A:D:

study, a large cohort study set up to look for toxicities in antiretrovirals, found an increased risk of myocardial infarction with boosted PIs, which was not seen with NNRTIs (Lundgren *et al.*, 2009).

Toxicity: Which NNRTI?

Most guidelines prefer efavirenz to nevirapine in most patients, for reasons of toxicity. Nevirapine can cause Stevens-Johnson syndrome (a potentially fatal severe rash) and fulminant hepatotoxicity. These severe early toxicities can be limited by restricting nevirapine to men with CD4 cell counts <400 cells/mm^3 and women with CD4 cell counts <250 cells/mm^3, where the risk is much lower (Boehringer Ingelheim Limited, 2007). Set against these relatively rare severe toxicities, nevirapine does not cause the same CNS side effects as efavirenz and for those who escape the early toxicities this may be an advantage. The other patient group where nevirapine is indicated (if CD4 cell count critieria are met) is women of childbearing age who may become pregnant. Efavirenz is currently contraindicated in these women due to teratogenicity in animal experiments and several retrospectively reported cases of teratogenicity in humans (Watts, 2007). The prospectively collected ART pregnancy registry has not found any evidence of a teratogenic effect so far.

Toxicity: Which PI?

As discussed previously, there are no randomised head-to-head comparisons of all the boosted PIs with all the others. However, where these exist it is possible to compare the adverse event profiles. In the ARTEMIS study (Ortiz *et al.*, 2008), darunavir 800 mg + ritonavir 100 mg was associated with significantly fewer grade 2–4 lipid elevations and less diarrhoea than lopinavir + ritonavir, which may relate to the higher ritonavir dose with lopinavir. Atazanavir + ritonavir was also better tolerated than twice daily lopinavir + ritonavir, in terms of diarrhoea and some lipid parameters in several studies (Johnson *et al.*, 2006; Molina *et al.*, 2008). However, atazanavir has its own particular toxicity, causing unconjugated hyperbilirubinaemia and jaundice in up to one-third of patients due to a harmless inhibition of UDP glucuronosyl transferase. Boosted saquinavir also caused less diarrhoea than lopinavir + ritonavir in a comparative study (Walmsley *et al.*, 2009), whereas fosamprenavir + ritonavir was associated with similar rates (Eron *et al.*, 2006). Indinavir + ritonavir is associated with kidney stones and is now uncommonly used (Youle, 2007b).

The D:A:D study finding, that cumulative exposure to a PI + ritonavir increases the risk of myocardial infarction, was broken down by PI (Lundgren *et al.*, 2009). The risk was statistically significant with lopinavir and with fosamprenavir. Darunavir and tipranavir were not included in the analysis.

Toxicity: Which NRTIs?

Traditionally, the NRTIs were associated with mitochondrial toxicity, leading to pancreatitis, lactic acidosis, neuropathy and lipodystrophy (Leake Date and Fisher, 2007). Stavudine is no longer recommended due to high rates of these problems. Didanosine is also implicated, particularly in neuropathy (Cherry *et al.*, 2006), and has also been linked to unexplained liver disease and is consequently not a preferred choice (Saifee *et al.*, 2008). The link between zidovudine and lipodystrophy (Dube *et al.*, 2007), which took longer to be demonstrated, has led clinicians and guidelines to move to newer drugs, such as abacavir and tenofovir, in naïve patients. Neither of these drugs is associated with lipodystrophy and both are well tolerated. However, the toxicity profiles are distinct.

Abacavir causes hypersensitivity reactions in a proportion (3–5%) of patients (Ruane and DeJesus, 2004). This reaction can be largely prevented by screening for an associated HLA type and excluding patients of that type from abacavir use (Mallal *et al.*, 2008). However, data from the D:A:D study found that abacavir use was associated with an increased risk of myocardial infarction (RR 1.9) (D:A:D Study Group, 2008). This risk seemed to disappear when the abacavir is stopped and the mechanism is as yet unexplained. The only other NRTI causing a similar increase in risk is didanosine and it is not seen with tenofovir (Lundgren *et al.*, 2009). Since the original results were published, there have been several further presentations looking at this and most (but not all) have shown a similar effect. There is much interest in the mechanism by which abacavir increases cardiovascular risk but it is not yet explained.

Of course, tenofovir is not without toxicity and has been associated with renal toxicity, including Fanconi's syndrome (proximal renal tubular acidosis), but this is rare in post-marketing surveillance (Nelson *et al.*, 2007). When it does occur, it is more common when co-administered with a PI and those patients with pre-existing renal problems are most at risk. There is also some data to suggest a detrimental effect of tenofovir on bone density, including in a randomised comparison with abacavir (Cooper *et al.*, 2009). The mechanism of this is not yet explained but theories include effects on phosphate metabolism via the renal tubular effect and some effect on the vitamin D pathway.

The toxicity profiles of lamivudine and emtricitabine are similar, with both being well tolerated, but emtricitabine can cause pigmentation on palms, which resolves on stopping the drug (Ruane and DeJesus, 2004).

Toxicity: Newer agents

In the STARTMRK studies, raltegravir was better tolerated than efavirenz, with fewer CNS adverse effects and fewer episodes of rash (Markowitz *et al.*, 2007). Maraviroc is also a well tolerated drug in clinical trials (Lieberman-Blum *et al.*, 2008). As these drugs are new, long-term side effects remain to be delineated and there have been concerns about the effect of maraviroc, in particular, as it blocks a human cellular receptor, although safety data to date is satisfactory. Rilpivirine has been shown to cause lower rates of rash and CNS effects than efavirenz (Santoscoy *et al.*, 2008) and it had entered phase III studies at the time of going to press. Boosted tipranavir was associated with higher rates of hepatic and lipid toxicity than comparator PIs in the RESIST studies, but these adverse effects rarely led to treatment discontinuation (and may be related to the higher dose of ritonavir used with tipranavir) (Youle, 2007b). Etravirine was well tolerated by treatment-experienced patients, with rash the main adverse effect seen (Madruga *et al.*, 2007).

12.1.6 Robustness or barrier to resistance

HIV evolves rapidly and can become resistant to antiretroviral treatments that are not fully suppressive (Deeks, 2006). The ease with which the virus can evolve resistance to a particular drug or class of drugs is variable and thought of as the barrier to resistance of that drug or regimen. Where clinicians are concerned about the likely adherence of a patient, they may choose regimens that are more robust, hoping to avoid development of resistance and preserve future options (Gazzard BG on behalf of the BHIVA Treatment Guidelines Writing Group, 2008). The main objective is always to ensure the regimen chosen is sufficiently potent to suppress the patient's virus, as this is the best way to avoid resistance.

Robustness: Boosted PI or NNRTI?

The main disadvantage of the first-generation NNRTIs is the ease with which HIV can evolve resistance to them. The virus requires only a single mutation in its genome to acquire high-level resistance to the whole class of drugs. Consequently, while efavirenz- or nevirapine-based therapy fails in only a small proportion of patients, when it does, resistance is likely to develop, both in clinical trials and cohort studies (van Leth *et al.*, 2004; Bannister *et al.*, 2008; Riddler *et al.*, 2008). Boosted PIs have a much higher barrier to resistance, with multiple mutations required and a more step-wise loss of drug sensitivity. When boosted PI regimens fail this often happens with no new resistance to the PI or NRTI components of their regimen (Ortiz *et al.*, 2008; Riddler *et al.*, 2008; Walmsley *et al.*, 2009).

Robustness: Which NNRTI?

Efavirenz and nevirapine are essentially equivalent in terms of development of resistance (Waters *et al.*, 2007). The newer, second-generation NNRTIs (etravirine and rilpivirine) are more robust and are active against many viruses which are resistant to first-generation drugs. (Ripamonti and Maggiolo, 2008; Johnson and Saravolatz, 2009) However, etravirine is used only in treatment-experienced patients and rilpivirine remains in phase III trials, so first-generation NNRTIs remain the drugs of choice for naïve patients.

Robustness: Which boosted PI?

In clinical trials, all the boosted PIs have been shown to have a high barrier to resistance. The second-generation PIs, darunavir and tipranavir, have activity against HIV resistant to other PIs but have not been shown to be more robust (Youle, 2007b).

Robustness: Which NRTIs?

Lamivudine and emtricitabine have a one-step resistance pathway, where a single mutation confers high-level resistance and are therefore fragile drugs. Zidovudine and stavudine are more robust, with a step-wise accrual of resistance over time. The development of resistance to other NRTIs is complex and can follow different pathways, with interactions between the NRTI drug pairs playing a role. There are also different resistance patterns seen in different HIV-1 subtypes (Geretti, 2006).

Robustness: Newer agents

Resistance to integrase inhibitors is still being characterised, but it is apparent that resistance can develop quickly and that there is cross-class resistance to the

Table 12.3 Licensed antiretroviral preparations.

Drug	Dosing frequency	Pills per dose	Pills per day
NRTI combination tablets			
Abacavir+Lamivudine	Once daily	1	1
Tenofovir + Emtricitabine	Once daily	1	1
Zidovudine + Lamivudine	Twice daily	1	2
NRTI + NNRTI combination tablets			
Tenofovir + Emtricitabine + Efavirenz	Once daily	1	1
Stavudine + Lamivudine + Nevirapine[*]	Twice daily	1	1
NNRTIs			
Efavirenz	Once daily	1	1
Nevirapine	Twice daily[a]	1	2
Boosted PIs			
Atazanavir + ritonavir	Once daily	1 atazanavir +1 ritonavir[b]	2
Darunavir + ritonavir	Once daily	2 darunavir + 1 ritonavir[b]	3
Fosamprenavir + ritonavir	Twice daily	1 fosamprenavir + 1 ritonavir[b]	4
Indinavir + ritonavir	Twice daily	1 indinavir 400 mg + 1 ritonavir[b]	4
Lopinavir + ritonavir combination tablet	Twice daily	2 combined tablets	4
Saquinavir + ritonavir	Twice daily	2 saquinavir + 1 ritonavir[b]	6

[*]This combination is available in many countries, produced by generic manufacturers.
[a]Nevirapine is commenced with a 200 mg once daily lead in dose for the first two weeks of therapy before increasing to bd. It is commonly used as 400 mg once daily in patients established on therapy for more than 12 weeks but is licensed as twice daily (Podzamczer *et al.*, 2009).
[b]100 mg capsule or heat stable tablet where available.

first-generation drugs (Evering and Markowitz, 2008). Clinicians view this class as more robust than NNRTIs but still more vulnerable than PIs.

Maraviroc and other CCR5 inhibitors target a human cellular receptor rather than a viral target. Resistance to these drugs has been seen via two different mechanisms, with the virus switching to use the alternative co-receptor (CXCR4) to enter CD4 cells in some cases and in others a change in the interaction with CCR5 to escape from the drug block (Fatkenheuer *et al.*, 2008; Gulick *et al.*, 2008).

12.1.7 Pill burden and dosing interval

The table above contains licensed antiretroviral preparations at the time of going to press and refers to licensed dosing for antiretroviral naïve patients. It is not exhaustive and includes only widely used drugs recommended in guidelines. Other combinations, particularly of NRTIs, are available in some parts of the world such as stavudine + lamivudine combination tablets produced by generic manufacturers. Other dosing regimens may also be used in treatment-experienced patients or off-licence and are not covered here.

When asked, patients generally prefer fewer pills, fewer times per day (Bartlett, 2002). The evidence that having one pill rather than two pills has a significant impact on adherence is, however, lacking. One advantage of fixed dose combination tablets is that it is impossible to take part of a regimen, which should minimise the risk of resistance (Table 12.3).

12.1.8   Cost

The issue of cost of antiretrovirals particularly affects lower income settings, where most HIV-infected individuals live. The WHO guidelines for antiretroviral treatment (World Health Organisation, 2006), which take a public health approach, recommend generic preparations which have been pre-qualified as these tend to be cheaper. The first-line recommendation is now zidovudine or tenofovir with lamivudine or emtricitabine plus efavirenz or nevirapine. However, in many countries, the cheaper generic combination of stavudine + lamivudine + nevirapine is still the first-line option as it is all they can afford.

In higher-income countries, cost pressures have previously had little impact on HIV drug choice, but this may change in the future as pressure on health care systems increases. Cost-effectiveness is established for ART in general (Beck *et al.*, 2008), but may become important particularly for newer medications in naïve patients, where older, cheaper options exist.

12.1.9   Neurological penetration

There is increasing interest in mild and moderate neurocognitive impairments in HIV-infected individuals. The prevalence of HIV-associated dementia is rare since the advent of antiretroviral therapy, but recent studies looking at milder effects have found that up to half of patients have some impairment (Heaton *et al.*, 2009). There is some evidence that impairment may be associated with ongoing HIV replication in the central nervous system (CNS) and that this may be attenuated by using medications which penetrate well into that compartment (Canestri *et al.*, 2009). Among the NRTIs, abacavir and zidovudine penetrate best into the CNS compartment while tenofovir has lower penetration. In the NNRTIs, nevirapine penetrates better than efavirenz but further data suggests that efavirenz levels in CSF may still reach therapeutic levels. In the boosted PI class, lopinavir + ritonavir has the best CNS penetration Letendre *et al.*, 2006).

This is an area of ongoing research and it is difficult to select regimens solely on this basis, but it may become more important in future and particularly for patients with neurocognitive dysfunction.

12.1.10   Co-morbidities and opportunistic infections

Other medical conditions, both HIV related and unrelated, may guide choice of antiretroviral regimen. A few examples are listed here:

- The increased relative risk of MI associated with abacavir is particularly important for patients with a moderate or high CVD risk where the absolute risk is high, and clinicians may avoid this drug in those individuals.
- Patients who have renal impairment may need to avoid tenofovir in case of renal toxicity.
- Hepatitis virus co-infection influences choice of NRTI, as tenofovir, lamivudine and emtricitabine are all active against Hepatitis B as well as HIV (Levy and Grant, 2006). In HCV co-infected individuals who need treatment for their hepatitis, careful ART selection is required to avoid or minimise toxicity and maximise chances of success (Soriano *et al.*, 2007).

- Patients requiring chemotherapy may need to avoid zidovudine to minimize risk of anaemia and there is evidence that PIs increase the risk of neutropenia (Bower *et al.*, 2008).

Drug–drug interactions will be discussed more fully below, but if an essential drug for an infection or medical condition, e.g. epilepsy, interacts with an antiretroviral, this may influence choice or regimen.

12.1.11   When to initiate therapy

In primary HIV infection there is currently no data to support initiation of ART and it is not recommended except in patients with severe symptoms such as meningoencephalitis. The results of a large randomised study looking at short-course ART in seroconverters are awaited. In chronic HIV infection, it has been clear for a number of years that in symptomatic patients and those with opportunistic infections or CD4 cell counts below 200 cells/mm^3 ART should be initiated. In asymptomatic patients with CD4 cell counts above 200 cells/mm^3, there has been debate for the last few years, particularly as there is no randomised controlled trial to guide practice. In the 2008 guidelines, both European and American, there was a shift to recommending earlier commencement of treatment (Clumeck *et al.*, 2008; Gazzard BG on behalf of the BHIVA Treatment Guidelines Writing Group, 2008; Panel on Antiretroviral Guidelines for Adult and Adolescents, 2008). This was based on evidence from cohort studies, suggesting that benefit, albeit small in absolute terms, can be gained by starting at 350 rather than 200 (Phillips *et al.*, 2007b). In addition, the availability of newer, more convenient and effective ART regimens and new classes of drug for those for whom initial therapy failed has addressed some of the issues that led to the previous conservative approach, namely that by starting earlier people would 'run out' of drugs sooner due to development of resistance and that the long-term toxicity of the medications was such that exposure should be limited. On this latter point, a key piece of evidence supporting earlier ART comes from the SMART study, a large multicentre randomised trial comparing continuous therapy with the aim of virological suppression with 'drug conservation' where therapy was stopped when CD4 cell count reached 350 and restarted when it fell to 250. The hypothesis was that those on continuous therapy would experience more drug side effects, offsetting the possible increase in opportunistic infections in the drug conservation arm. In fact, both AIDS and non-AIDS outcomes (renal disease, liver disease and cardiovascular disease) were significantly more common in the drug conservation arm and the trial was stopped early (El-Sadr *et al.*, 2006). A subgroup of the SMART study participants were off therapy at enrolment and this group allowed a comparison of immediate versus deferred therapy in those with CD4 >350. The immediate therapy group did better both in terms of AIDS and non-AIDS events, further evidence to support early treatment initiation (Emery *et al.*, 2008).

In some groups, ART is recommended at CD4 cell counts >350 cells/mm^3, for example hepatitis B co-infected patients or those at high risk of co-morbities (Gazzard, 2008). Recent cohort data has suggested that there may be benefit from starting therapy at CD4 cell counts >500 cells/mm^3 (Phillips *et al.*, 2007a; Kitahata *et al.*, 2008)and this hypothesis will be tested in a large, randomised controlled trial (the START study) which commenced in 2009.

For resource-poor countries, where the vast numbers requiring treatment necessitates a protocol-led treatment roll out, the recommendation changed to commencing therapy at CD4 cell count <350 cells/mm^3 in 2009, but this will take some time to implement (WHO 2009). The change from the previous recommended level of 200 cells/mm^3 follows developed world guidelines and a study in Haiti which found a significant reduction in morbidity and mortality when the earlier level is used. (Starting Antiretroviral Therapy Earlier Yields Better Clinical Outcomes. *NIH News* June 8, 2009.)

12.1.12   How do you know ART is working?

Monitoring is performed via blood tests to measure viral load (the quantity of virus per ml of blood) and CD4 cell count (measure of immune status) (see Chapter 1). Initially, it was believed that ART would completely eradicate the virus from the body, but we now know that viral replication persists in reservoir sites (such as the lymph nodes) even when the virus is undetectable in the blood by conventional assays (Marsden and Zack, 2009).

12.2   Drug interactions

12.2.1   Mechanism of drug interactions

Medications may interact by virtue of their effects. This can be synergistic such as zidovudine and lamivudine, producing additional benefit to the two agents given alone. It can also be antagonistic, such as zidovudine and stavudine. These drugs are activated by the same enzyme inside cells and therefore compete for it, reducing activity of both if co-administered. Drugs may also have overlapping toxicities which can work in an additive way, such as ribavirin (a hepatitis C treatment) and zidovudine, which both cause anaemia and given together cause more anaemia.

The absorption, metabolism, distribution and elimination of drugs are complex, incompletely understood and a rich source of drug interactions.

We will consider some examples of interactions involving HIV drugs at these points.

Absorption

Some drugs require an acid environment in the stomach for absorption, e.g. atazanavir. Antacid medications are therefore associated with a reduction in atazanavir levels that can be clinically significant. Didanosine is another drug which is sensitive to the effect of pH. To improve absorption, it is formulated as a tablet containing antacid, which should be taken 30 minutes before food, or as a capsule which is enteric-coated to minimise exposure to gastric acid. The capsules should be taken on an empty stomach 2 hours before or after food.

Metabolism

Many drugs are metabolised by the cytochrome P450 system in the liver, particularly the CYP3A4 enzyme. Medications can be substrates for particular enzymes, e.g. maraviroc is a substrate for CYP3A4. Enzymes can be induced (where the cells express increased levels of the enzyme) or inhibited by medications and some medications do both, e.g. efavirenz both induces and inhibits CYP3A4. This leads to pharmacokinetic interactions between different ART drugs and between ART drugs and other medications. This interaction is harnessed in ritonavir boosting of PIs: ritonavir is a potent inhibitor of the CYP3A4 enyzme and this is used to boost levels of other PIs by reducing their metabolism.

Other enzyme systems are also important for some ART drugs, such as UDP-glucuronosyltransferase 1A (UGT1A), which is inhibited by atazanavir and is responsible for the metabolism of raltegravir. P-glycoprotein (P-gp) is found in the lining of the gut, spleen and brain and is responsible for acting as a barrier and preventing the transportation of drugs or toxins into these areas. Drugs such as low-dose ritonavir which inhibit P-gp can, therefore, stop this mechanism working increasing amount of certain drugs and this is part of the boosting effect described above.

Elimination of medications can also occur in the kidney and an interaction between tenofovir and didanosine, where tenofovir leads to increased levels of didanosine, is thought to be mediated through tenofovir blocking excretion of didanosine at the renal tubule.

It is beyond the scope of this book to offer a comprehensive list of drug–drug interactions in HIV medicine but Table 12.4 lists some commonly encountered combinations. This is a fast-moving field and the safest approach is therefore always to check when giving a new medication to someone on ART, including prescription, over-the-counter and herbal preparations. There are also interactions with recreational drugs and therefore patients need to be made aware of the issues around interactions with non-prescribed drugs. Often patients will not regard items such as nasal spray or inhalers as medicines, even when asked about other sources of medicines or preparations. The website, www.hiv-druginteractions.org., is a useful resource for interaction information and tables can also be found in the US treatment guidelines (Panel on Antiretroviral Guidelines for Adult and Adolescents, 2008). HIV specialist pharmacists can also provide advice on how to manage or avoid potential drug–drug interactions and will have access to additional information sources.

12.3   Micronutrients used in HIV infection

Micronutrients may be used to prevent side effects of medications. Pyridoxine is co-administered with isoniazid, an essential component of TB treatment, to prevent neuropathy.

There have also been attempts to treat side effects of antiretroviral drugs, mainly neuropathy but also lipodystrophy, using micronutrients such as acetyl-L-carnitine and uridine-containing food supplements (Nucleomaxx) with varying degrees of success (Youle, 2007a; McComsey *et al.*, 2008).

A number of trials are underway using milk- and colostrum-based products designed to try to improve gut permeability, which is increased in HIV (Douek, 2007), with the aim of altering disease progression.

12.4   Food and drug interactions

Early ART drugs and regimens were notorious for being complex and requiring careful attention to food and liquid timing and consumption. Modern regimens are easier to take but some still require food for optimal absorption (Atazanavir + ritonavir) (BMS, 2009), Darunavir/ritonavir (Janssen-Cilag, 2009b), some require

Table 12.4 Examples of interactions with ART and commonly used drugs.

Drug name	Interaction with ART	Action required
Opportunistic infection drugs		
Erythromycin	Increased exposure with ritonavir (even at low boosting doses (Abbott Laboratories Limited, 2008).	Monitor, consider use of alternative such as azithromycin.
	Potential interaction with nevirapine (Boehringer Ingelheim Limited, 2007). suggest remove (not mentioned on 2009 SPC)	
Clarithromycin	Increased clarithromycin exposure with ritonavir (Abbott, 2008).	Monitor. Consider dose reduction of clarithromycin in renal impairment.
	Increased clarithromycin exposure and atazanavir exposure when co-administered without ritonavir (Bristol-Myers Squibb Pharmaceuticals Ltd, 2009a, 2009b).	Consider use of alternative such as azithromycin with NNRTIs.
	Reduced clarithromycin levels with NNRTIs (Boehringer Ingelheim, 2007; BMS, 2008a; Janssen-Cilag Ltd, 2009a).	Reduce dose maraviroc.
	Maraviroc likely to be increased (Pfizer Limited, 2009).	
Rifampicin	Reduces levels of NNRTIs and all boosted PIs (Boehringer Ingelheim, 2007; Roche Products Limited, 2008b; Abbott, 2009; BMS, 2009; Boehringer Ingelheim, 2009); GlaxoSmithKline (GSK) UK, 2009; Janssen-Cilag, 2009a; Janssen-Cilag Ltd, 2009b.	Increase dose efavirenz. Contraindicated with PIs, nevirapine (some increase dose) and etravirine.
	Reduces levels of raltegravir (Merck Sharp & Dohme (MSD) Limited, 2009).	
	Reduces levels of maraviroc (Pfizer, 2009).	Increase maraviroc dose.
Rifabutin	Ritonavir increases rifabutin level significantly. (Abbott, 2008) [77]	Do not administer with full dose ritonavir. Reduce rifabutin dose with low-dose ritonavir, i.e. all boosted PIs (to 150 mg three times per week).
	Efavirenz reduces rifabutin exposure (BMS, 2008a).	Increase rifabutin dose to 450 mg daily.
	Etravirine and rifabutin levels are reduced with co-administration (Janssen-Cilag, 2009a).	No dose adjustment is needed for either drug. Do not co-administer with boosted PI as there is a risk of significantly reduced etravirine exposure.

(Continued)

Table 12.4 (*Continued*).

Drug name	Interaction with ART	Action required
	Nevirapine increases rifabutin exposure in some patients. (Boehringer Ingelheim, 2007)	No dose adjustments are necessary but monitor for adverse effects.
Itraconazole	Ritonavir increases itraconazole exposure (Abbott, 2008).	Avoid high doses of itraconazole.
	Efavirenz, etravirine and nevirapine reduced itraconazole levels (Boehringer Ingelheim, 2007; BMS, 2008a; Janssen-Cilag Ltd, 2009a).	Consider alternative and monitor clinical effect.
	Maraviroc levels increased (Pfizer, 2009).	Reduce maraviroc dose.
Voriconazole	Ritonavir reduces voriconazole exposure (Abbott, 2008).	Avoid co-administration with boosted PIs unless likely risks/benefit to patient merit it.
	Efavirenz reduces voriconazole exposure and voriconazole increases efavirenz exposure (BMS, 2008a).	Increase voriconazole dose to 400mg bd and reduce efavirenz dose by 50% to 300 mg od.
	Co-administration with etravirine may increase levels of both drugs. (Janssen-Cilag L, 2009a)	No dose adjustment. Monitor.
	Co-administration with nevirapine may affect voriconazole metabolism (Boehringer Ingelheim, 2007).	No dose adjustment. Monitor.
Quinine	Increased quinine levels with ritonavir (Abbott, 2008).	May need to reduce quinine dose.
Antacids		
H2 receptor blockers	Reduced atazanavir levels (BMS, 2009).	Administer 12 hours apart from atazanavir.
Proton pump inhibitors	Reduced atazanavir levels by 95% (BMS, 2009).	Do not co-administer with atazanavir.
	Tipranavir reduces omeprazole levels (Boehringer Ingelheim, 2009). Saquinavir levels increased by lansoprazole (Roche, 2008b). Raltegravir levels increased with PPIs (MSD, 2009).	
Lipid lowering drugs		
Simvastatin	Levels increased by PIs leading to increased muscle toxicity (Abbott, 2008; Roche, 2008b); BMS, 2009; GSK, 2009.	Avoid co-administration.

(*Continued*)

Table 12.4   (*Continued*).

Drug name	Interaction with ART	Action required
Pravastatin	Levels increased when co-adminstered with boosted darunavir in a minority of subjects (Janssen-Cilag, 2009b). Efavirenz reduced pravastatin levels (BMS, 2008a).	Use lowest dose and titrate up.
Rosuvastatin	Increased plasma concentrations and reduced liver concentrations with ritonavir (Abbott, 2008).	Start with low dose and titrate up. Monitor effect.
Herbal medications		
St John's wort	Reduces concentrations of boosted PIs and NNRTIs (Boehringer Ingelheim, 2007; Abbott, 2008; BMS, 2008a, 2009; Roche, 2008b; Abbott, 2009; Boehringer Ingelheim, 2009); GSK, 2009; Janssen-Cilag, 2009a, 2009b.	Avoid co-administration.
Recreational drugs		
MDMA ("ecstasy")	Ritonavir may increase concentrations of MDMA (Henry and Hill, 1998; Harrington *et al.*, 1999).	Advise avoid or if cannot avoid, reduce dose.
Alcohol	Reduced tolerance in some patients with abacavir (BMS, 2009).	Warn patients.
Others		
Methadone	Ritonavir and NNRTIs can reduce methadone levels (Boehringer Ingelheim, 2007; Abbott, 2008; BMS, 2008a; Janssen-Cilag Ltd, 2009a). Etravirine does not appear to affect methadone levels (Janssen-Cilag, 2009a).	Monitor for withdrawal symptoms, increase dose as necessary over several days.
Sildenafil and other PDE5 inhibitors.	Ritonavir increases sildenafil concentrations (Abbott, 2008). Etravirine reduces sildenafil concentrations (Janssen-Cilag, 2009a).	Avoid or reduce sildenafil dose. Advise patient not to repeat dose for 72 hours
Warfarin	Ritonavir reduces effect of warfarin (Abbott, 2008).	Frequent INR monitoring initially.
	Efavirenz and Nevirapine have unpredictable effect on warfarin (Boehringer Ingelheim, 2007, BMS, 2008a). Etravirine may increase warfarin effect (Janssen-Cilag, 2009a).	Frequent INR monitoring initially.
Fluticasone (inhaled, or nasal)	Increased systemic absorption with ritonavir (Abbott, 2008).	Risk of steroid toxicity. Avoid, use alternative.

fasting pre- and post-dose (didanosine (BMS, 2008b)) and some can be taken without regard to food but there may be an impact on side effects if taken with a meal, e.g. efavirenz levels are greater if taken with a fatty meal with consequent increases in the severity of CNS effects for some patients (BMS, 2008a). Exactly how much food is required with a particular drug is often difficult to define and for some individuals these requirements can be onerous, particularly if they do not normally eat breakfast but are on twice-daily Darunavir/ritonavir or if they find fasting for 4 hours around a dose of didanosine capsules restrictive. Unboosted indinavir, which requires thrice-daily dosing on an empty stomach (no food for 2 hours before and 1 hour after) and 1 litre of water to be consumed per dose to limit renal toxicity, is rarely used now but may be the only PI available as a generic drug in some developing countries (MSD, 2008). This level of food restrictions is particularly difficult to comply with and requires significant lifestyle changes for many patients.

It may be useful for a dietician to discuss food requirements with patients and to suggest healthy ways of managing them to ensure optimal drug levels.

Many people with HIV still present late and need to take medications for opportunistic infections as well as antiretrovirals. This leads to increased pill burden but may also increase food restrictions, e.g. TB medications are often taken on an empty stomach.

12.5 Adherence

HIV is now a chronic manageable infection and infected individuals are expected to live for decades if they are able to adhere to medication (Antiretroviral Therapy Cohort Collaboration, 2008). Although newer regimens are thought to be more 'forgiving' than previously used combinations, adherence remains important. Past studies have shown that a greater than 95% adherence is needed to achieve the best results (Paterson *et al.*, 2000). Particularly in resource-rich settings where individualisation of therapy is possible within guidelines, fitting regimens to people's lives rather than trying to change their lives to fit the regimen should be possible (Bartlett, 2002) and simple measures can be employed anywhere in the world, e.g. treatment buddies and ART education and adherence support are a key part of many ART roll-out programmes worldwide. Many patients feel that they cannot, for example, switch the time of their dosing even if their routine changes, leading to difficulties such as having to take their medication at work where they have not disclosed their status. While emphasising the need to take every dose on time forever is important, clinicians should work with patients to identify potential difficulties and suggest solutions. One example of this tailoring of advice is timing of efavirenz dosing. For most people, taking efavirenz at night is best, but in a study of patients with CNS side effects who switched to morning dosing approximately half preferred this, whereas the others switched back (Skeie and Maeland, 2006). Explaining how to move doses safely, without compromising drug levels and 'giving permission' to make changes is an important part of consultations. This may be particularly important where patients travel frequently across time zones, where the advice for short trips may be to continue medications at the same (albeit inconvenient) times or to bring doses forward, resulting in too much rather than too little drug in a 24-hour period, as this approach is likely to be safest.

Another example where a pragmatic approach is needed is where a busy mother on a twice-daily regimen struggles frequently to take her morning medications as they need to be with food and she is occupied getting her children to school, not managing her own breakfast until later. This can be a particular difficulty where one or more children are also on ART. Dose time changes, switching to a once daily therapy or to a medication taken without regard to food can make her life much easier while improving her chances of maintaining virological suppression.

Even seemingly minor issues can make a big difference. Some people find that abacavir impacts on their tolerance to alcohol (Barber *et al.*, 2007). This may be trivial – you can choose not to drink at all – but if a glass of wine after work sometimes is important to them, this may impact on adherence. Changing to alternative drugs may make a big difference to quality of life.

A Cochrane review of interventions to help adherence to ART concluded that practical education and medication management interventions targeted at individuals were most likely to be beneficial (Rueda *et al.*, 2006).

12.5.1 Case study

Patient A-M was born in Burundi in 1963. She has been living in the UK since 1997 and was diagnosed with HIV infection in February 2001.

Medical conditions

Symptomatic HIV Disease
Hepatitis C infection with cirrhosis (diagnosed 2001)
Insulin-dependent diabetes mellitus since 1997
Hypertension (since 2003)

Past medical history

She started ART: zidovudine (AZT), lamivudine (3TC) efavrienz (EFV) November 2003 when CD4 down to 250 cells/mm^3 but changed to tenofovir (TDF)/3TC/EFV due to anaemia. Over the next 3 years her viral load remained undetectable and her CD4 count climbed to 502 cells/ mm^3 (27%).

A-M attended dietetic appointments infrequently. In July 2005 her diabetes was poorly controlled (blood glucose 27.9 mmol/L). Her reported dietary intake showed an intake high in fat/saturated fat, low in fruits and vegetables, and she reported a low activity level. Her BMI was 26.7 m^2. She was given dietary and lifestyle information and advice to help improve blood sugar levels, blood lipid levels, blood pressure and to reduce weight. A letter was sent to GP about arrangements for diabetes care.

This case illustrates that adherence is variable within the same patient. The patient is adhering well to her HIV medications but not to the measures required to control her diabetes. She is therefore at high risk of complications of diabetes.

She stopped taking HIV medication October 2006, which resulted in her viral load becoming detectable at 14,760 copies/ml, although her CD4 cell count remained high at 502 cells/ mm^3 (27%). Weight increased by 5 kg (BMI now 28).

What should A-M's doctor do next?

At this point a careful history is needed to explore why A-M stopped her medication and how she was taking it before she stopped. Was she experiencing side effects or is there some difficulty at home which is affecting her ability to adhere?

This will also give us some clues as to how likely it is that she has developed resistant HIV. If she was skipping doses before stopping, resistance may be even more likely. Once medication is stopped resistant virus becomes a minority species in the body and it is hard to detect resistance on testing. Clinicians may therefore have to construct a subsequent regimen with a best guess as to what will be effective.

The SMART study suggested that treatment interruption is associated with increased morbidity and mortality and it is therefore not recommended. However, when patients stop their medication for social or other reasons, it is often a good idea to try to resolve those issues before restarting to give the best chance of success.

Current medical history

Early 2007 she restarted ART and was taking the following medications while awaiting resistance test results:

ART

>Saquinavir (SQV) 2 gm nocte
>Ritonavir (RTV)100 mg nocte
>Didanosine (ddI) 400 mg daily
>Lamivudine (3TC) 300 mg daily

Other medication

>Metformin 500 mg daily
>Insulin Mixtard 30 bd
>Ramipril 10 mg daily
>Bendofluazide 2.5 mg daily
>Amlodipine 10 mg daily
>Pravastatin 40 mg daily

Why was this ART regimen chosen?
The previous regimen was NNRTI based and therefore, as there may now be NNRTI resistance, a boosted PI regimen is needed. This patient wanted a once-daily regimen and her clinician would be mindful of her lipid problems and diabetes, perhaps for that reason SQV was chosen, as it is a little more lipid-friendly than lopinavir/ritonavir or fosamprenavir/ritonavir. In a patient with cirrhosis it may be desirable to avoid Atazanavir as the usual (harmless) increase in bilirubin may make it difficult to monitor her liver.

Choosing an NRTI backbone in this patient is difficult. She is at risk of renal disease so TDF may be undesirable and risk of neuropathy may put clinicians off using ddI in the combination. There is also a co-toxicity with Metformin and ddI as both can cause lactic acidosis. If there was any chance of treating her hepatitis C, then ddI would be contraindicated because it interacts with Ribavirin, an important component of hepatitis C treatment. She has already tried AZT and developed anaemia. In 2009 we would wish to avoid abacavir, due to her high risk of cardiovascular disease, but that data was not yet available in 2007.

CD4 538 cells/ mm^3 VL detectable 330 copies/ml, blood pressure was 166/114, blood glucose was 20 mmols/L. Her doctor had written many letters over the years to different agencies about social issues such as immigration and benefits.

A-M next attended dietetic clinic June 2007. She presented with 13 kg weight loss and reported feeling unwell. She was still eating high-fat foods – chips and sausage – but increased her intake of vegetables and (she said) reduced oil in cooking, and ate fruit irregularly. She was seen by the dietitian 3 months later. Blood sugars had increased to 32 mmols/L in recent months, but she was now receiving care for diabetes at a specialist centre and blood sugar control had normalised.

Her drug regimen was quite complex and required careful planning in terms of timing of meals and medication. She found it difficult to take ddI on an empty stomach as she had to time insulin injections with regular mealtimes. Attempts to advise on this were limited as, when she did attend appointments, she seemed confused as to which tablets were for HIV, hypertension or diabetes and she was unable to state which medications she took for diabetes and hypertension. She denied that she was taking one of her antiretroviral medications and reported taking RTV am and SQV pm, which should be taken at the same time.

What measures might be suggested to help with adherence?
A-M has a complex medication regimen with multiple pills and insulin injections. She may benefit from a simple intervention such as a dosette box, which can be filled with help from pharmacy or a nurse specialist until she is confident on her own. If she has disclosed to any member of the household, they could be enlisted to help.

As A-M is from Burundi, it is likely that English is not her first language and this may make it especially difficult for her to cope with her complex medications.

In 2008 her medication was switched to Atazanavir/RTV, 3TC, ddI.

This would significantly reduce her pill burden from the ART from 7 to 4 per day. It is also a licensed PI dose.

Weight increased substantially to a BMI of 27. Patterns over the years showed evidence of a yo-yo effect in weight fluctuations. With considerable support, and input from members of the multidisciplinary team including doctor, clinical nurse specialist, centre based nurses, pharmacist, and dietitian, CD4 and viral load remained well controlled and considerable improvements were shown, over the years, in dietary intake, blood pressure, blood sugar levels and her blood lipid levels were well controlled on statins.

This case study helps illustrate the importance of multidisciplinary team work and considering individual patient requirements to promote good adherence.

12.6   Adherence and food

During dietetic consultations discussion points may include:

- What the patient would prefer: it is often the case that when asked why medication is taken at a particular time the response is 'because I was told to take it then'.
- When taking diet history it is useful to ask about timing of medication as well as meal patterns, especially if there are concerns about adherence. This may be particularly beneficial for those with irregular meal patterns, irregular working patterns, travel commitments, co-morbidities, chaotic lifestyles and those taking medications who have food restrictions or requirements, as this may highlight a reason for suboptimal virological control.
- If gastric problems are reported this may be exacerbated by the timing of food and medication. Taking medication with or after food (if not contraindicated, (see Table 12.5)) may help alleviate complaints such as bloating, nausea, and decreased appetite.

Table 12.5   Food requirements with antiretroviral drugs.

Drug	Food restriction	Reason
*Efavirenz (BMS, 2008a)	Empty stomach, preferably at bedtime. (However most patients take this without regard to food and only separate if they experience side effects)	Increased CNS effects due to increased absorption if taken with fatty meal.
*Efavirenz + Tenofovir + Emtricitabine (Atripla)(BMS, Atripla Summary of Product Characteristics)	Empty stomach, preferably at bedtime. As above	As above.
Tenofovir + didanosine	Taken with or without food.	Increased absorption when the two drugs taken together. Didanosine dose should be reduced.
Nevirapine (Boehringer Ingelheim, 2007)	Nil	
Atazanavir (unlicensed)	With food	
Atazanavir + ritonavir (BMS, 2009)	With food (studied with light meal and high-fat meal).	Improved absorption
Darunavir + ritonavir (Janssen-Cilag Ltd, 2009b)	With food – type of food does not matter.	Improved absorption
Fosamprenavir + ritonavir (GSK, 2009)	No restriction, however, advise patient to take with food if possible.	Reduced side effects associated with ritonavir
Indinavir (MSD, 2008)	1 hour before or 2 hours after meal, with water, min 1.5 l water per day	
Indinavir + ritonavir (MSD, 2008)	No restriction, however, still advise patient to take with 1.5 l water	
Lopinvir + ritonavir (Kaletra tablets) (Abbott, 2009)	No restriction, however, advise patient to take with food if possible	Reduced side effects associated with ritonavir
Saquinavir tablets + ritonavir (Roche, 2008b)	With or after food. (high-fat meal in studies, 46 g fat, 1000 calories)	Improved absorption
Tipranavir + ritonavir (Boehringer Ingelheim, 2009)	With food	Improves tolerability
Abacavir (GSK, 2008e) (and Kivexa (GSK, 2008c))	No restriction	
Didanosine		
Enteric-coated capsules (BMS, 2008b)	Two hours before or after food	Improved absorption (in US, SPC says no restriction for EC caps)
Dispersible or chewable tablets (BMS, 2007)	30 minutes before food	

(Continued)

Table 12.5 (*Continued*).

Drug	Food restriction	Reason
Emtricitabine (Gilead Sciences Ltd, 2009a)	No restriction	
Lamivudine (GSK, 2008b)	No restriction	
*Tenofovir (Gilead Sciences, 2009c) (and Truvada (Gilead Sciences, 2009b))	With food (light meal)	Improved absorption
Zidovudine (GSK, 2008d) (and Combivir (GSK, 2008a))	No restriction	
Raltegravir (MSD, 2009)	No restriction	
Maraviroc (Pfizer Limited, 2009)	No restriction	
Enfuvirtide (Roche, 2008a)	No restriction	Injected

*There is inconsistency in the SPC recommendations for tenofovir, Truvada, efavirenz and Atripla with regard to food advice. In practice, most pharmacists do not label Atripla to be taken on an empty stomach or Truvada to be taken with food.

Patients should liaise with pharmacy about changes in timing of medication. For patients taking medication two times a day it is important to maintain the same time interval if changes are made, i.e. 11–12 hours apart.

Healthy eating and lifestyle change should be promoted as nutrients are required to metabolise drugs in the body as well as well as to maintain health, prevent disease and promote good immune function.

Food insecurity, as well as worries about personal safety (Olupot-Olupot *et al.*, 2008), poverty, poor access to cooking, clean water, washing facilities and other social issues may affect adherence. It is important to liaise with other health professionals, and agencies to arrange additional support where possible.

12.7   Looking to the future

12.7.1   New drugs

Entry inhibitors

Vicriviroc, a CCR5 inhibitor with a long half-life when boosted with ritonavir, is currently in phase III trials in treatment-experienced patients after good results in a phase II b study (Zingman *et al.*, 2008). An earlier trial of this drug in treatment-naïve patients was halted due to inferior responses in the vicriviroc arm and it is not currently being investigated in this population, although the doses used in the halted study were lower than those being taken forward in experienced patients (Landovitz *et al.*, 2008).

There are two other CCR5 inhibitors which have shown promising results in very early stages of development, SCH532706 (Pett *et al.*, 2008) and INCB009471 (Cohen *et al.*, 2007). There are also two monoclonal antibodies directed against CCR5 under investigation for HIV treatment in phase I and II trials (Jacobson *et al.*, 2008; Lalezari *et al.*, 2008; Thompson *et al.*, 2009), which have shown good efficacy and safety results in early investigations.

Integrase inhibitors

Elvitegravir is an HIV integrase inhibitor which is currently in phase II/III trials (Shimura *et al.*, 2008). Levels are significantly boosted with ritonavir, allowing once-daily dosing, and it is being co-developed with a novel boosting agent, GS-9350, in a 'quad pill' with tenofovir and emtricitabine (Mathias *et al.*, 2009). Elvitegravir has a similar resistance profile to raltegravir and is unlikely to be effective against raltegravir-resistant virus (Grant and Zolopa, 2008). There is considerable interest in developing second-generation integrase inhibitors, which would be active against resistant virus, but none has come to clinical trials yet.

A new class of antiretroviral: maturation inhibitors

This new class of drug targets the gag-pro-pol polyprotein and blocks its cleavage into the correct constituents of mature viral particles (Martin *et al.*, 2008). This results in production of immature and non-infectious virus particles. The most studied member of the class, beviramat, has been slow in development, initially due to difficulties in formulation. More recently, it has been shown that naturally occurring gag polymorphisms, which occur at fairly high frequency in HIV-infected individuals, confer resistance to the drug (Van Baelen *et al.*, 2009).

12.7.2 New strategies

There is ongoing research into the best way to use available antiretroviral drugs. One strategy that has been studied is boosted PI monotherapy, which has been tried with lopinavir/ritonavir, atazanavir/ritonavir and in small trials with indinavir/ritonavir and saquinavir/ritonavir. There are two approaches to PI monotherapy, with some studies starting patients on it from the beginning of their treatment and others switching those with long-term virological suppression on ART. A review of studies to date suggests that boosted PI monotherapy is not as effective as conventional triple-drug therapy in naïve patients but is an option for fully suppressed patients to switch to for reasons of pill burden, cost or toxicity (Bierman *et al.*, 2009). It is also being investigated as a strategy for second-line ART in resource-limited settings.

12.7.3 Induction/maintenance

The use of induction/maintenance strategies, employing multiple drugs to suppress the HIV viral load and then simplifying the regimen while maintaining suppression, has been tested in several studies (Asboe *et al.*, 2007). The boosted PI monotherapy switch studies are a version of this strategy that has been quite successful (see the previous section). The Forte study randomised patients to nelfinavir/nevirapine/ddI/d4T for the first 24–32 weeks then dropping the PI if undetectable or standard treatment with ddI/d4T/nevirapine or to continuous four-drug treatment. The protocol was later amended to allow clinician choice of drugs within classes due to toxicity concerns. The induction/maintenance arm did lead to significantly fewer virological failures than the standard treatment arm (Asboe *et al.*, 2007). Other trials of 4 versus 3 drugs have not shown a benefit of adding an additional drug or class (Orkin *et al.*, 2005; Macarthur *et al.*, 2006). In addition, the efficacy, simplicity and low toxicity of current first-line regimens are such that such strategies may not be necessary in first-line therapy. However, it may be that a role for an induction-maintenance therapy emerges in second-line therapy, particularly in resource-poor settings.

12.7.4   Role of new classes in naïve patients: raltegravir and maraviroc

The current standard approach of 2NRTIs + NNRTI or boosted PI is clearly very successful and the role of new classes of drug in naïve patients is unclear. Raltegravir was non-inferior to efavirenz and demonstrated less toxicity in the STARTMRK studies, but it will be some years before the long-term follow-up data can match that of NNRTIs (Markowitz et al., 2007). Cost may limit use in practice even if a naïve licence is granted.

Maraviroc failed to demonstrate non-inferiority to efavirenz in the MERIT study, but in a subsequent reanalysis using an improved tropism test the non-inferiority criteria were met (Saag et al., 2007, Saag M et al., 2008). Side effects were less common in the maraviroc arm. At the time of publication, this drug was not licensed in treatment-naïve patients and use is limited to those with CCR5 tropic virus, necessitating costly testing. The role of this drug remains unclear, particularly in early treatment of HIV.

12.7.5   New uses of ART in prevention

The role of ART in preventing HIV infection is well established in the prevention of mother-to-child transmission and in post-exposure prophylaxis following occupational and sexual exposures. Studies of other prevention uses are ongoing, including pre-exposure prophylaxis where at-risk, HIV-negative individuals are given ART drugs to take to try and reduce HIV incidence (Paxton et al., 2007). The use of ART to prevent transmission of HIV during breastfeeding, either by treating the mother, the baby or both, has shown promising results so far (Coovadia and Kindra, 2008). This strategy was adopted by the WHO guidelines on PMTCT in 2009, with a recommendation that breastfeeding continues until 12 months of age where covered by antiretroviral therapy (WHO, 2009). Microbicides containing ART agents, used vaginally and rectally to prevent sexual transmission, are also being investigated, with clinical trials awaited.

There is interest in the role of treating HIV-infected individuals with ART for the public health benefit of reducing transmission (Wood and Montaner, 2007). This is controversial for individuals who don't need treatment yet for their own health and there is ongoing debate.

12.8   Conclusion

ART is an effective treatment for HIV and has transformed the outlook for infected patients. As in any chronic disease, maintaining adherence to therapy is challenging and a multidisciplinary approach, considering the whole patient, is required. The field moves quickly and further improvements in therapy and new uses of ART, e.g. in prevention, are likely to be developed in the next few years.

Acknowledgements

The author would like to thank:

Vivian Pribram, BA Hons, Bsc Hons, MSc, RD, Senior Specialist Dietitian, Department of Sexual Health and HIV, King's College Hospital NHS Foundation Trust, London

Clare Stradling, BSc MSc RD, Specialist Dietitian, Birmingham Heartlands HIV Service, Heart of England NHS Foundation Trust, Birmingham.

Rosy Weston, Senior HIV Pharmacist, Imperial College Healthcare NHS Trust, London.

References

Abbott Laboratories Limited. Norvir Summary of Product Characteristics. 2008.

Abbott Laboratories Limited. Kaletra Summary of Product Characteristics. 2009.

Antiretroviral Therapy Cohort Collaboration. Life expectancy of individuals on combination antiretroviral therapy in high-income countries: a collaborative analysis of 14 cohort studies. *Lancet* 2008; **372**:293–9.

Arribas JR, Pozniak AL, Gallant JE *et al.* Tenofovir Disoproxil Fumarate, Emtricitabine, and Efavirenz Compared With Zidovudine/Lamivudine and Efavirenz in Treatment-Naive Patients: 144-Week Analysis. *J Acquir Immune Defic Syndr* 2007; **7**: 74–78.

Asboe D, Williams IG, Goodall RL *et al.* A virological benefit from an induction/maintenance strategy: the Forte trial. *Antivir Ther* 2007; **12**:47–54.

Bannister WP, Ruiz L, Cozzi-Lepri A *et al.* Comparison of genotypic resistance profiles and virological response between patients starting nevirapine and efavirenz in EuroSIDA. *AIDS* 2008; **22**:367–76.

Barber TJ, Marett B, Waldron S *et al.* Are disulfiram-like reactions associated with abacavir-containing antiretroviral regimens in clinical practice? *AIDS* 2007; **21**:1823–4.

Bartlett JA Addressing the challenges of adherence. *J Acquir Immune Defic Syndr* 2002; **29** Suppl 1:S2–10.

Beck EJ, Mandalia S, Youle M *et al.* Treatment outcome and cost-effectiveness of different highly active antiretroviral therapy regimens in the UK (1996–2002). *Int J STD AIDS* 2008; **19**:297–304.

Berenguer J, Gonzalez J, Ribera E *et al.* Didanosine, lamivudine, and efavirenz versus zidovudine, lamivudine, and efavirenz for the initial treatment of HIV type 1 infection: final analysis (48 weeks) of a prospective, randomized, noninferiority clinical trial, GESIDA 3903. *Clin Infect Dis* 2008; **47**:1083–92.

Bierman WF, Van Agtmael MA, Nijhuis M *et al.* HIV monotherapy with ritonavir-boosted protease inhibitors: a systematic review. *AIDS* 2009; **23**:279–91.

Boehringer Ingelheim Limited. Viramune summary of Product Characteristics. electronic medicines compendium. 2007.

Boehringer Ingelheim Limited. Aptivus Summary of Product Characteristics. 2009.

Bower M, Collins S, Cottrill C *et al.* British HIV Association guidelines for HIV-associated malignancies 2008. *HIV Med* 2008; **9**:336–88.

(BMS)BRISTOL-MYERS SQUIBB PHARMACEUTICALS LTD. Videx Chewable or Dispersible tablet SPC. 2007.

(BMS)BRISTOL-MYERS SQUIBB PHARMACEUTICALS LTD. Sustiva Summary of Product Characteristics. 2008a.

(BMS)BRISTOL-MYERS SQUIBB PHARMACEUTICALS LTD. Videx Gastro-Resistant Capsules Summary of Product Characteristics. 2008b.

(BMS)BRISTOL-MYERS SQUIBB PHARMACEUTICALS LTD. (Atripla Summary of Product Characteristics) 2009a.

(BMS)BRISTOL-MYERS SQUIBB PHARMACEUTICALS LTD. Reyataz Summary of Product Characteristics. 2009b.

Canestri A, Lescure X, Jaureguiberry S *et al.* HIV-related meningoencephalitis in patients with optimally suppressed plasma HIV RNA receiving stable ART. *16th Conference on Retroviruses and Opportunistic Infections.* Montreal, Canada: 2009.

Cervia JS, Smith MA. Enfuvirtide (T-20): a novel human immunodeficiency virus type 1 fusion inhibitor. *Clin Infect Dis* 2003; **37:**1102–6.

Cherry CL, Skolasky RL, Lal L *et al.* Antiretroviral use and other risks for HIV-associated neuropathies in an international cohort. *Neurology* 2006; **66:**867–73.

Chesney MA, Ickovics JR, Chambers DB *et al.* Self-reported adherence to antiretroviral medications among participants in HIV clinical trials: the AACTG adherence instruments. Patient Care Committee & Adherence Working Group of the Outcomes Committee of the Adult AIDS Clinical Trials Group (AACTG). *AIDS Care* 2000; **12:**255–66.

Clumeck N, Pozniak A, Raffi F. European AIDS Clinical Society (EACS) guidelines for the clinical management and treatment of HIV-infected adults. *HIV Med* 2008; **9:**65–71.

Cohen C, Dejesus E, Mills A *et al.* Potent antiretroviral activity of the once-daily CCR5 antagonist INCB009471 over 14 days of monotherapy. *4th International AIDS Society Conference on HIV Pathogenesis, Treatment and Prevention;* Sydney, Australia, 2007.

Cooper D, Bloch M, Humphries A *et al.* Simplification with Fixed-dose Tenofovir/Emtricitabine or Abacavir/Lamivudine in Adults with Suppressed HIV Replication: The STEAL Study, a Randomized, Open-label, 96-Week, Non-inferiority Trial. *16th Conference on Retroviruses and Opportunistic Infections.* Montreal, Canada, 2009.

Coovadia H, Kindra G. Breastfeeding to prevent HIV transmission in infants: balancing pros and cons. *Curr Opin Infect Dis* 2008; **21:**11–5.

D:A:D STUDY GROUP Use of nucleoside reverse transcriptase inhibitors and risk of myocardial infarction in HIV-infected patients enrolled in the D:A:D study: a multi-cohort collaboration. *Lancet* 2008.

Daar E, Tierney C, Fischl M, *et al.* ACTG 5202: Final Results of ABC/3TC or TDF/FTC with either EFV or ATV/r in Treatment-naive HIV-infected Patients. 17th Conference on Retroviruses & Opportunistic Infections (CROI 2010). San Francisco. February 16–19, 2010. Abstract 59LB.

Deeks SG. Antiretroviral treatment of HIV infected adults. *BMJ* 2006; **332:**1489.

Dejesus E, Herrera G, Teofilo E *et al.* Abacavir versus zidovudine combined with lamivudine and efavirenz, for the treatment of antiretroviral-naive HIV-infected adults. *Clin Infect Dis* 2004; **39:**1038–46.

Douek D. HIV disease progression: immune activation, microbes, and a leaky gut. *Top HIV Med* 2007; **15:**114–7.

Dube MP, Komarow L, Mulligan K, *et al.* Long-term body fat outcomes in antiretroviral-naive participants randomized to nelfinavir or efavirenz or both plus dual nucleosides. Dual X-ray absorptiometry results from A5005s, a substudy of Adult Clinical Trials Group 384. *J Acquir Immune Defic Syndr* 2007; **45:**508–14.

El-Sadr WM, Lundgren JD, Neaton JD, Gordin F et.al CD4+ count-guided interruption of antiretroviral treatment. *N Engl J Med* 2006; **355:**2283–96.

Emery S, Neuhaus JA, Phillips AN *et al.* Major clinical outcomes in antiretroviral therapy (ART)-naive participants and in those not receiving ART at baseline in the SMART study. *J Infect Dis* 2008; **197:**1133–44.

Eron J JR, Yeni P, Gathe J JR *et al.* The KLEAN study of fosamprenavir-ritonavir versus lopinavir-ritonavir, each in combination with abacavir-lamivudine, for initial treatment of HIV infection over 48 weeks: a randomised non-inferiority trial. *Lancet* 2006; **368:**476–82.

Evering TH, Markowitz M. Raltegravir: an integrase inhibitor for HIV-1. *Expert Opin Investig Drugs* 2008; **17:**413–22.

Fatkenheuer G, Nelson M, Lazzarin A *et al.* Subgroup analyses of maraviroc in previously treated R5 HIV-1 infection. *N Engl J Med* 2008; **359:**1442–55.

Gazzard BG. British HIV Association Guidelines for the treatment of HIV-1-infected adults with antiretroviral therapy 2008. *HIV Med* 2008; **9:**563–608.

Gazzard BG on behalf of the Bhiva Treatment Guidelines Writing Group British HIV Association Guidelines for the treatment of HIV-infected adults with antiretroviral therapy. 2008.

Geretti AM. *Antiretroviral Resistance in Clinical Practice*, pp. 1–10. London, Mediscript Ltd.

GILEAD SCIENCES LTD. Emtriva Summary of Product Characteristics. 2009a.

GILEAD SCIENCES LTD. Truvada Summary of Product Characteristics. 2009b.

GILEAD SCIENCES LTD. Viread Summary of Product Characteristics. 2009c.

(GSK) GLAXOSMITHKLINE UK. Combivir Summary of Product Characteristics. 2008a.

(GSK) GLAXOSMITHKLINE UK. Epivir Summary of Product Characteristics. 2008b.

(GSK) GLAXOSMITHKLINE UK. Kivexa Summary of Product Characteristic. 2008c.

(GSK) GLAXOSMITHKLINE UK. Retrovir Summary of Product Characteristics. 2008d.

(GSK) GLAXOSMITHKLINE UK. Ziagen Summary of Product Characteristics. 2008e.

(GSK) GLAXOSMITHKLINE UK. Telzir Summary of Product Characteristics. 2009.

Grant P, Zolopa A. Integrase inhibitors: a clinical review of raltegravir and elvitegravir. *J HIV Ther* 2008; **13**:36–9.

Gulick RM, Lalezari J, Goodrich J *et al*. Maraviroc for previously treated patients with R5 HIV-1 infection. *N Engl J Med* 2008; **359**:1429–41.

Gulick RM, Ribaudo HJ, Shikuma CM *et al*. Triple-nucleoside regimens versus efavirenz-containing regimens for the initial treatment of HIV-1 infection. *N Engl J Med* 2004; **350**:1850–61.

Hammer SM, Squires KE, Hughes MD *et al*. A controlled trial of two nucleoside analogues plus indinavir in persons with human immunodeficiency virus infection and CD4 cell counts of 200 per cubic millimeter or less. *N Engl J Med* 1997; **337**:725–733.

Harrington RD, Woodward JA, Hooton TM, Horn JR. Life-threatening interactions between HIV-1 protease inhibitors and the illicit drugs MDMA and gamma-hydroxybutyrate. *Arch Intern Med* 1999; **159**:2221–4.

Heaton R, Franklin D, Clifford D *et al*. HIV-associated neurocognitive impairment remains prevalent in the era of combination ART: The CHARTER Study. *16th Conference on Retroviruses and Opportunistic Infections*. Montreal, Canada: 2009.

Henry JA, Hill IR. Fatal interaction between ritonavir and MDMA. *Lancet* 1998; **352**:1751–2.

Jacobson JM, Saag MS, Thompson MA *et al*. Antiviral activity of single-dose PRO 140, a CCR5 monoclonal antibody, in HIV-infected adults. *J Infect Dis* 2008; **198**:1345–52.

JANSSEN-CILAG LTD. Intelence Summary of Product Characteristics. 2009a.

JANSSEN-CILAG LTD. Prezista Summary of Product Characteristics. 2009b.

Jegede O, Babu J, Di Santo R *et al*. HIV type 1 integrase inhibitors: from basic research to clinical implications. *AIDS Rev* 2008; **10**:172–89.

Johnson LB, Saravolatz LD. Etravirine, a next-generation nonnucleoside reverse-transcriptase inhibitor. *Clin Infect Dis* 2009; **48**:1123–8.

Johnson M, Grinsztejn B, Rodriguez C *et al*. 96-week comparison of once-daily atazanavir/ritonavir and twice-daily lopinavir/ritonavir in patients with multiple virologic failures. *AIDS* 2006; **20**:711–8.

Kitahata MM, Gange SJ, Moore RD. Initiating rather than deferring HAART at a CD4 count between 351–500 cells/mm3 is associated with improved survival. *48th Annual ICAAC/IDSA 46th Annual Meeting*. Washington, DC: 2008.

Lalezari J, Yadavalli GK, Para M *et al*. Safety, pharmacokinetics, and antiviral activity of HGS004, a novel fully human IgG4 monoclonal antibody against CCR5, in HIV-1-infected patients. *J Infect Dis* 2008; **197**:721–7.

Landovitz RJ, Angel JB, Hoffmann C et.al. Phase II study of vicriviroc versus efavirenz (both with zidovudine/lamivudine) in treatment-naive subjects with HIV-1 infection. *J Infect Dis* 2008; **198**:1113–22.

Lapadula G, Costarelli S, Quiros-Roldan E *et al*. Risk of early virological failure of once-daily tenofovir-emtricitabine plus twice-daily nevirapine in antiretroviral therapy-naive HIV-infected patients. *Clin Infect Dis* 2008; **46**:1127–9.

Leake Date H, Fisher M. HIV infection. In: Walker R, ed. *Clinical Pharmacy and Therapeutics*, 4th edn. Oxford: Churchill Livingstone (Elsevier): 2007.

Letendre S, Capparelli E, Best B *et al*. Better Antiretroviral Penetration into the Central Nervous System Is Associated with Lower CSF Viral Load. *13th Conference on Retroviruses and Opportunistic Infection*. Denver, Colarado, USA: 2006.

Levy V, Grant RM. Antiretroviral therapy for hepatitis B virus-HIV-coinfected patients: promises and pitfalls. *Clin Infect Dis* 2006; **43**:904–10.

Lieberman-Blum SS, Fung HB, Bandres JC. Maraviroc: a CCR5-receptor antagonist for the treatment of HIV-1 infection. *Clin Ther* 2008; **30**:1228–50.

Lundgren JD, Reiss P, Worm S *et al*. Risk of Myocardial Infarction with Exposure to Specific ARV form the PI, NNRTI and NRTI Drug Classes: The D:A:D Study. *16th Conference on Retroviruses and Opportunistic Infections*. Montreal, Canada: 2009.

Macarthur RD, Novak RM. Reviews of anti-infective agents: maraviroc: the first of a new class of antiretroviral agents. *Clin Infect Dis* 2008; **47**:236–41.

Macarthur RD, Novak RM, Peng G et al. A comparison of three highly active antiretroviral treatment strategies consisting of non-nucleoside reverse transcriptase inhibitors, protease inhibitors, or both in the presence of nucleoside reverse transcriptase inhibitors as initial therapy (CPCRA 058 FIRST Study): a long-term randomised trial. Lancet 2006; 368:2125–35.

Madruga JV, Cahn P, Grinsztejn B et al. Efficacy and safety of TMC125 (etravirine) in treatment-experienced HIV-1-infected patients in DUET-1: 24-week results from a randomised, double-blind, placebo-controlled trial. Lancet 2007; 370:29–38.

Maitland D, Moyle G, Hand J et al. Early virologic failure in HIV-1 infected subjects on didanosine/tenofovir/efavirenz: 12-week results from a randomized trial. AIDS 2005; 19:1183–8.

Mallal S, Phillips E, Carosi G et al. HLA-B*5701 screening for hypersensitivity to abacavir. N Engl J Med 2008; 358:568–79.

Markowitz M, Nguyen BY, Gotuzzo E et al. Rapid and durable antiretroviral effect of the HIV-1 Integrase inhibitor raltegravir as part of combination therapy in treatment-naive patients with HIV-1 infection: results of a 48-week controlled study. J Acquir Immune Defic Syndr 2007; 46:125–33.

Marsden MD, Zack JA. Eradication of HIV: current challenges and new directions. J Antimicrob Chemother 2009; 63:7–10.

Martin DE, Salzwedel K, Allaway GP. Bevirimat: a novel maturation inhibitor for the treatment of HIV-1 infection. Antivir Chem Chemother 2008; 19:107–13.

Mathias A, Lee M, Callebaut C et al. A pharmaco-enhancer without anti-HIV activity. 16th Conference on Retroviruses and Opportunistic Infections. Montreal, Canada: 2009.

May M, Sterne JA, Sabin C et al. Prognosis of HIV-1-infected patients up to 5 years after initiation of HAART: collaborative analysis of prospective studies. AIDS 2007; 21:1185–97.

Mccomsey GA, O'riordan M, Setzer B et al. Uridine supplementation in HIV lipoatrophy: pilot trial on safety and effect on mitochondrial indices. Eur J Clin Nutr 2008; 62:1031–7.

(MSD)MERCK SHARP & DOHME LIMITED. Crixivan Summary of Product Characteristics. 2008.

(MSD)MERCK SHARP & DOHME LIMITED. Issentress Summary of Product Characteristics. 2009.

Mocroft A, Vella S, Benfield TL et al. Changing patterns of mortality across Europe in patients infected with HIV-1. EuroSIDA Study Group. Lancet 1998; 352:1725–30.

Molina JM, Andrade-Villanueva J, Echevarria J, et al. Once-daily atazanavir/ritonavir versus twice-daily lopinavir/ritonavir, each in combination with tenofovir and emtricitabine, for management of antiretroviral-naive HIV-1-infected patients: 48 week efficacy and safety results of the CASTLE study. Lancet 2008; 372:646–55.

Molina JM, Journot V, Furco A et al. Five-year follow up of once-daily therapy with emtricitabine, didanosine and efavirenz (Montana ANRS 091 trial). Antivir Ther 2007; 12:417–22.

Murphy EL, Collier AC, Kalish LA et al. Highly active antiretroviral therapy decreases mortality and morbidity in patients with advanced HIV disease. Ann Intern Med 2001; 135:17–26.

Nelson MR, Katlama C, Montaner JS et al. The safety of tenofovir disoproxil fumarate for the treatment of HIV infection in adults: the first 4 years. AIDS 2007; 21:1273–81.

Olupot-Olupot P, Katawera A, Cooper C et al. Adherence to antiretroviral therapy among a conflict-affected population in Northeastern Uganda: a qualitative study. AIDS 2008; 22:1882–4.

Orkin C, Stebbing J, Nelson M et al. A randomized study comparing a three- and four-drug HAART regimen in first-line therapy (QUAD study). J Antimicrob Chemother 2005; 55:246–51.

Ortiz R, Dejesus E, Khanlou H et al. Efficacy and safety of once-daily darunavir/ritonavir versus lopinavir/ritonavir in treatment-naive HIV-1-infected patients at week 48. AIDS 2008; 22:1389–97.

Panel on Antiretroviral Guidelines for Adult and Adolescents Guidelines for the Use of Antiretroviral Agents in HIV-1-infected Adults and Adolescents. Department of Health and Human Services: 2008.

Pappa K, Hernandez J, Ha B, Shaefer M, Brothers C, Liao Q. Abacavir/lamivudine (ABC/3TC) shows robust virologic responses in ART-naive patients for baseline (BL) viral loads (VL) of >100,000 c/mL and <100,000 c/mL by endpoint used in ACTG5202. XVII International AIDS Conference. Mexico City, Mexico: 2008.

Paterson DL, Swindells S, Mohr J et al. Adherence to protease inhibitor therapy and outcomes in patients with HIV infection. Ann Intern Med 2000; 133:21–30.

Paxton LA, Hope T, Jaffe HW. Pre-exposure prophylaxis for HIV infection: what if it works? *Lancet* 2007; **370**:89–93.

Pett S, Emery S et al. Safety and activity of SCH532706, a small molecular chemokine receptor 5 antagonist in HIV-1 infected individuals. *15th Conference on Retroviruses and Opportunistic Infections*. Boston, MA, USA: 2008.

PFIZER LIMITED Celsentri Summary of Product Characteristics. 2009.

Phillips AN, Gazzard B, Gilson R et al. Rate of AIDS diseases or death in HIV-infected antiretroviral therapy-naive individuals with high CD4 cell count. *AIDS* 2007a; **21**:1717–21.

Phillips AN, Gazzard BG, Clumeck N, Losso MH, Lundgren JD. When should antiretroviral therapy for HIV be started? *BMJ* 2007b; **334**:76–8.

Phillips AN, Pradier C, Lazzarin A et al. Viral load outcome of non-nucleoside reverse transcriptase inhibitor regimens for 2203 mainly antiretroviral-experienced patients. *AIDS* 2001; **15**:2385–95.

Podzamczer D, Olmo M, Sanz J et al. Safety of switching nevirapine twice daily to nevirapine once daily in virologically suppressed patients. *J Acquir Immune Defic Syndr*. 2009.

Rey D, Hoen B, Chavanet P et al. High rate of early virological failure with the once-daily tenofovir/lamivudine/nevirapine combination in naive HIV-1-infected patients. *J Antimicrob Chemother* 2009; **63**:380–8.

Riddler SA, Haubrich R, Dirienzo AG et al. Class-sparing regimens for initial treatment of HIV-1 infection. *N Engl J Med* 2008; **358**:2095–106.

Ripamonti D, Maggiolo F. Rilpivirine, a non-nucleoside reverse transcriptase inhibitor for the treatment of HIV infection. *Curr Opin Investig Drugs* 2008; **9**:899–912.

ROCHE PRODUCTS LIMITED. Fuzeon Summary of Product Characteristics. 2008a.

ROCHE PRODUCTS LIMITED. Invirase 500 mg Film-Coated Tablets Summary of Product Characteristics. 2008b.

Ruane PJ, Dejesus E. New nucleoside/nucleotide backbone options: a review of recent studies. *J Acquir Immune Defic Syndr* 2004; **37** Suppl 1:S21–9.

Rueda S, Park-Wyllie LY, Bayoumi AM et al. Patient support and education for promoting adherence to highly active antiretroviral therapy for HIV/AIDS. *Cochrane Database Syst Rev* 2006; **3**: CD001442.

Saag M et al. Reanalysis of the MERIT Study with the Enhanced Trofile Assay. *48th ICAAC*. Washington, D.C., USA: 2008.

Saag M, Ive P, Heera J, et al. A multicenter, randomized, double-blind, comparative trial of a novel CCR5 antagonist, maraviroc versus efavirenz, both in combination with Combivir (zidovudine [ZDV] / lamivudine [3TC]), for the treatment of antiretroviral naïve patients infected with R5 HIV-1: week 48 results of the MERIT study. *Fourth International AIDS Society Conference on HIV Treatment and Pathogenesis*. Sydney, Australia: 2007.

Saifee S, Joelson D, Braude J et al. Noncirrhotic portal hypertension in patients with human immunodeficiency virus-1 infection. *Clin Gastroenterol Hepatol* 2008; **6**:1167–9.

Santoscoy M, Cahn P, Gonsalez C et al. TMC278(rilipivirine), a next-generation NNRTI, demonstrates long-term efficacy and tolerability in ARV-naive patients: 96 week results of study C204. *AIDS 2008 – XVII International AIDS Conference*. Mexico City, Mexico: 2008.

Sax P, Tierney C, Collier A et al. ACTG 5202: shorter time to virologic failure (VF) with abacavir/lamivudine (ABC/3TC) than tenofovir/emtricitabine (TDF/FTC) as part of combination therapy in treatment-naive subjects with screening HIV RNA > 100,000 c/mL. *XVII International AIDS Conference*. Mexico City: 2008.

Shimura K, Kodama E, Sakagami Y et al. Broad antiretroviral activity and resistance profile of the novel human immunodeficiency virus integrase inhibitor elvitegravir (JTK-303/GS-9137). *J Virol* 2008; **82**:764–74.

Skeie L, Maeland A. Can efavirenz be taken in the morning? *Scand J Infect Dis* 2006; **38**:1089–91.

Smith K, Fine D, Patel P et al. Efficacy and Safety of Abacavir/Lamivudine Compared to Tenofovir/Emtricitabine in Combination with Once-daily Lopinavir/Ritonavir through 48 Weeks in the HEAT Study. *15th Conference on Retroviruses and Opportunistic Infections*. Boston, Mass, USA: 2008.

Soriano V, Barreiro P, Martin-Carbonero L et al. Update on the treatment of chronic hepatitis C in HIV-infected patients. *AIDS Rev* 2007; **9**:99–113.

Soriano V, Köppe S, Mingrone H, et al. Prospective comparison of nevirapine and atazanavir/ritonavir both combined with tenofovir DF/emtricitabine in treatment-naive HIV-1 infected patients: ARTEN study week 48 results. In: Program and abstracts of the 5th International AIDS Society Conference on HIV Pathogenesis, Treatment and Prevention; July 19–22, 2009; Cape Town, South Africa. Abstract LBPEB07.

Squires KE, Gulick R, Tebas P et al. A comparison of stavudine plus lamivudine versus zidovudine plus lamivudine in combination with indinavir in antiretroviral naive individuals with HIV infection: selection of thymidine analog regimen therapy (START I). AIDS 2000; 14:1591–600.

Thompson M, Lalezari J, Saag M et al. Weekly and Biweekly Subcutaneous PRO 140 Demonstrates Potent, Sustained Antiviral Activity. 16th Conference on Retroviruses and Opportunistic Infections. Montreal, Canada: 2009.

Van Baelen K, Salzwedel K, Rondelez E et al. HIV-1 Susceptibility to the Maturation Inhibitor Bevirimat Is Modulated by Baseline Polymorphisms in Gag SP1. Antimicrob Agents Chemother. 2009.

Van Leth F, Phanuphak P, Ruxrungtham K et al. Comparison of first-line antiretroviral therapy with regimens including nevirapine, efavirenz, or both drugs, plus stavudine and lamivudine: a randomised open-label trial, the 2NN Study. Lancet 2004; 363:1253–63.

Walmsley S, Avihingsanon A, Slim J et al. Gemini: A Noninferiority Study of Saquinavir/Ritonavir Versus Lopinavir/Ritonavir as Initial HIV-1 Therapy in Adults. J Acquir Immune Defic Syndr. 2009.

Walmsley S, Bernstein B, King M et al. Lopinavir-ritonavir versus nelfinavir for the initial treatment of HIV infection. N Engl J Med 2002; 346:2039–46.

Waters L, John L, Nelson M. Non-nucleoside reverse transcriptase inhibitors: a review. Int J Clin Pract 2007; 61:105–18.

Watts DH. Teratogenicity risk of antiretroviral therapy in pregnancy. Curr HIV/AIDS Rep 2007; 4:135–40.

Wood E, Montaner JS. When to initiate HIV antiretroviral therapy: do benefits other than survival deserve greater attention? J Acquir Immune Defic Syndr 2007; 45:131–2.

WORLD HEALTH ORGANISATION Antiretroviral Therapy for HIV Infection in Adults and Adolescents: Recommendations for a Public Health Approach. 2006 rev. Geneva, WHO Press: 2006.

WHO (World Health Organization), Rapid advice: antiretroviral therapy for HIV infection in adults and adolescents. November 2009 [electronic version]. Available at: http://www.who.int/hiv/pub/arv/rapid_advice_art.pdf. 2009.

Youle M. Acetyl-L-carnitine in HIV-associated antiretroviral toxic neuropathy. CNS Drugs 2007a; 21 Suppl 1:25–30; discussion 45–6.

Youle M. Overview of boosted protease inhibitors in treatment-experienced HIV-infected patients. J Antimicrob Chemother. 2007b.

Zingman B, Suleiman J et al. Vicriviroc, a next generation CCR5 antagonist, exhibits potent, sustained suppression of viral replication in treatment experienced adults: VICTOR-E1 48 week results. 15th Conference on Retroviruses and Opportunistic Infections. Boston, Massachusetts: 2008.

13 Healthy Eating and Well-Being

Vivian Pribram and Kirsten Foster

Key Points

- Non-communicable diseases (NCDs) such as heart disease, stroke, cancer, diabetes and chronic lung disease are responsible for about 35 million deaths each year.
- All these diseases share the same risk factors: tobacco use, unhealthy diets, physical inactivity and harmful use of alcohol.
- Healthy eating and a healthy lifestyle can help prevent ill health. Advice given to the general population is appropriate for people living with HIV when they are well.
- Good dietary intake and a healthy lifestyle may be particularly important for people living with HIV, as they may have a higher risk of ill health compared to people not infected with HIV.
- Factors that affect morbidity and mortality include age, ethnicity, sexual orientation, mental health, socio-economic status as well as lifestyle behaviours such as tobacco use, diet and physical activity level.
- Nutrition interventions should be tailored to individual circumstances and should help motivate and empower people to overcome barriers to lifestyle change.

13.1 Diet, lifestyle and disease prevention

At present NCDs such as heart disease, stroke, cancer, diabetes and chronic lung disease are responsible for about 35 million deaths each year, or 60% of all deaths worldwide, according to WHO. This is double the number of deaths from infectious diseases (including HIV, tuberculosis and malaria), maternal and perinatal conditions and nutritional deficiencies combined (WHO, 2005). Of the deaths from NCDs, 80% occur in low and middle income nations, many of which are worst affected by the burden of HIV disease. Chronic diseases also cause disability, often for decades, and impact negatively on quality of life. It is estimated that approximately half of the global burden of disease is caused by chronic diseases, as measured by DALYs (disability-adjusted life years) (WHO, 2005).

All these diseases share the same risk factors: tobacco use, unhealthy diets, physical inactivity and harmful use of alcohol. A substantial proportion of premature deaths from these causes can be prevented by affordable public health interventions, even in lower income countries, according to WHO experts (Zaracostas, 2009). According to WHO at least 2.7 million people die each year as a result of low fruit and vegetable consumption and 2.6 million die as a result of being overweight or obese (WHO, 2005).

An epic study, based on data from almost 900 000 participants, 57 prospective studies, and four continents, showed that obesity, as measured by BMI, is associated with increased total mortality in both men and women and in all age strata from 35 to 89 years. These results also confirm that the increased mortality due to high BMI is mainly from specific causes, such as ischaemic heart disease, stroke, diabetes, and liver disease. Thus, obesity shortens lifespan (Lopez-Jimenez, 2009).

WHO promotes population-wide interventions and, focusing on those at elevated risk, advises dietary changes, increased physical activity, weight reduction and avoiding smoking (Lipman, 2009). While successful prevention of NCD has been demonstrated (e.g. North Karelia Project in Finland), more research is needed on multifactorial interventions and the role of diet in prevention of chronic disease (Pomerleau et al., 2005). However, true causal connections between specific nutrients and these other disorders have been hard to establish, partly because most chronic diseases are highly multifactorial and partly because they have long latency periods. Additionally, the randomized controlled trial (RCT), which has become the gold standard for establishing the efficacy of pharmacologic agents, is poorly suited to the evaluation of nutritional effects, and the assigning of subjects to an intake that is inadequate, for lengthy periods, raises significant and probably insurmountable ethical problems (Heaney, 2006).

For information on healthy eating and prevention of obesity in children (see Chapter 6).

13.2   The importance of healthy eating for people living with HIV (PLHIV)

A higher prevalence of reduced bone mineral density, vitamin D deficiency, impaired glucose tolerance and cardiovascular disease risk has been reported in PLHIV compared to HIV-uninfected individuals. HIV infection itself and antiretroviral therapy (ART) can lead to a variety of metabolic disturbances that may increase risk for development of diabetes, coronary heart disease and bone fracture. Nutrition and lifestyle interventions may help prevent *onset* of metabolic side effects: limited evidence suggests that higher fibre diets are associated with a reduced risk of developing central fat deposition. Conventional lipid-lowering diets can prevent onset of antiretroviral-related dyslipidaemia and exercise is associated with a reduced incidence of both body-shape changes and insulin resistance. A small number of research trials have demonstrated that individualised dietary and lifestyle interventions can have a positive effect on dyslipidaemias, impaired glucose tolerance, diabetes and lipohypertrophy, but further research is needed on both preventions and treatment (see Chapters 10 for further information about these conditions). In addition to metabolic problems, higher rates of certain cancers have been reported among people with HIV (including Kaposi's sarcoma, non-Hodgkin's lymphoma, lung, skin, colorectal, prostate, cervical and anal cancers) (Deeks and Phillips, 2009). Renal failure is also associated with complications of HIV infection (see Chapter 19). Most of these conditions are also linked to lifestyle factors such as lack of exercise, smoking and malnutrition, particularly overnutrition. There is a high prevalence of overweight and obesity among PLHIV (particularly, among certain ethnic minorities such as Black African women in the UK). Prevalence of obesity among PLHIV was found to be 13% for men and 29% for women in a recent US study (Hendricks et al., 2006). Good nutrition helps support immune function and nutrients are needed to metabolise many of the drugs taken by PLHIV.

Despite these health risks, in resource-adequate regions with good access to ART, many people with HIV are leading long, healthy, active lives. In recent years, increasing attention has been paid to the needs of the growing ageing population of PLHIV. This is in contrast to the era before the availability of effective anti-HIV therapy, when HIV was an acute life-threatening condition without successful treatment options. At that time, health risks posed by long-term chronic conditions were not a major concern. It is now apparent that optimum nutrition and healthy lifestyle interventions may be particularly important for PLHIV to reduce morbidity, disease-related complications, adverse effects of treatment and to help people live long, active lives.

13.3   Factors that affect healthy eating and improved well-being among PLHIV

There are many socio-economic and other factors that exert an influence on health behaviours which should be taken into consideration when providing nutritional care.

13.3.1   Poverty and low income

Rates of malnutrition and food insecurity are very high in regions of the world where HIV is most endemic. In many cases, adequate food is unavailable and healthy eating is not an option (see Chapters 3 and 11). In contrast, obesity is increasing in most countries in the world, even in those in regions with high rates of undernutrition and HIV infection (e.g. sub-Saharan Africa).

While life expectancy rates continue to increase overall in the UK and early deaths from cancer, heart disease and other smoking-related diseases are declining, the gap in life-expectancy between rich and poor is widening. Messages about well-being and healthy lifestyles penetrate more rapidly into the middle class professional households than they do into low-income households, as it is easier to choose what to eat on a comfortable income (Bowcott, 2009). A US study showed risk of HIV infection and mortality related to HIV was higher among those on low incomes compared to wealthier PLHIV (Cunningham *et al.*, 2005). HIV can bring about low income due, for example, to ill health, uncertain immigration status, hate crime and discrimination The average income of people applying to the UK Crusaid Hardship Fund in 2005 was found to be £60 per week while 10% had no income at all. Many were living in substandard accommodation, unable to afford basic clothing and food (Crusaid, National AIDS Trust, 2006).

As large numbers of people living with HIV in the UK and other countries may have insufficient income to provide for basic needs, it is important to gain an understanding of the financial circumstances of service users in order to provide appropriate and realistic support around health promotion and lifestyle change. This may involve asking questions about income, housing, work, and cooking and food storage facilities. Dietitians can help by providing advice tailored for individual circumstances such as 'Healthy eating when money is in short supply' and 'Healthy eating without cooking facilities'.

13.3.2 Ethnicity

Sub-Saharan Africa remains the worst affected region globally with 22.0 million [20.5–23.6 million] adults and children living with HIV (see Chapter 1). In the USA, at the end of 2003, estimates indicated that 47% of the persons living with HIV were black, 17% were Hispanic, and 34% were white, with 2% made up of smaller groups (CDC, 2008).

Despite comprising less than 1% of the total UK population, in 2009, the total number of Black Africans diagnosed with HIV in the UK was similar to that of white people, who make up more than 90% of the population (AVERT, 2009). Black people in the UK are also more likely to present with advanced disease. People from the African and African Caribbean communities are at greater risk of high blood pressure and stroke than the general population, which increases the risk of heart attack and kidney disease. A healthy diet with plenty of fruits and vegetables, limited salt and saturated fat intake can help reduce risk of high blood pressure and stroke. Other measures include smoking cessation, moderate alcohol intake, regular physical activity (at least 30 minutes 5 times a week) (NHS, 2009) and avoiding or reducing stress where possible. (For more information see Section 13.5.)

People of African origin are particularly at risk of HIV-associated nephropathy (HIVAN), which can cause renal failure. HIVAN is the third most common cause of end-stage renal disease (ESRD) amongst African-Americans between the ages of 20 and 64 in the USA (see Chapter 19). Black African women in the UK were found to have the highest rate of obesity (39%) compared to all other ethnic groups included in the UK Health Survey (NHS, 2005).

13.3.3 Age

HIV affects people of all ages. With effective treatment and success in greatly reducing rates of vertical transmission, particularly in resource-adequate regions, the number of older adults living with HIV has increased. The scant data that exists suggests a high prevalence and incidence of HIV among individuals 50 years of age and over. Using UNAIDS data, prevalence in older individuals was found to be one-quarter to one-third that of the 15- to 49-year age group. Older individuals have a shorter time from diagnosis to onset of AIDS, reflecting both age-related faster progression to AIDS and doctors' failure to consider HIV as a diagnosis. Screening is less common for older adults, who are assumed not to be at risk (Schmid et al., 2009). Additionally, very little HIV prevention education is targeted at older people.

There is some evidence that major complications of treated HIV disease, including cardiovascular disease, cancer, renal and liver disease, bone disease and perhaps neurological complications affecting brain function, may occur at an earlier age in the HIV-infected population. Reasons for this are multifactorial such as natural ageing, drug-specific toxicity, lifestyle factors, persistent inflammation and perhaps residual immunodeficiency (Deeks and Phillips, 2009). Clinical management should include starting ART at an early stage (as risk of CVD and other co-morbidities is reduced by high CD4$^+$ T cell counts), screening for symptoms of CVD, cerebral vascular events and cancer; aggressive preventative care for CVD (Deeks and Phillips, 2009) and lifestyle advice such as good diet, increased physical activity, cessation of smoking and drug and alcohol misuse.

13.3.4   Sexual orientation

Sex between men who have sex with men (MSM) is thought to account for between 5 and 10% of global HIV infections, although the proportion of cases attributed to this mode of transmission varies considerably between countries. It is the predominant mode of HIV transmission in much of the developed world (UNAIDS, 2009). MSM accounted for 71% of all HIV infections among male adults and adolescents in 2005 in the US (CDC, 2007). In the UK, MSM accounted for 41% (2679/6566) of all new HIV diagnoses reported in 2007 (HPA, 2009a). Despite this there is limited data on health behaviours and health needs of men who have sex with men with HIV: many existing studies have focused largely on sexual health, risk behaviours and prevention of HIV and sexually transmitted infections.

Recent epidemiological data, from 14 countries, has shown risk of death among PLHIV on treatment with CD4s above 350 is higher than the general population, but the difference was marginal for MSM (Standard Mortality Rate (SMR) = 1.05) while heterosexual men and women as a group were found to have a risk of death three times higher (SMR = 3.04) than that of the general population. For intravenous drug users (IDUs), the risk was ten times greater (SMR = 10.21). The significant difference in SMR among subgroups of PLHIV suggests that there are factors, other than HIV, affecting mortality among PLHIV (Lodwick et al., 2008; Eggar, 2009). Clearly further studies are merited to identify differences in health and lifestyle behaviours between subgroups of PLHIV.

13.3.5   Injecting drug use

On average, one out of every ten new HIV infections is caused by injecting drug use, and in some countries and regions this percentage is much higher: over 80% of all HIV infections in Eastern Europe and Central Asia is related to drug use. Globally, around 16 million people inject drugs and 3 million of them are living with HIV (WHO, 2009b). Since the epidemic began, injecting drug use has directly and indirectly accounted for more than one-third (36%) of AIDS cases in the USA, with higher prevalence among adolescent and adult women, and African-American and Hispanic adults (CDC, 2002). HIV infection among injecting drug users (IDUs) has remained relatively uncommon in the UK, with around one in 75 IDUs currently infected with HIV. Surveillance data suggest that there have been raised levels of HIV transmission among IDUs in recent years (HPA, 2009a, 2009b). Non-injection drugs (such as 'crack' cocaine) also contribute to the spread of the epidemic when users trade sex for drugs or money, or when they engage in risky sexual behaviors that they might not engage in when not using (CDC, 2002).

The limited available data indicate that injection drug use further increases nutritional risk of PLHIV. The illicit drugs may interfere with nutrient absorption and erratic lifestyles may impair access to food and other essentials such as housing and social support. This may be further compounded by hepatitis co-infection, which also detrimentally affects nutritional status (see Chapter 20). Common nutritional disorders include weight loss and wasting, micronutrient deficiencies and metabolic abnormalities (Hendricks and Grobach, 2009). Dental decay also contributes to poor nutritional status. Constipation is common due to opiate drugs, methadone, or a low intake of dietary fibre. Clinicians should pay particular attention to nutritional status, lifestyle and socio-economic problems that may compromise access to food and dietary intake in this group of patients. Those who are unable to maintain both weight and an adequate daily nutritional intake may benefit from seeing a dietitian. Otherwise, basic healthy eating advice for intravenous drug users with HIV is the same as for the general population (Hendricks and Grobach, 2009).

13.4   Other lifestyle factors that influence health outcomes

13.4.1   Mental health

There is a high prevalence of depression and other mental health disorders among PLHIV. Together with drugs for treatment of mental health disorders, these can greatly affect nutritional intake and status (see Chapter 15, 'Mental Health').

13.4.2   Physical activity

It is recommended that individuals engage in adequate levels of physical activity throughout their lives to benefit their health. Different types and amounts of physical activity are required for different health outcomes: At least 30 minutes of moderate-intensity physical activity,[1] five days a week, reduces the risk of several common NCDs in adults:

- cardiovascular disease
- stroke
- type II diabetes
- colon cancer and
- breast cancer.

There is also evidence to suggest that increasing levels of various types of physical activity may benefit health through positive effects on

- hypertension
- osteoporosis and falls risk
- body weight and composition
- musculoskeletal conditions such as osteoarthritis and low back pain
- mental and psychological health by reducing depression, anxiety and stress and
- control over risky behaviours, particularly among children and young people (e.g. tobacco use, alcohol/substance use, unhealthy diet and violence).

More physical activity provides greater health benefits and may be required for weight control. School-aged youth should accumulate at least 60 minutes of moderate-to-vigorous intensity physical activity each day (WHO, 2009).

Those at most risk of sedentary lifestyles include women, older adults over 55, certain black and minority groups, young people after the age of 16 and people with disabilities. There is little data of physical activity levels based on sexual orientation

---

[1] Examples of moderate-intensity physical activity: brisk walking, gardening, dancing, housework and domestic chores, walking domestic animals and general building tasks.

in the UK (DH, 2009). PLHIV are at increased risk of having many of the conditions listed above, so benefits of regular physical activity may be even greater in this group compared to those without HIV infection (see Chapter 14, 'Exercise and Physical Activity and Long-Term Management of HIV').

13.4.3   Alcohol

Evidence suggests that small amounts of alcohol have a protective effect against CVD development. However, harmful alcohol use is an important contributor to the global disease burden. The health consequences include liver cirrhosis, pancreatitis and various cancers (WHO, 2005). For cancer prevention, the World Cancer Research Fund recommends not to drink alcohol at all and, if consumed at all, this should be limited to two units for men and one for women a day. If people do not drink, they should not be encouraged to do so and if they do drink alcohol, they should be encouraged to adhere to the recommended safe limits. In the UK recommended limits are up to 2–3 units per day for women, and up to 3–4 units for men spread throughout the week while avoiding binge drinking and having at least two alcohol-free days each week. Women are advised not to drink during pregnancy or while breastfeeding. If women do drink during pregnancy, a limit of no more than 1 or 2 units of alcohol, once or twice a week is advised (FSA, 2009).

Generally a unit is equal to:

- half a pint of normal strength (3–5% ABV) beer, lager or cider
- one 25 ml measure of spirits (40% ABV), such as vodka or whisky and
- one small 125 ml glass of wine (12–13% ABV) (WCRF, 2009).

13.4.4   Smoking

Tobacco use is the single most important health risk behaviour in the developed world, and an important cause of preventable premature death worldwide. Smoking can contribute to a wide range of diseases, including many types of cancer, chronic obstructive pulmonary disease, coronary heart disease, stroke, osteoporosis and peripheral vascular disease (Fagerström, 2002). This may be particularly important for people treated for HIV infection, who are at greater risk than non-HIV-infected individuals of cardiovascular disease, lung cancer and bone disease as well as many other HIV–related cancers and non-HIV-related malignancies (Deeks and Phillips, 2009). Smoking can also weaken the immune system, increasing the risk of certain opportunistic infections which may, in turn, affect nutritional intake. The benefits of smoking cessation may be even greater for PLHIV compared to the general population. In the UK there are many support services available to help people quit smoking. Recommended treatments that have been proven to be effective, either separately or combined, include:

- brief interventions by a GP and other practitioners working in a GP practice or the community (including advice, self-help materials and referral for more intensive support)
- individual behavioural counselling
- group behaviour therapy

- pharmacotherapies (e.g. nicotine replacement therapy (NRT), varenicline or bupropion)
- self-help materials
- telephone counselling and quit lines and
- mass media campaigns to get the stop-smoking message across (NICE, 2008).

13.5   Principles of healthy eating

The recommended Healthy Eating teaching tool in the UK is the 'Eatwell Plate' (Figure 13.1), developed by the Food Standards Agency (FSA). Alternative tools are used in other countries, e.g. the food pyramid, which applies the same principles. Box 13.1 provides practical tips for healthy eating (see also Table 13.1).

Box 13.1   Practical tips for healthy eating

- Base meals on starchy foods.
- Eat plenty of fruit and vegetables.
- Eat more fish
- Cut down on saturated fat and sugar.
- Try to eat less salt – no more than 6 grams a day.
- Drink plenty of water
- Don't skip breakfast.

The eatwell plate

Use the eatwell plate to help you get the balance right. It shows how much of what you eat should come from each food group.

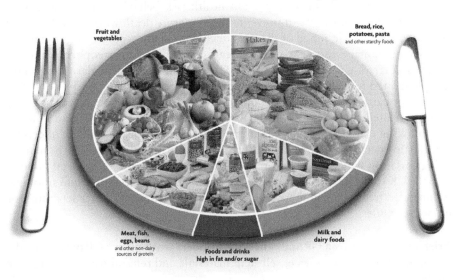

Figure 13.1 The FSA eatwell plate. Crown Copyright, 2007. Reproduced under the terms of the Click-Use Licence.

Table 13.1 Some of the starchy foods consumed in countries/regions of Africa; a thick porridge made from maize meal is common to many countries.

Region of Africa	Country	Staple food
North East Africa	Ethiopia/Eritrea	Injera (large 'pancake') Keja (bread)
	Sudan	Khibz (Arab bread) Kisrah (flat 'pancake') Rice Asida*
	Kenya	Ugali* Chapati Rice
	Uganda	Ugali* Matoke (green banana) Plantain Casssava Millet
Southern Africa	Zimbabwe	Sadza* Sorghum porridge Samp/Mashakada (whole maize grain)
	Malawi	Nsima* Rice
	South Africa	Mealiemeal Pap/phutu* Samp Mealies (corn on the cob)
	Botswana	Millet or sorghum porridge
Central African States	E.g. DRC, Congo, Cameroon	Plantain FuFu (cassava) Maize meal Rice
West Africa	E.g., Nigeria, Ivory Coast, Gambia	Gari (cassava) Isu/Iyan (yam) Jollof rice Plantain

From Kenley, 2006.
*Local name for maize meal porridge.

The eatwell plate is a pictorial representation of the types and proportions of foods needed to have a healthy and well-balanced diet. Foods are divided into five food groups, the size of the plate segment indicating how much of daily intake should come from each food group. This includes everything eaten during the day, including snacks (Box 13.2).

The eatwell plate is suitable for most people including people of all ethnic origins, people who are of a healthy weight or overweight and vegetarians. It does not apply to children under 2 years of age because they have different needs. Healthy eating messages and schematic models like The Balance of Good Health are not specifically intended for use among people with special dietary needs. It is often overlooked that people with a medical condition have one or more other co-morbidities and all of these conditions must be considered when dietary advice is provided. PLHIV who are unwell with HIV or other disorders, those with co-morbidities, such as renal, liver and cardiovascular diseases, and those at a high risk of ill health should be referred to a dietitian for nutritional advice.

Box 13.2   A step-wise approach to healthy eating using the eatwell plate

1. Food Groups: Introduce the food groups and the key nutrients for each group. Encourage regular meal patterns and selection of foods from all five food groups. This may be especially important for PLHIV to enhance medication adherence.
2. Variety and Choice: Promote eating a variety of foods and making better, healthier food choices within each food group, i.e. selecting foods which are lower in fat, salt and sugar more often, e.g. white and oily fish more often than fried and smoked fish.
3. Frequency: Encourage participants to eat from the big four food groups frequently and the smallest group occasionally, moving toward a dietary balance following the proportions of the eatwell plate.
4. Quantity: Discuss the number of portions per day for the five food groups in accordance with guidelines for a healthy diet, i.e. 5 a day for fruit and vegetables, 2–3 per day for dairy foods, etc. The amount of food/number of portions can be adjusted to individual client needs, e.g. for weight management and during pregnancy

(NHS Leeds *et al.*, 2009).

Meal pattern is an important component of healthy eating and regularly spaced meals are likely to provide varied and balanced nutritional intake (Hunt, 2007). Regular eating pattern may help with adherence for PLHIV taking anti-HIV medication.

13.5.1   Starchy foods

Foods in this group include bread, rice, potatoes, pasta, cereals, oats, noodles, yams, plantain, maize and millet. Beans and pulses can be eaten as part of this group.

Amount to be consumed: about one-third of total volume of food eaten

Main nutrients:

•   carbohydrate (starch)
•   fibre (especially insoluble fibre) and
•   calcium, iron and B vitamins.

Suggestions for service users:
- eat plenty of these foods
- include at least one starchy food with each main meal
- include wholemeal/wholegrain foods such as wholewheat breads, brown rice and high-fibre breakfast cereals as they contain more fibre and other nutrients than white or refined starchy foods
- avoid frying and adding too much fat to these foods (e.g. butter, margarine, dressings, mayonnaise and rich sauces such as cream or cheese.

Fibre

Fibre, or 'roughage', is only found in foods derived from plants, such as cereals, grains, seeds, pulses, fruit and vegetables. There are two types of fibre: soluble and insoluble.

Insoluble fibre (found in wholegrain foods) helps prevent constipation.
Soluble fibre may help to reduce the amount of cholesterol in the blood. Good sources of soluble fibre include oats, beans, peas, lentils, chickpeas, fruit and vegetables. (See Figures 13.2–13.5.)

Box 13.3–13.5 list the main nutrients of various food groups.

Box 13.3 Fruits and vegetables

Main Nutrients:

Vitamin C
Carotenes and other anti-oxidants
Folates
Fibre (especially soluble fibre)
Potassium

Amount: at least one-third of the total volume of food eaten
Suggestions for service users:

Eat plenty (at least 5 portions each day) and eat a wide variety. This can include fresh, frozen and canned fruit and vegetables and dried fruit.
Pulses and fruit juice can be included in this group as one portion, however much is consumed each day (Box 13.5 portion approximates).
Avoid: adding fat and rich sauces to vegetables and sugar/syrupy dressings to fruit.

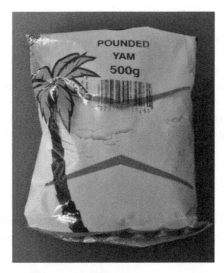

Figure 13.2 Pounded yam (Photo: V Pribram).

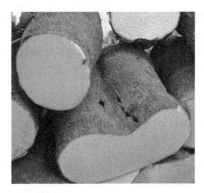

Figure 13.3 Fresh yams (Photo: Luis Luna).

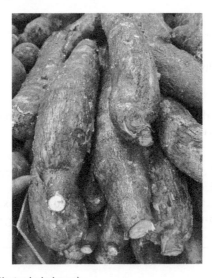

Figure 13.4 Cassava (Photo: Luis Luna).

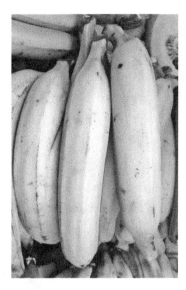

Figure 13.5   Plaintains (Photo: Luis Luna).

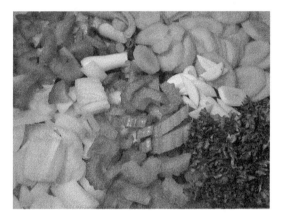

Figure 13.6   Raw vegetables (Photo: Luis Luna).

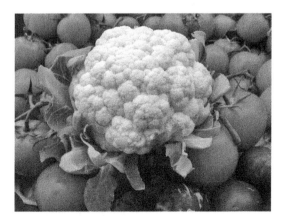

Figure 13.7   Cauliflower and tomatoes (Photo: Luis Luna).

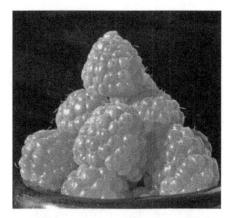

Figure 13.8   Raspberries (Photo: Luis Luna).

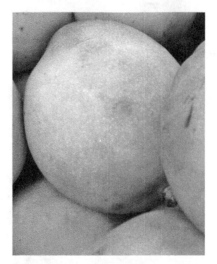

Figure 13.9   Mangoes (Photo: Luis Luna).

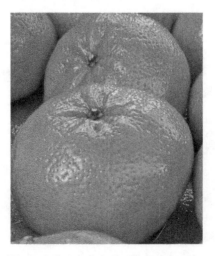

Figure 13.10   Mandarins (Photo: Luis Luna).

Box 13.4   Milk and dairy foods

Main nutrients:

Calcium, magnesium
Protein
Riboflavin and vitamin B12
Vitamins A, D (full-fat produce only)
Amount: about one-sixth of total volume of food eaten
Foods included in this group: milk, cheese, yoghurt and fromage frais
Foods *not* included in this group: butter, eggs and cream

Suggestions for service users:

Eat or drink moderate amounts and choose lower fat versions whenever you
    can
Check the amount of fat by looking at the nutrient information on the labels
Compare similar products and choose the lowest available

Box 13.5   Meat, poultry, fish, eggs, pulses, nuts and seeds

Main Nutrients:

Iron
Protein
B vitamins, especially B12
Zinc
Magnesium
Amount: about one-sixth of total volume of food eaten

Suggestions for service users:

- Eat moderate amounts and try to go for the leanest option whenever you
  can. For example, meat with the fat cut off, poultry without the skin and fish
  without batter. Cook these foods without added fat. As a general rule, the
  more white you can see on meat, the more fat it contains.
- Try to include beans and pulses as these are a good source of protein and
  naturally low in fat. This may include canned beans and pulses.

Box 13.6   Examples of portions of fruits and vegetables: one portion equals
approximately 80 g of these:

- One apple, banana, pear, orange or other similar-sized fruit
- Two plums or similar-sized fruit
- Half a grapefruit or avocado
- One slice of large fruit, such as melon or pineapple

- Three heaped tablespoons of vegetables (raw, cooked, frozen or tinned)
- Three heaped tablespoons of beans and pulses
- Three heaped tablespoons of fruit salad (fresh or tinned in fruit juice) or stewed fruit
- One heaped tablespoon of dried fruit (such as raisins and apricots)
- One handful of grapes, cherries or berries
- A dessert bowl of salad and
- A glass (150 ml) of fruit juice (however much you drink, fruit juice counts as a maximum of one portion a day).

Box 13.7 provides a list of some pulses.

Box 13.7 Pulses include the whole range of beans, peas and lentils such as:

- Baked beans
- Red, green, yellow and brown lentils
- Black eyed peas
- Garden peas
- Runner beans
- Chickpeas
- Broad beans
- Kidney beans
- Butter beans

Try eating at least two portions of fish a week, including one of oily fish (Box 13.7). Fish includes frozen, canned and dried fish

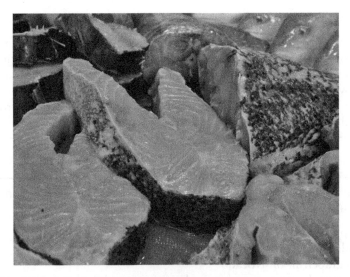

Figure 13.11 Salmon steaks (Photo: Luis Luna).

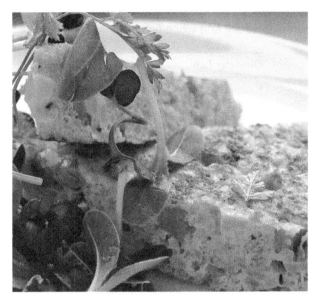

Figure 13.12 Vegetable omelette (Photo: Luis Luna).

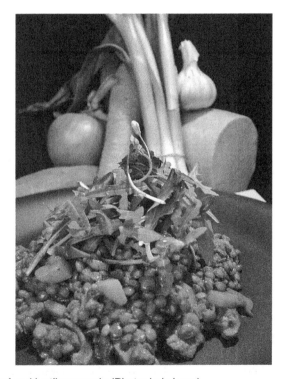

Figure 13.13 Beef and lentil casserole (Photo: Luis Luna).

Box 13.8   Examples of oily and white fish

Oily/fatty fish	White/non-oily fish
Salmon	Cod
Trout	Haddock
Mackerel	Plaice
Herring	Coley
Sardines	Whiting
Pilchards	Lemon sole
Kipper	Skate
	Halibut
Tuna (fish only)	Hake
Anchovies	Sea bream
Swordfish	Shark
	Tilapia
Carp	Turbot
Hilsa	Tinned tuna
Jack fish	Marlin
Katla	

There are recommendations for the maximum number of portions of oily fish we should be eating each week (a portion is about 140 g) due to risk of pollutants (Box 13.8).

Box 13.9

2 portions of oily fish	4 portions of oily fish
girls and women who might have a baby one day	other women
Women who are pregnant or breastfeeding	men and boys

Shark, marlin and swordfish: limit to one portion per week due to high levels of mercury.

• Try to avoid meat products with a high fat content (e.g. streaky bacon, salami sausages, beef burgers and pâté)

Nuts are a good source of fibre, protein, vitamins, minerals, essential fatty acids and monounsaturated fat, which can help reduce the amount of cholesterol in blood. As they have a high fat content it is best to eat in moderation ant to try to avoid salted nuts.

Seeds such as sunflower, pumpkin, poppy, sesame and flax contain protein, fibre and vitamins.

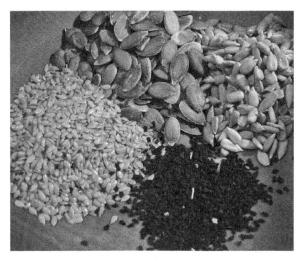

Figure 13.14   Seeds (Photo: Luis Luna).

13.5.2   Foods containing fat; foods and drinks containing sugar

Main nutrients: fat, including some essential fatty acids, but also some vitamins.

Some products also contain salt or sugar.
Amount: these foods should form only a small part of total food intake
Fat is high in calories so eating too much could lead to weight gain. Also excess
saturated fat could lead to raised blood cholesterol.

Foods that are high in saturated fat include:

- fatty cuts of meat and meat products such as sausages and pies
- butter, ghee and lard
- cream, soured cream, crème fraîche and ice cream
- cheese, particularly hard cheese
- pastries
- cakes and biscuits
- some savoury snacks like crisps
- some sweet snacks and chocolate and
- palm oil, coconut oil and coconut cream.

Other foods containing fat include:

Margarine, other spreading fats and low fat;
Spreads, cooking oils, oil-based salad dressings; and
Mayonnaise, puddings, rich sauces and gravies.

Foods and drinks containing sugar:

Soft drinks, sweets, jam and sugar, as well as foods such
as cakes, puddings, biscuits, pastries and ice cream.

Suggestions for service users:

- Use small amounts of foods like margarine, butter, other spreading fats (including low fat spreads), cooking oils, oil-based salad dressings and mayonnaise, and limit foods such as cakes, biscuits, pastries, ice cream and sweets;
- grill, bake, boil, poach or steam food, rather than adding extra fat, e.g. roasting;
- put more vegetables or beans in casseroles, stews and curries, and a bit less meat – drain or skim the fat off before serving;
- remove all visible fat from meat and skin and fat deposits on chicken;
- choose low fat alternatives when possible, e.g. reduced-fat/low-fat spreads and dairy product (such as skimmed or semi-skimmed milk rather than full-fat milk);
- cut down on foods and drinks containing sugar and these should be eaten mainly at mealtimes to reduce the risk of tooth decay; and
- check food labels to help you pick the foods with less added sugar or go for the low-sugar version (see Box 13.10).

Box 13.10   Check food labels for fat and saturated fat:

High fat is more than 20 g fat per 100 g
Low fat is 3 g fat or less per 100 g
High saturated fat is more than 5 g per 100 g
Low saturated fat is less than 1.5 g per 100 g
If the product is between these figures, it contains a medium level of fat

---

Salt

Eeating too much salt can raise blood pressure. People with high blood pressure are three times more likely to develop heart disease or have a stroke than people with normal blood pressure (NHS, 2008). Adults should have no more than 6 grams of salt a day (this equals about 2.5 grams of sodium). Evidence in general populations has shown that reduced salt diets can help lower blood pressure and that some groups are more sensitive to salt – such as people with type 2 diabetes and people of African and Caribbean origin (see Chapter 19).

Suggestions for service users:

Avoid adding salt to food and eating high salt foods like salty snacks, bacon, cheese, pickles, smoked fish, crips and savoury snacks.
Reduce or avoid salt in cooking. Try other ways of flavouring food such as using herbs, spices, mustard, onion, garlic or lemon juice.

Salt substitutes are not necessary for most people and are not suitable for people with renal disorders due to a high potassium content (Hunt, 2007; FSA, 2009) (see Box 13.11).

Box 13.11   Check labels for salt:

High is more than 1.5 g salt per 100 g (or 0.6 g sodium)
Low is 0.3 g salt or less per 100 g (or 0.1 g sodium)

If the amount of salt per 100 g is in between these figures, then that is a medium level of salt.

Vitamin and minerals

There are no specific recommendations for minerals and vitamin supplements for PLHIV that differ from the general population. PLHIV are advised to get all the nutrients they need from food. If individuals do wish to take vitamin and mineral supplements, one tablet a day providing a wide range of these nutrients is advised as opposed to taking large amounts of specific nutrients. For example, even doses of vitamin A (an antioxidant) above 1.5 mg/day over many years may decrease bone mineral density. Eating liver or liver products such as pâté once a week is likely to provide, on average, 1.5 mg of vitamin per day (see Chapters 7, 'Decreased Nutritional Status and Nutritional Interventions for People Living with HIV'). Vitamin D deficiency is now a major, worldwide concern and this may be even more prevalent among people with HIV (see Chapter 10).

13.6   Portion sizes and quantity of food required

Individuals differ in nutrient requirements and the amount of energy (calories) they require. Factors that may affect this include age, gender, physical activity level, and if they are overweight. For this reason information about portion sizes is not provided, other than for fruits and vegetables (FSA, 2009; Hunt, 2007)

13.7   Weight management for people living with HIV

Prevention and management of overweight and obesity are complex matters that are largely outside of the scope of this publication. Local and national guidelines should be used.

Evidence shows that a high intake of NSP (dietary fibre) promotes weight loss, while a high intake of energy-dense foods and, probably, increased consumption of sweetened drinks and large portion sizes promote weight gain (WHO, 2003). Nevertheless, a dietary approach alone is not sufficient. It is essential that any dietary recommendations are part of a multi-component intervention (NICE, 2006).

13.7.1   Assessment

Assessment should include:

- degree of overweight/obesity and health risk. Use BMI to classify degree of obesity and waist circumference to classify health risk if BMI less than 35 kg/m^2 (see Chapter 8, 'Nutritional Screening and Assessment')
- lifestyle and environmental factors
- co-morbidities
- willingness to change
- antiretrovirals or other drugs.

13.7.2   Weight reducing interventions

Weight reducing interventions should be:

- patient centred
- appropriate for the patient (e.g. in terms of age and cultural background) and
- delivered by trained professionals.

(NICE, 2006)

Multi-component interventions for PLHIV who are overweight, obese or gaining weight rapidly include:

- follow the healthy eating guidelines and improve the balance of their diet
- avoid eating and drinking more than they need
- become more physically active and
- seek advice from trained health care professionals such as their dietitian/qualified staff in their GP surgery.

There are a limited number of pharmacological treatments and surgical interventions available for those with very high degrees of obesity. There are potential interactions between antiretroviral and anti-obesity medication metabolised through the liver. PLHIV taking these medications are advised to speak to their pharmacist about this.

Motivational techniques and behavioural interventions may help bring about lifestyle change. These should be used by appropriately trained professionals. Strategies include:

- self-monitoring of behaviour and progress
- stimulus control
- goal setting
- slowing rate of eating
- ensuring social support
- problem solving
- cognitive restructuring (modifying thoughts)
- reinforcement of changes
- relapse prevention and
- strategies for dealing with weight regain.

13.7.3   Dietary advice

- Encourage people to improve their diet even if they do not lose weight, because there can be other health benefits.
- Tailor advice for individual food preferences and allow for flexible approaches to reduce calorie intake.
- Set realistic targets for weight loss: aim to lose 5–10% of original weight with a weekly maximum weight loss of 0.5–1 kg as rapid weight loss could result

in muscle wasting: particularly detrimental for PLHIV as untreated HIV is a muscle-wasting disease (see Chapter 7).
- Avoid using unduly restrictive and nutritionally unbalanced diets because they are ineffective in the long term and can be harmful.

Although evidence is limited, there are health concerns about some weight loss approaches such as long-term risk of renal and bone problems and cancer risk with 'high protein, low carbohydrate diet' and gallstones with very low calorie diets (VLDL). As PLHIV may already be at increased risk of such disorders, it is advisable for PLHIV to be referred to a dietitian for weight-reducing advice. Monitoring of weight reduction and maintenance can be checked at routine appointments with reinforcement of this advice by other clinical staff such as doctors and nurses. As PLHIV attend HIV treatment clinics regularly, this is an excellent opportunity for screening, identifying patients with excessive weight gain and trying to prevent this as much as possible. Training on weight management can be provided by dietitians in the clinical setting.

A conventional weight-reducing diet remains the most valuable intervention in the treatment of overweight and obesity, given considerations of safety, nutritional adequacy and efficacy and this usually results in 4–5 kg weight loss (Hankey, 2007).

Perceptions of ideal weight vary between cultures and ethnic groups. It is important to take a patient-centred approach and discuss concepts about ideal body size and shape while providing information about potential health and other benefits of weight loss (NICE, 2006).

Examples of weight reducing dietary advice for West African people:

There is a high incidence of diabetes, hypertension and obesity in the West African community in the UK. Weight-reducing advice is often needed. This includes:

- Reducing the amount of oil used in soups and stews. Palm oil and palm nut oil are often used. These are high in saturated fat. Alternative oils include vegetable, olive, sunflower and groundnut.
- Reducing the amount of peanut butter used in soups.
- Reducing the amount of fried foods such as fried fish or meat. Encourage stewing or baking instead.
- Portion sizes of green bananas, yams, ground rice and other starchy food is often substantial and may need to be reduced (Thaker, 2007).

13.7.4 Physical activity for weight management

Physical activity in addition to dietary intervention can offer opportunities for improved maintenance of weight loss, although physical activity programmes alone result in minimal weight loss (Hankey, 2007).

- Adults should:
  - take more exercise even if this does not lead to weight loss, as there are other health benefits (e.g. reduced risk of type 2 diabetes and cardiovascular disease)

- do at least 30 minutes of moderate-intensity physical activity on 5 or more days a week, in one session or several shorter ones lasting 10 minutes or more; 45–60 minutes may be needed to prevent obesity; people who have lost weight may need to do 60–90 minutes to avoid regaining weight
  - build up to the recommended levels, using a managed approach with agreed goals
  - reduce the time they spend inactive, such as watching television, or using a computer.
- Recommended types of physical activity include:
  - activities that can be incorporated into everyday life, such as brisk walking, gardening or cycling
  - supervised exercise programmes
  - other activities, such as swimming, walking a certain number of steps each day, or stair climbing.
- Take the person's current physical fitness and ability into account (NICE, 2006).

Practical advice to help clients achieve a healthy diet:

- Base meals on pasta, rice, potatoes, maize meal, bread, yam, etc. These provide energy and are cheap, filling options.
- Add one or two vegetables, salad items or fruit – fresh, tinned, frozen, dried and juice all count towards your five-a-day target.
- Include a small portion (75–120 g) of meat, fish, eggs, chicken, lentils or beans to meet protein needs.
  Low-cost ideas:
  - replace half the meat in meals with beans, lentils and chickpeas to make a larger amount of food without spending more.
  - try tinned fish as a filling for potatoes or in pasta dishes.
  - eggs – scrambled, boiled or as an omelette.
  - look for meat/fish on special offer, adapting your meal to suit.
- Include three portions of dairy products each day – if you are unable to tolerate milk, try soya alternatives with added calcium.

Shopping tips to make money go further:

- **Economy branded goods** – tinned tomatoes, pulses, cereals, etc. are just as good as known brand products, only much cheaper.
- **Special Offers and promotions** – look out for BOGOF (buy one get one free), 3 for 2 and other offers on your usual items. Store for later or share the saving with a friend. *Remember it's only a bargain if you would use it normally!*
- **Fresh and seasonal products** – get best value on fresh foods when they are in season, e.g. buy strawberries in June not at Christmas!
- **Larger sizes** – cost per portion is cheaper when things are bought in bulk. Buy frequently used foods like tea, coffee, rice and sugar in large packs and store or split the pack, sharing the cost between friends.
- **Reduced price items** – check at the end of the day or at reduced price points around supermarkets for these items. Check the use by date and buy only what can be safely consumed. Many items can be frozen on the day of purchase to use later.

- **Longer lasting or frozen foods** – buy long life, tinned or frozen foods when storage space for fresh food is insufficient. These foods can be just as nutritious and are useful to have in for days when you are not able to go to the shops.
- **Specialist ranges in local shops** – often local multicultural shops offer the best value on traditional foods, e.g. maize meal, rice and specialist vegetables. Get to know your local shops!

Source: Foster K, Leeds Community Nutrition and Dietetic Service (2009).

13.8 Summary

Improvements in dietary intake and other positive lifestyle changes may be of particular benefit to PLHIV. Potential outcomes include decreased morbidity and increased longevity. Studies of dietary and lifestyle interventions and behaviours in this population group are needed.

Acknowledgements

This chapter was reviewed by:

Alastair Duncan, BSc(Hons) MSc PGDipD RD, Principal Dietitian, HIV, Guy's and St. Thomas' Hospital NHS Foundation Trust, London
Deepa Kariyawasam BSc. RD, Senior Renal Dietitian, Department of Nutrition and Dietetics, King's College Hospital NHS Foundation Trust, London
Karen Klassen, BHEc(Hons), RD, HIV Specialist Dietitian, Imperial College Healthcare NHS Trust Honorary Research Associate, Imperial College, London

References

Lodwick R, Eggar M. *et al.* (Antiretroviral Cohort Collaboration (ART-CC). The ART cohort collaboration: life expectancy of individuals on combination antiretroviral therapy in high-income countries: a collaborative analysis of 14 cohort studies. *Lancet* 2008; 372:293–9.

AVERT. UK statistics by race, age and gender. Available at: http://www.avert.org/uk-race-age-gender.htm (June 2009). Accessed 2 August 2009.

Bowcott O. Life Expectancy Gap between rich and poor is widening. *The Guardian*, 4 July 2009; 16, UK.

CDC. Drug-Associated HIV Transmission Continues in the United States, Department of Health and Human Sciences, Centre for Disease Control and Prevention, 2008. 2002. Available at: http://www.cdc.gov/hiv/resources/Factsheets/idu.htm.

CDC. HIV/AIDS among Men Who Have Sex with Men, Fact Sheet, Department of Health and Human Sciences, Centre for Disease Control and Prevention. 2007. Available at http://www.cdc.gov/hiv/topics/msm/resources/factsheets/msm.htm. Accessed 4 aUG 2009.

CDC. HIV and AIDS in the United States: A Picture of Today's Epidemic, Department of Health and Human Sciences, Centre for Disease Control and Prevention. 2008. Available at: http://www.cdc.gov/hiv/topics/surveillance/united_states.htm. Accessed Aug 2009.

Crusaid, National AIDS Trust (NAT). Poverty and HIV: Findings from the Crusaid Hardship Fund, December 1 2006, London, UK. Available at: http://www.nat.org.uk/Media%20library/Files/PDF%20documents/HIV-Poverty-report.pdf. Accessed 2 August 2009.

Cunningham W *et al.* The effect of socioeconomic status on the survival of people receiving care for HIV infection in the United States. *J Health Care Poor Underserved* 2005; 6:655–676.

Deeks SG, Phillips AN. HIV infection, antiretroviral treatment, ageing, and non-AIDS related morbidity. *BMJ* 2009; 338a:3172.

DH leading in partnership with OGDs, Be Active Be Healthy: A Plan for Getting the Nation Moving, HM Government, Feb 2009, Gateway reference 10818. www.walkengland.org.uk/...Feb.../Be-Active-Be-Healthy.pdf

Eggar M. Oral presentation at 15th Annual Conference of the British HIV Association (BHIVA)1-3 April 2009, Liverpool Antiretroviral Cohort Collaboration (ART-CC), in press.

Fagerström K. The epidemiology of smoking: health consequences and benefits of cessation. *Drugs* 2002; **62**:1–9.

FSA (Food Stadards Agency). Eatwell. London. 2009. Available at: http://www.eatwell.gov.uk/info/aboutus/.

Hankey C. In: Thomas B, Bishop J, eds. *Management of Obesity and Overweight, Manual of Dietetic Practice*. Oxford: Blackwell Publishing, 2007.

Heaney RP. Nutrition, chronic disease, and the problem of proof. *Am J Clin Nutr* September 2006; **84**(3):471–2.

Hendricks K, Grobach S. Nutrition issues in chronic drug users living with HIV infection, Addiction Science and Clinical Practice. 2009. Available at: http://www.drugabuse.gov/PDF/ascp/vol5no1/Nutrition.pdf. Accessed 8 May 2010.

Hendricks KM, Willis K, Houser R, Jones CY. Obesity in HIV-infection: dietary correlates. *J Am Coll Nutr* 2006; **25**(4):321–31.

HPA. HIV data: Injecting Drug Users. 2009a. Health Protection Agency. Available at: http://www.hpa.nhs.uk/servlet/Satellite?childpagename=HPAweb%252FHPAwebPrinterFriendly&c=Page&p=1202115502904&pagename=HPAwebWrapper&cid=1202115502904.

HPA. MSM HIV Data, Health protection Agency, London UK, 2009b, Available at: http://www.hpa.org.uk/web/HPAweb&HPAwebStandard/HPAweb_C/1203928687610. Accessed 4 August 2009b.

Hunt P. In: Thomas B, Bishop J eds. *Healthy Eating, Healthy Lifestyle, Manual of Dietetic Practice*. Oxford: Blackwell Publishing, 2007.

Kenley D. Food from Home, Student Project, Leeds Community Nutrition & Dietetic Service, Leeds PCT, 2006.

Lippman SM, Hawk ET. Cancer prevention: from 1727 to milestones of the past 100 years. *Cancer Res.* 2009; **69**(13):5269–84.

Lodwick R, Porter K, Sabin CA *et al*. Age- and sex-specific death rates in ART-naive patients with CD4 count above 350 cells/mm3 compared with the general population. 15th Conference on Retroviruses and Opportunistic Infections. February 3–6, 2008. Boston. Abstract 141.

Lopez-Jimenez F. Speakable and unspeakable facts about BMI and mortality. *Lancet* 2009; **373**(9669):1083–96.

NHS. Prevalence of obesity by sex and ethnic group, 2004, adults aged 16 and over, England (Table). Source: Health Survey for England 2004. 2005. Available at: http://www.ic.nhs.uk/. Accessed 2 August 2009.

NHS. Blood pressure and stroke, NHS Choices, Your health, your choices. 2008. Available at: http://www.nhs.uk/Livewell/Blackhealth/Pages/Bloodpressureandstroke.aspx. Accessed 2 August 2009.

NHS. Leeds and Leeds Community Nutrition and Dietetic Service, Healthy Living Training Resource Pack, October 2009.

NICE (National Institute for Health and Clinical Excellence). *Obesity: The Prevention, Identification, Assessment and Management of Overweight and Obesity in Adults and Children*. London: CG43, 2006.

NICE (National Institute for Health and Clinical Excellence). Smoking Cessation Services. Public health guidance PH10, London, 2008.

Pomerleau J, Lock K, Knai C, McKee M. Interventions designed to increase adult fruit and vegetable intake can be effective: a systematic review of the literature. *J Nutr* 2005; **135**(10):2486–95.

Schmid GP, Williams BG, Garcia-Calleja JM *et al*. The Unexplored story of HIV and aging. *Bull World Health Org* 2009; **87**(3):161–244.

Thaker A. In: Thomas B, Bishop J, eds. *People from Black and Ethnic Groups, Manual of Dietetic Practice*. Oxford: Blackwell Publishing, 2007.

UNAIDS. Men who have sex with Men, UNAIDS. 2009. Available at: http://www.unaids.org/en/PolicyAndPractice/KeyPopulations/MenSexMen/. Accessed Aug 4 2009.

WCRF (World Cancer Research Fund). *Preventing Cancer Before it starts*. London: WCRF. 2009. Available at: http://www.wcrf-uk.org/preventing_cancer/.

WHO Benefits of Physical Activity, World Health Organization, Geneva. 2009. Available at: http://www.who.int/dietphysicalactivity/factsheet_benefits/en/index.html. Accessed 4 August 2009.

WHO. *Preventing Deaths from Chronic Diseases, A vital Investment.* Geneva: World Health Organization, 2005.

WHO. Injecting drug use (IDU) and prisons, World Health Organization, Geneva, 2009. Available at: http://www.who.int/hiv/topics/idu/en/index.html. Accessed 4 August 2009b.

WHO (World Health Organization). Diet, nutrition and the prevention of chronic disease. Technical Report Series 916. Geneva: WHO, 2003.

WHO/FAO. Diet, nutrition and the prevention of chronic diseases: report of a Joint FAO/WHO consultation, Geneva, 28 January – 1 February 2002. Geneva: WHO, 2002.

Zaracostas J. Non-communicable diseases must have greater priority, says WHO. *BMJ* 2009; **339**:b2857.

14 Exercise and Physical Activity and Long-Term Management of HIV

Joanna Lucy Bowtell and
Rebecca Weissbort

Key Points

- There are positive associations between physical activity levels and health status of patients living with HIV.
- Moderate intensity and duration exercise do not negatively affect virological or immunological markers, indeed there is some evidence to suggest that exercise may decrease viral load and increase CD4$^+$ count.
- Progressive resistance training programmes significantly increase lean body mass (LBM), muscle volume and strength, and are therefore an effective treatment, either singly or in combination with testosterone analogs, to counteract wasting syndrome or loss of LBM.
- Combined resistance and endurance exercise programmes have been shown to reduce body fat levels within both subcutaneous and visceral compartments, in addition to inducing favourable metabolic changes such as improved insulin sensitivity and improved blood lipid profiles.
- Exercise interventions improve psychological well-being and functional capacity, thus improving quality of life.

14.1 Introduction

Mortality from AIDS and the incidence of AIDS-defining illnesses has fallen steeply since the introduction of effective anti-HIV treatment with a protease inhibitor (PI) or a non-nucleoside reverse transcriptase inhibitor (NNRTI) in combination with two or more nucleoside reverse transcriptase inhibitors (NRTI). However, long-term use of antiretroviral treatment (ART) is limited by virological failure, the development of drug resistance and by the significant occurrence of drug toxicities. Approximately 40% of patients experience one or more adverse effects within 18 months of starting PIs (Easterbrook and Meadway, 2001) and, in addition, there are various NNRTI- and NRTI-specific side effects (White, 2001). The spectrum includes gastrointestinal problems, hepatic dysfunction, peripheral neuropathy, myopathy, renal toxicities, lactic acidosis, hypertension, hyperlipidaemia (primarily increased low-density lipoprotein (LDL) cholesterol, and triglycerides (TG), alongside reduced high-density lipoprotein (HDL)), insulin resistance, osteopaenia and body fat redistribution syndrome or lipodystrophy, which contributes to the major metabolic syndrome.

This atherogenic profile of elevated LDL, TG and reduced HDL, alongside increased visceral adiposity, is predicted to increase cardiovascular risk. There is considerable variability in the cardiovascular risk score derived when applying different risk tools, which suggests the need for caution in applying standard cardiovascular disease risk assessment tools to people living with HIV (PLHIV) (Garcia-Lazaro et al., 2007). Lima et al. (2009) found that amongst Framingham Risk Score, PRO-CAM, and National Cholesterol Education Programme (ATPIII), the Framingham Risk Score conferred greatest sensitivity. Nonetheless, many (Triant et al., 2007), although not all (Bozzette et al., 2003), studies have suggested an increased incidence of cardiovascular disease amongst PLHIV and those exposed to antiretroviral therapy. Brown et al. (2005) reported a fourfold higher incidence of diabetes mellitus in HIV+ men exposed to ART than in HIV-seronegative men. This effect is also evident amongst HIV+ children with 13.2% insulin resistance reported (Beregszaszi et al., 2005). Lipodystrophy is reported in up to 83% of patients after two years of antiretroviral therapy (Carr et al., 2003) and this is characterised by peripheral fat depletion, and/or central fat accumulation in the abdomen and in some cases enlargement of fat pads, e.g. buffalo hump or breast enlargement in women. The presence of these body composition changes affects long-term adherence to therapy (Duran et al., 2001), body image perception (Collins et al., 2002), and contributes to a poorer quality of life, particularly in the presence of other ART side effects (Blanch et al., 2002). Although drugs can be used to treat hyperlipidaemia (Manfredi and Chiodo, 2001), there are complications with drug interactions (statins in particular); and current strategies to manage body composition changes have only limited effectiveness.

The focus of this chapter is to consider the evidence supporting the use of exercise as an adjunct therapy to mitigate against the effects of HIV and the adverse effects of drug therapies.

Exercise has been defined as 'a sub-category of leisure-time physical activity in which planned, structured and repetitive bodily movements are performed to improve or maintain one or more components of physical fitness'. Whereas physical activity has been defined as 'any bodily movement produced by contraction of skeletal muscle that substantially increase energy expenditure' (Howley, 2001) and as such encompasses a broader range of activities. The next section will consider the evidence arising from observational studies in which the relationships between physical activity level and quality of life and immune function are explored; as well as factors affecting physical activity participation amongst this population.

Exercise can be split into two broad subcategories: resistance or strength training and aerobic or endurance training. Resistance training predominantly develops muscular strength, both through neural adaptations and in the longer term through hypertrophy (increased muscle fibre cross-sectional area), resulting in increased muscle mass. Progressive resistance training is based on the principle of overload such that progressively larger than normal loads are placed upon the exercising muscle inducing adaptation. This normally takes the form of using resistance machines or free weights within the gym setting, although this can involve counterbody weight activities in a less formalised setting. Endurance exercise is defined as muscle contraction against little or no resistance, which can be performed for prolonged periods of time and generally involves a greater total expenditure of energy. Endurance exercise can range from a brisk walk to running, cycling and swimming and can take place in a variety of settings. Endurance exercise induces cardiovascular, respiratory and metabolic adaptations as well as muscle-specific changes (including increased capillarisation and mitochondrial volume). The studies reviewed in the following sections consider the evidence derived from interventional studies, in which the effects of prescribed programmes of endurance and resistance exercise on immunological, metabolic parameters, body composition and quality of life are investigated. To support this analysis, a case study is presented detailing factors that should be considered in prescribing exercise for individual patients.

14.2 Observational studies

Several studies involving PLHIV have now demonstrated positive associations between health status and regular participation in physical activity. Mustafa *et al.* (1999) assessed correlations between self-reported physical activity and HIV disease progression in 415 individuals (156 HIV^+, 259 HIV^-) from the Longitudinal Aids Impact Study (851 homosexual men in New York, 1985–1991). On entry to the study, individuals were asked, 'How many times a week do you engage in physical exercise?' Those that responded 3–4 times per week or more were categorized as physically active and others as physically inactive. After one year follow-up those who were physically active at baseline had a slower decline in $CD4^+$, a lesser risk of progression to AIDS and lower AIDS mortality. This protective effect declined with the duration of follow-up, however there were a number of confounding factors, not least that changes in physical activity over the follow-up period were not considered. More recently Bopp *et al.* (2004) measured physical activity over a 3-day period using wrist accelerometers in 66 HIV^+ patients, and found an inverse relationship between viral load and physical activity level, but no relationship between $CD4^+$ cell counts and physical activity. The authors suggest that by lowering viral load values, physical activity may prolong the asymptomatic period of HIV disease, decreasing the incidence of opportunistic infection and delaying the initiation of treatment.

Gavrila *et al.* (2003) assessed the relationship amongst physical activity, diet and metabolic changes in 120 HIV^+ subjects (89% male). Physical activity level was assessed by questionnaire, and blood lipid profile, insulin resistance (HOMA) and body composition data (DEXA, L4 CT scan) were available for 94% of subjects. Inverse relationships were found between total physical activity and fasting TG, borderline significance with insulin resistance, and a positive relationship between total physical activity and LBM. Ramirez-Marrero *et al.* (2004) also found that physically active (≥ 300 kcal/d) Hispanic PLHIV from Puerto Rico ($n = 68$) had healthier body composition as measured by lower body mass index and less subcutaneous trunk and limb fat (skinfold thickness) than those who were less active. In addition, physically active individuals had higher life satisfaction scores but there was no difference in $CD4^+$ cell counts between physically active and less active or inactive subjects.

Fillipas *et al.* (2008) asked ambulatory PLHIV attending an infectious diseases clinic in Melbourne, Australia, to complete a short Physical Activity Questionnaire (PAQ) to quantify their levels of physical activity. One in four PLHIV ($n = 191$) and one in three HIV– people ($n = 70$) were not meeting the ACSM physical activity recommendations (30 minutes of moderate activity on 5 days per week, or 20 minutes of vigorous activity on 3 days per week). Clingerman (2003) assessed physical activity behaviour in a sample of PLHIV ($n = 78$) recruited from an infectious disease clinic and a community service organization in the USA. As for Fillipas *et al.* (2008), walking was the preferred form of activity and 53% of the sampled population completed 30 minutes of walking per day on 5 days per week. However, only 28.2% identified that they met the moderate physical activity recommendations and in common with the rest of the US population, 26.9% did not participate in any leisure-time physical activity. Levels of physical activity were also positively correlated with income and total functional social support from friends. The degree of social support and self-efficacy are key determinants of physical activity participation and other healthy behaviours, thus use of 'buddying' and other systems providing social support should be considered in order to maximize participation rates.

There are however a number of limitations to such descriptive, correlational study design, not least that such studies use questionnaires to assess physical activity level, and are therefore entirely dependent on the accuracy of recall of the amount and intensity of previous physical activities completed. As observed in other populations, Ramirez-Marrero *et al.* (2008) recently raised significant concerns with regard to over-reporting of activity amongst Hispanic PLHIV, using such measurement tools. In addition, no causal relationships can be determined from such data. For instance, the observed inverse relationship between viral load and physical activity participation may merely be a consequence of more severe disease symptoms or accelerated disease progression, limiting physical activity participation. Alternatively, those participating in more physical activity may have lower viral load levels, leading to fewer symptoms and less disability than those PLHIV participating in lower levels of physical activity. Evidence from exercise training studies would support the latter conclusion. The subsequent sections of this chapter will therefore evaluate the evidence derived from interventional studies where PLHIV have participated in chronic endurance and/or resistance exercise programmes.

14.3   Effect of exercise on immunological parameters

The relationship between exercise and immune function has been modelled as a J-shaped curve (Nieman and Nehlsen-Cannarella, 1994), with regular moderate intensity and duration exercise associated with a reduced incidence of infection compared with a completely sedentary state. However, prolonged bouts of strenuous exercise cause a temporary depression of various aspects of immune function lasting 3–24 hours after exercise, with more pronounced effects after continuous, prolonged (>1.5 hours) moderate- to high-intensity (55–75% VO_2max) exercise performed without food intake (for a detailed review, see Gleeson, 2007). In the light of this, prolonged (>1.5 hour) and/or very high-intensity exercise are/is contraindicated for HIV⁺ patients; in addition exercise should not be completed in the fasted state, to avoid the potential for temporary suppression of various aspects of immune function including neutrophil respiratory burst, lymphocyte proliferation and monocyte antigen presentation.

However, Smith *et al.* (2004) measured the response to a novel antigen (keyhole limpet haemocyanin) challenge in sedentary and physically active young and older men, and found that regular physical activity was able to counteract the age-related decline in primary antibody and memory T-cell response. In addition to this improvement in immune response, there is good evidence that regular physical activity has an anti-inflammatory effect. Regular physical activity is associated with lower mitogen-stimulated inflammatory cytokine production, lower skeletal muscle inflammatory protein content, lower adipokine production and lower serum levels of C-reactive protein (Gleeson *et al.*, 2006). Since such blood markers of inflammation are strongly associated with cardiovascular and metabolic disease including insulin resistance (for a recent review, see Wei *et al.*, 2008), and HIV$^+$ patients are at increased risk for these conditions; physical activity should on balance exert beneficial effects, particularly since there is no evidence that exercise further compromises immune function in HIV$^+$ patients.

Roubenoff *et al.* (1999a) investigated the acute phase and viral load response to a single 15-minute bout of step exercise in 25 HIV$^+$ patients, designed to replicate the effects of a first training session at the initiation of an exercise programme. There was a mild acute phase response with a tendency for increased circulating neurophil counts but there was no increase in HIV RNA, indeed there was a small but statistically significant reduction in viral load 2 hours after exercise, although this was not deemed to be clinically significant.

CD4$^+$ count and viral load before and after completion of endurance, resistance or combined exercise programmes have been reported in many of the interventional studies (Stringer *et al.*, 1998; Bhasin *et al.*, 2000; Grinspoon *et al.*, 2000; Smith *et al.*, 2001; Rojas *et al.*, 2003; Driscoll *et al.*, 2004a; Fillipas *et al.*, 2006; Terry *et al.*, 2006). None of these studies have shown statistically significant alterations in these markers of disease progression, although some suggest tendencies for increased CD4 count. Using meta-analysis O'Brien *et al.* (2004) combined data from three studies comparing the effects of interval aerobic exercise with a non-exercising control group and found a 70 cells/mm^{-3} increase in CD4$^+$ count, which, although not statistically significant, may be clinically important. The stability of immunological and virological parameters during moderate-intensity endurance, resistance or combined exercise programmes indicates that exercise is a safe therapy for patients with HIV.

14.4 Effect of exercise on wasting

Although death from HIV and AIDS wasting has been dramatically reduced by antiretroviral therapy, some studies suggest that weight loss remains a significant complication. Wanke *et al.* (2000) found that 18% of patients in a cohort of HIV$^+$ subjects in Boston lost more than 10% of their body weight over serial visits and 21% had a sustained loss of more than 5% body weight for 1 year. In a subset (166 male HIV$^+$ patients; 43% on ART) of participants from the Tufts Nutrition for Healthy Living Study, followed up for 8 months on average, a relatively small proportion experienced classical AIDS wasting (2%) (Roubenoff *et al.*, 2002a). However, more than one-third of PLHIV lost ≥ 1 kg of LBM, and 12% of men lost $>5\%$ of LBM, in the presence of elevated resting metabolic rate. There was a positive relationship between loss of LBM and cytokine production (tumour necrosis factor, TNF-α; and interleukin 1β, IL-1β check) by peripheral blood mononuclear cells; and TNF-α was positively associated with resting energy expenditure. Few of the men in this study were hypogonadal and there was no direct relationship between serum testosterone and loss of LBM in this population, but serum testosterone was inversely associated with cytokine production. TNF-α has also been linked with the lipodystrophy syndrome (Ledru *et al.*, 2000) since it has been linked with insulin resistance, reduced lipoprotein lipase activity and increased triglyceride synthetase activity. More recently, Maher *et al.* (2002) found that a polymorphism in the promoter region of the TNF-α gene is a determinant of HIV-related lipodystrophy. Interestingly, elderly subjects experienced reduced skeletal muscle TNF-α gene and protein expression in parallel with increased resting muscle protein synthesis in response to a resistance training programme (Greiwe *et al.*, 2001).

One of the primary adaptations in response to resistance training is an increase in muscle mass (hypertrophy) induced by significant elevations in muscle protein synthesis and smaller increases in muscle protein breakdown such that a positive muscle protein balance is achieved (for a review see, Bowtell, 2007). Hence, it is feasible that resistance exercise will counteract loss of LBM. A number of studies have investigated the effects of resistance exercise in PLHIV upon body weight, LBM, muscle area/volume as well as muscle strength and, hence, physical capacity either singly (Roubenoff and Wilson, 2001; Yarasheski *et al.*, 2001; Lindegaard *et al.*, 2008); or in combination with whey protein consumption (Agin *et al.*, 2001), androgen therapy (Sattler *et al.*, 1999; Bhasin *et al.*, 2000; Grinspoon *et al.*, 2000), or creatine supplementation (Sakkas *et al.*, 2009).

Roubenoff and Wilson (2001) found that an 8-week progressive intensive resistance exercise programme resulted in significant gains in LBM and muscle strength, particularly in those with AIDS wasting (2.8 versus 1.4 kg gain in LBM). Yarasheski *et al.* (2001) found that a 16-week progressive resistance training programme resulted in significant gains in trunk and limb lean mass as assessed by DEXA, and increases in thigh muscle cross-sectional area as assessed by MRI, with concomitant increases in muscle strength. Lindegaard *et al.* (2008) found that a 16-week progressive resistance training programme resulted in significant increases in LBM (DEXA) and muscle strength. Other studies employing resistance exercise in combination with endurance exercise have found significant gains in muscle strength and LBM, muscle area or limb circumference (Roubenoff *et al.*, 1999b; Jones *et al.*, 2001; Dolan *et al.*, 2006; Robinson *et al.*, 2007). Fourteen weeks of progressive resistance training increased muscle strength, fat free mass (DEXA) and skeletal muscle (MRI) and body cell mass in HIV+ women, but these effects were not enhanced when combined with consumption of 1g/kg whey protein per day (Agin *et al.*, 2001). Sakkas *et al.* (2009) found that 13 weeks of progressive resistance training resulted in significant increases in muscle strength, thigh cross-sectional area (MRI) and LBM (DEXA). Half of the participants (*n* = 17) received creatine monohydrate supplementation during the resistance training programme, which resulted in significantly greater gains in LBM (versus placebo). However, this did not translate into greater hypertrophy (no difference between groups in thigh cross-sectional area gains) or functional benefits (no difference between groups in muscle strength gains). Sattler *et al.* (1999) compared testosterone therapy alone with testosterone plus progressive resistance exercise and found similar increases in body cell mass and muscle cross-sectional area in both groups but LBM gains were greater in the combined treatment group. Both Bhasin *et al.* (2000) and Grinspoon *et al.* (2000) assessed the effects of testosterone analogs and exercise, either singly or in combination, in HIV+ men. In both studies exercise resulted in significant increases in LBM and muscle area or volume as well as improved muscle strength. Bhasin *et al.* (2000) did not find additive effects when combining testosterone and exercise, whereas the Grinspoon *et al.* (2000) study was not sufficiently powered to address this question. Since the long-term administration of testosterone may be associated with adverse metabolic effects, such as reduced HDL and insulin resistance, exercise alone would seem the better long-term option. The evidence supporting the anabolic effects of resistance exercise for patients with or without existence of wasting is compelling, with the associated benefits of improved physical function (Roubenoff and Wilson, 2001). Indeed, Beaston-Blaakman *et al.* (2007) recently concluded that nutrition counselling plus progressive resistance training was a more cost-effective treatment for AIDS wasting than nutrition counselling alone or in combination with oxandralone.

In addition to the loss of muscle mass, an increased prevalence of osteopaenia and osteoporosis has been reported for PLHIV particularly post-introduction of ART. Brown and Qaqish (2006) conducted a meta-analysis of studies and found a 15% prevalence of osteoporosis in PLHIV in an Australian population of PLHIV 3% had osteoporosis and 20% osteopaenia (Carr *et al.*, 2001); whereas more recently Cazanave *et al.* (2008) reported a 53.7% prevalence of osteopaenia and 26.8% prevalence of osteoporosis amongst 492 patients representative of the Aquitane cohort. Potential causes of osteoporosis include a direct effect of HIV upon osteogenic cells, persistent activation of pro-inflammatory cytokines and drug toxicity. In addition, the associations between visceral adiposity, peripheral fat loss and bone demineralisation found in some studies suggest that there may be common mechanisms in action. However, our understanding of the pathophysiology of bone demineralisation in PLHIV is still poor. In addition, there is excellent evidence from healthy and osteoporotic populations that weight-bearing exercise is able to reverse or slow the rate of bone loss, since mechanical forces transmitted through the bone induce remodelling at the site of loading. There is as yet no such evidence in PLHIV indeed Roubenoff *et al.* (1999b) found no significant change in bone density (DEXA) after 16 weeks of resistance training. However, longer duration studies (at least 6 months) with larger study populations are required to allow sufficient time for detectable changes in bone mineral density to occur.

14.5   Management of metabolic disturbances with exercise programmes

Metabolic disturbances experienced by PLHIV include dyslipidaemia (hypertriglyceridaemia, high total cholesterol with or without elevated LDL, and low HDL), hyperinsulinaemia and adipose tissue redistribution. Lipodystrophy is characterised by peripheral lipoatrophy, and/or abdominal lipohypertrophy, and in some cases enlargement of fat pads, e.g. buffalo hump or breast enlargement. Fat loss typically from the subcutaneous depots may result from cell atrophy, apoptosis or cell de-differentiation. Fat accumulation in the visceral area may result from adipogenesis, lipogenesis and increased uptake of systemic lipid. However, since dyslipidaemia can occur without obvious lipoatrophy and insulin resistance, it has been suggested that these are either mechanistically independent or perhaps dyslipidaemia precedes fat redistribution and insulin resistance and as such can be used as a sensitive early marker of disease (Oh and Hegele, 2007).

The pathogenesis of these metabolic disturbances is complex (for a recent review, see (Oh and Hegele, 2007)). In brief, the increased levels of inflammatory cytokines associated with HIV infection result in reduced lipoprotein lipase activity, thus increasing blood concentration of triglyceride-rich lipoproteins, reducing HDL formation due to reductions in cholesterol efflux from peripheral cells and increasing HDL breakdown due to increased activity of phospholipase A2 and endothelial lipase. HDL catabolism is also enhanced due to abnormal triglyceride enrichment of HDL particles. ART has been suggested to inhibit the binding of retinoic acid to CRABP-1, due to the high degree of homology between HIV-1 protease and the retinoic acid binding domains of cytoplasmic retinoic-acid binding protein type 1 (CRABP-1). CRABP-1 binds with intracellular retinoic acid and presents it to cytochrome P450 3A isoforms, which catalyses its conversion to cis-9-retinoic acid.

Cis-9-retinoic acid is the sole ligand for retinoid X receptor (RXR) which functions as a heterodimer in adipocyte nuclei with peroxisome-proliferator-activated receptor type gamma (PPAR-γ). Ligand binding to RXR or PPAR-γ inhibits adipocyte apoptosis, and upregulates adipocyte differentiation and proliferation. Carr et al. (1998) hypothesised that HIV protease inhibitors inhibit the binding of retinoic acid to CRABP-1, thus reducing RXR activity, and reducing differentiation and increasing peripheral adipocyte apoptosis which would be expected to contribute to lipoatrophy. The resulting increased free fatty acid spillover is suggested to increase triglyceride synthesis in the liver contributing to the increase in blood triglyceride concentration. In the muscle, fatty acid oxidation is compromised due to mitochondrial depletions relating to drug-related inhibition of mitochondrial DNA polymerase γ, leading to mitochondrial DNA depletion, respiratory chain dysfunction and reduced energy production. In combination, with increased free fatty acid spillover, this likely contributes to intramyocellular fat accumulation which has been linked to insulin resistance.

The beneficial effects of exercise on cardiovascular risk factors, including blood lipid profile (reduced blood concentrations of triglyceride, total cholesterol and LDL, as well as increased HDL), blood pressure, insulin sensitivity and body fat levels are well-established from both epidemiological and interventional studies. Exercise is recommended as an adjunct therapy for patients with diabetes and cardiovascular disease, and it is also an effective preventive tool in those at increased risk of these conditions. There is growing evidence to support the beneficial effects of exercise, both endurance and resistance, in counteracting the metabolic syndrome (body fat redistribution, dyslipidaemia and insulin resistance) experienced by many HIV$^+$ patients. In a cross-sectional study of HIV$^+$ patients on long-term ART, the level of physical activity was the only independent predictor for the presence of lipid redistribution (Domingo et al., 2003). There is also direct evidence from interventional studies, where HIV$^+$ patients have completed endurance, resistance or combined training programmes, that total body fat can be reduced in response to exercise. Although not all studies have demonstrated this effect (Grinspoon et al., 2000; Yarasheski et al., 2001), but presence of lipid distribution was not an inclusion criterion in either of these studies.

The effect of endurance exercise on body composition was assessed in four studies, three of which showed favourable changes in body fat levels: reduced% body fat using skinfold measurements and reduced waist:hip ratio (Smith et al., 2001; Terry et al., 2006) or reduced truncal fat (Thoni et al., 2002). However, Lindegaard et al. (2008) found that 16 weeks of resistance training ($n = 10$) resulted in significant reductions in total, trunk and limb fat mass (DEXA), but the small reductions observed after 16 weeks of endurance training ($n = 8$) did not achieve statistical significance. Agin et al. (2001) found that fat mass (measured using both DEXA and MRI) was reduced after 14 weeks of resistance training, whereas those receiving a whey protein supplement alone or in combination with resistance training experienced increases or no change in fat mass, respectively. Roubenoff et al. (2002b) reported dramatic reductions in total body fat (28%, DEXA) and visceral fat (52%, L4-L5 CT scan) in a male HIV$^+$ patient with peripheral lipoatrophy and central lipohypertrophy, after a 4-month combined diet with endurance and resistance exercise programme. Engelson et al. (2006) recently demonstrated that an energy restriction diet combined with an endurance and resistance exercise programme induced significant waist circumference and total body fat (DEXA) reductions in obese female HIV$^+$ patients

(BMI > 30 kg.m^{-2}). Although there was a very high dropout rate in this study, with only 18 out of 39 women completing the study (this was not due to adverse events, with only one dropout due to unrelated ear infection). Interestingly, Dolan *et al.* (2006) recently conducted a randomized controlled trial in which HIV$^+$ women with evidence of fat redistribution were randomized to a supervised home exercise programme (endurance and resistance) versus normal activity, which achieved far better adherence rates (only 1 dropout from each group). However, although exercisers experienced significant reductions in waist circumference, abdominal and total fat did not change. Three other studies employing combined exercise programmes in a single group pre- and post-training design without control group found significant reductions in trunk and total body fat (DEXA, Robinson *et al.*, 2007; Roubenoff *et al.*, 1999b) or percentage body fat (skinfold measurements, Jones *et al.*, 2001). Driscoll *et al.* (2004a, 2004b) compared the effect of metformin versus metformin plus combined exercise in HIV$^+$ patients with fat redistribution. Patients in the exercise and metformin group tended to achieve greater reductions in abdominal and thigh subcutaneous and visceral fat deposits (abdominal and mid-thigh CT scan), than those receiving metformin alone. In addition to the favourable effects on body composition, insulin sensitivity was increased to a greater degree in those who combined exercise with metformin.

In their cross-sectional study of PLHIV, Gavrila *et al.* (2003) found a strong tendency for an inverse association between insulin resistance and total or endurance exercise. Sattler *et al.* (2002) also found that markers of insulin sensitivity (fasting glucose and insulin, HOMA-IR and QUICKI) were improved in PLHIV receiving nandralone and performing resistance exercise for 12 weeks. Perhaps, surprisingly no significant change occurred in the nandralone only group as previous studies have demonstrated worsening of insulin sensitivity with androgen therapy. Until recently (Lindegaard *et al* 2008), no other studies have demonstrated any significant effects of endurance (Thoni *et al.*, 2002; Terry *et al.*, 2006), resistance (Yarasheski *et al.*, 2001) or combined exercise (Dolan *et al.*, 2006; Engelson *et al.*, 2006) on insulin sensitivity, although the measures used (fasting insulin and glucose concentration) may not have been sufficiently sensitive. Lindegaard *et al.* (2008) employed euglycaemic hyperinsulinameic clamps to quantify peripheral insulin sensitivity in PLHIV before and after 16 weeks of either progressive endurance ($n = 8$) or resistance ($n = 10$) training. Insulin mediated glucose disposal was significantly improved after both forms of training, and these changes were found to be independent of the significant reductions in total, trunk and limb fat. Interestingly, both Dolan *et al.* (2006) and Driscoll *et al.* (2002) have reported exercise-induced increases in CT anterior thigh muscle attenuation, which is indicative of reduced muscle adiposity. In the latter study there was a correlation with fasting insulin, and a number of studies have now implicated intramyocellular lipid in the development of insulin resistance. Skeletal muscle is responsible for approximately 75% of insulin-stimulated glucose uptake, and hence one might expect that exercise, which exerts such a profound effect on skeletal muscle metabolism, will modulate insulin sensitivity. Acute exercise exerts an insulin-like effect by triggering Glut 4 translocation to the sarcolemma, thus facilitating glucose uptake. In addition, exercise training has been shown to increase Glut 4 gene and protein expression, as well as insulin receptors and other proteins implicated in the insulin cell-signalling pathway.

Unsurprisingly, since insulin has an important regulatory role in lipid as well as carbohydrate and protein metabolism, dyslipidaemia is also characteristic of the metabolic syndrome. Acute exercise causes activation of the lipoprotein lipase enzyme, which is responsible for lipolysis, and chronically increases gene and protein expression. This is one of the putative mechanisms by which it is thought that exercise engenders a less atherogenic lipid profile. However, dyslipidaemic PLHIV seem to experience smaller benefits than other dyslipidaemic populations, perhaps due to interaction with their drug regimes. Several studies found that fasting blood lipid profile was not altered by endurance (Terry *et al.*, 2006), or combined exercise programmes (Driscoll *et al.*, 2004a, 2004b; Dolan *et al.*, 2006; Engelson *et al.*, 2006). However, several studies have demonstrated significant reductions in blood triglycerides in response to endurance (Thoni *et al.*, 2002), resistance (Yarasheski *et al.*, 2001) or combined exercise (Jones *et al.*, 2001; Roubenoff *et al.*, 2002b). Interestingly, the significant training-induced increases in HDL concentrations observed in other populations do not seem to occur with HIV$^+$ patients, with the exception of the Grinspoon *et al.* (2000) study, perhaps due to drug interactions, although, more recently, Lindegaard *et al.* (2008) directly compared the effects of endurance and resistance training on blood lipid profile in PLHIV with confirmed lipodystrophy. Endurance training resulted in significant reductions in total cholesterol, LDL and free fatty acids and significant increase in HDL; whereas resistance training resulted in significant reductions in TG and free fatty acids as well as significant increase in HDL.

The mechanisms by which exercise interventions induce favourable metabolic changes in PLHIV with fat redistribution have not yet explicitly been established, and this would require large-scale and complex interventional studies. However, the exercise literature provides some strong clues. Endurance and resistance exercise reduce inflammatory cytokine production (Gleeson, 2007), which should result in decreased reactive oxygen species production, improved processing of blood lipids and increased muscle protein synthesis. Interestingly, Lindegaard *et al.* (2008) demonstrated that 16 weeks of endurance training resulted in reductions in a number of inflammatory markers (C-reactive protein, TNF-α, IL6 and IL18), whereas the same duration of resistance training only reduced IL18 concentration in PLHIV. Endurance exercise increases endogenous antioxidant capacity including glutathione, which is depleted in PLHIV. In addition, endurance training increases mitochondrial volume and hence oxidative capacity of muscle, and increases insulin sensitivity. However, there is evidence that the oxidative capacity of adolescents and adults with HIV is impaired, with peak VO$_2$ 15–40% lower than that predicted for sedentary age-matched HIV-seronegative controls (for a review, see (Cade *et al.*, 2004)). In addition, the ventilatory threshold appears to occur at low exercise intensities. The ventilatory threshold is defined as the point at which the rate of increase in carbon dioxide exceeds that of oxygen uptake, presumably due to excess carbon dioxide production from buffering of hydrogen ions. It is thus reflective of an increased dependency of the muscle upon non-oxidative metabolism (lactate production and phosphocreatine breakdown) due to insufficiency of the oxidative pathways. Potential mechanisms include mitochondrial abnormalities as evidenced by decreased cytochrome-*c*-oxidase and lactic acidosis; reduced oxygen extraction into the muscle as demonstrated by a reduced arterio-venous oxygen difference during peak exercise impaired muscle glucose uptake due to reduced Glut 4 function; cardiac abnormalities and possibly pulmonary ventilation limitations; and anaemia. These factors that determine the individual's capacity for exercise must be considered when reaching an appropriate exercise prescription.

In addition, in the last few years concerns have emerged regarding the cardiotoxic effects of ART. Schuster *et al.* (2008) found that there was an increased prevalence of resting left ventricular diastolic dysfunction (abnormal relaxation and filling pattern) and reduced left ventricular functional indices (reduced ejection fraction and peak systolic velocity). These factors may also contribute to the reduced exercise tolerance amongst this population and may suggest the need for systematic non-invasive assessment of cardiac function.

14.6   Effect of exercise on quality of life and physical capacity

Although ART has revolutionized the treatment of HIV, such that HIV mortality and incidence of AIDS-defining illness have fallen steeply since its introduction, there is a high prevalence of adverse effects that can significantly impinge upon quality of life. Prior to the introduction of ART, fatigue, anorexia, wasting, cough, pain, night sweats and fever were the most commonly reported physical symptoms, accompanied by anxiety, worrying, fear, depression and sadness. In one study, 80% of PLHIV reported depression and anxiety (Horwath, 2002); fatigue was also reported consistently in more than 50% of populations of PLHIV (Breitbart *et al.*, 1998). Post-introduction of ART, depression, anxiety and fatigue remain amongst the patients' most commonly reported symptoms. Symptoms of HIV are compounded by ART adverse effects, which include nausea and vomiting, diarrhea, skin rashes, fat redistribution and neuropathy; all of which significantly impact upon quality of life. Body image, self-esteem, social functioning and bodily comfort are all impaired in the presence of fat redistribution (Collins *et al.*, 2002).

There is good evidence from studies amongst other clinical populations that exercise interventions are able to counteract many of the commonly reported adverse effects of ART and HIV. Fatigue experienced by cancer, cardiovascular disease, chronic fatigue syndrome and fibromyalgia patients has been successfully counteracted by aerobic exercise interventions. Most commonly, exercise programmes comprise aerobic exercise at 60–85% maximum heart rate, 3–5 times per week for 8 to 12 weeks, although as little as 10 minutes of brisk walking has been shown to reduce fatigue in healthy individuals (Thayer, 1987). This may be of importance, since the ability of PLHIV experiencing adverse effects, to commit to regular exercise may be compromised. Several studies with PLHIV have demonstrated that exercise training increases time to fatigue during an incremental exercise test on the treadmill, for example Smith *et al.* (2001), but this is more indicative of improved physical capacity rather than general sensations of fatigue. Lox *et al.* (1995) found that both endurance and resistance exercise programmes improved perceived physical ability and physical self-efficacy; and more recently Dolan *et al.* (2006) found that a home-based progressive endurance and resistance training programme resulted in improved self-reported energy and appearance.

Neuropathic pain is also a significant factor in impaired quality of life for PLHIV with 31% patients commonly experiencing pain in one study (Newshan *et al.*, 2002). There is some evidence to suggest that both endurance and resistance exercise alters perceptions of pain and pain tolerance. Certainly, exercise is one of the self-care strategies adopted by PLHIV to counteract neuropathic pain (Nicholas *et al.*, 2007), however, the optimal exercise prescription to achieve this effect is not yet clear.

Nor is there any direct evidence amongst a population of HIV$^+$ patients that such strategies are successful.

Intense exercise has been shown to induce nausea in healthy individuals, especially when in warm environments. However, moderate-intensity cycle exercise has been shown to decrease nausea experienced by breast cancer patients undergoing chemotherapy versus control and placebo groups (Lee and Dodd, 2007). As yet no data are available regarding the effects of exercise on nausea experienced by PLHIV.

There is a large body of evidence demonstrating the efficacy of exercise in reducing anxiety and moderate depression in a broad range of clinical populations, including cardiovascular disease, diabetes, breast cancer, chronic obstructive pulmonary disease, fibromyalgia and multiple sclerosis. In addition, exercise is able to increase positive mood state and well-being. There are a small number of studies in which the effects of exercise interventions on indicators of psychological state, such as depressed mood and anxiety in PLHIV have been measured (for a detailed review, see (Ciccolo *et al.*, 2004)). The majority of these studies have found significant psychological benefits (Lox *et al.*, 1995; 1996; Wagner *et al.*, 1998; Neidig *et al.*, 2003) with two exceptions. Endurance, resistance and combined training programmes have been shown to improve depressive symptoms and depressed mood (Neidig *et al.*, 2003), increase positive well-being and life satisfaction whilst reducing perceived distress (Lox *et al.*, 1995) and increase psychological well-being (Wagner *et al.*, 1998) relative to non-exercising controls. However, Terry *et al.* (1999) found no significant change in depression scores assessed using the Montgomery-Asberg Depression Rating Scale (MADRS) after 12 weeks of either moderate- or high-intensity endurance exercise. It has been suggested that this clinical measure of depression rather than depressed mood may not be appropriate. Rojas *et al.* (2003) found no effect of 16 weeks of moderate intensity endurance and resistance exercise on depression, anxiety or global severity index measured using the Symptom Checklist revised versus a control. In fact, both control and exercise groups experienced significant improvements in all measures over the intervention period. The authors suggest that the control group's involvement in self-help groups as part of the 'control' intervention may have achieved a similar effect to the exercise intervention.

Many studies have demonstrated the positive impact of endurance and/or resistance exercise programmes upon quality of life (Laperriere *et al.*, 1990; Rigsby *et al.*, 1992; Macarthur *et al.*, 1993; Lox *et al.*, 1996; Stringer *et al.*, 1998; Wagner *et al.*, 1998; Agin *et al.*, 2001; Roubenoff and Wilson, 2001; Rojas *et al.*, 2003; Engelson *et al.*, 2006; Fillipas *et al.*, 2006), likely arising from improvements in psychological well-being (decreased depressed mood and anxiety), self-efficacy (Fillipas *et al.*, 2006), cognitive function (Fillipas *et al.*, 2006), as well as favourable changes in body composition and perceived improvements in physical appearance (Dolan *et al.*, 2006).

14.7 Exercise prescription for people living with HIV/AIDS

Good practice in designing an exercise programme for PLHIV involves a thorough and detailed approach. Clinicians should always refer PLHIV to an established medical referral programme with a signed and mutually agreed Service Level Agreement (SLA). This ensures seamless care and referral to a safe facility with qualified exercise professionals, who are competent to deal with the wide range of conditions a patient might be facing. There may of course be exceptions to this in the case of PLHIV who are currently well and/or who already exercise regularly and are able to adjust their training according to their changing status.

Basic guidelines that characterise a good referral programme include:

- Good communication structure between referring clinician and the exercise facility
- A robust and recorded assessment process for PLHIV
- A set 'course' of exercise which will typically be over a period of roughly 12 weeks in duration
- A risk assessment criteria stating which patients are suitable to be referred
- Fully qualified personnel. Membership of the Register of Exercise Professionals is the industry agreed standard, and this organisation (website link available at http://www.exerciseregister.org/) can provide guidelines on the level of qualification necessary to work with this patient group
- Confidentiality procedures in place at the facility. These may include a membership system that enables patients' access to the facility without their status being revealed and systems for keeping patient information secure and available to approved personnel only.
- Adequate attention and supervision given to patients whilst exercising
- Exercise prescription that takes into account the referrer's intentions, medication, current medical condition (including side effects), medical history/treatment and patient goals.

The fundamental principles underpinning all exercise prescription are that it should be safe and effective.

14.8   Practical considerations for exercise prescription

Prior to reaching an appropriate exercise prescription, baseline assessment of physical fitness and functional capacity are recommended, as well as consideration of medical history. This information is also useful in tracking the patient's response to the exercise programme, which can provide good motivation to encourage patients' compliance. Fitness components generally include cardiorespiratory endurance, body composition, flexibility, muscle endurance and strength and different protocols can be adopted depending upon the patient's status and the desired outcomes. The research reviewed in the earlier sections of this chapter supports the prescription of a combination of progressive resistance training and cardiovascular endurance training, and the American College of Sports Medicine (ACSM) provides recommendations for exercise prescription and programming for this patient group (Schmitz et al., 2002). However, the initiation of an exercise programme requires significant alteration to the patient's routine, and the exercise professional and patient must take into account any change in the patient's health status which may vary on a day-to-day basis. To this end, exercise professionals and/or those wishing to exercise must use their judgement in determining how much and what exercise to take part in.

Medication and side effects must be taken into account when prescribing exercise, with timing of medication also impacting upon the exercise prescription. In some ways long-term side effects, such as peripheral neuropathy and lipodystrophy, are easier to deal with, from an exercise prescription point of view. For example, a patient with peripheral neuropathy may be directed away from aerobic activity such as treadmill walking/ running. There are several alternatives that may be available within the gym environment such as arm cycling, swimming or stationary cycling ensuring that foot pedals are loosened to avoid discomfort. If a person living with HIV suffers with lipodystrophy, it would make sense to prescribe a programme that includes aerobic activity for the enhancement of cardiovascular health and to improve blood lipids, whilst also using strength training to build up the legs and gluts to give the impression of bulk in those areas where wasting has occurred. Sensitivity and ability to make adaptations are essential. For example, if a dorsocervical fat pad (buffalo hump) is evident, prone exercise such as sit-ups may be uncomfortable or impossible. Alternatives are always available such as offering physical supports to maintain spinal alignment or substitution of exercises that use the same muscle groups but from a different position. It is rare for PLHIV to present with one simple condition and the skill of the instructor becomes apparent when prescribing exercise for multiple conditions.

Figure 14.1 shows examples of various exercises that may be undertaken in the gym environment.

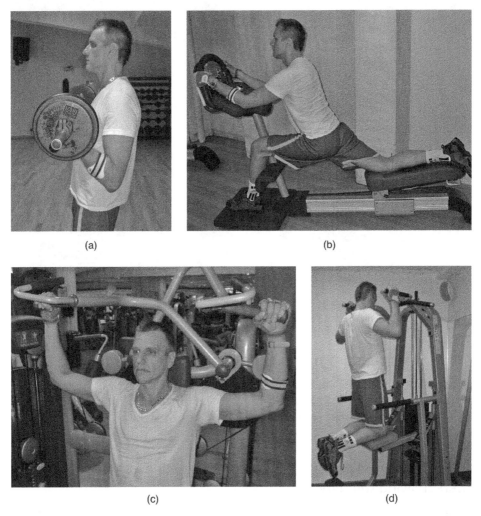

(a)   (b)

(c)   (d)

Figure 14.1   (a) Bicep curl; (b) hip flexor stretch; (c) overhead press; (d) pull ups; (e) seated rower; (f) sit-up on a core stability ball. (g) treadmill walking; (h) tricep extension. All photos taken with permission by Nelson Lafraia.

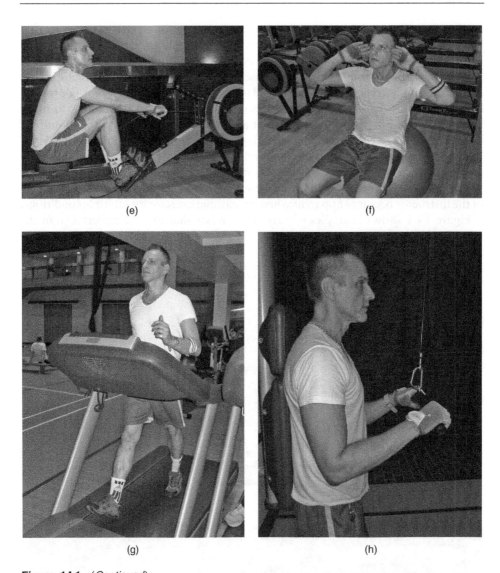

(e)

(f)

(g)

(h)

Figure 14.1 (*Continued*)

14.9 Exercise programme for a patient living with HIV

Case study 14.1 is a case study providing an overview of an exercise programme for a patient living with HIV, and demonstrates the pitfalls and realities of working with a patient over a long time period, including the necessity to incorporate adaptability within the programme.

Case study 14.1   Assessment and exercise prescription for a person living with HIV

A is 45 years old and has been living with HIV for 15 years. He had pneumonia three times several years ago and has been hospitalized with opportunistic infections, including septicaemia. He is on combination therapy and reacts severely to the medication. His symptoms include: night sweats, peripheral neuropathy, lipodystrophy, hyperlipidaemia, borderline diabetes and osteoporosis (affecting particularly hips and ribs).

Initial assessment

Prior to commencing the exercise programme, assessment of A's physical fitness revealed the following:

Blood Pressure 150/100 mmHg
Weight 61 kg
Body fat percentage under 10% (estimated from skinfold thickness measurements)
Cardiovascular fitness was poor (assessed via 6-minute walk test)
Flexibility was poor (assessed via sit and reach test)
Muscle strength was poor (assessed as maximum weight lifted for one repetition using good form, one repetition maximum, 1 RM).

Exercise prescription: 0–2 months

Training took place 3 days per week with importance placed on the need for recovery between sessions, with each session lasting 45–60 minutes in total.

Strength training: focus was on major muscle groups to build up general strength, using resistance machines. Free weights were used for arms only, as core strength was poor. In each training session, 1–3 sets of 8–12 repetitions per set were completed for 6 to 8 different exercises at 60–65% 1RM. A started with 1 set per exercise and over the 2 months this was progressively increased to achieve 3 sets per exercise by the end of the 2 months.

Cardiovascular: stationary bike was prescribed because of A's peripheral neuropathy, which made weight-bearing exercise painful. Pain on walking was one factor that led to the his lack of desire to exercise previously. In this early phase of training, A completed low-intensity steady state cardiovascular exercise to gently build fitness and confidence. This consisted initially of a 5-minute warm-up, followed by 5 minutes at the target intensity of 65–70% HRmax (age-predicted maximum heart rate), followed by a 5-minute cool down. A was also encouraged to use rate of perceived exertion, i.e. how hard the exercise subjectively feels, to judge the appropriate intensity. Over the first two months, the duration of training at the target intensity was progressively increased to 10 minutes and then the intensity increased to 70–75% HRmax.

Exercise prescription: 2–6 months

Exercise made A feel great and for the first time, in a long time, he felt he had taken some control over his body. He was finally doing something positive for himself and this made him feel much better, however, this overenthusiasm led him to overtrain. In addition, whilst he was training without his fitness instructor, his technique suffered and as a consequence he developed some minor musculoskeletal injuries. For these reasons, and also to continue the positive effects of training, his prescription was altered once he had recovered from the minor injuries and was able to train again. Training frequency was increased to 4 days per week, with each session lasting 60–85 minutes, including yoga and flexibility work.

Strength training: the focus was on performing slow and controlled movements using resistance machines. Specific scapula and core stability exercises were completed at the end of each workout to help improve posture which was poor, and to reduce the risk of injury which may be associated with poor core stability. As shoulders were drawn forwards, scapular exercises were introduced in order to begin to straighten posture and to give a more confident appearance. In each training session, 2–3 sets of 12–15 repetitions per set at 60–65% 1RM were completed for eight different exercises, using a split routine (training different body parts on different days with 2 days recovery between sessions for each body part) to ensure sufficient recovery for muscles to adapt between sessions.

Cardiovascular: consisting initially of a 5-minute warm-up, followed by 10 to 15 minutes at the target intensity, followed by a 5-minute cool down. The target intensity was alternated between 65 and 70, and 70–75% HRmax. In addition, to introduce some variety and some higher intensity work, A completed 5-minute bursts on the elliptical trainer at 80–85% HRmax.

Exercise prescription: more than 6 months

Once A had become more accustomed to the exercise programme and his technique improved, no more injuries occurred. It usually takes time not only for the body to adapt, but also for the patient to learn to 'listen' to their own body regarding exercise and daily living:

- Frequency: 4–5 days; 2 complete rest days every week
- Intensity: 3–4 sets, 10–12 reps to failure or fatigue at 80–85% 1RM [N.B. A wanted to build muscle bulk, hence lower repetitions and higher weight]
- Duration: 45 minutes to 1 hour
- Type: weights (including free weight) and cardiovascular sessions now include interval training.

Present condition:

- CD4 count healthy
- Viral load undetectable
- No hospitalizations for over a year
- Lipodystrophy visible effects are much better, due in part to exercise, but also surgery, 'new fill' and exercise compliance
- Improved blood lipid profile: higher HDL, lower LDL and TG
- Great improvements in body composition, with improved body mass and muscularity
- Fewer bone fractures and a greater range of movement
- Increased energy levels have also meant the patient has returned to full-time employment
- Blood pressure: 128/94 mmHg
- Weight: 80 kg
- Body fat percentage: 18%
- CV fitness is good
- Muscle strength is good

Clearly, the case study in Box 14.1 is a complex case and many factors must be considered to successfully achieve these long-term changes, which had enormous benefits not only for the physical appearance of this patient but also his mental health. Cardiovascular training must begin gently whilst teaching techniques for the patient to assess their own exercise intensity relative to their heart rate response. Resistance training began on fixed machines and progressed to using different systems of strength training to focus on areas of weakness and also to build strength and size of muscles. This was particularly important in this case because the patient had significant lipodystrophy.

14.10 Conclusion

Systematic reviews of randomised controlled trials have clearly demonstrated that PLHIV are able to increase muscle strength and cardiovascular fitness in response to progressive resistance exercise and/or endurance exercise, in analogous fashion to seronegative individuals. Randomised controlled trials published since then and those studies employing less rigorous designs, e.g. single group before and after studies, corroborate these findings. Considering the safety of moderate exercise interventions, it is clear therefore that the benefits derived in terms of functional capacity alone are sufficient to advocate the prescription of individualised exercise programmes for people living with HIV. When taking into account the additional benefits that have been clearly demonstrated and those that remain to be proven, but for which there are reasonable mechanistic hypotheses, the case for exercise is compelling. PLHIV should be advised to increase their levels of physical activity and, where possible, referred to participate in structured exercise which enables appropriate monitoring, support and advice to be provided, as well as social support which increases adherence to exercise.

References

Agin D, Gallagher D, Wang J, Heymsfield SB, Pierson RN, Kotler DP. Effects of whey protein and resistance exercise on body cell mass, muscle strength, and quality of life in women with HIV. *AIDS* 2001; **15**(18):2431–40.

Beaston-Blaakman A, Shepard DS, Stone N, Shevitz AH. Cost-effectiveness of clinical interventions for AIDS wasting. *AIDS Care-Psychol Soc-Med Aspects of AIDS/HIV* 2007; **19**:996–1001.

Beregszaszi M, Dollfus C, Levine M *et al.* Longitudinal evaluation and risk factors of lipodystrophy and associated metabolic changes in HIV-infected children. *J Acquir Immune Defic Syndr* 2005; **40**(2):161–8.

Bhasin S, Storer TW, Javanbakht M *et al.* Testosterone replacement and resistance exercise in HIV-infected men with weight loss and low testosterone levels. *J Am Med Assoc* 2000; **283**(6):763–70.

Blanch J, Rousaud A, Martinez E *et al.* Impact of lipodystrophy on the quality of life of HIV-1-infected patients. *J Acqu Immun Defic Syndr* 2002; **31**(4):404–407.

Bopp CM, Phillips KD, Fulk LJ, Dudgeon WD, Sowell R, Hand GA. Physical activity and immunity in HIV-infected individuals. *AIDS Care-Psychol Soc-Med Aspects AIDS/HIV* 2004; **16**(3):387–93.

Bowtell JL. Protein and amino acid requirements for sport and exercise nutrition. In: MacLaren D, Spurway N, eds. *Advanced Topics in Sport and Exercise Physiology: Sport and Exercise Nutrition and Metabolism*. Amsterdam: Elsevier, 2007.

Bozzette SA, Ake CF, Tam HK, Chang SW, Louis TA. Cardiovascular and cerebrovascular events in patients treated for human immunodeficiency virus infection. *New Engl J Med* 2003; **348**(8):702–710.

Breitbart W, McDonald MV, Rosenfeld B, Monkman ND, Passik S. Fatigue in ambulatory AIDS patients. *J Pain Symptom Manage* 1998; **15**(3):159–67.

Brown TT, Cole SR, Li XH *et al*. Antiretroviral therapy and the prevalence and incidence of diabetes mellitus in the Multicenter AIDS Cohort Study. *Arch Intern Med* 2005; **165**(10):1179–84.

Brown TT, Qaqish RB. Antiretroviral therapy and the prevalence of osteopaenia and osteoporosis: a meta-analytic review. *AIDS* 2006; **20**(17):2165–74.

Cade WT, Peralta L, Keyser RE. Aerobic exercise dysfunction in human immunodeficiency virus: A potential link to physical disability. *Phys Ther* 2004; **84**(7):655–64.

Carr A, Emery S, Law M, Puls R, Lundgren JD, Powderly WG. An objective case definition of lipodystrophy in HIV-infected adults: a case-control study. *Lancet* 2003; **361**(9359):726–35.

Carr A, Miller J, Eisman JA, Cooper DA. Osteopaenia in HIV-infected men: association with asymptomatic lactic acidemia and lower weight pre-antiretroviral therapy. *AIDS* 2001; **15**(6):703–709.

Carr A, Samaras K, Chisholm DJ, Cooper DA. Pathogenesis of HIV-1-protease inhibitor-associated peripheral lipodystrophy, hyperlipidaemia, and insulin resistance. *Lancet* 1998; **351**(9119):1881–3.

Cazanave C, Dupon M, Lavignolle-Aurillac V *et al*. Reduced bone mineral density in HIV-infected patients: prevalence and associated factors. *AIDS* 2008; **22**, 395–402.

Ciccolo JT, Jowers EM, Bartholomew JB. The benefits of exercise training for quality of life in HIV/AIDS in the post-ART era. *Sports Med* 2004; **34**(8):487–99.

Clingerman EM. Participation in physical activity by persons living with HIV disease. *J Assoc Nurses AIDS Care* 2003; **14**(5):59–70.

Collins EJ, Burgoyne RW, Wagner CA, Halman MH, Walmsley SL. The impact of lipodystrophy on health related quality of life, body image, mood, self-esteem and medication compliance. *Antivir Ther* 2002; **7**(3):73.

Dolan SE, Frontera W, Librizzi J *et al*. Effects of a supervised home-based aerobic and progressive resistance training regimen in women infected with human immunodeficiency virus – A randomized trial. *Arch Intern Med* 2006; **166**(11):1225–31.

Domingo P, Sambeat MA, Perez A, Ordonez J, Rodriguez J, Vazquez G. Fat distribution and metabolic abnormalities in HIV-infected patients on first combination antiretroviral therapy including stavudine or zidovudine: role of physical activity as a protective factor. *Antiviral Therapy* 2003; **8**(3):223–31.

Driscoll SD, Meininger GE, Lareau MT *et al*. Effects of exercise training and metformin on body composition and cardiovascular indices in HIV-infected patients. *AIDS* 2004a; **18**(3):465–73.

Driscoll SD, Meininger GE, Ljungquist K *et al*. Differential effects of metformin and exercise on muscle adiposity and metabolic indices in human immunodeficiency virus-infected patients. *J Clin Endocrinol Metab* 2004b; **89**(5):2171–8.

Duran S, Saves M, Spire B *et al*. Failure to maintain long-term adherence to highly active antiretroviral therapy: the role of lipodystrophy. *AIDS* 2001; **15**(18):2441–44.

Easterbrook P, Meadway J. The changing epidemiology of HIV infection: new challenges for HIV palliative care. *J R Soc Med* 2001; **94**(9):442–8.

Engelson ES, Agin D, Kenya S *et al*. Body composition and metabolic effects of a diet and exercise weight loss regimen on obese, HIV-infected women. *Metab Clin Exp* 2006; **55**(10):1327–36.

Fillipas S, Bowtell-Harris CA *et al*. Physical activity uptake in patients with HIV: Who does how much?. *Int J STD AIDS* 2008; **19**:514–8.

Fillipas S, Oldmeadow LB, Bailey MJ, Cherry CL. A six-month, supervised, aerobic and resistance exercise program improves self-efficacy in people with human immunodeficiency virus: A randomised controlled trial. *Aust J Physiother* 2006; **52**(3):185–90.

Garcia-Lazaro M, Roman AR *et al*. Variability in coronary risk assessment in HIV-infected patients. *Med Clin* 2007; **129**:521–4.

Gavrila A, Tsiodras S, Doweiko J *et al*. Exercise and vitamin E intake are independently associated with metabolic abnormalities in human immunodeficiency virus- positive subjects: A cross-sectional study. *Clin Infect Dis* 2003; **36**(12):1593–601.

Gleeson M. Immune function in sport and exercise. *J Appl Physiol* 2007; **103**(2):693–9.

Gleeson M, McFarlin B, Flynn M. Exercise and Toll-like receptors. *Exerc Immunol Rev* 2006; **12**:34–53.

Greiwe JS, Cheng B, Rubin DC, Yarasheski KE, Semenkovich CF. Resistance exercise decreases skeletal muscle tumor necrosis factor alpha in frail elderly humans. *FASEB J* 2001; **15**(2):475–82.

Grinspoon S, Corcoran C, Parlman K *et al.* Effects of testosterone and progressive resistance training in eugonadal men with AIDS wasting – A randomized, controlled trial. *Ann Intern Med* 2000; **133**(5):348–55.

Horwath E. Psychiatric and neuropsychiatric manifestations of HIV infection. *J Int Assoc Phys AIDS Care (Chic Ill)* 2002; **1** Suppl 1:S1–15.

Howley ET. Type of activity: resistance, aerobic, anaerobic and leisure-time versus occupational physical activity. *Med Sci Sports Exerc* 2001; **33**:S364–369.

Jones SP, Doran DA, Leat PB, Maher B, Pirmohamed M. Short-term exercise training improves body composition and hyperlipidaemia in HIV-positive individuals with lipodystrophy. *AIDS* 2001; **15**(15):2049–2051.

Laperriere AR, Antoni MH, Schneiderman N *et al.* Exercise intervention attenuates emotional distress and natural-killer-cell decrements following notification of positive serologic status for Hiv-1. *Biofeedback Self Regul* 1990; **15**(3):229–42.

Ledru E, Christeff N, Patey O, de Truchis P, Melchior JC, & Gougeon ML. Alteration of tumor necrosis factor-alpha T-cell homeostasis following potent antiretroviral therapy: contribution to the development of human immunodeficiency virus-associated lipodystrophy syndrome. *Blood* 2000; **95**(10):3191–8.

Lee JY, Dodd M. Exercise during adjuvant cancer treatment decreased nausea at the end of treatment in breast cancer patients. *Oncol Nurs Forum* 2007; **34**(2), 549.

Lima EMO, Gualandro DM, Yu DC *et al.* Cardiovascular prevention in HV patients: Results from a successful intervention programme. *Atherosclerosis* 2009; **204**:229–32.

Lindegaard B, Hansen T, Hvid T *et al.* The effect of strength and endurance training on insulin sensitivity and fat distribution in human immunodeficiency virus-infected patients with lipodystrophy. *J Clin Endocrinol Metab* 2008; **93**(10):3860–869.

Lox CL, McAuley E, Tucker RS. Exercise as an intervention for enhancing subjective well-being in an Hiv-1 population. *J Sport Exerc Psychol* 1995; **17**(4):345–62.

Lox CL, McAuley E, Tucker RS. Aerobic and resistance exercise training effects on body composition, muscular strength, and cardiovascular fitness in an HIV-1 population. *Int J Behav Med* 1996; **3**(1):55–69.

MacArthur RD, Levine SD, Birk TJ. Supervised exercise trainign improves cardiopulmonary fitness in HIV-infected persons. *Med Sci Sports Exerc* 1993; **25**(6):684–8.

Maher B, Alfirevic A, Vilar FJ, Wilkins EL, Park BK, Pirmohamed M. TNF-alpha promoter region gene polymorphisms in HIV-positive patients with lipodystrophy. *AIDS* 2002; **16**(15):2013–2018.

Manfredi R, Chiodo F. Disorders of lipid metbolism in patients with HIV disease treated with antiretgroviral agents: frequency, relationship with administered drugs, and role of hypolipidemic therapy with bezafibrate. *J Infect* 2001; **42**:181–8.

Mustafa T, Sy SF, Macera CA *et al.* Association between Exercise and HIV Disease Progression in a Cohort of Homosexual Men. *Ann Epidemiol* 1999; **9**:127–31.

Neidig JL, Smith BA, Brashers DE. Aerobic exercise training for depressive symptom management in adults living with HIV infection. *J Assoc Nurses AIDS Care* 2003; **14**(2):30–40.

Newshan G, Bennett J, Holman S. Pain and other symptoms in ambulatory HIV patients in the age of highly active antiretroviral therapy. *J Assoc Nurses AIDS Care* 2002; **13**(4):78–3.

Nicholas PK, Kemppainen JK, Canaval GE *et al.* Symptom management and self-care for peripheral neuropathy in HIV/AIDS. *AIDS Care-Psychol Soc-Med Aspects AIDS/HIV* 2007; **19**(2):179–89.

Nieman DC, Nehlsen-Cannarella SL. The immune response to exercise. *Semin Hematol* 1994; **31**, 166–79.

O'Brien K, Nixon S, Tynan AM, Glazier RH. Effectiveness of aerobic exercise in adults living with HIV/AIDS: Systematic review. *Med Sci Sports Exerc* 2004; **36**(10):1659–66.

Oh J, Hegele RA. HIV-associated dyslipidaemia: pathogenesis and treatment. *Lancet Infect Dis* 2007; **7**:787–96.

Ramirez-Marrero FA, Rivera-Brown AM, Nazario CM, Rodriguez-Orengo JF, Smit E, Smith BA. Self-Reported Physical Activity in Hispanic Adults Living With HIV: Comparison With Accelerometer and Pedometer. *J Assoc Nurses in AIDS Care* 2008; **19**(4):283–94.

Ramirez-Marrero FA, Smith BA, Melendez-Brau N, Santana-Bagur JL. Physical and leisure activity, body composition, and life satisfaction in HIV-positive Hispanics in Puerto Rico. *J Assoc Nurses AIDS Care* 2004; **15**(4):68–77.

Rigsby LW, Dishman RK, Jackson AW, Maclean GS, Raven PB. Effects of exercise training on men seropositive for the human immunodeficienct virus-1. *Med Sci Sports Exerc* 1992; **24**(1):6–12.

Robinson FP, Quinn LT, Rimmer JH. Effects of high-intensity endurance and resistance exercise on HIV metabolic abnormalities: A pilot study. *Biol Res Nurs* 2007; **8**(3):177–85.

Rojas R, Schlicht W, Hautzinger M. Effects of exercise training on quality of life, psychological well-being, immune status, and cardiopulmonary fitness in an HIV-1 positive population. *J Sport Exerc Psychol* 2003; **25**(4):440–455.

Roubenoff R, Grinspoon S, Skolnik PR *et al.* Role of cytokines and testosterone in regulating lean body mass and resting energy expenditure in HIV-infected men. *Am J Physiol Endocrinol Metabol* 2002a; **283**(1):E138–E145.

Roubenoff R, Schmitz H, Bairos L *et al.* Reduction of abdominal obesity in lipodystrophy associated with human immunodeficiency virus infection by means of diet and exercise: Case report and proof of principle. *Clin Infect Dis* 2002b; **34**(3):390–93.

Roubenoff R, Skolnik PR, Shevitz A *et al.* Effect of a single bout of acute exercise on plasma human immunodeficiency virus RNA levels. *J Appl Physiol* 1999a; **86**:1197–201.

Roubenoff R, Weiss L, McDermott A *et al.* A pilot study of exercise training to reduce trunk fat in adults with HIV-associated fat redistribution. *AIDS* 1999b; **13**(11):1373–5.

Roubenoff R, Wilson IB. Effect of resistance training on self-reported physical functioning in HIV infection. *Med Sci Sports Exerc* 2001; **33**(11):1811–7.

Sakkas GK, Mulligan K, DaSilva M *et al.* Creatine fails to augment the benefits from resistance training in patients with HIV infection: a randomized, double-blind, placebo-controlled study. *PLoS One* 2009; **4**(2):e4605.

Sattler FR, Jaque SV, Schroeder ET *et al.* Effects of pharmacological doses of nandrolone decanoate and progressive resistance training in immunodeficient patients infected with human immunodeficiency virus. *J Clin Endocrinol Metab* 1999; **84**(4):1268–76.

Sattler FR, Schroeder ET, Dube MP *et al.* Metabolic effects of nandrolone decanoate and resistance training in men with HIV. *AJP – Endocrinol Metab* 2002; **283**(6):E1214–E1222.

Schmitz HR, Layne JE, Roubenoff R. Exercise and HIV Infection. In: Myers JN, Herbert WG, Humphrey R, eds. *ACSM's Resources for Clinical Exercise Physiology*. Philadelphia, PA: Lippincott Williams & Wilkins, 2002.

Schuster I, Thöni GJ, Edérhy S *et al.* Subclinical cardiac abnormalities in human immunodeficiency virus–infected men receiving antiretroviral therapy. *Am J Cardiol* 2008; **101**:1213–7.

Smith BA, Neidig JL, Nickel JT, Mitchell GL, Para MF, Fass RJ. Aerobic exercise: effects on parameters related to fatigue, dyspnea, weight and body composition in HIV-infected adults. *AIDS* 2001; **15**(6):693–701.

Smith TP, Kennedy SL, Fleshner M. Influence of age and physical activity on the primary in vivo antibody and T cell-mediated responses in men. *J Appl Physiol* 2004; **97**(2):491–8.

Stringer WW, Berezovskaya M, O'Brien WA, Beck CK, Casaburi R. The effect of exercise training on aerobic fitness, immune indices, and quality of life in HIV$^+$ patients. *Med Sci Sports Exerc* 1998; **30**(1):11–6.

Terry L, Sprinz E, Ribeiro JP. Moderate and high intensity exercise training in HIV-1 seropositive individuals: a randomized trial. *Int J Sports Med* 1999; **20**(2):142–6.

Terry L, Sprinz E, Stein R, Medeiros NB, Oliveira J, Ribeiro JP. Exercise training in HIV-1-infected individuals with dyslipidemia and lipodystrophy. *Med Sci Sports Exerc* 2006; **38**(3):411–7.

Thayer RE. Energy, tiredness, and tension effects of a sugar snack versus moderate exercise. *J Pers Soc Psychol* 1987; **52**(1):119–25.

Thoni GJ, Fedou C, Brun JF *et al.* Reduction of fat accumulation and lipid disorders by individualized light aerobic training in human immunodeficiency virus infected patients with lipodystrophy and/or dyslipidemia. *Diabetes Metab* 2002; **28**(5):397–04.

Triant VA, Lee H, Hadigan C, Grinspoon SK. Increased acute myocardial infarction rates and cardiovascular risk factors among patients with human immunodeficiency virus disease. *J Clin Endocrinol Metab* 2007; **92**(7):2506–12.

Wagner G, Rabkin J, Rabkin R. Exercise as a mediator of psychological and nutritional effects of testosterone therapy in HIV$^+$ men. *Med Sci Sports Exerc* 1998; **30**(6):811–17.

Wanke CA, Silva M, Knox TA, Forrester J, Speigelman D, Gorbach SL. Weight loss and wasting remain common complications in individuals infected with human immunodeficiency virus in the era of highly active antiretroviral therapy. *Clin Infect Dis* 2000; **31**(3):803–805.

Wei YZ, Chen KM, Whaley-Connell AT, Stump CS, Ibdah JA, Sowers JR. Skeletal muscle insulin resistance: role of inflammatory cytokines and reactive oxygen species. *Am J Physiol-Regul Integr Comp Physiol* 2008; **294**:R673-R680.

White AJ. Mitochondrial toxicity and HIV therapy. *Sex Transm Infect* 2001; **77**:158–73.

Yarasheski KE, Tebas P, Stanerson E *et al.* Resistance exercise training reduces hypertriglyceridemia in HIV-infected men treated with antiviral therapy. *J Appl Physiol* 2001; **90**(1):133–38.

15 Mental Health

Shirley Hamilton and Christian Lee

Key Points

- Symptoms of mental disorders and side effects of the medications used to treat these disorders may contribute to nutritional problems.
- The prevalence of HIV in people with serious mental disorders is higher than the general population and people who are HIV positive are more likely to have mental health problems than the general population.
- Medication, education and psychological therapies, such as cognitive behavioural therapy, have proven effective in treating various types of mental health disorders.
- Managing clients' who have mental health problems and HIV infection can be challenging for health professionals. Collaborative input between mental health and HIV services (including dietitians) can result in positive outcomes.
- A referral should be made to a dietitian in cases of decreased nutritional status and other nutrition related problems.
- Appropriate weight programmes (including exercise and diet) for clients with chronic mental health problems are strongly encouraged to reduce obesity and improve quality of life.

15.1 Introduction

The actual number of psychiatric patients with HIV is not known. However, there is evidence that HIV prevalence in the chronic psychiatric population is higher than the general population (Cournos *et al.*, 1991), and HIV infection has been shown to be more frequent among people with mental health problems. It is estimated that half of HIV-infected patients will have a co-morbid mental health problem such as depression or anxiety (Green and Smith, 2004).

Left undiagnosed and untreated, mental health disorders can jeopardise the physical health of an individual living with HIV. For example, untreated psychiatric problems can reduce adherence to medical treatments and may lead to an increase in behaviours that increase the risk of HIV infection (Treisman *et al.*, 2001). Non-adherence to antiretrovirals due to psychiatric problems can be reversed if the mental health disorder is treated (Basu *et al.*, 2005).

15.2 Mental disorders and nutrition

Symptoms associated with mental illness can bring about a decline in nutritional status as in the case of the following:

- weight loss and poor appetite often seen in depression (Isaac *et al.*, 2008)

- increased requirements and irregular eating patterns seen in patients with mania
- increased prevalence of obesity in the chronically mentally ill – primarily as a side effect of atypical antipsychotic medications that increase appetite and decrease physical activity
- adverse effects from medications to treat an illness (e.g. anorectic action or appetite stimulation seen with certain antipsychotic medication)
- adverse effects such as appetite suppression from use of tobacco and recreational drug use, which can be higher in the mental health population
- lower body mass index (BMI) associated with drug use and the socio-economic status of a patient (e.g. access to food and homelessness (Quach *et al.*, 2008).

15.3   Acute cognitive impairment

Acute cognitive impairment, such as delirium, is common in people who are severely immunosuppressed due to HIV infection. The cause of delirium can be due to:

- opportunistic infections including, toxoplasmosis, lymphoma, tuberculosis, CMV, herpes zoster and cryptococcal meningitis
- Wernicke-Korsakoff syndrome
- hepatic encephalopathy
- peripheral neuropathy
- adverse effects of HIV medications
- adverse effects of medications prescribed to treat complicated infections, e.g. pneumonia may be treated with steroids (which can cause confusion)
- metabolic encephalopathies, such as hypoglycaemia and dehydration
- drug and alcohol intoxication or withdrawal and
- vitamin deficiencies – niacin and thiamine (Maggi *et al.*, 2005).

Box 15.1   Signs and symptoms of acute cognitive impairment (delirium)

- Acute Onset
- Impaired concentration, attention and memory
- Disorientation
- Agitation/irritability
- Hallucinations (usually visual)
- Delusions (usually persecutory and involving caregivers)
- Sleep disturbance

Acute cognitive impairment is classified as a medical emergency requiring, hospitalisation for treatment of the underlying aetiology. The symptoms associated with delirium (Box 15.1) may be treated using antipsychotic agents such as haloperidol and sedatives. Wernicke encephalopathy and Korsakoff's psychosis, especially seen in chronic alcoholism, are best treated initially by parenteral administration of B vitamins followed by oral administration of thiamine in the longer term (Royal Pharmaceutical Society of Great Britain, 2008).

15.4   Delirium and nutrition

The patient may refuse food or fluids due to symptoms of delirium such as lack of motivation, confusion, delusional content, disorganisation and agitation. Management would include:

- staff observation and recording of oral intake
- prompts by nursing staff to encourage food and fluid intake
- initial nutritional assessment carried out by nursing staff and if appropriate referral to dietitian for follow-up assessment and interventions
- involvement of a dietitian for nutritional assessment
- correction of dehydration, if present
- correction of malnutrition, if present
- consideration of nasogastric feeding if nutritional requirements are not met over a prolonged period of time with oral intake alone (see Chapter 8, 'Nutritional Screening and Assessment'; (NICE, 2006)
- considering testing for thiamine, B12 and folate deficiencies, if no obvious aetiology for delirium, and supplementing appropriately (Buchman *et al.*, 2005) and
- being aware of the risk of refeeding syndrome in this group and monitoring appropriately.

It is important to note that Wernicke-Korsakoff is easy to misdiagnose as the symptoms can often be mistaken for being drunk. As such, patients with chronic high alcohol intake, exhibiting these symptoms, should automatically be treated for Wernicke-Korsakoff syndrome as a prophylactic measure (Thomson *et al.*, 2002).

15.5   Chronic cognitive impairment

Progressive Multifocal Leukoencephalopathy (PML), central nervous system (CNS) lymphoma and HIV-associated dementia (from mild to severe) may cause chronic cognitive impairment. Chronic high alcohol intake can also complicate the deleterious effects of HIV-associated cognitive impairment. Chronic cognitive impairment has a poor prognosis (Panther and Libman, 2005).

Box 15.2   Signs and symptoms of chronic cognitive impairment – dementia

- Insidious
- Subcortical similar to Parkinson's
- Triad of impairments of cognition, affect, motor performance and behaviour
- Impaired short-term memory, especially retrieval
- Poor concentration and slowed thinking
- Poor balance, clumsiness and poor handwriting
- Apathy
- Emotional liability
- Disinhibition
- Social withdrawal
- Progresses to more severe cognitive impairment or chronic inactive 'burnt out' state

---

The first choice of treatment for HIV-associated dementia is the use of antiretro-viral therapy. Successful antiretroviral treatment can sometimes reverse cognitive deficits associated with a severely compromised immune system (Treisman *et al.*, 2001; Maggi *et al.*, 2005). Psychiatric medications may be used to stabilise affective or behavioural symptoms, including antidepressants and antipsychotics. These medications would be initiated in small doses and gradually increased, due to the negative interactions that can occur between antipsychotics/ antidepressants with antiretrovirals (Maggi *et al.*, 2005).

15.6   Chronic cognitive impairment and nutrition

The nutritional impact from chronic cognitive impairment depends largely on the severity of the impairment. The nutritional problems that potentially could occur in response to a client with the above symptoms are:

- difficulty shopping, preparing and cooking food
- poor planning and organisational skills leading to a diet that is not nutritionally balanced
- inadequate diet and fluid intake and
- difficulty eating food due to impaired motor skills and dysphagia.

Management includes the intervention of appropriate support services to maintain quality of life. The amount and type of support could vary and would also depend on the severity of the client's condition. There is a range of nutritional interventions which may include:

- being supported in the community by neighbours, family or services
- assistance with shopping
- provision of prompts to eat
- meals on wheels and
- nursing care, ranging from weekly visits to 24-hour care.

A referral to a dietitian may be useful in helping to manage and monitor these interventions. An urgent referral is recommended if the patient has unintentionally lost 3% of their body weight in one month, 5% or more of their body weight within the last 3 months, or 10% loss in the last 6 months (BAPEN, 2003).

15.7   Depression

Depression is the most common mental health disorder among PLHIV (people living with HIV) (Clark and Everall, 1997; Valente, 2003). More than 50% of people who are HIV positive suffer from a major depression (Ciesla and Roberts, 2001; DeSilva *et al.*, 2001; Savetsky *et al.*, 2001; Morrison *et al.*, 2002; Stolar *et al.*, 2005).

- Depression associated with HIV often results from the neuropsychiatric aspects of HIV immunosuppression. Injecting drug use may be a cause of depression in some people (DeSilva *et al.*, 2001; Valente, 2003). The potential for depression in people with HIV can be increased by factors such as side effects of medication, nutritional imbalances, history of depression, poor social support, and progression of HIV disease (Valente, 2003). A co-morbid diagnosis of depression leads to poor quality of life for people living with HIV. Other issues associated with depression in this group include:

- non-adherence to HIV medications
- delayed access to treatment and
- propensity of physical decline and functioning in people with AIDS.

There are conflicting reports of effects of depression on the immune system, some found that depression causes an accelerated progression of HIV while other studies have shown no relationship (Lyon and Younger, 2001). The effect of depression on poor adherence to treatment should not be underestimated.

Box 15.3   Signs and symptoms of depression

- Depressed mood
- Diminished pleasure/interest in activities
- Weight loss or weight gain
- Insomnia or hypersomnia
- Fatigue
- Feelings of worthlessness/hopelessness
- Feelings of excessive guilt
- Diminished ability to concentrate
- Indecisiveness
- Recurrent thoughts of death
- Suicidal ideation (with or without plan)
- Five of the above symptoms must have been present during the same two-week period and be a change from past functioning. Either depressed mood or/and diminished pleasure must be present.

15.8   Depression and nutrition

Depression can influence food consumption in a variety of different ways. Lack of interest in food can lead to weight loss, undernutrition and anorexia (Fava, 2000; Abayomi and Hackett, 2004; McQuire, 2007). This may be further influenced by poor motivation and disinterest in preparing and cooking balanced meals. In some cases, the client may feel so worthless and hopeless that they feel they don't deserve food. The client may also refuse fluids in addition to food causing dehydration and constipation (McQuire, 2007).

Alternatively, a depressed client may binge or comfort eat, in particular carbohydrates and chocolate, which can lead to excessive weight gain (Kazes *et al.*, 1994; Benton and Donohoe, 1999). There is a lower exercise level among those diagnosed with depression, which can also contribute to weight gain (Wurtman, 1993). Side effects of some of the serotonin reuptake inhibitors (SSRIs) include anorexia, vomiting and nausea (Abayomi and Hackett, 2004) (see Box 15.3). Weight gain is another side effect of antidepressants (Christensen and Somers, 1996) and this often unde-sirable effect may lead to non-concordance with therapy. Alternatively, weight gain following antidepressant treatment may be a sign of recovery from depression and may be viewed positively by patients (Fava, 2000).

15.9 Management of depression

Although depression is recognisable and treatable, it continues to be under-identified and undertreated by many health care professionals (Treisman *et al.*, 2001). Tak-ing this into consideration, it is important that HIV clinicians are able to identify depression by using appropriate effective screening tools which can encourage early intervention and treatment. A referral can be made to the local mental health team who will carry out a full mental state examination to confirm depression and iden-tify any other existing psychiatric symptoms, in addition to suicide risk, which is essential. Often there can be difficulty separating the diagnosis of depression from a medical illness associated with HIV (Valente, 2003). For example, fatigue and listlessness in depression may resemble symptoms associated with advanced HIV disease.

Antidepressants are a common form of treatment, in particular SSRIs (Treisman *et al.*, 2001; Elder *et al.*, 2005). It can often take 2–6 weeks for antidepressants to produce the desired therapeutic effect. This should be explained to the client as treatment failure has been associated with poor dosing and not using it for long enough (Basu *et al.*, 2005). In spite of their effectiveness, antidepressant medications carry the risk of side effects and drug–drug interactions with many medications including antiretrovirals (Treisman *et al.*, 2001).

To effectively treat depression a combination of treatments are used such as cog-nitive behavioural therapy, counselling, education, pharmacotherapy, good dietary intake, exercise and self management tools (Valente, 2003; Stolar *et al.*, 2005). Al-though controversial, the use of electroconvulsive therapy (ECT) can be used as a last resort, with proven efficacy (Valente, 2003).

Investigations are under way on the treatment of depression with therapeutic use of Omega-3 essential fatty acids containing eicosapentanoic acid (EPA) and docosahexanoic acid (DHA) (Freeman *et al.*, 2006, 2008; Hallahan *et al.*, 2007). Epidemiological studies have shown that countries with high fish consumption have significantly lower incidences of major depression than those countries with lower fish consumption (Hibbeln, 1998, 2009; Tanskanen *et al.*, 2001). However, if Omega-3 is used as a treatment modality, a purified, pharmaceutical-grade fish oil supplement is recommended, as opposed to increasing fish in the diet, as a high fish intake (> 4 portions of oily fish per week, for not-at-risk individuals) increases the risk of toxicity from heavy metals, PCBs and dioxins (Committee on Toxicity Report, 2008). The beneficial Omega-3 is eicosapentanoic acid from cold water fish, rather than the shorter chained omega-3 alpha linolenic acid (ALA), which is poorly converted to EPA in the body (max. 10% conversion rate, Goyens *et al.*, 2005). It is important to use fish oil rather than cod liver oil to avoid hypervitaminosis A (Tables 15.1 and 15.2).

Table 15.1 Interactions between HIV medications with antipsychotic neuroleptic and anticonvulsant medications.

Anticonvulsants	Atazanavir	Darunavir	Fosamprenavir	Indinavir	Lopinavir	Nelfinavir	Ritonavir	Saquinavir	Tipranavir	Delavirdine	Efavirenz	Etravirine	Nevirapine
Carbamazepine	■	■	■	■	■	■	■	■	■	●	■	●	■
Clonazepam	■	■	■	■	■	■	■	■	■	■	■	■	■
Ethosuximide	■	■	■	■	■	■	■	■	■	■	■	■	■
Gabapentin	◆	◆	◆	◆	◆	◆	◆	◆	◆	◆	◆	◆	◆
Lamotrigine	■	◆	◆	■	■	◆	■	◆	◆	◆	◆	◆	◆
Levetiracetam	◆	◆	◆	◆	◆	◆	◆	◆	◆	◆	◆	◆	◆
Oxcarbazepine	■	■	■	■	■	■	■	■	■	■	◆	■	■
Phenobarbital (Phenobarbitone)	■	●	■	■	■	■	■	■	■	●	■	●	■
Phenytoin	■	●	■	■	■	■	■	■	■	●	■	●	■
Valproate (Divalproex)	■	◆	◆	■	■	■	■	◆	■	◆	◆	◆	■
Vigabatrin	◆	◆	◆	◆	◆	◆	◆	◆	◆	◆	◆	◆	◆

Antipsychotics/Neuroleptics	Atazanavir	Darunavir	Fosamprenavir	Indinavir	Lopinavir	Nelfinavir	Ritonavir	Saquinavir	Tipranavir	Delavirdine	Efavirenz	Etravirine	Nevirapine
Chlorpromazine	■	■	■	■	■	■	■	■	■	■	◇	◇	◇
Clozapine	■	■	■	○	■	■	■	■	■	◇	◇	◇	◇
Haloperidol	■	■	■	■	■	■	■	■	■	■	■	■	■
Olanzapine	■	■	■	■	■	■	■	■	■	■	■	■	■
Perphenazine	◇	◇	◇	◇	◇	◇	■	◇	◇	◇	◇	◇	◇
Pimozide	○	○	○	○	○	○	○	○	○	○	○	■	■
Quetiapine	■	■	■	■	■	■	■	■	■	■	■	■	■
Risperidone	◇	■	◇	◇	◇	◇	■	◇	◇	◇	◇	◇	◇
Sulpiride	◇	◇	◇	◇	◇	◇	◇	◇	◇	◇	◇	◇	◇
Thioridazine	◇	■	◇	◇	◇	◇	■	◇	◇	◇	◇	◇	◇

○ These drugs should not be coadministered

■ Potential interaction that may require close monitoring, alteration of drug dosage or timing of administration

◇ No clinically significant interaction expected

Tables modified with permission from the University of Liverpool www.hiv-druginteractions.org.

Table 15.2 Possible nutritional side effects of most commonly used antidepressant drugs in clients who have HIV.

Drug	Generic name	Possible side effects affecting nutrition
Selective Serotonin	Citalopram	Weight loss/gain
Reuptake inhibitors (SSRIs) – first-line medication in depressed HIV-positive clients due to their effectiveness and tolerance.	Escitalopram Fluoxetine Fluvoxamine Paroxetine Sertraline	Nausea/vomiting Diarrhoea Taste disturbances Anorexia Dyspepsia Abdominal pain GI upset SIADH (Syndrome of inappropriate antidiuretic hormone secretion leading to hyponatraemia)
Tricyclic	Amitriptyline Clomipramine Doxepine Imipramine	Dry mouth Constipation or diarrhoea (rarely) Nausea/vomiting Weight gain Increased appetite Changes in blood glucose SIADH Oedema GI upset
Serotonin and noradrenaline reuptake inhibitors (SNRIs) – not much data relating to their use in HIV clients	Venlafaxine	Weight loss/gain Increased cholesterol Constipation/diarrohoea Nausea/vomiting Dry mouth GI disturbances Taste disturbances Dyspepsia SIADH
Noradrenergic and specific serotonergic – not much data relating to use in HIV clients	Mirtazepine	Oedema Weight Gain Increased appetite Nausea Diarrhoea Dry mouth Stomatitis (rare) Oral hypaesthesia (rare) Mouth oedema (rare)
RIMA (Reversible Inhibitors of Monoamine Oxidase type A)	Moclobemide	Nausea Dry Mouth Constipation Diarrhoea

15.10 Suicide

Suicidal ideation occurs frequently among PLHIV (Clark and Everall, 1997; Frey *et al.*, 1997; Basu *et al.*, 2005). Suicidal ideation may increase at different stages of HIV disease, such as notification of HIV-positive result, death or loss of a loved one and diagnosis of AIDS-defining illness (Clark and Everall, 1997). Clients who misuse substances and/or have a diagnosis of personality disorder are suggested to be at an increased risk of suicide (Kalichman *et al.*, 2000). Other risk factors for suicidal behaviour inlcude:

- male gender between the ages of 15 and 30 years old
- history of previous suicide attempts or self harm
- having a mental health disorder
- co-morbidity of substance misuse and mental health problems
- recent stressful events including loss and death of a loved one (Elder *et al.*, 2005).

15.11   Management of suicidal ideation

It is important to directly ask the patient about suicidal ideation, for instance, 'Have you been having thoughts about killing yourself? Do you have a plan in place to kill yourself? What steps have you been taking towards doing this?' (Elder *et al.*, 2005). A proper suicide screening should include past psychiatric history (especially suicide attempts or friend/family history of suicide), mental status evaluation (psychotic symptoms, especially command hallucinations), a review of major life stressors (especially losses), current levels of financial and social support, patient beliefs about personal disease progression and future, and a discussion about any specific suicidal plans. A contract should be established with the patient, specifying an emergency plan to be implemented in the event that the patient experiences increased suicidal ideation. An emergency psychiatric assessment is necessary when a patient has clear intention to act on suicidal ideations' (Basu *et al.*, 2005, p. 2059).

15.12   Mania

Symptoms of mania include forced speech, grandiosity, irritability, verbosity, distractibility, disinhibition, psychomotor agitation and abnormal elevation of mood that lasts for at least one week (Elder *et al.*, 2005).

There is little data detailing the prevalence of mania in people with HIV. However, it is generally believed that the risk of mania increases as HIV disease progresses. Mania may result from central nervous system toxicity or pathology or, if the client has a history (personal or family), mania may suggest an affective disorder. Lithium is the drug of choice used to treat mania. However, it must be used with caution, with close monitoring of lithium levels to avoid the person developing toxicity with dehydration, due to vomiting and diarrhoea, which may be a direct effect of the antiretrovirals (Stolar *et al.*, 2005). It is important to be aware that patients diagnosed with bipolar conditions have been shown to have a tendency to use prescribed mood stabilisers at a higher dose than prescribed because of their impatience with the slow onset of action (Kemppainen *et al.*, 2004).

15.13   Mania and nutrition

Patients with mania feel that they have a diminished need for sleep and food, their eating patterns may become erratic and their energy expenditure may increase due to increased activity (Australasian Society for HIV Medicine, 2004). Due to these

Table 15.3 Possible nutritional side effects of most commonly used mood stabilisers in clients who have HIV.

Drug	Generic name	Possible side effects affecting nutrition
Mood stabilisers	Lithium carbonate	Nausea/vomiting
Lithium salts –	Lithium citrate	Weight gain
Used for treatment of mania and prophylactic treatment of recurrent mood disorders.		Dehydration
Used for young people with personality disorders with cyclothymia.		Increased thirst
		Electrolyte imbalance
		(Reduced dietary intake)
		(Loss of appetite)
		Oedema
		Polyuria
		Metallic taste
		Hyperglycaemia
		Hypothyroidism
		Toxic effects (caused by sodium depletion)
		Excess salivation

factors a patient with mania may experience weight loss (McQuire, 2007) (Table 15.3).

15.14   Anxiety

PLHIV commonly suffer from anxiety disorders, in particular, anxiety around deterioriation, loss and death. Symptoms of anxiety in an individual can vary in range and effect, from being mild to debilitating (Andreasen and Black, 2001; Basu et al., 2005). Symptoms of anxiety include feeling restless, fatigue and irritable with difficulties in concentrating and sleeping. Muscle tension, hyperarousal and excessive worry are also signs of anxiety (Bourne, 2000). Anxiety or panic attacks include sensations of chest pain, sweating, palpitations, hyperventilation, shortness of breath, tingling, nausea and headaches (Basu et al., 2005). Vomiting and diarrhoea may also occur. The individual may become unnecessarily fearful and phobic. This may result in someone becoming obsessive about health, preoccupied with checking for body signs of illness and frequent requests for tests. Often presentations and complaints of somatic symptoms may actually be an anxiety disorder (Andreasen and Black, 2001). Increased suicidal risk can occur with severe anxiety (Basu et al., 2005). There are a variety of different anxiety disorders including obsessive compulsive disorder, generalised anxiety disorder, substance induced anxiety disorder, anxiety disorder due to a medical condition, phobias and post-traumatic stress disorder (Bourne, 2000).

15.14.1   Post-traumatic stress disorder (PTSD)

PTSD may result from exposure to and/or witnessing an unusually traumatic event (Basu et al., 2005, p. 2063). It is well reported that many people with HIV infection have faced high rates of abuse and violence, thus increasing their risk of PTSD (Basu *et al.*, 2005). *Note*: Receiving a diagnosis of HIV can also serve as a PTSD trigger as one's survival is threatened.

People often suffer many of the similar body symptoms that are associated with hyperarousal of the autonomic nervous system during and after a traumatic incident. Symptoms of hyperarousal include increased heart rate, palpitations, 'jumpiness' and hyper-vigilance. When chronic, symptoms include sleep disturbances, sexual dysfunction and decreased appetite (Rothschild, 2000). In response, the patient may avoid situations or activities that remind him/her of the traumatic event, become detached and isolated from other people, and have a foreshortened sense of the future (Basu *et al.*, 2005).

15.14.2   Panic disorder

A panic attack is a sudden feeling of physiological arousal that occurs unexpectedly. It can occur in response to thinking about and/or encountering a much feared situation. However, it can also occur out of nowhere for no easily discernable reason. People can learn to cope and manage with panic attacks over time (Bourne, 2000). In addition to symptoms already described for anxiety, choking sensations, shortness of breath, nausea, dizziness, shaking and hot or cold flushes occur as intermittent panic attacks, during which fear and somatic symptoms will peak within 10 minutes and generally resolve within a half-hour if the patient is left untreated in a calm environment. To meet the Diagnostic and Statistical Manual of Mental Disorders IV (DSM-IV-TR) criteria of panic disorder, a patient must worry persistently, over a 1-month period, about experiencing a panic attack or display important behavioural changes connected to the attack (Basu *et al.*, 2005).

15.14.3   Anxiety and nutrition

Symptoms associated with anxiety can impact on nutrition in a variety of ways. An individual who is suffering with anxiety attacks may be experiencing choking sensations, nausea, vomiting or even diarrhoea. These symptoms may cause a patient to become nutritionally compromised and a referral to a dietitian should be made if there is any concern.

15.14.4   Management of anxiety

To evaluate a diagnosis of an anxiety-related disorder, it is important to obtain the patient's psychiatric history, medication (prescribed drugs) history and substance misuse (non-prescribed drugs) history. Other events need to be assessed, such as exposure to domestic violence and other possible traumatic and arousing events. Even a person's dietary habits, such as caffeine intake, need to be evaluated (Basu *et al.*, 2005).

There are many prescribed drugs (usually SSRIs) that can be used to treat anxiety. However, anxiety-reducing drugs are not always required. For a list of drugs that can be used to treat anxiety, refer to Table 15.3. Lifestyle changes, including reducing caffeine and substance use, and initiating exercise can all reduce anxiety. Further benefits for patients with anxiety are counselling, stress management (relaxation and problem-solving techniques) support and cognitive behavioural therapy (which may help with distorted thinking), which can be implemented (Bourne, 2000; Andreasen and Black, 2001).

Benzodiazepines may be used for the treatment of anxiety. However, they should be used for a brief time for acute anxiety because of tolerance, misuse and dependency issues that may occur, especially with an individual who has a history of addiction (Blalock *et al.*, 2005).

15.15   Psychosis

Schizophrenia (psychosis) is one of the most severe mental health disorders. It is characterised by severe changes in a person's thinking, mood, and behaviour, which can result in considerable compromised interpersonal and occupational functioning. It usually manifests in people between the ages of 18 and 24 years. Studies suggest that immigrant status is a risk factor for schizophrenia, especially within the African-Caribbean population in England (McDonald and Murray, 2000; Selten *et al.*, 2007). However, the reasons for such cultural differences in diagnoses of schizophrenia remain unknown.

Psychotic symptoms during the course of HIV infection constitute a known complication. New-onset psychosis, diagnosed usually by exclusion of other psychoses, is characterized by a distinct constellation of symptoms and a varied clinical course, and has been linked to putative neurotransmitter pathology in cortical neurones (Sabhesan *et al.*, 1998). Common symptoms include vivid hallucinations, bizarre delusions (persecutory, grandiose and somatic), and disorganised speech and behaviour. One study revealed that agitation, anxiety, thought disorder and cognitive impairment were also experienced. Usually patients had been psychotic for a period of time, varying between days to months, before presentation. Patients who fit this category, who have more than one risk factor for AIDS should have HIV omitted as the cause of their symptoms (Andreasen and Black, 2001).

In the acute phase of schizophrenia symptoms include:

- delusions (paranoid/persecutory or grandiose)
- ideas of reference
- hallucinations (most common auditory, however, may involve all five senses)
- incoherence
- thought broadcasting
- blunted affect
- anhedonia
- incongruent affect
- catatonia
- agitation
- hostility

In the chronic phase of schizophrenia symptoms include:

- lack of motivation
- social and emotional withdrawal
- limited conversational skills
- disordered thinking
- fear and anxiety
- difficulty forming relationships

- poor insight
- poor personal hygiene
- inadequate nutritional intake
- inability to cope with daily living tasks

There can be many difficulties associated with medications prescribed for HIV with individuals who have serious mental health problems. For example, fluctuation and severity of psychiatric symptoms; interactions between the HIV medications and psychiatric medications; poor insight; deficits in cognition; substance abuse; and the differential diagnosis of psychiatric symptoms. It is difficult for clients to achieve full medication adherence, despite using blister packs or dosette boxes, and is hard to determine whether non-compliance is deliberate or not. In contrast, there were benefits of incorporating HIV medicines into the client's daily structure, by using reminder signs and calendars. An essential factor for this client group was having support (from family/carers/services) to assist with filling reminder pillboxes. It has been reported that non-white (African-American) participants tended to depend more on visual reminders and cues (Kemppainen *et al.*, 2004).

15.15.1   Psychosis and nutrition

The symptoms of schizophrenia may determine dietary intake and may affect the ability to interact and communicate with a health care professional (McQuire, 2007). Patients may have difficulty understanding the connection between weight, diet and exercise (Beebe, 2008) (Table 15.4).

15.15.2   Management of psychosis

Early intervention to assess and plan treatment for the client and deliver the appropriate interventions is very important to avoid crisis (Frey *et al.*, 1997).

Antipsychotic medication, mainly atypical antipsychotics due to their tolerability in HIV clients, are effective in treating symptoms of psychosis including hallucinations and delusions (Andreasen and Black, 2001). Caution has to be taken when prescribing antipsychotics because people with HIV/AIDS are at an increased risk of developing extrapyramidal side effects (EPSE – is only a side effect of typical anticpsychotics; atypical antipsychotics do not cause EPSE). (See Table 15.5.) As an atypical antipsychotic, Olanzepine is known to be at lower risk of causing EPSE and therefore is often used (Stolar *et al.*, 2005). Atypicals generally increase appetite and decrease physical activity and lead to 30–40% of patients experiencing undesirable weight gain.

Cognitive behavioural therapy has proven to be effective when used with patients who have schizophrenia, e.g. a client who hears 'voices' may discover that they can be dulled by listening to music through headphones (Elder *et al.*, 2005)

PLHIV and mental health problems have specialised needs and require the input of psychiatrist services with knowledge and expertise of the co-morbidities (Clark and Everall, 1997). Furthermore, it is important that people with HIV have integrated health and social care that are culturally appropriate and individually tailored to meet the clients' need, and that mental health and other HIV services work collaboratively (Green and Smith, 2004). Case management is recommended as a way of improving treatment, care and medication adherence in clients with serious mental illness in combination with HIV (Sullivan *et al.*, 2006).

Table 15.4 Effects of psychotic symptoms on diet.

Symptom	Example	Effect on diet
Delusions	May believe that food is being poisoned	Avoid certain foods
Hallucinations	May hear voices telling them that they are not allowed to eat or drink and therefore respond to this	Dehydration Dry mouth Weight loss Deficiency in vitamins Constipation
Agitation	May be preoccupied with psychotic symptoms making it difficult for the dietitian to form a rapport	Difficult for dietitian to assess nutritional needs and problems
Poor insight	May not believe they have an illness and that their symptoms are not 'real' and may think that their diet is fine	Difficult for dietitian to identify problems and manage.
Withdrawal	May not leave the house to go shopping for food	Inadequate fluid and food intake
Inability to cope with daily tasks	May lack the ability, due to cognitive impairment, to budget, shop and prepare meals	Weight loss Weight Gain (if eating high carbohydrate diet)
Irrational thinking	Thought blocking may occur, causing the patient to stop suddenly and normal associations between words and ideas may break down. This causes difficulty in communicating	Difficulty for dietitian to assess and manage and maintain.
Impaired memory	May forget that they have already eaten, and as such constantly seek out food, or completely forget to eat, believing that they have eaten when they haven't	$\uparrow\downarrow$ dietary intake $\Rightarrow$ impaired nutritional status

Table 15.5 Possible nutritional side effects of most commonly used psychotropic drugs in clients who have HIV.

Drug	Generic name	Possible side effects affecting nutrition
Antipsychotics Atypical – used for psychotic disorders and mania. Drug of choice as they cause less extra-pyramidal side effects and tardive dyskinesia than other drugs.	Olanzepine Risperidone Quetiapine Amisulpiride Ziprasidone Clozapine (not used if client is on protease inhibitors)	Increased appetite and weight gain (more evident in olanzepine and clozapine) Hyperglycaemia Diabetes Constipation Dry mouth Excess salivation Dysphagia Impairment of intestinal peristalsis Increased triglyceride levels GI upset

Table 15.6 Description of extrapyramidal side effects of antipsychotic medications.

Extrapyramidal side effects	Characteristics
Acute dystonic reaction	Painful muscle spasms in back, head and torso, which can have rapid onset and last from minutes to hours
Akathisia	Feeling restless, legs ache and unable to stay still
Parkinsonism	Excess salivation, shuffling gait and mask-like facial expression
Tardive dyskinesia	Involuntary movements of lips, tongue and feet, usually in response to prolonged use of traditional antipsychotic medication, such as largactil
Neuroleptic malignant syndrome	Potentially fatal. Severe extrapyramidal side effects, hyperthermia, clouding of consciousness and rigid muscles
Seizures	Low risk

It is highly recommended that in mental health facilities, a means of identifying patients at high risk of HIV should be implemented and evaluated (Kelly *et al.*, 1992; Ayos-Mateos *et al.*, 1997). This should include routine assessment of HIV risk behaviours, offers of HIV testing and counselling and HIV prevention programmes for those with high risk (Carey *et al.*, 2004) (Tables 15.5 and 15.6).

Extrapyramidal side effects are treated by antiparkinsonian medication, such as procyclidine. Support and reassurance is necessary to alleviate the patient's fear. In more severe cases of EPS, hospitalisation may be required (Elder *et al.*, 2005).

15.16 Socio-economic factors for mental health/HIV clients affecting nutrition

Groups from low socio-economic standing are disproportionately affected by mental health and HIV (Kelly, 1997; Dembling *et al.*, 2002; Skapinakas *et al.*, 2006; Weich *et al.*, 2007). People diagnosed with mental health conditions living in the community often have poor diets due, largely, to low incomes. Therefore, they are less likely to buy fruit and vegetables and may have skills deficits in activities of daily living (Abayomi and Hackett, 2004).

Population groups who have recently emigrated from other regions, such as PLHIV in the UK from African countries, may be more likely to have many additional social issues to face, such as housing, employment, income, poor health, poverty and immigration. In such cases, treatment issues have been shown to be a lower priority than daily living issues such as having enough money to buy food, clothes and pay for housing (Green and Smith, 2004). People from lower socio-economic groups may be less likely to access and adhere to treatment (Weich *et al.*, 2007).

Examples of some possible nutritional problems that may occur as a result of socio-economic issues include:

- Poor dentition due to medications, recreational drugs, poor hygiene, poor food choices and difficulty accessing dental services (Nikias *et al.*, 1975; AIHW, 2001).
- Missing teeth and ill-fitting dentures which impair eating and lower body mass index (Ficher and Johnson, 1990; Sheiham *et al.*, 2002).

- Food purchasing behaviours of socio-economically disadvantaged groups are least in accordance with dietary guidelines (Nolan *et al.*, 2006).
- The use of tobacco/recreational drugs can decrease appetite and increase metabolism at the same time (e.g., methamphetamines).
- Homelessness may lead to impaired nutritional status due to limited access to food stores and cooking facilities.

15.17 Personality disorders

There are various types of personality disorders, but within the HIV population borderline personality disorder is one of the most frequent, followed by narcissistic and antisocial personality disorders. Personality disorder and HIV are at times linked, as personality disorders are associated with impulsivity that, in turn, is connected to high-risk behaviours (Millon *et al.*, 2000). Clinical signs of borderline personality disorder include emotional instability, impulsivity, substance and alcohol misuse, deliberate self-harm, low self-esteem and inability to form stable relationships (Clark and Everall, 1997; Andreasen and Black, 2001).

Often clinicians can find patients with personality disorders frustrating and stressful, possibly due to the seemingly irrational and self-destructive behaviour that can often be displayed (Treisman *et al.*, 2001; Perseius *et al.*, 2007). It is important and effective to set firm, consistent and clear clinical boundaries with the service user, to have a clearly written care plan and to provide regular support (Clark and Everall, 1997; Millon *et al.*, 2000; Treisman *et al.*, 2001).

15.18 Dual diagnosis

Dual diagnosis can be defined as the combination of substance abuse (including alcohol) and a mental health disorder (Elder *et al.*, 2005). It is estimated that almost 50% of people with severe mental disorders also have a substance use disorder. These symptoms often overlap making diagnosis and treatment more difficult. One disorder may remain undetected and untreated and may exacerbate each other. People with dual diagnoses often experience medical problems, more severe symptoms, poor adherence to treatment, increased relapse, increased risk of suicide and higher rates of service use. Social consequences can include homelessness, violence (perpetrator or victim), being incarcerated and increased risk of contracting HIV (Parry *et al.*, 2007).

There have been few published studies on the subject of double diagnosis and triple diagnosis. It can potentially be very difficult to differentiate between signs and symptoms related to HIV, psychiatric disorder and illicit substance misuse, grouping some cases, especially with people who are reluctant to engage with services and are normally late presenters (Clark and Everall, 1997). The importance of working as a multidisciplinary team using an integrated approach is highly suggested and effective in providing treatment (Kwasnik *et al.*, 1997; Tilley and Chambers, 2006).

The provision of education to deal with substance use (including alcohol) and HIV prevention is highly important. Similarly, cooperative efforts between addictions specialists, psychiatrists and infectious disease personnel must be established to address the 'triple diagnoses' in these patients to better care for a complicated medical presentation (Goforth *et al.*, 2004 p. 181).

15.18.1   Education

Education assists the patients, caregivers, family, etc. to understand the limitations of the disorder, to retain a sense of control, alleviate fears and anticipate future needs (Frey *et al.*, 1997).

Educational programmes for people with mental health problems were one of the first methods used, with some success, to promote HIV prevention (Kelly, 1997).

15.19   Nutritional management of patients with HIV/mental health issues

The general recommendation for a patient with asymptomatic, non-advanced HIV and mental health issues would be to follow a healthy diet, as with the general population. This should include a variety of foods from the five food groups (fruits, vegetables, grains and cereals, meat and alternatives, and dairy foods) with minimal additional fat and sugar (see Chapter 13, 'Healthy Eating and Well-Being'). A referral should be made to a dietitian if there are circumstances such as:

- decreased nutritional status such as weight loss, poor appetite, nausea, diarrhoea and vomiting related to factors such as illness, and side effects of medication
- inability to maintain or access a healthy diet
- avoidance of food groups due to paranoia, leading to nutritional deficiencies (although rarely seen)
- obesity due to a variety of reasons including increased appetite from medication, making poor food choices and a sedentary lifestyle.

Management of these symptoms are covered in other chapters of this text book (e.g. Chapters 7 and 9).

Ideally, a weight programme involving exercise and diet tailored to meet individual needs should be implemented at the beginning of antipsychotic treatment and this should be monitored during the course of the treatment (Malhi, 2003). However, it is important to recognise cognitive limitations (such as reduced attention span and memory) of people with chronic mental health issues when delivering education about diet and exercise (Beebe, 2000). Weight loss goals for patients who have experienced weight gain as a side effect of antipsychotic medication need to be more modest than weight loss goals for the general population. The primary goal should always be weight maintenance with the secondary goal of 5–10% weight loss over 6–12 months, rather than the more ambitious 3–6 months, often seen in general weight-loss programmes. This is due primarily to the double-edged side effect of the antipsychotic medications increasing appetite and lowering physical activity. Also, it is important to take into account that many people living with HIV/AIDS see weight loss as an AIDS-defining illness and as such are less likely to be responsive to weight loss advice, as they would associate any weight loss as a negative.

Acknowledgements

This chapter was reviewed by:

Stuart Gibson, PhD CPsychol, Clinical Psychologist, CASCAID (HIV Mental Health Service), South London & Maudsley NHS Foundation Trust.

The authors would also like to thank Dr Melissa Corr, Psychiatrist, Royal Prince Alfred Hospital, Sydney, Australia, Mr. Wand, Nurse Practitioner, Consultation Liaison, Royal Prince Alfred Hospital, Sydney, Australia, and Antoinette Ackerie, Dietitian HIV, Royal Prince Alfred Hospital, Sydney, Australia, for their support and input.

References

Abayomi J, Hackett A. Assessment of malnutrition in mental health clients: nurses. *J Adv Nurs* 2004; **45**(4):430–437.

Andreasen NC, Black DW. *Introductory Textbook of Psychiatry*, 3rd edn. Arlington, VA: American Psychiatric Publishing, 2001.

AIHW Dental Statistics and Research Unit. Oral health and access to dental care- the gap between deprived and privilege in Australia. Research report. 2001. Available at http://www.adelaide.edu.au/spdent/dsru/pub-frame.htm. Cited on 15th. May 2008.

Australasian Society for HIV Medicine. In: Hoy J, Lewin S eds. *HIV Management in Australasia: A Guide for Clinical Care*. Sydney, Australia: Australasian Society for HIV Medicine. 2004.

Ayos-Mateos JL, Montanes F, Lastra I, Picazo De La Garza JJ, Ayuso-Gutierrez JL. HIV infection in psychiatric patients: an unlinked anonymous study. *Br J Psychiatry* 1997; **170**:181–185.

BAPEN. *Malnutrition Universal Screening Tool: MUST*. Redditch, UK: British Association for Parenteral and Enteral Nutrition, 2003.

Basu S, Chwastiak LA, Bruce RD. Clinical management of depression and anxiety in HIV-infected adults. *AIDS* 2005; **19**:2057–2067.

Beebe HL. Obesity in schizophrenia: screening, monitoring, and health promotion. *Perspect Psychiatr Care* 2008; **44**(1):25–31.

Beebe, D.W. (2000). The attention to body shape scale. In: Maltby J, Lewis CA, Hill AP, eds., *Commissioned Reviews on 250 Psychological Tests*. Lampeter, Wales: Edwin Mellen Press, 2000: 11–13.

Benton D, Donohoe RT. The effects of nutrients on mood. *Public Health Nutr* 1999; **2**(3a):403–409.

Blalock AC, Sharma SM, McDaniel JS. Anxiety disorders and HIV disease. In: Citron K, Brouillette MJ, Beckett A, eds. *HIV and Psychiatry: A Training and Resource Manual*, 2nd edn. Cambridge, UK: Cambridge University Press, 2005.

Bourne EJ. *The Anxiety & Phobia Workbook*, 3rd edn. California, USA: New Harbinger Publications, 2000.

Carey MP, Carey KB, Maisto SA, Schroder KEE, Vanable PA, Gordon CM. HIV risk behaviour among psychiatric outpatients: association with psychiatric disorder, substance use disorder, and gender. *J Nerv Ment Dis* 2004 April; **192**(4):289–296.

Christensen L, Somers S. Comparison of nutrient intake among depressed and nondepressed individuals. *Int J Eat Disord* 1996; **20**(1):105–109.

Ciesla JA, Roberts JE. A meta-analysis of risk for major depressive disorder among HIV-positive individuals. *Am J Psychiatry* 2001; **158**:725–730.

Clark BR, Everall IP. What is the role of the HIV liaison psychiatrist? *Genitourin Med* 1997; **73**:568–570.

Committee on Toxicity of Chemicals in Food. Consumer Products and the Environment: Statement on Organic Chlorinated and Brominated Contaminants in Shellfish, Farmed and Wild Fish, 2008. Available at: http://cot.food.gov.uk/pdfs/cotstatementfishsurveys.pdf.

Cournos F, Empfield M, Horwath E *et al*. HIV seroprevalence among patients admitted to two psychiatric hospitals. *Am J Psychiatry* Spring 1991; **148**(9):1225–1229.

Dembling BP, Rovnyak V, Mackey S, Blank M. Effect of geographic migration on SMI prevalence estimates. *Menalt Health Serv Res* 2002; **4**(1):7–12.

DeSilva KE, Le Flore DB, Marston BJ, Rimland D. Serotonin syndrome in HIV-infected individuals receiving antiretroviral therapy and fluoxetine. *AIDS* 2001; **15**:1281–1285.

Elder R, Evans K, Nizette DP. *Psychiatric and Mental Health Nursing*. Sydney, NSW: Elsevier Australia, 2005.

Essock SM, Dowden S, Constantine NT, *et al*. & the Five-Site Health and Risk Study Research Committee. Blood-borne infections and persons with mental illness: risk factors for HIV,

Hepatitis B and Hepatitis C among persons with severe mental illness. *Psychiatry Serv* 2003; 54:836–841.

Fava M. Weight gain and antidepressants. *J Clin Psychiatry* 2000; **61**(suppl. 11):37–41.

Ficher J, Johnson MA. Low body weight and weight loss in the aged. *J Am Diet Assoc* 1990; 90:1697–1706.

Freeman MP, Davis M, Sinha P, Wisner KL, Hibbeln JR, Gelenberg AJ. Omega-3 fatty acids and supportive psychotherapy for perinatal depression: a randomized placebo-controlled study. *J Affect Disord* 2008 Sep; **110**(1–2):142–148. Epub 2008 Feb 21.

Freeman MP, Hibbeln JR, Wisner KL *et al.* Omega-3 fatty acids: evidence basis for treatment and future research in psychiatry. *J Clin Psychiatry* 2006 Dec; **67**(12):1954–1967. Review. Erratum in: J Clin Psychiatry. 2007 Feb; 68(2):338.

Frey D, Oman K, Wagner WR. Delivering mental health services to the home. In: Winiarski M, ed. *HIV Mental Health for the 21st Century*. New York: New York University Press, 1997: 224–240.

Goforth HW, Lupash DP, Brown ME, Tan J, Fernandez F. Role of Alcohol and substances of abuse in the immunomodulation of human immunodeficiency virus disease a review. *Addict Disord Treat* 2004; 3(4):174–182.

Goyens PL, Spilker ME, Zock PL *et al.* Compartmental modeling to quantify alpha-linolenic acid conversion after longer term intake of multiple tracer boluses. *J Lipid Res* 2005; **46**:1474–83

Green G, Smith R. The psychosocial and health care needs of HIV-positive people in the United Kingdom :a review. *HIV Med* 2004; 5(1):5–46.

Hallahan B, Hibbeln JR, Davis JM, Garland MR. Omega-3 fatty acid supplementation in patients with recurrent self-harm. Single-centre double-blind randomised controlled trial. *Br J Psychiatry* 2007 Feb; **190**:118–22.

Hibbeln JR. Fish consumption and major depression. *Lancet* 1998 Apr 18; **351**(9110):1213.

Hibbeln JR. Depression, suicide and deficiencies of omega-3 essential fatty acids in modern diets. *World Rev Nutr Diet* 2009; **99**:17–30. Epub 2009 Jan 9.

Kalichman SC, Heckman T, Kochman A, Sikkema, K, Bergholte J. Depression and thoughts of suicide among middle-aged and older persons living with HIV-AIDS. *Psychiatr Serv* 2000 July; 51(7):903–907.

Kazes M, Danion JM, Grange D *et al.* Eating behaviour and depression before and after antide-pressant treatment: a prospective, naturalistic study. *J Affect Disord* 1994; 30:193–207.

Kelly JA. HIV risk reduction interventions for persons with severe mental illness. *Clin Psychol Rev* 1997; **17**(3):293–309.

Kelly JA, Murphy DA, Bahr GR *et al.* AIDS/HIV risk behaviour among the chronic mentally ill. *Am J Psychiatry* 1992; **149**(7):886–889.

Kemppainen JK, Levine R, Buffum M, Holzemer W, Finley, P, Jenses P. Antiretroviral adherence in persons with HIV/AIDS and severe mental illness. *J Nerv Ment Dis* 2004; **192**(6):395–404.

Kwasnik BC, Moynihan RT, Royle MH. HIV mental health services integrated with medical care. In: Winiarski M, ed. *HIV Mental Health for the 21st Century*. New York: New York University Press, 1997.

Liverpool HIV Pharmacology Group, HIV Drug Interactions, University of Liverpool, 2009: Available at: http://www.hiv-druginteractions.org/.

Lyon DE, Younger JB. Purpose in life and depressive symptoms in persons living with HIV disease. *J Nurs Sch* 2001; 33(2):129–133.

Maggi JD, Rourke SB, Halman M. Cognitive disorders in people living with HIV disease. In: Citron K, Brouillette MJ, Beckett A, eds. *HIV and Psychiatry: A Training and Resource Manual*, 2nd edn. Cambridge, UK: Cambridge University Press, 2005.

Malhi GS. Editorial: weight gain: gained by waiting? *Acta Psychiatr Scand* 2003; **108**:249–251.

McDermott BE, Sautter FJ Jr., Winstead DK, Quirk T. Diagnosis, health beliefs, and risk of HIV infection in psychiatric patients. *Hosp Community Psychiatry*1994; 45(6):580–585.

McDonald C, Murray RM. Early and late environmental risk factors for schizophrenia. *Brain Res Rev* 2000; 31:130–137.

McQuire, S. Mental Illness. In: Thomas B, Bishop J, eds. & The British Dietetic Association. *Manual of Dietetic Practice*, 4th edn. Oxford, UK: Blackwell Publishing, 2007.

Millon T, Davis R, Millon C, Escovar L, Meagher S. *Personality Disorders in Modern Life*. New York: John Wiley & Sons, 2000.

Morrison MF, Petitto JM, Ten Have T et al. Depressive and anxiety disorders in women with HIV infection. Am J Psychiatry 2002 May; 159(5):789–796.

NICE (National Institute for Health and Clinical Excellence). Nutritional Support in Adults: Oral Nutrition Support, Enteral Tube Feeding and Parenteral Nutrition. Clinical Guideline 32. London, 2006.

Nikias MK, Fink R, Shapiro S. Comparisons of poverty and no poverty groups on dental status, needs and practices. J Public Health Dent 1975; 35(4):237–259.

Nolan M, Williams M, Rikard-Bell G, Mohsin M. Food insecurity in three socially disadvantaged localities in Sydney, Australia. Health Promot J Aust 2006 December; 17(3):247–254.

Panther LA, Libman H. Medical overview. In: Citron K, Brouillette MJ, Beckett A, eds. HIV and Psychiatry: A Training and Resource Manual, 2nd edn. Cambridge, UK: Cambridge University Press, 2005.

Parry CD, Blank MB, Pithey AL. Responding to the threat of HIV among persons with mental illness and substance abuse. Curr Opin Psychiatry 2007; 20:235–241.

Perseius KI, Kaver A, Ekdahl S, Asberg M, Samuelsson M. Stress and burnout in psychiatric professionals when starting to use dialectal behavioural therapy in the work with young self-harming women showing borderline personality symptoms. J Psychiatr Ment Health Nurs 2007; 14:635–643.

Quach LA, Wanke CA, Schmid CH et al. Drug use and other risk factors related to a lower body mass index among HIV-infected individuals. Drug Alcohol Depend 2008 May; 95(1):30–36.

Rothschild B. The Body Remembers: The Psychophysiology of Trauma and Trauma Treatment. New York: W.W. Norton & Company, 2000.

Royal Pharmaceutical Society of Great Britain. British National Formulary, 56, London, 2008

Sabhesan S, Edwin T, Nammalvar N, Nageswari A. New-onset psychosis in AIDS. Indian J Psychiatry. 1998 Oct; 40(4):383–5

Savetsky J, Sullivan L, Clarke J, Stein M, Samet JH. Evolution of depressive symptoms in human immunodeficiency virus infected patients entering primary care. J Nerv Ment Dis 2001 February; 189(2):76–83.

Selten JP, Cantor-Grae E, Kahn RS. Migration and schizophrenia. Curr Opin Psychiatry 2007; 20:111–115.

Sheiham A, Steele JG, Marcenes W, Finch S, Walls AWG. The relationship between oral health status and Body Mass Index among older people: a national survey of older people in Great Britain. Br Dent J 2002; 192:703–706.

Skapinakas P, Weich S, Lewis G, Singleton N, Araya R. Socio-economic position and common mental disorders. Br J Psychiatry 2006; 189:109–117.

Stolar A, Catalano G, Hakala SM, Bright RP, Fernandez F. Mood disorders and psychosis in HIV. In: Citron K, Brouillette MJ, Beckett A, eds. HIV and psychiatry: A Training and Resource Manual, 2nd edn. Cambridge, UK: Cambridge University Press, 2005.

Sullivan G, Kanouse D, Young AS, Han X, Perlman J, Koegel P. Co-location of health care for adults with serious mental illness and HIV infection. Community Ment Health J 2006; 42(4):345–361.

Tanskanen A, Hibbeln JR, Hintikka J, Haatainen K, Honkalampi K, Viinamäki H. Fish consumption, depression, and suicidality in a general population. Arch Gen Psychiatry 2001; 58(5):512–3.

Thomson AD, Cook CCH, Touquet R, Henry JA. The Royal College of physicians report on alcohol: guidelines for managing WERNICKE'S encephalopathy in the accident and emergency department Oxford. J Med Alcohol Alcohol 2002; 37(6):513–521.

Tilley S, Chambers M. Perceived facilitators and barriers to the implementation of an advanced practice: nursing intervention for HIV regimen adherence among the seriously mentally ill. J Psychiatr Ment Health Nurs 2006; 13:626–628.

Treisman GJ, Angelino AF, Hutton HE. Psychiatric issues in the management of patients with HIV infection. J Am Med Assoc 2001; 286(22):2857–2864.

Valente SM. Depression and HIV disease. J Assoc Nurses AIDS Care 2003; 14(2):41–51.

Weich S, Nazareth I, Morgan L, King M. Treatment of depression in primary care. Br J Psychiatry 2007; 191:164–169.

Wurtman JJ. Depression and weight gain: the serotonin connection. J Affect Disord 1993; 29:183–192.

16 Complementary and Alternative Therapy

Charle Maritz, Sharon Byrne
and Vivian Pribram

Key Points

- The use of complementary and alternative therapy (CAT), including nutritional supplements, has grown over the past decades during the time of the HIV pandemic.
- While the majority of CAT is generally safe, herbal remedies are of particular concern because of potential interactions with antiretroviral therapy and other medications which may have serious consequences for treatment success.
- High doses of some vitamins and minerals can cause harmful effects.
- Patients should be actively encouraged to disclose their use of CAT to health care professionals and clinicians should ask about use of herbal remedies, vitamins and minerals and alternative treatments as part of routine practice.

16.1   Introduction

Complementary and alternative therapy (CAT) is a broad term, encompassing many unconventional practices including relaxation techniques, spiritual healing, massage, herbal remedies and dietary supplementation.

CAT comprises two components, namely:

- Complementary medicine, which is used in addition to conventional medicine
- Alternative medicine, which is used in place of conventional medical therapy.

There are many different types of CAT. Common therapies include:

- manipulative therapies (osteopathy and chiropractic)
- acupuncture
- herbal remedies (treatment based on plant or plant extracts)
- homeopathy
- hypnosis and relaxation therapies (e.g. yoga and t'ai chi)
- massage therapies
- nutritional therapies.

In therapeutic systems more than one type of therapy may be combined (e.g. Chinese medicine may use herbal remedies and acupuncture; and Ayurveda may include massage, fasting, herbal remedies and exercise (Thomas, 2007).

Nutritional therapies may have an effect on dietary intake and nutritional status. Assessment and information provided by a dietitian is important to help ensure nutritional intake and status is not compromised and to provide information on potential benefits and harm so that informed decisions can be made.

16.2   Safety and regulation of CAT therapy

While some vitamin and mineral preparations are licensed by the Medicines and Healthcare Products Agency (MHPA) in the UK, many CAT products are subject to less stringent rules and regulations than imposed on over-the-counter and prescription medicines.

Most vitamins, mineral and other supplements sold are classified as 'unlicensed preparations' and are treated like food products. They are controlled under food legislation by the Food Standards Agency (FSA) and regulated by the local trading standards authorities.

The public may use unlicensed products for therapeutic purposes, although companies are not required to demonstrate their efficacy before marketing, nor are these products subject to prior approval. The main requirements for food-related products are safety and labelling according to EU guidelines. Companies are not allowed to make medicinal claims, however, health claims and functional claims are allowed.

As these products are natural, it is not possible to patent them, so unlike pharmaceutical companies who can 'own' a drug for a given patent time and charge a high price for it, natural products can be owned by lots of companies whose prices must be competitive and do not incorporate research costs. The reduced limitations in regulatory control of these products has resulted in a lack of evidence-based research regarding CAT's pharmacology, pharmacokinetics, drug interactions, efficacy and safety (Piscitelli *et al.*, 2000). Thus, there is inadequate data from research studies on the safety and efficacy of CAT, including herbal and natural health products/dietary supplements and drug interactions (Wheaton *et al.*, 2005; NIH, 2006).

In the UK the Herbal Medicines Advisory Committee was set up in 2005 to advise the Medicines and Healthcare Products Regulatory Agency about the safety issues related to herbal medicines. The establishment of this agency should enable access to better information about usage and safety of herbal medicines for both patients and health care professionals and it should bring about stricter control over the supply of herbal products.

16.3   Use of CAT

The use of complementary and alternative therapy (CAT), including nutritional supplements, has grown over the past decades during the time of the HIV pandemic (Eisenberg *et al.*, 1998; NIH 2006; Eberhardie, 2007). It is estimated that 80% of the world's population use some form of CAT as part of their primary health care (Launso, 1995). CAT therapy is commonly used by people living with chronic diseases for which there is no cure and/or for which conventional medical therapy is only partially effective (Cassileth *et al.*, 1984; Cronan *et al.*, 1989; Burstein *et al.*,

1999). These therapies are often used in conjunction with conventional therapies (Eisenberg *et al.*, 1998). Although the majority of CAT is safe to use, particularly in the massage and movement systems, there are potential problems with herbal remedies and interactions with conventional medicines. This is discussed in more detail later in Section 16.13.

16.4   Factors influencing use of CAT

Within the UK the most popular types of CAT are herbal medicine and homeopathy. Several factors are known to influence the choice to use CAT. These include:

* dissatisfaction with conventional medical therapy
* the desire to have more control over decisions about one's health
* cultural beliefs
* cultural background
* ethnicity and
* media reports and celebrity behaviour.

(Astin, 1998; Eliason *et al.*, 1999; Tang *et al.*, 2005; Ritchie, 2007).

While *some therapies* are often used in combination with conventional treatments, it has also been shown that some individuals engage in self-care practices using CAT exclusively as an alternative to conventional medicine. This may potentially place them at risk of delayed diagnosis with possible serious consequences (Klepser and Klepser, 1999). A well-known public misconception is that because a product is 'natural' it is safe, and free from side effects and drug interactions (RPSGB, 2006). Some herbal remedies have been shown to be unsafe or potentially unsafe, and individuals using these products may therefore be at risk of both herb- and disease-related problems that are largely preventable (Klepser and Klepser, 1999).

16.5   CAT use in HIV

When HIV first emerged, little was known of the disease, so effective treatment was not available. At this time, people living with HIV (PLHIV) primarily used CAT that allegedly had antiviral or immunostimulatory properties (Swanson *et al.*, 2000). Now that effective treatment is widely available, in areas where cost is not an overriding limiting factor, antiretroviral therapy (ART) and prophylactic medications for opportunistic infections (OIs) have increased the life expectancy for PLHIV (Maat *et al.*, 2001). While this is an excellent outcome, PLHIV have also had more time to experience the side effects associated with ART as well as the disease itself (Portillo *et al.*, 2005). It has been estimated that the use of CAT is higher among PLHIV than the general population (Piscitelli and Gallicano, 2001). The use of CAT among PLHIV reported in various studies is shown in Table 16.1. Interestingly, the advent of effective ART has not led to a decrease in CAT use in PLHIV.

CAT used by PLHIV may take the form of meditation, massage, acupuncture, spiritual healing and other non-pharmacological therapies, but it has been found to be particularly associated with dietary supplements, vitamins and herbal remedies (Piscitelli *et al.*, 2000). Much of the CAT used by PLHIV has been found to be

Table 16.1 Reported prevalence studies of complementary/alternative medicines and use of ART in HIV-positive patients.

Study	Country	Sample size	CAT use (%)
Josephs *et al.*, 2007	USA	914	16
Bica *et al.*, 2003	USA	642	60
Hsiao *et al.*, 2003	USA	2466	53
Furler *et al.*, 2003	Canada	104	89
Wiwanitkit, 2003	Thailand	160	95
De Visser *et al.*, 2002	Australia	924	55
Colebunders *et al.*, 2003	Europe	517	63*
Duggan *et al.*, 1989	USA	191	67
Barton *et al.*, 1989	UK	190	38
Anderson *et al.*, 1993	USA	184	40

*Only vitamins and minerals surveyed.

related to lifestyle issues such as reducing stress, good nutritional intake, and regular exercise (Mills *et al.*, 2005). CAT use has been shown to provide relief of disease symptoms, and to help manage ART-related side effects and increase the sense of hope and empowerment among PLHIV (Astin, 1998; Fairfield *et al.*, 1998).

16.6   Reasons for CAT use among PLHIV

Studies have shown that many PLHIV explore CAT therapy as a way to achieve relief from symptoms related to HIV and, in some cases, to inhibit viral activity (Kotler, 2000; Wu *et al.*, 2001). The more the symptoms experienced, due to disease progression or drug side effects, the more likely the individual is to use CAT (Visser *et al.*, 2000)

The opportunity to manage certain symptoms of HIV disease may not only improve patient well-being but also influence immune status and integrity in this population (Swanson *et al.*, 2000). Ladenheim *et al.* (2008) found most patients took antioxidants or immune stimulants for the benefit of the immune system, while others used herbal medicines and supplements to counter detrimental effects of the disease, such as muscle wasting, HIV-induced neuropathy or associated CNS effects such as cognitive deficiency, sleep problems and loss of energy.

Other commonly reported reasons for CAT therapy use include: nausea, insomnia, dermatological problems, weakness and depression, weight loss and diarrhoea (Eisenberg *et al.*, 1993; Sparber *et al.*, 2000).

Primary reasons for use of acupuncture and massage were found to be pain, depression and stress (Calabrese *et al.*, 1998). In summary, study results suggest that PLHIV turn to CAT in the hope of reducing symptoms associated with HIV, managing the side effects of drug therapy, maximising quality of life, slowing disease progression and as a way to better cope with their illness (Pawluch *et al.*, 2000; Piscitelli and Gallicano, 2001; Fawzi, 2003). Notably, in the era of effective ART, most people living with HIV in the UK choose CAT to complement ART, not to replace it (Visser and Grierson, 2002).

16.7   Information sources about CAT

Sources of information on CAT for PLHIV are varied. They include CAT providers (alternative health practitioners), friends' recommendations, the internet pharmacists, physicians, books, resources from HIV Service Organisations, and health food stores (Targ, 2000).

16.8   Disclosure of CAT use

Despite the potential risks involved in the use of CAT, there is evidence that physician–patient disclosure and dialogue about CAT use is infrequent (Bica *et al.*, 2003). A study on US adult PLHIV found that 72% of patients did not inform their physician about their CAT use (Kotler, 2000). These patients reported symptoms that included diarrhoea, nausea and vomiting, and hypertension. The physicians prescribed allopathic treatments without knowing the full context of their patients' symptoms and CAT use (Targ, 2000). The main reason for non-disclosure was that the patient thought it was not important and would not affect their ART. This is why it is crucial that there is an open dialogue between physician/pharmacist and the patient.

16.9   Evidence for the use of CAT

Despite the widespread use of CAT among PLHIV, the effectiveness of some of these therapies has not been established. In a systematic review of 2005, Mills *et al.* found

Table 16.2   Herbal products with harmful effects.

Product	Toxicity
Borage	Potential for hepatotoxicity and veno-occlusive disease due to toxic pyrrolizidine alkaloids. Can obtain alkaloid-free preparations.
Calamus	May contain beta-isoasarone, which is carcinogenic and also associated with nephrotoxicity and convulsions
Chaparral	Acute hepatitis, kidney and liver failure
Coltsfoot	May contain pyrrolizidine alkaloids which can cause hepatotoxicity and veno-occlusive disease
Comfrey (oral use), acceptable typically for short periods	Hepatotoxicty and veno-occulsive disease
Ephedra	Increased blood pressure, arrhythmias, psychosis and heart failure
Germander	Hepatitis and liver cell necrosis
Kava	Hepatotoxicity and liver failure
Golden ragwort	May contain pyrrolizidine alkaloids which can cause hepatotoxicity and veno-occulsive disease
Sassafras (amounts used in food are safe)	Hallucinations, vomiting, tachycardia, stupor, paralysis, diaphoresis and hot flushes

Adapted from Tyler (1996), and Therapeutic Research Faculty (2000).

that there were shortcomings in methodology of studies and most were small. The results of the review suggested that stress management and using cognitive behavioural techniques proved to be an effective way to increase quality of life, while data was insufficient to demonstrate effectiveness for all other treatments. The beneficial effects of stress management were primarily on subjective symptoms, such as anxiety and depression. The review authors highlighted serious concern about the lack of evidence supporting the use of natural health products and the potential for serious adverse effects and drug interactions with HIV medications. A number of alternative products have been reported to either have antiviral or immune-stimulating effects. Dextran sulphate, SPV-30, high dose vitamin C, compound Q, and curcumin have claims of activity and in some cases data suggesting activity are available (Elion and Cohen, 1997). While some in vitro studies have demonstrated potential interactions between ART and African potato and Goldenseal, clear risks in the use of St John's wort and high-dose garlic supplements have been shown (Mills *et al.*, 2005).

16.10   Dietary supplements

Five categories of dietary supplements have been identified into which most supplements fit:

1. Single or combined vitamins and minerals
2. Organic compounds that are normal body metabolites but not recognised as essential nutrients because they are synthesised endogenously, e.g. glucosamine, S-adenosylmethionine, L-carnitine and ubiquinone 10
3. Natural extracts that may contain bioactive substances (e.g. garlic (*Allium sativum* L.), soya bean (*Ginkgo biloba* L.), ginseng (*Panax* spp.))
4. Natural fats and oils such as fish oil and evening primrose (*Oenothera biennis* L.) oil
5. Antioxidants, which span the other categories listed[2]; thus, vitamin E, β-carotene, lycopene, Se, ubiquinone 10 and extracts of green tea and milk thistle (*Silybum marianum* (L.) Gaertner) are all marketed as antioxidants (Webb, 2007).

16.11   Dietary supplement use among PLHIV

Studies of micronutrient supplementation and requirements in HIV infection are discussed in Chapter 7: 'Decreased Nutritional Status and Nutritional Interventions for People Living with HIV'.

People living with HIV, as with other individuals, are encouraged to meet daily recommended nutritional requirements from food where possible. There is no routine recommendation for micronutrient supplementation in the UK. As with the general population or other groups of people living with acute and chronic illness, PLHIV may require nutritional supplementation for a variety of reasons such as:

*   an identified vitamin or mineral deficiency (e.g. iron, vitamin D and thiamine)
*   increased physiological needs (e.g. during infancy, childhood and pregnancy)

- increased nutritional losses as a result of gastrointestinal disease or resection, side effects of drug treatment
- poor appetite and or swallowing difficulties
- restrictive dietary intake (whether prescribed or self-imposed) and
- high risk of disorders such as osteoporosis or rickets (Thomas, 2007).

In cases where individuals choose to supplement their dietary intake with micronutrients, UK dietitians generally recommend a broad spectrum multivitamin, mineral tablet and discourage mega-dosing (consumption of high doses of specific micronutrients/dietary supplements at many times the reference nutrient intake (RNI)), as this can lead to overdosing and the occurrence of adverse effects. Large doses of some vitamins and minerals can be toxic and can also cause unpleasant side effects (e.g. vomiting, abdominal cramping and diarrhoea) (Thomas, 2007).

While the threshold between the safe upper limits may be small in some cases and overt toxicity is rare, the long-term consequences of excessively high intake may be significant in some cases. There are interactions as micronutrients function as part of an intricate network of absorption mechanisms, transport systems and metabolic pathways. For example, a high intake of iron can impair the absorption of zinc, resulting in a deficiency and a high intake of vitamin E could disturb the antioxidant/pro-oxidant pathway and pose potential risks (Thomas, 2007).

The size of the safe intake range for each nutrient will vary and in a few cases may be very small. Certain nutrients such as vitamin A and manganese have known and potentially serious adverse effects at high intakes, whereas others such as iron or vitamin C may have more minor adverse effects that are readily reversible and may only be associated with supplement intake. The risk of harm occurring from taking dietary supplements will depend on the safe intake range of the nutrient concerned, the susceptibility of the individual, and the likely intake of the same nutrient from other supplements or the rest of the diet. Although multivitamins, multiminerals and similar terms are commonly used, they have no standard scientific, regulatory or marketplace definitions. Yet, actual vitamin and mineral amounts often deviate from label values. Thus, the term 'multivitamins and multiminerals' can be applied to products that vary widely in their composition and characteristics. Systematic information on the bioavailability and bioequivalence of vitamins and minerals in marketed products and on potential drug interactions is scarce (Yetley, 2007). In many cases, the available database for the safety of nutrients is very limited because the studies, where available, were not designed to assess adverse effects but may have detected problems when they occurred. Further information on the safety of nutrients could be obtained through careful experimental design (Mulholland and Benford, 2007).

16.12   Knowledge of drug–CAT interactions

Little is known of CAT–drug interactions due to limited research on this subject. However, the majority of CAT can be used safely alongside ART (see Table 16.4).

Caution is required when using herbal products and ART due to potential interactions. Interactions between herbs and drugs are based on the same pharmacokinetic

Table 16.3 Potential toxicity of some vitamins and minerals in common use as CAT.

Dietary supplement	Possible adverse effects
Beta-carotene	Long-term intake of greater than 7 mg/day may increase the risk of lung cancer. Beta-carotene supplements should not be taken by people who smoke (Thomas, 2007)
Nicotinic acid	50 mg doses of nicotinic acid can cause skin flushing and other reversible side effects such as gastrointestinal problems. Prolonged intake of higher doses may cause liver dysfunction. It is recommended that supplemental intakes of nicotinic acid do not exceed 17 mg/day (Thomas, 2007)
Vitamin A	Chronic toxicity usually occurs from intakes in excess of 7500–1500 micrograms retinol equivalent (RE)/day but adverse effects may result from prolonged intake of 1500–3000 microgram RE/day. Large amounts can cause liver and bone damage, vomiting and headache. Retinol-containing supplements should be avoided by people consuming liver more than once per week and older adults at risk of osteoporosis. Pregnant women should not take supplements containing vitamin A before consulting their doctors on medicinally advised vitamin A, as high intakes are potentially teratogenic
Vitamin C	Doses above 1000 mg per day may lead to gastrointestinal side effects like diarrhoea and abdominal pain. The possibility that high vitamin C intake may increase oxalate excretion and increase the risk of renal stones remains uncertain. People who choose to take vitamin C supplements that significantly increase requirements (500 mg-1 g/day) may well be advised not to take them for longer than a few weeks and then to reduce the level of intake gradually. Special care is needed if taking Indinavir (Crixivan)
Vitamin E	A safe upper limit for supplemental intake has been set at 540 mg α-tocopherol/day. Special care is needed if patients are taking anticoagulants or have haemophilia as it interacts with vitamin K and has an anticoagulant effect
Vitamin B_6	More than 200 mg per day associated with irreversible neurological damage. Doses as low as 50 mg per day have been associated with peripheral sensory neuropathy. It is recommended that supplementary intakes do not exceed 10 mg per day (Thomas B)
Calcium	More than 1500 mg per day may cause abdominal pain and diarrhoea (Thomas, 2007)
Iron	More than 17 mg/day may cause constipation, nausea, abdominal pain (Thomas, 2007)
Magnesium	More than 400 mg/day may cause osmotic diarrhoea (Thomas, 2007)
Manganese	Manganese is neurotoxic at high levels of intake. It is recommended that supplemental intakes should not exceed 4 mg per day. It should not exceed 0.5 mg per day in older adults. (Thomas, 2007)
Nickel	Nickel-containing products may cause a skin rash in sensitive individuals (Thomas, 2007)
Phosphorus	More than 250 mg per day may cause mild stomach upsets in sensitive individuals. Long-term excessive intake may be detrimental to bone health (Thomas, 2007)
Zinc	High intakes have been linked with copper and iron deficiency and gastrointestinal side effects (Thomas, 2007) It is recommended that supplemental zinc intake does not exceed 25 mg/day
Selenium	The safe upper limit for selenium has been set at 450 microgram/day, so a maximum of 350 microgram/day should be consumed in supplemental form. Chronic toxicity may result in adverse effects on the nervous system and a condition called selenosis

From Thomas (2007).

Table 16.4 CAT that can be used safely with ART drugs.

Yoga
Homeopathy
Reflexology
Massage therapies, including aromatherapy
Bach flower remedies
Osteopathy and chiropractic techniques
Acupuncture
Tai Chi
Spiritual healing
Stress management
Meditation

and pharmacodynamic principles as drug–drug interactions. Clinically important interactions involve effects on drug metabolism via the cytochrome P450 isoenzymes (CYP450), glucuronidation, p-glycoprotein (a transporter protein), metabolism and other possible mechanisms, e.g. impaired hepatic function. Many antiretroviral drugs such as protease inhibitors, non-nucleoside reverse transcriptase inhibitors (NNRTIs) and Maraviroc are predominantly metabolised through the cytochrome P450 3A4 (CYP3A4) oxidative metabolic pathway. PIs, are also substrates for drug transporters such as p-glycoprotein. Some herbs have been shown to affect the serum levels of ART drugs through their effects on CYP3A4 metabolism and p-glycoprotein (Mills *et al.*, 2005) (see Table 16.5).

The long-term success of ART depends upon maintaining inhibitory concentrations of active drug to suppress viral replication. Drugs or herbs that induce the CYP450 enzymes, in particular the 3A4 isoenzyme, or increase the activity of p-glycoprotein may result in reduced serum levels of ART drugs that could cause treatment failure and the development of ART drug resistance. Drugs or herbs that inhibit the CYP450 enzymes, especially 3A4 or p-glycoprotein, may result in high serum levels of ART which may increase side effects. In many cases the interactions are theoretical and little is known on how such potential interactions demonstrated in vitro might be translated into clinically significant effects in vivo. St. John's wort illustrates how results obtained in vitro may not reflect what happens in vivo. In vitro St. John's wort has been found to inhibit CYP 2C9, CYP2D6 and CYP3A4 (Budzinski *et al.*, 2000; Garson *et al.*, 2000; Obach, 2000). However, in vivo it is a potent enzyme inducer causing a significant reduction in the levels of PIs, NNRTIs and Maraviroc and it is contraindicated with all the drugs in these classes (Piscitelli *et al.*, 2000). This is the only herb that is included in any product datasheet. More research is needed to establish the clinical significance of other herbs with ART. So far the known interactions are confined to the drug classes: protease inhibitors, non-nucleoside reverse transcriptors and Maraviroc. To date the nucleoside reserve transcriptors, fusion inhibitors and Raltegravir have not shown any interactions with herbal medicines.

16.13 Herbal remedies

Table 16.6 includes herbal products for which there is no evidence of interaction with antiretroviral medication.

Table 16.5 Commonly used herbal remedies, their purpose for use and known interactions.

Herbal remedy	Purpose for use	Known interactions with ART treatment	Outcome	References
St. John's wort (*hypericum*)	Depression, anxiety and/or sleep disorders	Induces CYP3A4, CYP1A2, CYP2C9 in the liver and P-glycoprotein. Indinavir (PI) and Nevirapine (NNRTI) levels significantly reduced	Co-administration is contraindicated with all PIs, NNRTIs and Maraviroc, as St. John's wort is expected to substantially decrease drug concentrations which may result in suboptimal levels	Piscitelli *et al.* (2000), Maat *et al.* (2001); see University of Liverpool (2009) SPC for all PIs, NNRTIS and Maraviroc
Echinacea	Prevent colds, flu and other infections. Stimulate immune system to help fight infections	Causes inhibition of CYP1A2 and intestinal CYP3A activity and induction of hepatic CYP3A activity	As both inhibition and induction take place, the magnitude and direction of the interaction cannot be predicted	G (Gorski *et al.*, 2004)
Garlic (*Allium sativum*)	Beneficial cardiovascular effect. The most common use in terms of HIV. Antibiotic properties	In vitro can induce CYP3A4, CYP2C9 and CYP 2D6. In vivo study did show reduction in unboosted Saquinavir levels. Possibly caused by induction of gut mucosal CYP450 3A4. P-glycoprotein effects are also possible.	Decreased unboosted Saquinavir levels. Difficult to compare with boosted PIs, but caution should be advised.	See University of Liverpool (2009), Dalvi (1992), Foster *et al.* (2001) Piscitelli *et al.* (2002)
Milk thistle (*Silybum marianum*)	Hepato-protective effects and therefore typically used for liver diseases such as cirrhosis and hepatitis.	In vitro potential inhibitor of CYP2C9 and CYP3A4 which may lead to increased levels of PIs, NNRTIs and Maraviroc but in vivo studies have shown no effects on the levels of Indinavir and other CYP3A4 substrates.	In vivo did not affect Indinavir levels, so would expect it not to affect the levels of other PIs. However, as there is no available clinical data, caution is advised when using with other PIs NNRTIs and Maraviroc.	Disenzo *et al.* (2003), Mills *et al.* (2005) and Natural medicines database
Sutherlandia (*Frutescens*)	Antioxidant and anti-inflammatory potentials	In-vitro early inhibition of CYP3A4 and P-glycoprotein expression but then followed by induction with prolonged therapy resulting in potentially decreased drug levels.	Potentially decreased drug levels of PIs NNRTIs and Maraviroc.	Mills *et al.* (2005)

Herb	Use	Mechanism/in vitro	Potential interaction	Reference
African potato (*Hypoxis*)	Immunostimulant	In vitro early inhibition of CYP3A4 and P-glycoprotein expression, but then followed by induction with prolonged therapy, resulting in potentially decreased drug levels	Potentially decreased drug levels of PIs, NNRTIs and Maraviroc	Mills *et al.* (2005)
Cats Claw (*Uncaria tomentosa*)	GI complaints, Immunostimulant	In vitro may inhibit CYP 3A4. No reported interactions.	Potential to increase levels of PIs, NNRTIs and Maraviroc. Caution advised in extrapolating in vitro data to clinical situations	Medscape (2002)
Goldenseal (*Hydrastis canadensis*)	Immunostimulant	In vitro may inhibit CYP 3A4. No reported interactions	Potential to increase levels of PIs, NNRTIs and Maraviroc Caution advised in extrapolating in vitro data to clinical situations.	Medscape (2002)
Gingko biloba	Dementia, including Alzheimer's, conditions associated with cerebral vascular insufficiency, especially in the elderly, including memory loss.	Possible CYP3A4 or P-gp induction. A study looked at Lopinavir (boosted with ritonavir) levels when administered with gingko and found no reduction in boosted Lopinavir levels. There is a case report of a possible interaction with Efavirenz, leading to reduced Efavirenz levels in a patient taking *Gingko biloba*.	Gingko is unlikely to reduce exposure of boosted PIs but unboosted PIs may be affected. It is advised to avoid use of *Gingko biloba* and NNRTIs following this case report. As there is no available data on Maraviroc, it would be advisable to avoid using *Gingko biloba* with Maraviroc	Robertson *et al.* (2008), Wiegman *et al.* (2009)

Table 16.6 Herbal products for which there is no known evidence of interaction with antiretroviral medication.

Astragalus	Ipriflavone (synthetic isoflavone)
Avena sativa	Marshmallow
Berberis vulgaria	Melatonin
Bitter orange	Passiflora
Chamomile	Poria Cocos
Citrus reticulate	Raspberry leaf
Co-enzyme Q10	Sage
Crataegus	Saw Palmetto
Ganoderma lucidem	Skull cap
Ginger	Valerian
Glucosamine	Vervain
Green tea	Willow
Gurana	

From Stargrove *et al.* (2008).

16.14   Addressing patients' use of CAT

It is unrealistic to ask patients not to use CAT, since many will continue to do so without informing their health care professional, which can be a perilous situation. Many patients believe that these products do indeed provide benefit and are important adjunctive therapies to their ART regimen. Patients should be actively encouraged to disclose information about CAT to health care professionals.

1. All health care providers should perform a complete drug history. Patients should be asked specifically about their use of CAT.
2. It is important not to alienate patients by making them feel that they are not being taken seriously or that they are being criticised for their use of CAT. Research has shown that patients may feel deprived of their autonomy if their health care professionals are insensitive when addressing their use of CAT (Werneke *et al.*, 2004).
3. Pharmacists should check for other medications including herbal remedies when working in adherence clinics and when dispensing ART drugs.
4. If unsure of an interaction, ask the HIV pharmacist.

16.15   Conclusions

The use of CAT is widespread among PLHIV, even in the era of effective ART, although there is a lack of knowledge of the efficacy and safety of CAT. This lack of data is mostly due to limited funding and research in this field and shortcomings in methodology of existing studies.

As a result clinicians and patients do not have access to good quality evidence to inform clinical decision-making. As shown in Table 16.4, much of CAT is generally safe for PLHIV taking ART. Herbal remedies are of particular concern because of potential interactions with ART and other medications, which may have serious consequences for treatment success. In the absence of evidence, clinicians should discuss the use of specific CAT with patients and ensure that patients are aware of likely benefits or harm to enable them to make an informed decision. While values and beliefs need to be respected, the potential for important adverse effects and drug interactions needs to be conveyed to patients (Mills *et al.*, 2005). The most important element in managing CAT use is that patients should be actively encouraged to disclose their use of CAT to health care professionals. Clinicians such as doctors, nurses, pharmacists and dietitians should ask about use of herbal remedies, vitamins and minerals and alternative treatments as part of routine practice. The establishment of the Herbal Advisory Committee is hopefully the first of many steps in the right direction to help establish more evidence for the safety and efficacy of CAT. Further large, well-designed studies are needed so that more is known of benefits and potential harmful effects of CAT.

References

Anderson W, O'Connor B, MacGregor R, Schwartz J. Patient use and assessment of conventional and alternative therapies for HIV infection and AIDS. *AIDS* 1993; 75:561–4.

Astin J. Why patients use alternative medicine: results of a national study. *JAMA* 1998; 279:1548–53.

Barton SE, Hawkins DA, Jadresic DM, Gazzard BG. Alternative treatments for HIV infection. *BMJ* 1989; 298:1519–20.

Bica I, Tang A, Skinner S *et al.* Use of complementary and alternative therapies by patients with human immunodeficiency virus disease in the era of highly active antiretroviral therapy. *J Altern Complement Med* 2003; 9(1):65–76.

Budzinski JW, Foster BC, Vandenhoek S *et al.* An in vitro evaluation of human cytochrome P450 3A4, inhibition by selected commercial herbal extracts and tinctures. *Phytomedicine* 2000; 7:273–82.

Burstein H, Gelber S, Guandagnoli E, Weeks J. Use of alternative medicine by women with early-stage breast cancer. *N Engl J Med* 1999; 340:1733–9.

Calabrese C, Wenner C, Reeves C, Turet P, Standish L. Treatment of human immunodeficiency virus positive patients with complementary and alternative medicine: a survey of practitioners. *J Altern Complement Med* 1998; 4(3):281–7.

Cassileth B, Lusk E, Strouse T, Bodenheimer B. Contemporary unorthodox treatments in cancer medicine. A study of patients, treatments and practitioners. *Ann Intern Med* 1984; 101:105–7.

Colebunders R, Dreezen C, Florence E, Pelgrom Y, Schrooten W. The use of complementary and alternative medicine by persons with HIV infection in Europe. *Int J STD AIDS* 2003; 14(10):672–4.

Cronan T, Kaplan R, Posner L, Blumberg E, Kozin F. Prevalence of the use of unconventional remedies for arthritis in a metropolitan community. *Arthritis Rheum* 1989; 32:1604–7.

Dalvi RR. Alterations in hepatic phase I and phase II biotransformation enzymes by garlic oil in rats. *Toxicol Lett* 1992; 60:299–305.

de Visser R, Grierson J. Use of alternative therapies by people living with HIV/AIDS in Australia. *AIDS Care* 2002; 14(5):599–606.

DiCenzo R, Shelton M, Jordan K *et al.* Coadministration of milk thistle and indinavir in healthy subjects. *Pharmacotherapy* 2003; 23:866–70.

Duggan J, Peterson WS, Schutz M, Khuder S, Charkraborty J. Use of complementary and alternative therapies in HIV-infected patients. *AIDS Patient Care STDs* 2001; 15(3):159–67.

Eberhardie C. Nutritional supplements and the EU: is anyone happy? *Proc Nutr Soc* 2007; 66:508–11.

Eisenberg D, Davis R, Ettner S, Appel S, Wilkey S, Rompay MV. Trends in alternative medicine use in the United States 1990–1997. *JAMA* 1998; 208:1569–75.

Eisenberg D, Kessler R, Foster C, Norlock F, Calkins D, Delbanco T. Unconventional medicine in the United States – prevalence, costs, and patterns of use. *N Engl J Med* 1993; 329: 1200–204.

Eliason B, Huebner J, Marchand L. What physicians can learn from consumers of dietary supplements. *J Fam Prac* 1999; 48:459–63.

Elion RA, Cohen C. Complementary Medicine and HIV Infection. *Primary Care* 1997; 24(4):905–19.

Expert Group on Vitamins and Minerals (EVM). *Safe Upper Limits for Vitamins and Minerals.* London: FSA, 2003.

Fairfield K, Eisenberg D, Davis R, Libman H, Philips R. Patterns of use, expenditures and perceived efficacy of complementary and alternative therapies in HIV-infected patients. *Arch Intern Med* 1998; 158(20):2257–64.

Fawzi W. Micronutrients and human immunodeficiency virus type 1 disease progression among adults and children. *CID* 2003; 37:S112–16.

Foster BC, Foster MS, Vandenhoek S *et al.* An in-vitro evaluation of human cytochrome P450 3A4 and P-glycoprotein inhibition by garlic. *J Pharm Sci* 2001; 4:176–84.

Furler MD, Einarson TR, Walmsley S, Millson M, Bendayan R. Use of complementary and alternative medicine by HIV-infected outpatients in Ontario, Canada. *AIDS Patient Care STDs* 2003; 17(4):155–68.

Garson SW, Hill-Zabala GE, Roberts SH *et al.* Inhibitory effect of methanolic solution of St. John's wort *(Hyperieum perforatum)* on cytochrome P450 3A4 activity in human liver microsomes. *Clin Pharmacol Ther* 2000; 67:99.

Gorski JC, Huang S-M, Pinto A *et al.* The effect of Echinacea (Echinacea purpurea root) on cytochrome P450 activity in vivo. *Clin Pharmacol Ther* 2004; 75:89–100.

HIV Drug interactions. University of Liverpool. [Online] Available at http://www.hiv-druginteractions.org./frames.asp?drug/drg_main.asp. Accessed on 21 July 2007.

Hsiao AF, Wong MD, Kanouse DE *et al.* Complementary and alternative medicine use and substitution for conventional therapy by HIV-infected patients. *J Acquir Immune Defic Syndr* 2003; 33(2):157–65.

Jeff MJ, Gregory P, Batz F, Hitchen K, Burson S, Shaver K, Palacioz K, eds. *Natural Medicines-Comprehensive Database*, 3rd edn. Stockton, CA: Therapeutic Research, 2000:1530 p.

Josephs JS, Fleishman JA, Gaist P, Gebo KA. Use of complementary and alternative medicines among a multistate, multisite cohort of people living with HIV/AIDS. *HIV Med* 2007; 8:300–305.

Klepser T, Klepser M. Unsafe and potentially safe herbal therapies. *Am J Health Syst Pharm* 1999; 56:125–38.

Kotler DP. Nutritional alterations associated with HIV infection. *JAIDS* 2000; 25:S81–7.

Ladenheim D, Horn O, Werneke U *et al.* Potential health risks of complementary alternative medicines in HIV patients. *HIV Med* 2008; 9:653–9.

Launso L. People choose alternative therapies: the consequences for future pharmacy practice. *J Soc Adm Pharm* 1995; 12:43–52.

Maat MD, Hoetelmans R, Mathot R *et al.* Drug interactions between St. John's wort and nevirapine. *AIDS* 2001; 15(3):420–21.

Mills E, Cooper C, Seely D, Kanfer I. African herbal medicines in the treatment of HIV: Hypoxis and Sutherlandia. An overview of evidence and pharmacology. *Nutr J* 2005; 4(19).

Mills E, Montori V, Perri D, Phillips E, Koren G. Natural health products-HIV drug interactions: a systematic review. *Int J STD AIDS* 2005; 16(3):181–6.

Mills E, Wilson K, Clarke M *et al.* Milk thistle and indinavir: a randomized controlled pharmacokinetics study and meta-analysis. *Eur J Clin Pharmacol* 2005; 61(1):1–7.

Mulholland CA, Benford DJ. What is known about the safety of multivitamin-multimineral supplements for the general healthy population? Theoretical basis for harm. *Am J Clin Nutr* 2007; 85(1):318S–22.

NIH State-of-the-Science Panel*. National institutes of health state-of-the-science conference statement: multivitamin/mineral supplements and Chronic disease prevention. *Ann Intern Med* 2006; 145(5):364–71.

Obach RS. Inhibition of human cytochrome P450 enzymes by constituents of St. John's wort, an herbal preparation used in the treatment of depression. *Pharmacol Exp Ther* 2000; 294:88–95.

Pawluch D, Cain R, Gillett J. Lay constructions of HIV and complementary therapy use. *Soc Sci Med* 2000; 51:251–64.

Piscitelli S, Burnstein A, Chaitt D, Alfaro R, Fallon J. Indinavir concentrations and St. John's wort. *Lancet* 2000; 355(9203):547–8.

Piscitelli S, Burnstein A, Welden N, Gallicano K, Fallon J. The effect of garlic supplements on the pharmacokinetics of saquinavir. *Clin Infect Dis* 2002; **34**:234–8.

Piscitelli S, Gallicano K. Interactions among drugs for HIV and opportunistic infections. *N Engl J Med* 2001; **344**:984–96.

Portillo CJ, Rivero-Mendez M, Corless IB. Quality of life of ethnic minority persons living with HIV/AIDS. *J Multicult Nurs Health* 2005; **11**(1):31–7.

Ritchie MR. Use of herbal supplements and nutritional supplements in the UK: who at do we know about their pattern of usage? *Proc Nutr Soc* 2007; **66**:479–82.

Robertson S, Davey RT, Voell J, Formentini E, Alfaro R, Penzak S. Effect of Ginkgo biloba extract on lopinavir, midazolam and fexofenadine pharmacokinetics in healthy subjects. *Curr Med Res Opin* 2008; **24**:591–9.

(RPSGB) Royal Pharmaceutical Society of Great Britain. [Online] Available at www.rpsgb.org.uk. Assessed on 22 November 2006.

Sparber A, Wootton J, Bauer L et al. Use of complementary medicine by adult patients participating in HIV/AIDS clinical trials. *J Altern Complement Med* 2000; **6**(5):415–22.

Stargrove MB, Treasure J, McKee DL. *Herb, Nutrient, and Drug Interactions: Clinical Implications and Therapeutic Strategies*. St. Louis: Mosby/Elsevier, 2008.

Swanson B, Keithley J, Zeller J, Cronin-Stubbs D. Complementary and alternative therapies to manage HIV-related symptoms. *J Assoc Nurses AIDS Care* 2000; **11**(5):40–60.

Tang A, Lanzilotti J, Hendricks K et al. Micronutrients: current issues for HIV care providers. *AIDS* 2005; **19**(9):847–62.

Targ E. CAT and HIV/AIDS: the importance of complementarity. *Altern Ther* 2000; **6**(5):30–3.

Thomas B. *Complementary and Alternative Therapies, Manual of Dietetic Practice*. 4th ed., Oxford: Wiley Blackwell, 2007.

Tyler VE. What pharmacists should know about herbal remedies. *J Am Pharm Assoc* 1996; NS**36**:29–37.

University of Liverpool. Welcome to www.hiv-druginteractions.org www.hiv-druginteractions.org. 2009.

Visser Rd, Ezzy D, Bartos M. Alternative or complementary? Nonallopathic therapies for HIV/AIDS. *Altern Ther* 2000; **6**(5):44–52.

Visser Rd, Grierson J. Use of alternative therapies by people living with HIV/AIDS in Australia. *AIDS Care* 2002; **14**(5):599–606.

Webb GP. Nutritional supplements and conventional medicine; what the physician should know. *Proc Nutr Soc* 2007; **66**:471–8.

Werneke U, Earl J, Seydel C, Horn O. Potential health risks of complementary alternative medicines in cancer patients. *Br J Cancer* 2004; **26**:408–13.

Wheaton A, Blanck H, Gizlice Z, Reyes M. Medicinal herb use in a population-based survey in adults: prevalence and frequency of use, reasons for use, and use among their children. *Ann Epidemiol* 2005; **15**:678–85.

Wiwanitkit V. The use of CAM by HIV-positive patients in Thailand. *Complementary Therapies in Medicine* 2003; **11**(1):39–41.

Wu J, Attele A, Zhang L, Yuan C. Anti-HIV activity of medicinal herbal remedies: usage and potential development. *Am J Chin Med* 2001; **29**(1):69–81.

Wiegman D-J, Brinkman K, Franssen EJF. Interaction of *Gingko biloba* with efavirenz. *AIDS* 2009; **23**:1184–5.

Yetley EA. Multivitamin and multimineral dietary supplements: definitions, characterization, bioavailability, and drug interactions. *Am J Clin Nutr* 2007; **85**(1):269S–76.

17 Food and Water Safety

Louise Houtzager

Key Points

- People living with HIV infection (PLHIV) have an increased risk of contracting food- and waterborne diseases and need to take additional precautions with food and water.
- Food-borne illnesses can be caused by toxic chemicals as well as microorganisms.
- There are better outcomes and lower risks of food-borne illness in PLHIV with good immune function.
- The likelihood of contracting food- and waterborne illnesses can be reduced if care is taken in food handling and with choices of food and water.
- When food- and waterborne infections do occur, it is important for PLHIV to see a health worker without delay in order to minimise illness and avoid weight loss and nutritional impairment.

17.1   Introduction

Food-borne disease is a problem in both developing and developed countries. People living with HIV infection (PLHIV) have an increased risk of contracting food and waterborne diseases and need to take additional precautions with food and water safety. Food and water safety relates to all measures that are taken to ensure food and water will not cause harm to people when consumed.

There are more than 200 known diseases that are transmitted through food (Mead *et al.*, 1999). The World Health Organization (WHO) estimates that 1.8 million people die each year as a result of diarrhoeal diseases, with most cases being attributable to contaminated food and water (WHO, 2006).

Food- and waterborne illnesses are caused by pathogenic microorganisms and/or toxic chemicals. The likelihood of contracting food- and waterborne illnesses can be reduced if care is taken with food handling and in choices of food and water. This chapter discusses food and water safety issues for PLHIV, details some of the common causes of food- and waterborne illnesses and offers strategies to prevent illness resulting from consumption of contaminated food or water.

17.2   Why food and water safety is important for PLHIV

HIV infection progressively damages the immune system and increases the risk of food- and waterborne illnesses, particularly in people with advanced-stage disease (AIDS). Infections transmitted through food and water contribute significantly to morbidity and mortality in PLHIV (Hayes *et al.*, 2003).

High rates of cryptosporidiosis, salmonellosis, campylobacteriosis, toxoplasmosis and listeriosis occur in PLHIV with severely compromised immunity (WHO Clinical Stage 4 AIDS) (Alterkruse *et al.*, 1994; Smith, 1997) Campylobacter infections, for example, are 40 times more common in the setting of HIV infection (Sorvillo *et al.*, 1991) and a 20 times higher incidence of Salmonellosis has been reported (Celum *et al.*, 1987).

Infection with some pathogens that rarely cause illness in healthy people can have serious outcomes in people with a compromised immune system. Listeriosis in people with AIDS, if untreated, has a case fatality rate of 70% (Alterkruse *et al.*, 1994). *Cryptosporidium parvum* has been reported to cause 10–20% of cases of AIDS-associated diarrhoea (Morris and Potter, 1997). Food-borne disease may also lead to malnutrition. Malnutrition and HIV infection have an additive effect in damaging the immune system and in combination contribute to more rapid disease progression.

There are better outcomes and lower risks of food-borne illness in PLHIV with good immune function such as those in early stage of HIV, or responsive to antiretroviral therapy (ART) compared to those with advanced disease (Hoffman *et al.*, 2005).

Most importantly, the likelihood of contracting food- and waterborne illnesses can be reduced if care is taken in food handling and with choices of food and water.

Barriers to acceptance of food safety recommendations among PLHIV should be considered in patient education and counselling. Some barriers reported amongst PLHIV include (Hoffman *et al.*, 2005):

- a lack of understanding of the importance of food and water safety and knowledge of safe food and water practices
- willingness to take risks
- resistance to change
- feelings that someone else should control food-related risks (e.g. food processors and inspectors)
- being 'overwhelmed' by having to make changes to their diets for food safety reasons, because these recommendations are added on to an already complicated health care regimen.

Depending on the health beliefs of a client, the following strategies may be useful for motivated PLHIV to change behaviours related to food and water safety:

- provide statistics and explain that PLHIV are more at risk of food-borne illness
- state that food-borne illness can result in long-term health problems and even death
- correct any misinformation on food preparation and microorganisms (pathogens)
- provide education and information on how to prepare and eat and drink safely
- give suggestions for substitutes for high-risk foods.

Food service staff, dietitians and other health care professionals working with PLHIV should be familiar with the different causes of food- and waterborne illnesses and the recommended strategies for prevention described within this chapter.

17.3   Causes of food- and waterborne illness in PLHIV

17.3.1   Microorganisms

Microorganisms are so small that they can only be seen with a microscope. It takes 1 million microorganisms to cover the head of a pin. There are different types of microorganisms. Bacteria, viruses, yeasts, moulds and parasites are all microorganisms. Some are good and help digest food or are used in making food such as cheese and yoghurt. Others may cause food to spoil, while pathogens (dangerous organisms) make people sick and can even kill. Some common bacteria and parasites infecting PLHIV are described in Section 17.3.2.

Smell, taste and appearance are not good indicators of whether food will make people sick. Dangerous food-borne microorganisms do not always change the look of food but can still cause food poisoning. Spoilage microorganisms do not usually cause illness but change the smell, taste and appearance of food. The difference between food poisoning and spoilage is summarised in Box 17.1.

Box 17.1   The difference between food poisoning/food-borne disease and spoilage

Spoilage occurs in the natural breakdown of food. It is usually caused by the enzymes found in food, though it may be caused by some types of microorganisms. Eating spoiled food does NOT necessarily make people sick. Eating contaminated food CAN make people sick. Some foods that appear spoiled and are contaminated with toxins that can cause illness include: bread with green mould (which produces mycotoxins); mouldy or damaged apples (which may contain a toxin called patulin); and the green on potatoes (if glycoalkaloid content is high).

Food poisoning or food-borne disease is caused by eating food contaminated by certain microorganisms or chemicals. They can, but do not always, change the smell, taste or appearance of food.

Microorganisms are everywhere but are mostly found in faeces, soil and water, pests, domestic and farm animals and people (e.g. in the mouth, hands and fingernails). According to WHO (2002), there have been significant increases in the last few decades in the incidence of diseases caused by microorganisms transmitted primarily by food, including pathogens such as *Salmonella* spp., *Campylobacter* spp., *Escherichia coli* and parasites such as *Cryptosporidium* (WHO, 2002).

Foods contaminated with pathogenic microorganisms can lead to infection and illness in two main ways:

1. Consumption of the contaminated food under conditions that allow the survival of the pathogen or its toxin, e.g. when a meat or poultry product is consumed raw or undercooked.
2. Through cross-contamination in the kitchen or other food-handling areas. For example, when raw chicken or beef with a microorganism-contaminated exterior (e.g. *Salmonella* spp.) contaminates a person's hands, a cutting board, counter-top, or kitchen utensil, which then comes into contact with cooked products or

foods consumed raw, such as salad. For some pathogens, such as *Salmonella*, it is likely that more cases of illness result from cross-contamination than from direct consumption of undercooked product.

17.3.2   Common parasites, bacteria and viruses that may cause food-borne illness in PLHIV

Parasites

Cryptosporidium parvum
Cryptosporidiosis is an intestinal disease of humans and animals caused by the protozoan parasite *Cryptosporidium parvum*. Although water treatment processes to remove *Cryptosporidium* are improving and detection methods for identifying the parasite in water are becoming more sensitive, outbreaks of cryptosporidiosis continue in the human population (Jenkins, 2005).

Cryptosporidium predominately causes gastrointestinal disease (acute and chronic diarrhoeal syndrome) in immunocompromised patients with HIV infection. It is clear that those with low CD4 counts under 200 cells/µl and especially under 100 cells/µl are at greater risk for an acute illness from *Cryptosporidium*. However, PLHIV with higher CD4 counts may recover from cryptosporidiosis (with or without significant symptoms) but not clear the parasite completely, allowing it to cause serious illness later in the presence of advanced immune suppression.

Infection in humans usually occurs via consumption of faecally contaminated water or food, person-to-person or animal-to-person contact or contact with environmental sources (e.g. contaminated swimming water). Unpasteurised cow's milk is the food most commonly associated with food-borne cryptosporidiosis, while other foods to which infection has been attributed include fresh pressed apple juice, salad, raw meat and frozen (uncooked) tripe.

Characteristics of cryptosporidial disease in PLHIV are often related to CD4 count. Patients with CD4 counts >180 cells/µl tend to have acute diarrhoea with abdominal cramping, anorexia, fever and vomiting lasting 7–10 days. Patients with CD4 cell counts <180 cells/µl usually experience a chronic diarrhoeal syndrome of watery voluminous stools associated with weight loss.

Diagnosis of cryptosporidiosis requires a specific request for the laboratory to assess the stool for *Cryptosporidium*, as routine stool examinations are unable to detect this small parasite. The most effective way to treat chronic cryptosporidiosis is to improve immune function with ART. Symptomatic and dietary management is described in Chapter 9.

Prevention

The US Centers for Disease Control and Prevention (CDC) advices that during waterborne outbreaks (or other situations in which a community boil-water advisory is issued), immunocompromised persons should **boil water for 1 minute** to eliminate the risk of acquiring cryptosporidiosis. Using submicron, personal-use filters (e.g. home water filters) or high-quality bottled water also can reduce the risk of transmission. However, boiling water is the most reliable method of killing *Cryptosporidium* oocysts.

Toxoplasma gondii (T. gondii)

Toxoplasma gondii is a protozoan parasite of warm-blooded animals and humans. However, only members of the cat family are definitive hosts for the organism (Jones *et al.*, 2003).

Nearly one-third of the human population worldwide has been exposed to *T. gondii* (Hill *et al.*, 2006). Infection in humans generally occurs either by ingesting viable tissue cysts in raw or undercooked meat or by ingesting oocysts shed in the faeces of a cat occurring through exposure to cat litter or soil (e.g. from gardening or unwashed fruits or vegetables). Acute infections in pregnant women can transmit the organism to the foetus and cause severe illness (e.g. mental retardation, blindness and epilepsy).

After acute infection, *T. gondii* persists in tissue cysts in humans, particularly in brain, skeletal muscles and heart, for life. Development of cell-mediated immunity after acute infection with *T. gondii* results in control but not eradication of the infection. Immunoglobulin (Ig) G antibodies to *T. gondii* appear early after infection.

A chronically infected individual who develops defects in cell-mediated immunity is at risk for reactivation of the infection (Luft and Remington, 1992). Toxoplasmosis in this setting manifests primarily as toxoplasmic encephalitis, typically with multiple mass lesions in the brain. Loss of vision and neurological conditions including seizures and weakness are common presentations. A definitive diagnosis of cerebral toxoplasmosis can only be made by histological examination of the affected brain tissue. A presumptive diagnosis can be made by neuroimaging, with MRI being more sensitive than CT. The diagnosis in other organ systems is by microscopic examination of tissue samples.

Clinical presentation of toxoplasmosis typically occurs in PLHIV when the CD4 cell count is less than 100 cells/μl (Luft and Remington, 1992). Toxoplasmosis was found to be the most frequent severe neurologic infection among PLHIV with advanced disease in a large cohort in the United States, even after the advent of antiretroviral therapy (Jones *et al.*, 1999). However, like other opportunistic infections, the number of diagnoses of toxoplasmosis has declined with ART use. Prophylaxis and treatments are available for toxoplasmosis.

Prevention

Primary prevention of acquisition of *T. gondii* infection is by avoiding consumption of undercooked meat and practising good food hygiene to prevent ingestion of oocysts shed in the faeces of a cat. Tissue cysts present in meat are rendered nonviable by heating to 67°C, freezing to −20°C or by gamma-irradiation. *T. gondii*-seronegative, HIV-infected persons (or those with unknown serology) should be instructed about measures to prevent acquisition of *T. gondii* infection. Box 17.2 describes prevention strategies for infection with *T. gondii* (Figure 17.1).

Giardia

Giardia lamblia (= *intestinalis*) is a parasite that inhabits the small intestines of humans and other mammals. This protozoan parasite is one of the two most significant waterborne pathogens around the world (*Cryptosporidium* being the other). The main symptoms of infection are watery diarrhoea and abdominal cramps. It causes up to 5% of acute diarrhoeal illnesses in patients with HIV infection (Kelly, 2006).

Box 17.2   Prevention of *T. Gondii* infection (Hughes *et al.*, 2000)

- A food thermometer should be used to measure the internal temperature of cooked meat to ensure that meat is cooked all the way through.
- Meat products should only be consumed if well cooked (no pink inside). Meats should be cooked to an internal temperature of 85°C. The specific minimum temperatures for different meats to be cooked to before eating include:
  - ○ beef, lamb, veal roasts and steaks – at least 65°C
  - ○ pork, ground meat, and wild game – at least 71°C.
  - ○ whole poultry (in the thigh) – at least 82°C to ensure poultry is well done.
- Fruits and vegetables should be peeled or thoroughly washed before eating.
- Hands should be washed thoroughly before commencing all food preparation.
- Cutting boards, dishes, counters, utensils and hands should always be washed with hot soapy water after they have contacted raw meat, poultry, seafood, or unwashed fruits or vegetables.
- Patients should avoid contact with materials that may be contaminated with cat faeces; and gloves should be worn during gardening. After gardening or contact with soil or sand, wash hands thoroughly.
- Handling cat litter boxes should be avoided.
- Cat faeces should be disposed of daily to avoid maturation of oocysts, and litter box can be cleaned by exposure to boiling water for 5 minutes.
- Cats should be fed only canned or dried commercial food or well-cooked table food, not raw or undercooked meats.

Giardia lamblia is transmitted via the faecal-oral route, including person-to-person, food- and waterborne transmission. Food-borne transmission occurs via raw foods or foods contaminated after cooking. Incidents of food-borne infection caused by *Giardia* have been attributed to fruit salad, sandwiches, fresh vegetables,

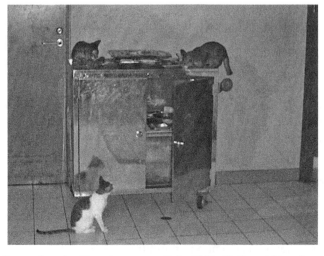

Figure 17.1   Cats, a host for *Toxoplasma gondii* (by Philip Melling, Albion Street Centre). With permission from Philip Melling, the Albion Street Centre.

noodle salad and home-canned salmon (Smith, 1993) In each of these giardiasis incidents, the implicated foods appear to have been contaminated by an infected food handler.

The symptoms and treatment of giardiasis are the same for people with or without HIV infection. Symptoms of nausea, vomiting, abdominal pain, bloating and non-bloody diarrhoea usually occur after an incubation period of 7–10 days, although this may be up to several weeks. Symptoms of giardiasis often last 1 week but may last 2–6 weeks and longer. In some instances diarrhoea may not occur. Diagnosis is from microscopy of stool samples. Rarely, biopsy is also required. Treatment is usually a single dose of oral Tinidazole (2 g) or Metronidazole (250–400 mg) tds for 7 to 10 days.

Prevention

A summary of recommendations by the US CDC for prevention of giardiasis appears in Box 17.3.

Box 17.3   Tips to avoid giardiasis

1. Practice good hygiene as described in Section 17.3.
2. Avoid water that might be contaminated.
    - Do not swallow recreational water, e.g. from lakes and rivers.
    - Do not drink untreated water from shallow wells, lakes, rivers, springs, ponds and streams.
    - Do not drink untreated water during community-wide outbreaks of disease caused by contaminated drinking water.
    - Do not use untreated ice or drinking water when travelling or living in countries where the water supply might be unsafe.

If you are unable to avoid using or drinking water that might be contaminated, you can make the water safe to drink by doing one of the following:

Heat the water to a rolling boil for at **least 1 minute.**
OR
Use a filter that has an absolute pore size of 1 micron or smaller, or one that has been rated for 'cyst removal'.

If you cannot heat the water to a rolling boil or use a recommended filter, then chemically treat the water by chlorination or iodination. Note: using chemicals may be less effective than boiling or filtering because the amount of chemical required to make the water safe is highly dependent on the temperature, pH and cloudiness of the water.

3. Avoid food that might be contaminated.
    - Wash and/or peel all raw vegetables and fruits before eating.
    - Use safe, uncontaminated water to wash all food that is to be eaten raw.
    - Avoid eating uncooked foods when travelling or living in countries with minimal water treatment and sanitation systems.
4. Avoid faecal exposure during sexual activity.

Modified from: United States, Centers for Disease Control and Prevention, National Center for Infectious Diseases, Division of Parasitic Diseases (2004) Giardiasis Factsheet.

Cyclospora

Cyclospora cayetanensis, another protozoan parasite, infects epithelial cells of the small intestine and induces diarrhoea. In both immunocompetent and immunosuppressed PLHIV it causes profuse watery diarrhoea and biliary disease (Pape *et al.*, 1994; Sifunetes-Osornio *et al.*, 1995). In PLHIV with CD4 counts <100 cells/μl, it can cause a more prolonged diarrhoeal illness.

Cyclospora is transmitted by food and water and is more prevalent in tropical climates. It has been associated with food-borne infection in the USAs via raspberries, basil and pesto sauce made from basil (Herwaldt and Ackers, 1997; Lopez *et al.*, 2001; Ho *et al.*, 2002).

Faecal-oral transmission is likely but has not been defined. Humans are the only known host for *Cyclospora* (Kelly, 2006).

Diagnosis of *Cyclospora* is by specific laboratory tests that are not routinely done on stool examinations. Three or more specimens may be required for accurate diagnosis. Treatments are available for patients with chronic infection. In some instances PLHIV that do not achieve immune recovery (CD4 >200 cells/μl) with ART, maintenance therapy may be required.

Prevention

Prevention is by avoiding contaminated food and water. Refer to food safety guidelines in Section 17.3.

Bacteria

Salmonella

PLHIV have a higher risk of salmonellosis than that of HIV-uninfected persons. *Salmonella* infection can occur at any CD4 count, however, recurrent *Salmonella* infection is an indicator of immune deficiency and is an AIDS-defining illness.

The symptoms of salmonellosis are more severe in PLHIV in whom diarrhoea is accompanied by abdominal pain, distension, nausea and fever (Kelly, 2006) and occur within 6–48 hours of ingestion of contaminated food.

Any raw food of animal origin, such as meat, poultry, milk and dairy products, eggs, seafood, and some fruits and vegetables, may carry *Salmonella* bacteria. The bacteria can survive and cause illness if meat, poultry and egg products are not cooked to a safe minimum internal temperature, or if fruits and vegetables are not thoroughly washed. Cross-contamination of food preparation equipment with *Salmonella* can also cause Salmonella enteritis when contaminated food is ingested.

Diagnosis is made by isolation of *Salmonella* spp. in stool culture. Treatment is available with duration of therapy dependent on the severity of infection. (See Chapter 9 for symptomatic control and management of diarrhoea and nausea.)

Prevention

Safe food handling practices are necessary to prevent *Salmonella* infection. Refer to Section 17.4 for safe food handling practices. Avoidance of high-risk foods for PLHIV is advised. Specifically, they should avoid consuming:

- unpasteurised milk and products made from unpasteurised milk
- raw or undercooked chicken, other poultry and meats
- raw or lightly cooked eggs
- dishes prepared with raw or lightly cooked eggs, including home-made mayonnaise, hollandaise sauce, home-made ice cream/soufflé/mousse and egg nogg.

Note: Most commercially prepared foods are made with pasteurised eggs and are safe. Pasteurised eggs can also be purchased for home cooking.

Shigella

Shigella spp. cause enteritis more frequently amongst PLHIV and it has a more severe clinical course than in the general population (Kelly, 2006). After a 1–7-day incubation period, bloody watery diarrhoea, fever, abdominal pain and nausea may develop.

The predominant mode of transmission is by oral/anal contact or ingestion of contaminated food and water.

Diagnosis is by stool culture. Treatment is available and may be required for a longer period of time in PLHIV. (See Chapter 9 for symptomatic control and management of diarrhoea and nausea.)

Prevention

Refer to Section 17.4 for safe food and water practices to prevent shigella and other food-borne illnesses.

Campylobacter

Campylobacter infections are more common in PLHIV than the general community. After a 2- to 6-day incubation period, diarrhoea, fever and abdominal pain develop. Less commonly, nausea and vomiting occur.

Infection usually follows ingestion of contaminated food and water. Undercooked poultry is the most common cause of infection, though outbreaks have occurred with ingestion of contaminated milk or water.

Diagnosis is by specialised microbiological culture techniques on stool samples. All PLHIV are recommended to have antibiotic treatment for campylobacter enteritis given the risk of prolonged and recurrent illness. (See Chapter 9 for symptomatic control and management of diarrhoea and nausea.)

Prevention

Refer to Section 17.4 for safe food and water practices to prevent infection with *Campylobacter* and other food-borne illnesses. PLHIV should be advised to avoid eating undercooked poultry and follow the guidelines in Section 17.4.

Escherichia coli (E. coli)

Escherichia coli are a large and diverse group of bacteria affecting both PLHIV and the general community. Although most strains of *E. coli* are harmless, others can cause disease. Some strains of *E. coli* can cause diarrhoea, while others cause urinary tract infections, respiratory illness and pneumonia, and other illnesses.

The symptoms of *E. coli* infections vary for each person but commonly include severe stomach cramps, diarrhoea (often bloody) and vomiting. If there is fever, it usually is not very high (less than 38.5°C). Most people recover within 5–7 days.

Exposures that result in illness include consumption of contaminated food, consumption of unpasteurised (raw) milk, consumption of water that has not been disinfected, contact with cattle, or contact with the faeces of infected people. Some foods are considered to be at such a high risk of contamination with *E. coli* O157 that health officials recommend people avoid them completely. These foods include unpasteurised (raw) milk, unpasteurised apple cider and soft cheeses made from raw milk.

The diagnosis of *E. coli* is by stool culture. There is no specific antimicrobial treatment, however it is important to drink a lot of fluids to avoid dehydration. (See Chapter 9 for symptomatic control and management of diarrhoea.)

Prevention

Refer to Section 17.4 for safe food and water practices to prevent *E coli* and other food-borne illnesses.

Listeria monocytogenes

Infection with certain types of *Listeria* bacteria can cause serious illness (i.e. listeriosis) in people who have a compromised immune system. PLHIV have been reported to have 60- to more than 150-fold increased risk of infection, especially if they have CD4 <50–100 cells/µl (Jurado *et al.*, 1993). Pregnant women and people over the age of 65 are also at higher risk.

Listeria monocytogenes is found in soil and water. *Listeria* is widespread in nature and the most common food sources are raw vegetables, unpasteurised milk, meats, fish and poultry (Schlech, 2000). Vegetables can become contaminated from the soil and animals can carry the bacterium and thereby contaminate foods of animal origin such as meats and dairy products. Processed foods may be contaminated after processing, such as with soft cheeses and cold cuts of meat from a delicatessen. *Listeria* is killed by pasteurisation and cooking; however, in certain ready-to-eat foods such as hot dogs and deli meats, contamination may occur after cooking but before packaging.

Listeriosis can be caused by eating foods that are contaminated with *Listeria* even if the food is stored in a refrigerator. Unlike other bacteria, *Listeria* can still grow at temperatures less than 5°C. *Listeria* may be present in raw foods or may contaminate food after it has been cooked or processed.

Food histories taken in a study of PLHIV in the United Stated showed that over 50% had consumed undercooked meat, poultry or fish 1 month before *Listeria* diagnosis (Mascola *et al.*, 1991).

Listeriosis can cause fever, headache, fatigue and, occasionally, nausea and diarrhoea. In more serious forms, listeriosis leads to meningitis and septicaemia. Often systemic infections (bacteremia, endocarditis and central nervous system infections) may be preceded by gastroenteritis.

In pregnant women symptoms may be mild but can lead to miscarriage, premature birth and, in rare cases, still birth.

Diagnosis involves analysis of blood and cerebral spinal fluid. Antibiotic treatments are available.

Table 17.1 Foods with a higher risk of *Listeria* contamination and safer alternatives.

Food type	High-risk foods	Safer option
Cold meats	Unpackaged and packaged sliced ready-to-eat cold meats from sandwich bars and supermarkets	Home-cooked meats stored in the refrigerator and used within 24 hours of cooking
Cold cooked chicken	Purchased ready-to-eat cold chicken.	Home-cooked or hot takeaway chicken. Ensure chicken is cooked right through
Dairy	Soft, semi-soft and surface ripened cheeses, e.g. brie, camembert, feta and blue	Hard cheese (cheddar, tasty). Processed cheese
	Soft-serve ice cream	Pasteurised dairy products (e.g. milk, yoghurt, custard and packaged frozen ice cream)
	Unpasteurised dairy products	
Salads	Pre-packaged or pre-prepared salads from salad bars and smorgasbords	Home-made freshly prepared salad from thoroughly washed vegetables and fruit, or canned or similar packaged foods
		Note: Store salads and canned vegetables at less than 4°C and use within the day of preparation
Seafood	Raw oysters, sashimi, sushi and other smoked and ready-to-eat seafood. Cooked ready to eat peeled prawns, e.g. in prawn cocktails	All freshly cooked seafood. Any leftovers should be stored in the fridge and used within a day of cooking
Pate	All types	

Prevention

ART with immune reconstitution may decrease risk of infection. PLHIV should be advised to follow the food safety guidelines in Section 17.4 and avoid foods that have higher risk of *Listeria* contamination, shown in Table 17.1.

Viruses

Hepatitis A
Hepatitis A is a liver disease caused by the hepatitis A virus. Hepatitis A is usually spread from person to person by putting something in the mouth (even though it might look clean) that has been contaminated with the faeces of a person with hepatitis A. Transmission may be via uncooked foods (salads), shellfish from contaminated waters, contaminated drinking water or sexual contact.

Some people infected with hepatitis A get little or no symptoms at all and children are more likely than adults to show no symptoms of infection. In more severe cases, hepatitis A can cause:

- loss of appetite
- nausea and vomiting
- weight loss
- fever and malaise

- pain in the liver (under the right rib cage)
- jaundice (when the urine becomes darker than normal and the eyes and skin go yellow).

On average, signs and symptoms appear 4 weeks after infection (range 2–7 weeks). More marked symptoms may last for several weeks but full recovery is usual. People with hepatitis A can pass it on to others from 2 weeks before they show symptoms to 1 week after they become jaundiced.

Hepatitis A is diagnosed by a blood test looking for specific antibodies of the virus. There is no specific antiviral treatment for hepatitis A.

Prevention

Hepatitis A vaccine is the best protection. It has a protective antibody response rate of 99% in persons who are not immunocompromised. The response rate is less in PLHIV but still warrants vaccination.

Good personal hygiene is a key strategy for the prevention of hepatitis A. For example: hands should be thoroughly washed with soap and hot running water for at least 10 to 15 seconds:

- before preparing food
- between handling raw and ready-to-eat foods
- before eating
- after going to the toilet or after changing nappies
- after handling used condoms or after contact with the anal area.

Note: In situations where there is no running water such as picnics, bushwalking or sport meetings, commercially prepared alcohol-based hand rubs are an excellent substitute for soap and water. These alcohol preparations should be rubbed into the hands for 10 to 15 seconds or until the alcohol has evaporated.

17.3.3   Toxic chemicals

Microorganisms are not the only cause of food-borne illness. People also get sick following exposure to poisonous chemicals including:

- natural toxins, e.g. aflatoxins
- incorrectly used food additives
- metals and environmental pollutants
- chemicals used for treating animals
- chemicals used for cleaning
- improperly used pesticides.

Note: Poisoning is the term used to describe sickness resulting from chemical contamination.

PLHIV are not known to have any different risk or outcomes from chemical food poisoning. However, some chemicals have harmful effects on the liver. For PLHIV co-infected with hepatitis C and/or B or who have abnormal liver function due to

ART, other medications or alcohol, any further damage to the liver by toxins from food should be avoided.

Examples of harmful toxins in foods

Aflatoxins

Aflatoxins are one of the most potent toxic substances occurring naturally. They are a group of closely related mycotoxins produced by fungi *Aspergillus flavus* and *A. parasiticus*. Aflatoxicosis is poisoning resulting from ingestion of aflatoxins in contaminated food. Diet is the major way through which humans are exposed to aflatoxins. Exposure to large doses (>6000 mg) of aflatoxin may cause acute toxicity with lethal effect, whereas exposure to small doses for prolonged periods is carcinogenic. Aflatoxins may be both carcinogenic and hepatotoxic, depending on the duration and level of exposure.

In Kenya, acute aflatoxin poisoning has been reported to result in liver failure and death in up to 40% of cases (Lewis *et al.*, 2005).

Food products contaminated with aflatoxins include cereal (maize, sorghum, pearl millet, rice and wheat), oilseeds (groundnut, soybean, sunflower and cottonseed), spices (chillies, black pepper, coriander, turmeric and ginger), tree nuts (peanuts, almonds, pistachio, walnuts and coconut) and milk. Agricultural practices and food processing are not always adequate to achieve low concentrations of these in foods.

Aflatoxicosis in humans has been reported in many countries in Asia and Africa, where environmental conditions favour aflatoxin contamination. A study in West Africa showed a significant correlation between the level of aflatoxin exposure in neonatal stages and stunting of growth in children (Gong *et al.*, 2002).

In developing nations, many people are exposed to aflatoxins through food grown at home. Inadequate harvesting and storage techniques allow for the growth of aflatoxin-producing fungus and home-grown crops are not routinely tested for the presence of aflatoxins. As a result, an estimated 4.5 billion people living in developing countries may be chronically exposed to aflatoxins through their diet. Good agricultural practices should be followed using local guidelines for prevention of chemical contamination of food (Bhat *et al.*, 1997).

Prevention

Tips to avoid aflatoxicosis at home:

- Purchase cereals and spices and nuts from vendors who use clean and dry packaging.
- Do not purchase foods that appear discoloured and mouldy.
- Always discard mouldy nuts and other mouldy foods.
- Store all nuts and grains in containers without moisture.

Bacillus cereus

Bacillus cereus (*B. cereus*) is a spore-forming bacteria found naturally in a wide range of food. When a food is heated under normal cooking conditions, the *B. cereus* cells are usually destroyed, however, the spores of *B. cereus* are much more resistant to cooking temperatures and can remain viable in the food.

Common sources of B. cereus

B. cereus spores are naturally occurring in soil and therefore may be found in a wide range of foods including:

- dry soups
- spices and seasonings
- dried dairy products
- infant formulas
- rice – fried rice is a common cause of food poisoning due to *B. cereus*, because of the long period between boiling the rice and consumption after frying.

B. cereus prefers to grow at temperatures between 30 and 37°C, although it can grow at temperatures up to 55°C and in some cases down to 5°C.

There are two types of food poisoning that are associated with *B. cereus*: diarrhoeal illness and emetic illness.

1. *Diarrhoeal illness*: Diarrhoeal illness will produce symptoms of abdominal pain and watery diarrhoea. Nausea and vomiting can occur but are less frequently seen with this type of poisoning. These symptoms will present 8–16 hours after ingestion of the food, and last for 12 to 24 hours.
2. *Emetic illness*: The primary symptoms of emetic illness are nausea and vomiting lasting between 6 and 24 hours. Onset is typically more rapid than the diarrhoeal illness with symptoms beginning 0.5–5 hours after food consumption. This quick onset of symptoms is due to the presence of a preformed toxin produced by bacterial growth in the food. Heating a food that contains *B. cereus* toxin will not destroy the toxin.

This type of emetic food poisoning is commonly associated with starchy foods, such as rice and pasta that have been incorrectly cooled after cooking.

Prevention

Food poisoning with *B. cereus* in PLHIV can be prevented by:

- Keeping cold prepared foods under refrigeration (5°C) until ready to be served.
- Keeping hot foods at a temperature greater than 60°C.
- Avoiding preparing foods too far in advance.
- Ensuring foods to be eaten hot at a later time are cooled (within 30 minutes), covered and stored below 5°C after cooking. Separating large quantities of food into smaller containers may aid the food to cool in an acceptable time frame.

For information on other toxins in foods refer to the Food Standards Agency website, including www.food.gov.uk/multimedia/pdfs/naturaltoxins.

17.4 Management and prevention of food-borne illness

Recommendations for people experiencing food-borne illness are summarised in Box 17.4. Section 17.4 outlines food safety guidelines.

Box 17.4   Recommendations for people experiencing food-borne illness

- Many people have mild symptoms and recover within a few days. However, if symptoms persist for more than 3 days or are very severe medical advice should be sought.
- A doctor should be consulted immediately if symptoms include blood or mucus in the diarrhoea.
- People at risk of dehydration such as infants and the elderly should seek medical advice as early as possible.
- People with diarrhoea and vomiting should stay home from work or school and drink plenty of fluids.
- As a precaution, people with any food-borne or gastrointestinal illness should not prepare food for 48 hours after their symptoms have finished.

17.4.1   Food and water safety guidelines

PLHIV should follow the Five Keys to Safer Food (WHO, 2006) developed by the World Health Organization or the advice of their local government food safety authority. Figure 17.2 is WHO's client resource 'Five Keys to Safer Food'. A copy of the five keys to safer food manual is available at: www.who.int/foodsafety/publications/consumer/5keys/en/index.html.

Section 17.4.2 describes the key points for preventing food-borne illness under these five strategies for safer food. A useful website for PLHIV living in the UK is: http://www.eatwell.gov.uk/keepingfoodsafe/.

17.4.2   Guidelines for prevention of food-borne illness in developed and developing countries

Keep clean

Most food poisoning can be prevented by following some basic rules of hygiene.

Disposal of faeces
Many of the microorganisms responsible for food poisoning are spread through faeces. PLHIV should be advised to:

- use a latrine and keep it clean and free from flies
- keep the surroundings clean and
- wash clothes, bedding and surfaces that may have been contaminated with faeces in hot water with soap.

Personal hygiene recommendations include to:

- Always wash hands with clean water and soap before, during and after preparing food or eating. Dry hands on a clean cloth or towel. (See Figure 17.3 for the recommended hand washing procedure.) Hands should also be washed after:
  ○ visiting the toilet or changing a babies nappy
  ○ handling raw meat or poultry
  ○ handling rubbish

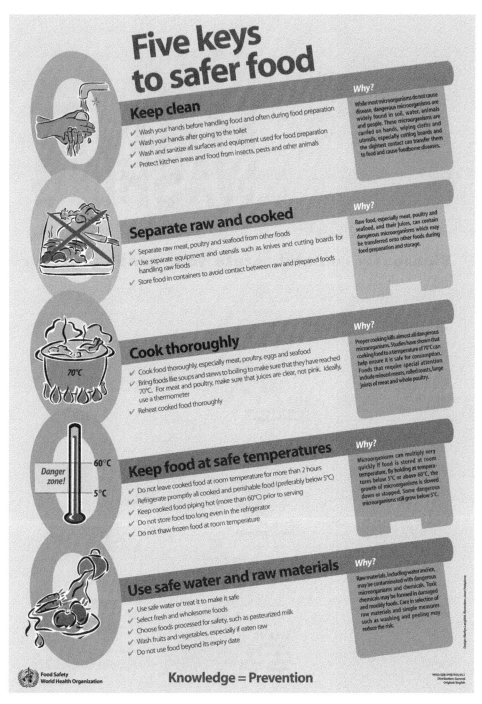

Figure 17.2 Five keys to safer foods. With permission from Department of Food Safety, Zoonoses and Foodborne Diseases (FOS), WHO.

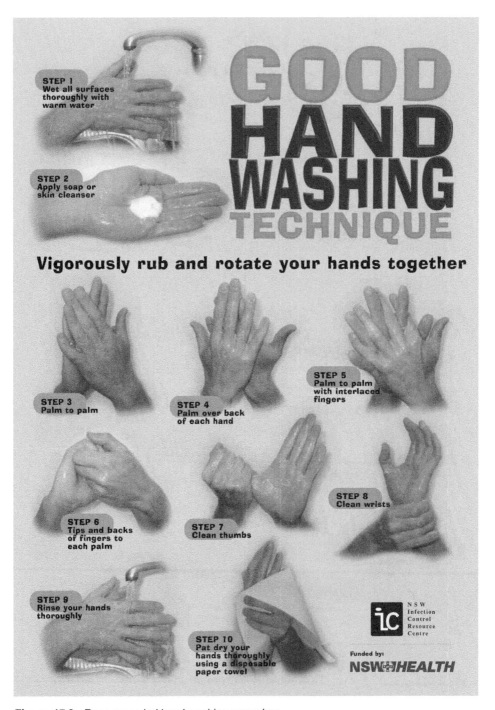

Figure 17.3 Recommended hand washing procedure.

- handling chemicals
- playing with pets
- smoking and
- blowing your nose.

- Cover all cuts and wounds to prevent contamination of food during preparation and handling.
- Use safe clean water from protected sources such as treated piped water supplies, boreholes, gravity feed schemes and protected wells. If the water is not from a protected source, it should be boiled before consumption. Care must be taken during collection and storage to use clean containers to prevent contamination. Water containers in the home can easily become contaminated by dirty cups and hands that have not been washed. When people drink contaminated water, they will become sick.

If slaughtering of animals is practised in the home, PLHIV should:

- keep the slaughtering area clean and separate from food preparation areas
- change clothes and wash hands and equipment after slaughtering and
- keep live animals away from the food-growing, preparation and storage areas.

Hygiene in the food preparation area
PLHIV or people preparing food for PLHIV should always:

- wash hands before handling food and often during food preparation (see personal hygiene above and Figure 17.3)
- sanitise all surfaces and equipment used for food preparation (including cutting boards, wiping clothes, benches and knives)
- use boiling water or a sanitising solution (e.g. 5 ml of household bleach and 750 ml of water)
- use clean dishes and utensils to store, prepare, serve and eat food
- wash vegetables and fruit with clean water
- cover food to prevent flies, insects and dust from contaminating the food
- protect kitchen areas and food from insects, pests, pets and other animals and
- keep rubbish in a covered bin (and empty it regularly) so as to minimise offensive smells and attracting flies.

Separate raw and cooked food

Advice to PLHIV should include:

- store raw and cooked food in separate containers, thus avoiding contact between them (i.e. cross-contamination)
- in the refrigerator, store raw meat, seafood and poultry below cooked or ready-to-eat foods
- use separate equipment and utensils such as knives and cutting boards for handling raw foods
- always use clean plates for either raw or cooked foods
- do not eat cooked food from plates used to prepare raw food without washing in boiled water first.

Cook thoroughly

Microorganisms multiply more quickly in warm food. Storing food in a refrigerator or cool place slows down this growth. Cooking on a high heat can kill most microorganisms.

Food should be:

- served immediately after cooking. (To avoid microorganisms multiplying, food should not be left standing at room temperature before eating)
- covered and stored in containers away from insects, rodents and other animals
- stored in a cool place or refrigerator where available, especially fresh meats, chicken, fish and dairy foods
- cooked thoroughly (without overcooking vegetables)
  - ○ wet dishes like soups and stews should be brought to boiling point to ensure that a temperature of 70°C has been reached
  - ○ the juices from meat and poultry should be clear, not pink. Ideally, a thermometer should be used to check food temperatures
- discarded after cooking if there are leftovers unless they can be kept in a refrigerator or in a cool place. (Leftovers should not be kept for more than 1 day)
- reheated ONCE only and at a high temperature.

Eggs should be hard-boiled. Soft-boiled eggs, raw eggs, cracked eggs or any foods containing raw eggs are to be avoided by PLHIV.

Keep food at safe temperatures

Advice to PLHIV should include:

- do not leave cooked food at room temperature for more than 2 hours (30 minutes in hot climates)
- refrigerate promptly all cooked and perishable food (preferable below 5°C)
- keep hot food above 60°C before serving (5–60°C is the temperature at which most bacteria prefer to grow).

Note: When microwaves are used to thaw food, they can leave warms spots where microorganisms can grow. Food thawed in a microwave should be cooked promptly.

Use safe water and raw materials

Advice to PLHIV should include:

- use safe water (i.e. free from microorganisms or toxins) or treat it to make it safe
- select fresh foods that do not appear spoiled
- choose foods processed for safety, e.g. pasteurised milk
- wash fruit and vegetables with clean water
- do not use food beyond its expiry date.

17.4.3 Safe water

Drinking water in the UK is safe. However, on rare occasions tap water may become contaminated and in these instances all water should be boiled before drinking, being used in cooking or made into ice. Boiled water should only be stored in refrigeration for up to 24 hours then discarded. For PLHIV who are visiting or living in countries where there is poor hygiene and sanitation, all water should be treated.

Guidelines for making water safe in countries with poor hygiene and sanitation

ALL FLUIDS CONSUMED should be prepared with SAFE WATER. Beverages that may contain contaminated water include fresh juices and any drinks with ice. These should be avoided unless clean disinfected water was used in the production of these drinks and ice. All hot beverages made from boiled water and carbonated bottled beverages, pasteurised or canned juice, sports beverages and pasteurised, boiled or sterilised milk are normally safe.

Boil

Boiling water is the most effective way to kill microorganisms. Water should be brought to a rolling boil for at least 1 minute (though 2–10 minutes is recommended by some agencies) then cooled without the addition of ice (which may not be safe).

Disinfect

If water cannot be boiled, it can be disinfected with chemicals after it is filtered. Chlorine and iodine are the most commonly used chemicals for disinfecting water. WHO (2005) recommend the use of a product which combines chlorine disinfection with coagulation flocculation (i.e. chemical precipitation) to disinfect water. These products remove significant numbers of protozoa, in addition to killing bacteria and viruses (WHO, 2005).

   Box 17.5 describes a recommended procedure to disinfect small quantities of water (Infection Control Working Group, 2002).

Box 17.5   Procedure to disinfect small quantities of water

1. Prepare a stock solution of 1% concentration:
    – 15 g calcium hypochlorite (70%) OR 33 g bleaching powder or chlorinated lime (30%) OR sodium hypochlorite (liquid bleach) 357 ml (3.5%); 313 ml (4.0%), 250 ml (5.0%)
2. Mix and wait for 30 minutes
3. Pour the clear chlorine stock into another container for storage and use (always keep in cool, dark place)
4. To disinfect water that is clear and has light colour, add three drops of the stock solution to each litre of water. If the colour of the water is darker (like tea), add six drops of the stock solution to each litre of water
5. After adding the chlorine solution to the water, mix the water thoroughly and wait for 30 minutes before using the water
6. Use clean containers for storage and wash at least weekly

Note: Chemical disinfection is not effective in killing some protozoa including *Cryptosporidium parvum* and *Giardia lamblia*.

Filter
A water treatment device can be used if it has been certified to remove protozoa such as *Cryptosporidium parvum and Giardia lamblia*. A size of 1 micron or less for the filter media pore is recommended to ensure removal of *Cryptosporidium* and *Giardia* in clear water.

WHO (2005) recommend that unless water is boiled, a combination of technologies should be used to ensure safe drinking water, e.g. filtration followed by chemical disinfection (WHO, 2005). Alternatively, bottled water in sealed, tamper-proof containers and bottled by certified brands should be used.

Store water in clean containers
Clean water should be stored in containers with a narrow mouth, a lid and a spigot (or ideally a tap) to prevent recontamination. All water storage vessels should be intact with no cracks and leaks. Containers should be washed using boiled water (or chlorine solution) at least once per week or more often if they become dirty.

For more information on water safety, refer to resources available on the World Health Organization website (www.who.int).

17.4.4   Special food safety considerations in resource-poor settings

UK food safety standards for the home may not always be realistic for PLHIV without access to adequate cooking facilities and accommodation and for those in resource-poor settings. Local health care workers should modify the recommendations above when required. An example can be found in Chapter 11, 'Community Interventions in Resource-Limited Settings'.

17.4.5   Food and water safety information for food service providers

Hazard Analysis Critical Control Point (HACCP) guidelines should be followed by all organisations providing food to the community. HACCP is a framework for preventing food-borne illness. The actions to be taken if critical limits are exceeded may be different for PLHIV and others with a compromised immune system. When the status of clients is unknown, all clients should be considered immunocompromised and the highest level of food safety precautions implemented. For example, in the hospital food service setting, salads and sandwiches may be given a critical limit of being used within 4 hours. This may be extended in lower-risk groups if food safety can be ensured but never exceeded for PLHIV.

The Food Standards Agency (www.food.gov.uk) can provide information and links for food service providers and individuals on food safety and HACCP.

Note: Normal crockery and cutlery should be used for PLHIV in hospital as there is no risk of HIV transmission through sharing eating utensils (i.e. do not use disposables on the basis of HIV infection).

17.5   Conclusion

Following food and water safety guidelines will help reduce food-borne illness in PLHIV. When food- and waterborne infections do occur it is important for PLHIV to see a health worker without delay in order to minimise illness and avoid weight loss and nutritional impairment. The recommendations for symptom control and management in Chapter 9 may be of assistance but should not replace appropriate medical management.

Acknowledgements

The author would like to thank:

Philip Melling former CNC – Infection Control; Infection Prevention & Control Unit; The Albion Street Centre, Sydney, Australia for review and contributions to this chapter; **WHO, Department of Food Safety, Zoonoses and Foodborne Diseases** for the use of the "Five keys to safer food" and Amy Goodwin, HIV Specialist Dietitian, Nutrition and Dietetic Therapy Service Cardiff and the Vale NHS Trust.

References

Alterkruse S, Hyman F, Klontz K, Timbo B, Tollesfson, L. Food borne bacterial infections in individual with the human immunodeficiency virus. *South Med J* 1994; 87:169–73.

Bhat RV, Shetty PH, Amruth RP, Sudersham RV. A food-borne disease outbreak due to consumption of mouldy sorghum and maize containing fumonisin mycotoxins. *J Toxicol Clin Toxicol* 1997; 35:249–55.

Celum CL, Chaisson RE, Rutherford GW, Barnhart JL, Echenberg DF. Incidence of salmonellosis in patients with AIDS. *J Infect Dis* 1987; 156:998–1002.

Gong YY, Cardwell K, Hounsa A *et al*. Dietary aflatoxin exposure and impaired growth in young children from Benin and Togo: cross sectional study. *Br Med J* 2002; 325:20–21.

Hayes C, Elliot E, Krales E, Downer G. Food and water safety for persons infected with human immunodeficiency virus. *Clin Infect Dis* 2003; 36(Suppl 2):S106–S9.

Herwaldt BL, Ackers ML. An outbreak in 1996 of cyclosporiasis associated with imported raspberries. *N Engl J Med* 1997; 336:1548–56.

Hill DE, Benedetto SM, Coss C, Mccrary JL, Fournet VM, Dubey JP. Time and temperature effects on T. gondii tissue cysts in enhanced meats; the effect of time and temperature on the viability of Toxoplasma gondii tissue cysts in enhanced pork loin. *J Food Prot* 2006; 69:1961–5.

Ho AY, Lopez AS, Eberhart MG *et al*. Outbreak of cyclosporiasis associated with imported raspberries, Philadelphia, Pennsylvania, 2000. *Emerg Infect Dis* 2002; 8:783–8.

Hoffman EW, Bergmann V, Shultz JA *et al*. Application of a five step message development model for food safety education materials targeting people with HIV/AIDS. *J Am Diet Assoc* 2005; 105:1597–604.

Hughes JM, Colley DG, Lopez A *et al*. Preventing Congenital Toxoplasmosis. *CDC MMWR Recommendations and Reports* 2000; 49(RR02):57–75.

Infection control working group Water Disinfection. *Infection control manual for Health facilities*. Hospital services directorate, Ministry of Health, Fiji, in association with the Australian Government-funded Fiji Health Management Reform Project, 2002: 59.

Jenkins M. Present and future control of cryptosporidiosis in humans and animals. Review Article. *Expert Review of Vaccines* 2005; 3:669–71.

Jones L, Hanson DL, Dworkin MS *et al*. Surveillance for AIDS-defining opportunistic illnesses, 1992–1997. *MMWR Morb Mortal Wkly Rep CDC Surveill Summ* 1999; 48(SS-2):1–22.

Jones JL, Kruszon-Moran D, Wilson M. Toxoplasma gondii infection in the United States, 1999–2000. *Emerg Infect Dis* [serial online] 2003 Nov [cited 150408]. Available at http://www.cdc.gov/ncidod/EID/vol9no11/03–0098.htm, 2003.

Jurado RL, Farley MM, Pereira E *et al*. Increased risk of meningitis and bacteremia due to Listeria monocytogenes in patients with human immunodeficiency virus infection. *Clin Infect Dis* 1993; 17:224–7.

Kelly M. Gastrointestinal and oral infections. *HIV Management in Australia, A Guide to Clinical Care*. Sydney: Australasian Society for HIV Medicine, Inc, 2006: 178–86.

Lewis L, Onsongo M, Njapau H *et al.* Aflatoxin contamination of commercial maize products during an outbreak of acute aflatoxicosis in eastern and central Kenya. *Environ Health Perspect* 2005; 113:1763–7.

Lopez AS, Dodson DR, Arrowood MJ *et al.* Outbreak of cyclosporiasis associated with basil in Missouri in 1999. *Clin Infect Dis* 2001; 32:1010–17.

Luft BJ, Remington JS. Toxoplasmic encephalitis in AIDS. *Clin Infect Dis* 1992; 15(2):211–22.

Mascola L, Enguidanos R, Lieb L, Sorvillo F. Public health implications of listeriosis in HIV-infected persons: a formidable food borne pathogen. *International Conference on AIDS*. 1991; 7: 348 (abstract no. M.C.3203).

Mead PS, Slutsker L, Dietz V *et al.* Food related illness and death in the United States. *Emerg Infect Dis* 1999; 5(5):607–25.

Morris JG, Potter M. Emergence of new pathogens as a function of changes in host susceptibility. *Emerg Infect Dis* 1997; 3:435–41.

Pape JW, Verdier RI, Boncy J, Johnson WD. Cyclospora infection in adults infected with HIV Clinical manifestations, treatment, and prophylaxis. *Ann Intern Med* 1994; 121:654–7.

Schlech WF. Foodborne listeriosis. *Clin Infect Dis* 2000; 31:770–75.

Sifunetes-Osornio J, Porras-Cortes G, Bendall RP, Morales-Villarreal F, Reyes-Teran G, Ruiz-Palacios GM. Cyclospora cayetanensis infection in patients with and without AIDS: biliary disease as another clinica manifestation. *Clin Infect Dis* 1995; 21:1092–7.

Smith J. Long term consequences of food borne toxoplasmosis: Effects on the unborn, the immuno-compormised, the elderly and the immunocompetent. *J Food Protect* 1997; 60:1595.

Smith JL. Cryptosporidium and Giardia as agents of food borne disease. *J Food Protect* 1993; 56:451–6.

Sorvillo FJ, Lieb LE, Waterman SH. Incidence of campylobacteriosis among patients with AIDS in Los Angeles County. *J Acquir Immune Defic Syndr* 1991; 4:598–602.

WHO. *WHO Global Strategy for Food Safety, Safer Food for Better Health*. Geneva: World Health Organization, 2002.

WHO. *WHO Preventing Travellers' Diarrhoea: How to Make Drinking Water Safe Sustainable Development and Healthy Environments, Water, Sanitation and Health*. Geneva: World Health Organization, 2005.

WHO. *Five Keys to Safer Food Manual*. Geneva: World Health Organization, 2006.

Section 5
THE NUTRITIONAL MANAGEMENT OF HIV AND CO-MORBIDITIES

18 The Nutritional Management of Patients Living with Tuberculosis and HIV Co-Infection

Louise Houtzager, Tim Barnes and Kirilee Matters

Key Points

- The incidence of TB is increasing globally. WHO estimates that 9.27 million new cases of TB occurred in 2007 of which an estimated 1.37 million (14.8%) were HIV-positive. It is estimated that there were 456,000 deaths from TB among HIV-positive people and this accounts for 23% of the estimated 2 million HIV deaths that occurred in 2007 (WHO, 2009).
- TB most commonly affects the lungs. The symptoms of pulmonary TB include cough, fever, shortness of breath, anorexia, weight loss, night sweats, chest pain, fatigue and exhaustion.
- TB treatment requires taking multiple drugs without interruption for extended periods of time (e.g. 6 months) to kill the organism causing TB infection and prevent the development of resistance to the drugs being used.
- There is a clear relationship between TB infection and nutrition. Malnutrition can predispose people with TB to develop disease and TB disease can result in secondary malnutrition.
- TB and HIV both impact on the clinical course of each other. HIV not only increases the risk of acquiring TB but significantly increases the likelihood of latent disease becoming active and treated disease relapsing. TB accelerates the progress of HIV infection and is a major cause of morbidity and mortality.
- The short-term goals of nutritional therapy in TB and HIV include optimizing nutritional intake, attaining and maintaining ideal body weight, restoring lean body mass, the provision of nutrients according to daily requirements and preventing further nutrient deficiencies.
- More research is required into the role of specific micronutrients in the pathogenesis and treatment of TB in HIV infection and the role of generic vitamin and mineral supplementation in the treatment of TB.

18.1 Tuberculosis

Tuberculosis (TB) is an infectious disease caused by the bacteria *Mycobacterium tuberculosis*. The mycobacteria that cause TB are versatile, slender, rod-shaped, aerobic Gram-positive organisms that are not capable of forming spores (Mattson Porth, 2007). They contain an outer waxy lipid capsule that makes them resistant to destruction, detergents, disinfectants and common antibacterial agents (Murray et al., 2005).

TB can infect any organ in the body, however, the lungs are most frequently infected. Transmission occurs when infectious people (those with active TB) cough, sneeze or spit spreading the TB organisms into the air. Non-infected people inhale the bacteria which penetrate the alveolar spaces of the lungs (Mattson Porth, 2007). The symptoms of pulmonary TB include fever, weight loss, night sweats, cough with or without production (sometimes there is blood present), anorexia, chest pain, fatigue and malaise.

In most cases the body can fight the bacteria with a cell-mediated response involving the proliferation of antigen-specific lymphocytes and cytokines. In immunocompromised people, the TB organisms are more able to multiply, increasing the progression of infection to active TB (Johnson and Ellner, 1999). In these circumstances, TB is also more likely to spread to other parts of the body (Murray et al., 2005).

The gold standard for the diagnosis of TB includes the detection of acid-fast bacilli (AFB) on microscopic examination of sputum or tissue samples, followed by culture and drug sensitivity testing (BHIVA, 2005). Whilst detection of AFB on microscopic smears is fast (test results are usually available within one day), culture and antibiotic sensitivity testing takes many weeks and may not be accessible for many patients.

Long periods of treatment and high levels of adherence are necessary to achieve a cure for TB (Paton et al., 2004). A period of isolation is often recommended for the first two weeks of treatment after which it is considered that the patient is no longer infectious (Mandal et al., 2004). In many situations patients with TB are not able to be isolated, potentially furthering the spread of the disease.

18.2 Epidemiology

According to WHO (2009) in 2008, there were an estimated 9.4 (range, 8.9–9.9 million) million incident cases (equivalent to 139 cases per 100 000 population) of TB globally. This is an increase from the 9.3 million TB cases estimated to have occurred in 2007. Most of the estimated number of cases in 2008 occurred in Asia (55%) and Africa (30%), with small proportions of cases in the Eastern Mediterranean Region (7%), the European Region (5%) and the Region of the Americas (3%). WHO estimates a worldwide increase in TB of up to 40% over the next 20 years. Reasons for this include population growth, migration patterns and the increase in HIV infection. Migration patterns of persons from regions of high TB incidence, such as sub-Saharan Africa and South East Asia, to the UK may increase UK TB incidence. There were an estimated 11.1 million (range, 9.6–13.3 million) prevalent cases of TB in 2008 (1 equivalent to 164 cases per 100 000 population (WHO 2009).

The World Health Organisation (WHO) declared TB as a global emergency in 1993 and the disease remains a leading cause of morbidity and mortality. TB incidence continues to increase in England, Wales and Northern Ireland. A total of 8497 TB cases were reported in 2006, a rate of 14.0 per 100,000 population (HPA, 2007). TB rates in London remain the highest in the UK and some London boroughs have rates comparable to developing countries (DoH, 2004).

TB is typically a disease of poverty and deprivation. It thrives in communities where overcrowding, poor nutrition, low education, limited access to health care and poor

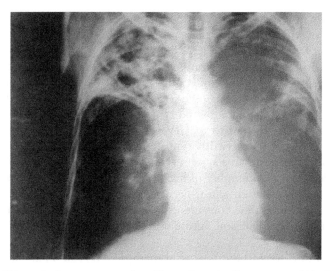

Figure 18.1   Tuberculosis as seen on chest X-ray. From the Department of Health and Human Services.

housing are common (Carballo *et al.*, 1998). The disease mainly affects those who are migrants, homeless, young, elderly, immunocompromised (particularly those with HIV infection), or users of illicit drugs and/or excess alcohol (Murray *et al.*, 2005).

In the UK in 2006, 72% of TB cases occurred amongst people who were not born in the UK (HPA, 2007). Compared to the indigenous population, migrants may be more likely to end up in overcrowded, non-hygienic living conditions, more conducive to the spread of TB and they may also have poorer access to health services. (Carballo *et al.*, 1998).

In 2008, an estimated 1.3 million (range, 1.1–1.7 million) deaths, including 0.5 million (range, 0.45–0.62 million) deaths among women, occurred among HIV-negative incident cases of TB. This is equivalent to 20 deaths per 100 000 population. There were an estimated 0.5 million deaths among incident TB cases who were HIV-positive (WHO, 2009). Worldwide, 11.4 million people are co-infected with TB and HIV (WHO, 2006) and this figure is increasing. TB is a common cause of death in those living with HIV and an estimated 50% of HIV deaths globally are due to TB. Thirteen million people living with HIV are at risk of developing TB and, in some regions of Africa, up to 80% of adult TB patients are HIV co-infected. The late diagnosis of TB and untreated HIV in many settings results in one-third of these co-infected patients dying within weeks of initiating treatment of their TB (Figure 18.1).

18.3   The relationship between tuberculosis and HIV

TB and HIV are closely interlinked, and are referred to as co-infection. TB/HIV co-infection prevalence is particularly high in sub-Sahara Africa, Asia and India, where there are also high rates of poverty and malnutrition (Schwenk and Macallan, 2000).

TB infected persons who are HIV positive are up to 50 times more likely to develop active TB than those who are HIV negative. TB infection accelerates the progress of HIV infection whilst HIV infection is the most potent risk factor for rapid TB disease progression (Pratt, 2003), reactivation of latent TB and for the relapse of treated TB.

Many people infected with HIV in developing countries develop TB as the first manifestation of AIDS, and TB in these people is almost certain to be rapidly fatal if undiagnosed or left untreated (WHO, 2007).

TB causes chronic immune activation and an increase in HIV viral load, facilitating progression of HIV infection (Collins et al., 2002). With increasing immune suppression (reducing CD4 count), there is an increased risk of opportunistic infection, including disseminated/non pulmonary TB and mortality (Collins et al., 2002).

Diagnosis of TB in the context of HIV is often difficult. In more advanced HIV disease, there is a decreased sensitivity using microscopy to detect AFB in sputum smears, as a weakened immune system reduces sputum production which contains AFB. Thus, despite a high number of bacilli in lung tissue, a person with advanced HIV disease may be sputum smear-negative (Mugusi et al., 2006). This reduces diagnosis accuracy and is time-consuming. Due to the reduced inflammatory response there is also less lung cavitation, meaning a chest X-ray may appear near normal (Pratt, 2003).

The optimal time to start antiretroviral therapy (ART) in a patient being treated for TB is not agreed upon. When to start ART still depends on a patients CD4 count. There are arguments for and against starting ART immediately and it is up to the managing physician to make a clinical decision on the timing of therapy. There is risk involved in delaying ART in a patient with advanced HIV disease as ongoing immunosuppression could lead to opportunistic infection but there is also the risk that concomitant HIV and TB treatment may have to be discontinued altogether due to toxicity, drug interactions, adherence issues and/or side effects (BHIVA, 2005). Additionally, starting ART for HIV in the first 1–2 months of anti-TB treatment may increase the risk of immune reconstitution inflammatory syndrome (IRIS) (BHIVA, 2005). WHO states that these concerns should not cause too much of a delay to starting TB or HIV treatment (WHO, 2007). Generally, if the CD4 is very low (e.g. <100 cells/microL), then once the person is established on TB therapy for 2 to 4 weeks, consideration should be given to the introduction of ART. At higher CD4 counts there may be the argument to defer ART until the end of the 2-month induction period.

BHIVA (2005) HIV treatment guidelines include the recommendation that those with a CD4 count consistently greater than 200 cells should wait until their anti-tuberculosis therapy is completed before starting HIV therapy. WHO strongly suggest that treatment for both HIV and TB start without delay (WHO, 2007).

18.4   Medical issues

18.4.1   TB treatment

TB treatment involves taking multiple drugs without interruption to kill the bacteria and prevent them from becoming resistant to one or more TB drugs (BNF, 2007). The aim of treatment is to cure the person of TB as well as minimise the transmission of the bacteria (BHIVA, 2005).

In the UK there is National Institute of Clinical Excellence (NICE) and British Thoracic Society (BTS) guidance on the management of TB and the former includes HIV. There are also BHIVA (British HIV Association) treatment guidelines for TB/HIV co-infection. WHO guidelines also provide recommendations on standard TB treatment although each country will usually have a national TB program based on current WHO recommendations. (WHO, 2003).

Standard TB chemotherapy is quadruple therapy consisting of rifampicin, isoniazid, ethambutol and pyrizinamide and dosage is based on weight.

- Rifampicin (RIF, R) initial phase and continuation phase, 10 mg/kg once daily.
- Isoniazid (INH, H) initial phase and continuation phase, 5 mg/kg once daily.
- Pyrazinamide (PZA, Z) initial phase only, 25 mg/kg once daily.
- Ethambutol (EMB, E) initial phase only 15 mg/kg once daily.
- It is recommended to take the entire regimen on an empty stomach, e.g. early in the day, 1 hour before food. However, a small meal may be taken if required to reduce side effects.

This is the recommended combination as it is the most effective in the treatment of TB even in the case of TB/HIV co-infection (Maartens and Wilkinson, 2007). All four drugs are used for the initial phase which lasts 2 months. Rifampicin and isoniazid are continued for the continuation phase which lasts 4 months. In active meningeal TB, patients should be offered a treatment regimen lasting 12 months with the initial phase for 2 months (BNF, 2007). Corticosteroids should be started at the same time as anti-TB therapy in meningeal or pericardial TB. Streptomycin is used as an additional drug in retreatment of TB.

A common side effect of isoniazid is peripheral neuropathy, which is more likely to occur where there are pre-existing risk factors such as diabetes, alcohol dependence, chronic renal failure, malnutrition and HIV infection. Pyridoxine (vitamin B6) 10–25 mg daily may be given prophylactically from the beginning of treatment.

There are potential drug interactions between ART and TB therapy due to shared metabolic pathways, as Rifampicin is a powerful inducer of cytochrome P450 enzymes. The alternative use of rifabutin may overcome some of the difficulties in co-administration of rifampicin with protease inhibitors and non-nucleosides, however, the high cost of the drug makes it unavailable in many countries. When Rifabutin is not available, Efavirenz is recommended instead of Nevirapine and Protease Inhibitors are preferably not used. Rifampicin causes significant decreases in all Protease Inhibitors and increased liver toxicity is likely. If modified doses of Protease Inhibitors are used careful monitoring of liver enzymes is required.

Overlapping toxicity profiles may exist, including peripheral neuropathy with stavudine and isoniazid, or rash with non-nucleoside reverse transcriptase inhibitors (NNRTIs) and rifampicin. These situations require more careful monitoring (BHIVA, 2005). Significant drug interactions exist with many other non HIV medicines (ATS 2003).

Patients with poor drug adherence, those who are homeless or have drug or alcohol dependencies may benefit from directly observed therapy (DOT), where drugs are given supervised three times a week (BNF, 2007) (see Appendix 14).

18.4.2   TB resistance

TB resistance develops most commonly when those on TB treatment do not adhere to the recommended dosage regimen or they are infected with a strain of multi-drug resistant (MDR) TB. This may include stopping treatment early, missing or skipping doses or neglecting to take one or more of the prescribed medications. Inadequate dosing frequently enables the bacteria to become resistant to a certain drug (BNF, 2007). Resistance to TB therapy has to be considered and addressed at a local level.

Multi-drug resistant TB is a form of TB that is resistant to two or more of the primary drugs (isoniazid and rifampicin) used for treatment. MDR-TB is a serious and expanding public health concern (WHO, 2007). Treatment of MDR TB depends on Drug Susceptibility Testing results and surveillance. BTS guidelines should be consulted for guidance on management.

Extensively Drug Resistant TB (XDR-TB) is a strand of MDR-TB, which, is resistant to any fluoroquinolone and at least 1 of 3 injectable second-line drugs and it also demonstrates resistance to isoniazid and rifampicin. XDR-TB is increasingly prevalent in developing countries.

Treatment of both MDR-TB and XDR-TB remains a challenge in health care settings. The best treatment is prevention of drug resistance.

18.4.3   Prevention

The efficient diagnosis and treatment of people with TB offers the best protection against the spread of the disease. In some cases, immunisation has played a role in preventing TB but the vaccination does not offer full protection. The Bacille Calmette-Guerin (BCG) vaccine provides some protection but the duration of protection is variable. The vaccine does not reduce the transmission of TB (Maartens and Wilkinson, 2007). (See Appendix 15).

18.5   Nutrition, HIV infection and TB

18.5.1   Nutritional status can affect susceptibility to TB and outcomes of TB treatment in PLHIV

Protein-energy malnutrition is an important determinant in susceptibility to infection, particularly HIV and TB co-infection. This is apparent in developing countries where the prevalence of infectious diseases is high (Schaible and Kaufmann, 2007). The hormone leptin, which is a central mediator connecting nutrition and immunity, is reduced in people with protein-energy malnutrition. Body fat and leptin concentrations are correlated, with leptin levels quickly decreasing with fasting. Animal studies have shown that leptin-deficient mice are more susceptible to TB, suggesting that leptin may provide a level of protection against TB. More research in this area is required (Schaible and Kaufmann, 2007).

18.5.2   Factors affecting nutritional status in PLHIV with co-infection with TB

Malnutrition may predispose to TB but TB also causes malnutrition. Social and biological factors contribute to malnutrition in PLHIV and TB.

Social

TB can be highly stigmatised and, in combination with HIV, may reduce economic productivity, decrease individual and/or family food production and reduce access of PLHIV to food, leading to food insecurity and subsequent malnutrition.

Biological

Active TB is associated with malnutrition cachexia, weight loss and low serum concentrations of leptin. Leptin regulates satiety and has a vital role in activating and stimulating various immune cells (Schaible and Kaufmann, 2007). TB can therefore reduce appetite and lead to inadequate dietary intake.

HIV and TB co-infection is also associated with anaemia and hypoalbuminaema (Swaminathan *et al.*, 2008).

Protein-energy malnutrition and low body mass index (BMI) is common in adults presenting with TB and HIV infection (van Lettow *et al.*, 2003). In developing countries, between 30 and 80% of TB patients are undernourished at diagnosis and moderate-to-severe undernutrition is associated with increased mortality (Zachariah *et al.*, 2002; Ockenga *et al.*, 2006). Active TB increases energy expenditure and the combination of both TB and HIV infections results in a greater decrease in body cell mass and fat mass than HIV infection alone (Paton *et al.*, 2004).

Various micronutrient deficiencies have been noted in people with TB and HIV but more research is required to determine the role in prevention and treatment of the infection (Table 18.1).

Data supports the protective role of vitamin D in TB (Schwenk and Macallan, 2000). Research has shown that vitamin D boosts anti-TB immunity. Vitamin D has no direct impact on TB bacteria but regulates the immune response by inducing interleukin-10. Interleukin-10 is a cytokine with anti-inflammatory and immune-stimulating properties. Cytokines are known to be down regulated in TB and HIV infection (Martineau *et al.*, 2005).

Table 18.1   Specific micronutrients and TB infection.

Nutrient	Role in TB infection
Vitamin A	The role of vitamin A in infection is well documented (Ambrus and Ambrus, 2004). Vitamin A deficiency has been noted in children and adults with HIV and TB infection
Vitamin D	Vitamin D deficiency has been observed in those infected with TB
Vitamin B complex	No difference seen in those with and without TB
Vitamin E	Prior to the introduction of effective ART, plasma serum levels were low
Vitamin C	May have a protective role against TB
Iron	Anaemia is prevalent among adults with pulmonary TB infection, but it is unclear whether it is related to other chronic diseases and it is important to distinguish between iron deficiency anaemia and anaemia of chronic infection (Ambrus and Ambrus, 2004).
Zinc	Zinc deficiency results in reduced T4 helper cell population and a decrease in killer cell activity, failure to thrive and anorexia (Ambrus and Ambrus, 2004).

Source: van Lettow *et al.* (2003).

Martineau *et al.*'s research group conducted a randomised controlled trial with 202 patients with active TB in East London, UK. The participants were assigned to either a single dose of vitamin D or a placebo. Blood levels of both 25-hydroxy-vitamin D and the TB bacteria levels were measured at baseline, day 7 and day 49. The research has shown that mycobacterial immunity was stronger in the vitamin D supplemented group. This research has raised the issue of whether routine vitamin D should be prescribed for people with TB. More research is required to determine if vitamin D deficiency can predispose someone to TB or whether vitamin D deficiency can occur as a consequence of TB.

In a study conducted by Kassu *et al.* (2006), it was demonstrated that TB patients had lower concentrations of iron, zinc and selenium, and higher concentrations of copper compared with those without TB. Zinc deficiency may be implicated in the activation of TB, as it plays a role in decreasing production of cytokines involved in immune system regulation. Plasma concentrations of copper are known to increase as a result of infection and inflammation. Low serum iron concentrations may be associated with inflammation. More research is required to determine if anaemia is related to TB. This study raises the question of routine nutritional supplementation in TB (Kassu, 2006).

18.6   Nutrition screening

The malnutrition universal screening tool (MUST) used in the UK may help identify those at risk of malnutrition. The tool is linked to a care plan outlining quick and effective dietary changes or referral for specialist advice (BAPEN, 2007). (See Chapter 8, 'Nutritional Screening and Assessment'.)

18.7   Nutrition assessment: special considerations in TB

To determine the most appropriate nutritional support in PLHIV with TB, it is important to distinguish between depletion of muscle mass (wasting) and peripheral fat loss (lipoatrophy) (Ockenga *et al.*, 2006). A study of PLHIV with TB in India found that weight loss was associated with loss of fat in female patients and loss of body cell mass in male patients. Anthropometry and bioelectrical impedance analysis (BIA) are simple field tools which can be used to assess body composition in PLHIV with TB.

18.7.1   Symptom identification

TB can increase the production of inflammatory cytokines (van Lettow *et al.*, 2003), which leads to reduced appetite, weight loss and diarrhoea resulting in wasting. A detailed nutrition assessment should include presence, duration and severity of symptoms.

18.7.2   Micronutrient status

Micronutrient deficiencies have been noted in some studies of people with TB infection. Assessment of micronutrient status may be required when deficiencies are suspected.

18.8   Nutritional treatment/intervention

The short-term goals of nutritional therapy in TB and HIV include optimising nutritional intake, attaining and maintaining ideal body weight, restoring lean body mass (LBM), decreasing functional impairment from undernutrition (incapacity to work and muscular fatigue), improving tolerance to ART, the provision of nutrients according to daily requirements, preventing further nutrient deficiencies and improving quality of life (Ockenga *et al.*, 2006).

Treatment of TB wasting may consist of anti-TB therapy and nutritional support. Most patients will gain weight after starting antibacterial therapy but this alone may not be enough to restore weight and normalise BMI (Schwenk and Macallan,y 2000).

Patients often report reduced oral intake while taking TB medications as well as adverse side effects from taking TB medications on an empty stomach. Both of these issues will impact on nutritional status. Liaising with other members of the multidisciplinary team is essential to ensure both TB medication adherence and nutritional intake. If gastrointestinal side effects are present (ie nausea, stomach pain, poor appetite) medicines may be given with small meals or at night before sleeping. Smaller meals more often are encouraged and half portions of supplements may encourage appetite and intake.

18.8.1   Supplements

Oral nutrition supplements were found to be preferable with regard to weight gain and muscle strength in patients with TB who had lost weight. Research shows that patients who receive early nutritional support show greater weight gain, increased LBM and grip strength (Paton *et al.*, 2004).

Lower carbohydrate diets or supplements are not recommended for PLHIV with active pulmonary TB, especially when underweight. There is inadequate evidence to support their use in this patient population and may contribute to reduced kilojoule intake.

Micronutrient supplementation has been shown to increase weight in patients with pulmonary TB (Range *et al.*, 2005). Routine micronutrient supplementation should be considered in view of TB-associated weight loss and HIV. Advice on levels of micro- and macronutrients may be required in some cases if there is a risk of excessive use of multivitamins and minerals.

Texture medication may be required depending on individual symptoms, including fatigue as a result of difficulty in breathing. If oral diet and optimal use of nutritional supplements, do not promote optimum nutritional intake enteral feeding may be appropriate. Enteral feeding is indicated during acute infections, sustained poor oral intake or established undernourishment and can provide either supplementary or full nutritional requirements (Ockenga *et al.*, 2006). Nasogastric feeding is an ideal short-term option, while for long-term nutritional support a percutaneous endoscopic gastrostomy (PEG) should be considered. Standard feeds with fibre allow for normal bowel function and higher energy feeds give more calories in less volume. In gastrointestinal patients, elemental and semi-elemental feeds may be used in situations where malabsorption is a clinical issue. Parenteral nutrition should only be used when the gastrointestinal tract is not functioning.

18.8.2 Resource-poor settings

Providing food assistance to PLHIV with food insecurity as an incentive to complete TB treatment can improve compliance. Food by prescription (FBP) programming may also be appropriate for PLHIV who are malnourished. FBP programming aims to improve health and/or treatment outcomes in patients who are clinically malnourished, by providing short-term, individual nutritional supplementation with a specialised commodity. Nutrition counselling is recommended to be provided to all patients receiving food support in these settings.

18.9 Recommendations

Research into the nutritional aspects of TB is limited with even less specifically addressing nutrition in HIV and TB co-infection. More research is required into the role of specific micronutrients in the pathogenesis and treatment of TB. The role of generic vitamin and mineral supplementation in the treatment of TB should be investigated.

Nutrition guidelines for TB and nutrition should be developed when there is a greater evidence base to support both new and current practice.

Before being immunised with BCG, a tuberculin skin test (called Heaf) is preformed to test previous exposure to the TB bacteria. If there is no reaction, it shows that there has been no contact with TB or the BCG vaccine and immunisation is indicated. A positive reaction can indicate previous or current infection with TB and vaccination is not indicated. A tuberculin skin test and BCG vaccinations are not recommended for those with HIV as BCG is a live vaccine and could cause illness (DOH, 2007). A more effective vaccine is required to greatly improve TB control. Vaccinologists are involved in developing novel vaccines in animal studies, which are in phase I and II clinical trials (Maartens and Wilkinson, 2007).

Acknowledgements

The authors would like to thank Jennifer Swan, HIV specialist pharmacist, Newham University Hospital, Rebecca Wilkins, Clinical Nurse Specialist (HIV), Newham Primary Care Trust and Jason Bower, Regional HIV Specialist Pharmacist, Secretariat of the Pacific Community.

References

Ambrus JL Sr, Ambrus JL Jr. Nutrition and infectious diseases in developing countries and problems of acquired immunodeficiency syndrome. *Exp Biol Med* 2004; 229:464–72.

ATS, CDC, and Infectious Diseases Society of America. Treatment of tuberculosis. *MMWR* 2003; 52 (No. RR-11). http://www.cdc.gov/mmwr/PDF/rr/rr5211.pdf Errata – http://www.cdc.gov/mmwr/preview/mmwrhtml/mm5351a5.htm

British Association of Parenteral and Enteral Nutrition (BAPEN). *The MUST Report. Nutritional Screening of Adults: A Multidisciplinary Responsibility.* UK: BAPEN, 2007.

British HIV Association (BHIVA). *BHIVA Treatment Guidelines for TB/HIV Infection.* London: BHIVA, 2005.

British National Formulary (BNF). *British National Formulary.* London: BMJ Publishing Group, 2007.

Carballo M, Divino JJ, Zeric D. Migration and health in the European Union. *Trop Med Int Health* 1998; 3(12):936–44.

Collins KR, Quinones-Mateu ME, Toossi Z, Arts EJ. Impact of Tuberculosis on HIV-1 replication, diversity, and disease progression. *AIDS Rev* 2002; 1(4):165–76.

Department of Health (DOH). *Stopping Tuberculosis in England. An Action Plan from the Chief Medical Officer.* London: DOH, 2004.

Department of Health (DOH). 2007. http://www.dh.gov.uk/en/Policyandguidance/Healthand-socialcaretopics/Greenbook/DH_4097254. Accessed on 29 October 2007.

Health Protection Agency (HPA). *Tuberculosis in the UK: Annual Report on Tuberculosis Surveillance and Control in the UK.* London: Health Protection Agency Centre for Infections, 2007. Available at http://www.hpa.org.uk/infections/topics_az/tb/menu.htm. Accessed on 12 July 2007.

Johnson JL, Ellner JJ. *Clinical Infectious Diseases.* Oxford: Oxford University Press, 1999.

Kassu A, Yabutani T, Mahmud ZH *et al.* Alterations in serum levels of trace elements in tuberculosis and HIV infections. *Eur J Clin Nutr* 2006; 60:580–86.

Maartens G, Wilkinson RJ. Tuberculosis. *Lancet* 2007; 370(9604):2030–43.

Mandal BK, Wilkins EGL, Dunar EM, Mayon-White RT. *Infectious Diseases.* Oxford: Blackwell Publishing, 2004.

Martineau A *et al.* Effect of vitamin D supplementation on anti-mycobacterial immunity: a double-blind randomised placebo-controlled trial in London tuberculosis contacts. *Int J Tuberc Lung Dis* 2005; 9(11 supp 1):S173.

Mattson Porth C. *Essentials of Pathophysiology.* London: Lippincott Williams & Wilkins, 2007.

Mugusi F, Villamor E, Urassa W, Saathoff E, Bosch RJ, Fawzi WW. HIV co-infection, CD4 cell counts and clinical correlates of bicillary density in Pulmonary tuberculosis. *Int J Tuberc Lung Dis* 2006; 10(6):663–9

Murray PR, Rosenthal KS, Pfaller MA. *Medical Microbiology.* Philadelphia, USA: Elsevier Mosby, 2005.

Ockenga J *et al.* ESPEN guidelines on enteral nutrition: wasting in HIV and other chronic infectious diseases. *Clin Nutr* 2006; 25:319–29.

Paton NI, Chua YK, Earnest A, Chee CB. Randomized controlled trial of nutritional supplementation in patients with newly diagnosed tuberculosis and wasting. *Am J Clin Nutr* 2004; 80:460–65.

Pratt RJ. *HIV and AIDS: A Foundation for Nursing and Healthcare Practice.* 5th edn., London: Arnold, 2003.

Range N *et al.* The effect of micronutrient supplementation on treatment outcome in patients with pulmonary tuberculosis: a randomized controlled trial in Mwanza, Tanzania. *Trop Med Int Health* 2005; 10(9):826–32.

Schaible UE, Kaufmann SHE. Malnutrition and infection: complex mechanisms and global impacts. *PLoS Med* 2007; 4(5).

Schwenk A, Macallan D. Tuberculosis, malnutrition and wasting. *Curr Opin Clin Nutr Metab Care* 2000; 3:285–91.

Swaminathan S, Padmapriyadarsini C, Sukumar B *et al.* Nutritional status of persons with HIV infection, persons with HIV infection and tuberculosis, and HIV-negative individuals from southern India. *Clin Infect Dis* 2008; 46(6):946–9.

van Lettow M, Fawzi WW, Semba RD. Triple trouble: the role of malnutrition in tuberculosis and human immunodeficiency virus co-infection. *Nutr Rev* 2003; 61:81–90.

WHO Report. Global tuberculosis control: a short update to the 2009 report, Geneva, 2009. Available at http://www.who.int/tb/publications/global_report/2009/update/en/index.html. Accessed on 12 May 2009.

World Health Organization (WHO). *Treatment of Tuberculosis: Guidelines for National Programmes*, 3rd edn. Geneva: WHO/CDS/TB/2003.313 World Health Organization, 2003. Available at http://whqlibdoc.who.int/hq/2003/WHO_CDS_TB_2003.313_eng.pdf. Accessed on 31 August 2009.

World Health Organization (WHO). The 5 Elements of DOTS. 2007. Available at http://www.who.int/tb/dots/whatisdots/en/index4.html. Accessed on 30 June 2007.

19 The Nutritional Management of Patients Living with HIV and Renal Disease

Deepa Kariyawasam

Key Points

- HIVAN is the third most common cause of end-stage renal disease (ESRD) amongst African-Americans between the ages of 20 and 64 in the United States.
- Renal failure may be present in two forms: acute (short term) or chronic.
- Dietary treatment depends on the stage of kidney disease, nutritional status and modality of treatment.
- The symptoms of poor renal function, e.g. nausea and anorexia, as well as patients adhering to dietary restrictions during periods of insufficient intake can contribute to malnutrition.
- Increased losses of protein during renal replacement therapy necessitate higher protein requirements.
- All patients with HIV should have estimated glomerular filtration rate (eGFR) and proteinuria measures at baseline. Certain patient groups are advised to be screened annually, e.g. people of African origin, those with CD4 < 200 cells/uL or HIV RNA levels >4000 copies/ml, and those with diabetes, hypertension or hepatitis C virus.

19.1 Introduction

Renal failure can occur in people living with HIV (PLHIV) due to many reasons. Renal failure may become present in either of two forms: acute or chronic. Acute renal failure (ARF) also known as acute kidney injury (AKI) is a short-term loss of renal function which may be caused by sepsis, dehydration or nephrotoxic agents (including antiretroviral therapy). Chronic renal failure (CRF) is a long-term decline in renal function. The single most common cause of CRF in PLHIV is HIV-associated nephropathy (HIVAN) (Winston *et al.*, 1998). HIVAN is the third most common cause of end-stage renal disease (ESRD) amongst African-Americans between the ages of 20 and 64 in the United States. The deterioration in renal function in HIVAN is caused by an inflammatory process in the glomeruli of the kidney, and it is found almost exclusively in the black population. HIVAN is caused by the direct effect of HIV-1 on renal cells (Herman and Klotman, 2003). Despite HIVAN being the most common cause of CRF in this patient group, the incidence of HIVAN is decreasing while the use of antiretrovirals is increasing (Blower *et al.*, 2003). HIVAN is not the sole cause of renal failure in PLHIV as other conditions such as diabetes, hypertension, vascular disease and nephrotoxic drugs can also lead to the development of chronic kidney disease (CKD) in patients with a background of HIV. Those who tend to develop HIVAN tend not to have been diagnosed with HIV prior to the diagnosis of HIVAN and therefore have a high viral load and low CD4 count, whereas those that have non-HIVAN CKD tend to have been diagnosed with HIV for longer and are more likely to be on ART on diagnosis of CKD.

19.2 Presentation and symptoms

The features of HIVAN are similar to the features found in nephrotic syndrome, such as proteinuria, hypoalbuminaemia, oedema and hypercholesterolaemia, although the latter two characteristics may not always be present. People with HIVAN are likely to have a high viral load, fatigue, malaise, anorexia and pruritis. Due to the high viral load, they may also have other symptoms associated with this. Some of the features of advanced HIV disease may exacerbate weight loss in conjunction with the poor appetite and nausea associated with uraemia.

19.3 Screening

Guidelines suggest that all PLHIV should have estimated glomerular filtration rate (eGFR) and proteinuria measures at baseline. Certain patient groups are advised to be screened annually, e.g. people of African origin, those with CD4 < 200 cells/uL or HIV RNA levels >4000 copies/ml, and those with diabetes, hypertension or hepatitis C virus. People with proteinuria greater than or equal to 1+, or those with eGFR less than 60 are advised to be referred to a nephrologist (Gupta *et al.*, 2005).

19.4 Diagnosis

HIVAN is usually diagnosed by the presence of proteinuria (>3.5 g/24 hours), along with large echogenic kidneys on ultrasound, and is confirmed by renal biopsy. Renal biopsy will also help differentiate between HIVAN and other causes of CKD (e.g. hypertension and diabetes). Serum creatinine itself may be a poor marker of renal function, as levels may be low in malnourished people with reduced muscle mass. In these patients the low body mass should be borne in mind when interpreting eGFR. If HIVAN is caught early, the progression may be reversed or halted in some cases, while others may develop end-stage renal disease and require dialysis. The treatment to halt the progression of HIVAN is antiretroviral treatment (ART) and ACE inhibitors, which work by reducing the capillary pressure in the glomeruli (Wei *et al.*, 2003). Since the advent of effective combination anti-HIV treatment, the prognosis for people with HIVAN has improved. If the CKD is due to another co-morbidity, e.g. diabetes or hypertension, then gaining good control of these conditions can help limit the progression of CKD.

19.5 Classification of chronic kidney disease

Chronic kidney disease is classified into five stages, regardless of its cause:

Stage 1 GFR >90: normal kidney function but urine findings, structural abnormalities or genetic trait indicate kidney disease
Stage 2 GFR 60–89: mildly reduced kidney function

Stage 3 GFR 30–59: moderately reduced kidney function
Stage 4 GFR 15–29: severely reduced kidney function
Stage 5 GFR < 15: very severe, end-stage kidney disease (ESKD) or end-stage renal
   failure (ESRF)

19.6 Treatment

Treatment for HIVAN is dependent on the stage of kidney disease. ART and ACE inhibitors can help to halt progression as well as steroids. ACE inhibitors can help reduce proteinuria and also reduce the decline in creatinine clearance. People who have reached ESRF will need to be treated with renal replacement therapy. The progression to ESRF can be rapid, occurring over only a few weeks to months. In the UK 56% of people with HIVAN developed ESRF after a median of 4.2 years of which 35% developed ESRF in less than 3 months (Post *et al.*, 2008).

19.7 Methods of renal replacement therapy

19.7.1 Haemodialysis

Blood is filtered extracorporeally via an artificial membrane. Haemodialysis is carried out either in the centre or at home. Home haemodialysis may not always be available in all units and may not be suitable for some patients. People with cramped living accommodation may not be suitable for home haemodialysis, as the equipment and machine can take up large amounts of space. Haemodialysis is usually carried out for approximately 4 hours, three times per week. The time of treatment is dependent on the patient's residual renal function and muscle mass.

19.7.2 Peritoneal dialysis

A catheter (Tenckhoff) is placed into the peritoneal cavity and solutes are removed by diffusion against a concentration gradient produced by the glucose in the dialysate bag. The peritoneum acts as a dialysis membrane and the dialysate with the solutes is then drained out several hours afterwards. This is a daily process.

Peritoneal dialysis may be done continuously or be automated. Continuous ambulatory peritoneal dialysis (CAPD) is carried out by infusing a bag into the peritoneal cavity, and leaving it to dwell for 6 to 8 hours before draining it out and then replacing it with a new bag. This is done throughout the day and 3–4 bags may be used over the course of a 24-hour period.

Automated peritoneal dialysis (APD) is a type of dialysis whereby a machine drains in and out several doses of dialysate overnight automatically. Some patients may also have another bag indwelling during the day. The choice between APD or CAPD is dependent on the state of the patient's peritoneal membrane and lifestyle.

Peritoneal dialysis is carried out by the patient at home and thus patients need to have good dexterity and be able to lift the dialysis bags. People who live in cramped living accommodations (such as small bedsits, hostels) may not be suitable for this type of dialysis because of the amount of room needed to store the dialysis bags. Good hygiene is also essential to help prevent episodes of peritonitis. If patients are assessed to be suitable for this treatment, then those with HIV on PD and HD have similar survival rates. The peritonitis rates between HIV-infected patients and non-HIV-infected patients is no different (Kimmel *et al.*, 1993).

19.8   Renal transplantation

Renal transplantation is also an option and the number of transplants being carried out in the HIV population is increasing. UK transplant guidelines suggest the factors that need to be considered prior to listing a patient for renal transplant. Some of the criteria suggested are:

- a life expectancy of at least 5 years
- CD4 count >200 cells/mm^3 for at least 6 months
- undetectable HIV viraemia (<50 copies/ml) for at least 6 months
- adherence and stable ART regimen for 6 months (Brook, 2005).

19.8.1   Nutritional considerations for chronic kidney disease stages 1–3

Stage 1–3 CKD does not usually lead to uraemic symptoms and thus appetite is not usually affected but oral intake may be limited due to the symptoms caused by advanced HIV disease or other co-morbidities. If patients are complaining of poor appetite or unintentional weight loss, the primary aim is to meet nutritional requirements.

For adequately nourished patients with good appetite and stable weight, the main nutritional aims are to ensure good control of blood sugar and blood pressure, as diabetes and hypertension may contribute to impaired renal function. These patients are unlikely to require any electrolyte restriction other than sodium restriction. Occasionally, patients on ACE inhibitors and angiotensin receptor blockers may develop mild hyperkalaemia and may need to consider restricting their potassium intake slightly, but this is usually done on an individual basis rather than routinely.

Controlling blood pressure

Good blood pressure control has been shown to slow the progression of renal dysfunction. Evidence from the general population has shown that reduced salt diets can help lower blood pressure and that some groups are more sensitive to salt – such as people of African and Caribbean origin and people with type 2 diabetes (Luft and Weinberger, 1997). One of the dietary approaches found to help lower blood pressure is the DASH (Dietary Approaches to Stop Hypertension) diet. The DASH diet, which is rich in fruit, vegetables and low-fat dairy products, lowers blood pressure more than a reduced salt (Na < 100 mmol/day) diet alone (Sacks *et al.*, 2001). The DASH diet, due to its higher potassium content, will not be suitable for people with very poor renal function but may be beneficial for those with only slightly decreased kidney function and well controlled potassium levels. A reduction in salt would nonetheless be beneficial for all patients, despite their level of kidney function. Evidence in the UK has shown that in black populations, most of the salt is added at home in cooking or at the table. This is in contrast to white Europeans, where most of the salt in the diet comes from processed foods (data from CASH). People of African and Caribbean origin may add salt in a variety of ways. Examples include salt, monosodium glutamate seasonings (MSG), Maggi/Oxo cubes and jerk seasoning. These salt-based seasonings should be reduced and other herbs and spices should be encouraged instead.

Achieving good glycaemic control

People with diabetes should ensure that their blood glucose levels are well controlled with diet or diet and medication as good management of blood glucose levels can help reduce the risk of progression of renal disease among people with diabetes.

19.8.2   Nutritional considerations for CKD stage 4

The symptoms of uraemia will occur at this stage and patients may suffer from nausea, taste changes and anorexia as a result. Patients can also be acidotic and this has been found to lead to muscle loss in renal patients (Reaich et al., 1995). Correction with a bicarbonate supplement such as sodium bicarbonate is advisable when bicarbonate levels are low.

Potassium, salt, phosphate moderation and nutrition support are dietetic treatments often needed during stage 4 CKD (see Table 19.1).

Protein requirements vary depending on the stage of kidney disease. European guidelines suggest 0.6–1.0 g protein per kg IBW for pre-dialysis, 1–1.2 g/kg IBW for HD patients and 1.2–1.5 g/kg IBW for PD patients (James and Jackson, 2002). Historically, and in some developing countries, low-protein diets are still being followed, but in the UK and the United States, 0.8–1.0 g/kg IBW is the level that most dietitians will aim for with pre-dialysis patients. The reason for avoiding low-protein diets is to prevent malnutrition. Some evidence suggests that low-protein diets can slow the progression of chronic kidney disease, but this has to be considered in conjunction with the risks of malnutrition. Many patients, as they develop uraemia, spontaneously decrease their intake of protein and thus it is important to ensure they are receiving adequate amounts. Patients who are taking only 0.6–0.8 g/kg protein per day need to ensure that at least 50% is from high biological value proteins.

19.8.3   Nutritional considerations for CKD stage 5

Patients will either be treated with renal replacement therapy or may be conservatively managed (no dialysis). The decision for conservative management or dialysis is based on the patient's long-term prognosis and choice. The majority will be started on dialysis and the symptoms of uraemia, such as anorexia and nausea, will improve as dialysis is established. Acidosis is also improved as bicarbonate is added to the dialysis. Those who choose to be conservatively treated will still receive medication, such as anti-emetics, iron and erythropoiesis-stimulating agents, to help keep them symptom free. Patients who choose to be conservatively managed may have many years to live and therefore dietary restrictions, such as potassium moderation, may be appropriate if the patient is eating well and has room for dietary improvement.

Table 19.1 Nutritional requirements for CKD stages 4–5.

Modality	Energy	Protein	Phosphorous	Potassium	Sodium	Fluid
HD	30–35 kcal/kg IBW*	1–1.2 g/kg IBW	1000–1400 mg/d (32–45 mmol/d)	2000–2500 mg/d (50–65 mmol/d)	1800–2500 mg/d (80–110 mmol/d)	500 mls + 24 hr urine output
PD	30–35 kcal/kg IBW* (this includes the calories absorbed from PD)	1–1.2 g/kg IBW Peritonitis = 1.5 g/kg IBW†	1000–1400 mg/d (32–45 mmol/d)	2000–2500 mg/d (50–65 mmol/d)	1800–2500 mg/d (80–110 mmol/d)	800 mls + 24 hr urine output
Pre-dialysis	30–35 kcal/ kg IBW*	0.6–1.0 g/kg IBW‡	600–1000 mg/d (19–32 mmol/d)	2000–2500 mg/d (50–65 mmol/d)	1800–2500 mg/d (80–110 mmol/d)	Only restrict if oedematous or medically indicated

*30 kcal/kg IBW should be considered for the elderly and those with limited mobility.
†Peritoneal dialysis patients with peritonitis have large protein losses and therefore will benefit from a higher intake of protein.
‡Pre-dialysis patients who are receiving less than 0.8 g protein/kg IBW should be monitored regularly by an experienced renal dietitian due to the risk of malnutrition.

Adapted from James and Jackson (2002), with permission.
IBW = ideal body weight.

19.9   Nutritional issues on dialysis

Problems with eating may occur if patients on dialysis develop infections. Common infections found in renal patients are line infections (haemodialysis patients) and peritonitis (PD patients). In addition to these infections, which can also occur in the non-HIV dialysis population, the HIV patient with end-stage renal failure is immunocompromised and therefore more susceptible to infections. As the infection is treated with antibiotics, appetite will be likely to improve. To limit the risk of infection, patients undergoing PD are taught good hygiene practices. Those who undergo haemodialysis are encouraged to have dialysis via a fistula rather than a line due to the reduced risk of infections with a fistula.

19.9.1   Nutritional issues specific to peritoneal dialysis

Patients on peritoneal dialysis may also find that they feel full more quickly due to the volume of fluid in the abdominal cavity, and also since glucose absorption from the dialysate can dull the appetite. Some patients, concerned about body image, may have difficulty adjusting to the presence of dialysis fluid in the peritoneum and therefore may feel that they need to adjust what they are eating to compensate for the slightly distended abdomen.

19.9.2   Nutritional issues specific to haemodialysis

Patients who have in-centre haemodialysis and require hospital transport may spend a large part of their day in transport or on the dialysis machine; as a result the time to fit in meals may be limited. They should be encouraged to bring their own food to the dialysis centres (if this practice conforms with the Renal Unit procedures). Some haemodialysis units do specify a no-food rule during dialysis. The reasons for this include infection risk as well as the risk of aspiration due to a drop in blood pressure caused by the shift of blood to the splanchnic regions (Barakat *et al.*, 1993). The evidence for not eating on dialysis is limited and therefore each patient should be assessed on an individual basis, as many can tolerate eating on dialysis and, in many UK units, it is common practice for patients to eat on HD.

19.10   Nutritional assessment

Anthropometry such as weight and height may be sufficient for euvolaemic patients, but for those who are fluid overloaded, assessing weight may be problematic as patients may not always be aware of their dry weight. Fluid-overloaded patients may benefit from subjective global assessment (SGA) as a nutritional assessment. Subjective global assessment looks at the patient's weight change, GI symptoms, trend of current intake and fat and muscle stores. Multifrequency, multisegmental body composition machines can also be used for analysis of fat and muscle mass. Multifrequency bioelectrical impedance analysers can differentiate between extracellular and intracellular water (Earthman *et al.*, 2007) and hence the amount of excess fluid can be estimated.

When assessing the oral intake of haemodialysis patients, consider taking a diet history for both HD and non-HD days, as patients tend to eat less on dialysis days due to the time spent travelling (Burrowes *et al.*, 2003).

19.11   Nutritional requirements

The nutritional requirements for people with renal failure are dependent on the stage of kidney function and modality of treatment. The main nutrients to consider are calories, protein, potassium, sodium, phosphate and fluid.

Renal failure per se does not appear to increase energy requirements, but patients on PD can absorb 40–60% of glucose from the dialysis bags, depending on the type of peritoneal dialysis and membrane characteristics (McCann, 2002). Energy requirements from food should therefore be amended in patients on PD. Protein requirements are raised in dialysis patients due to the increased losses of protein during dialysis. PD patients can lose approximately 10 g protein per day and during peritonitis lose a further 50% (Bannister *et al.*, 1987; Lindholm and Bergstrom 1988). The ratio of calories to protein therefore needed for a patient on PD is quite different to a patient on HD. Some patients on PD manage to maintain their weight inadvertently, as their appetite drops due to the glucose absorption and the volume of PD fluid. The protein intake of these patients needs to be monitored to ensure that they have not decreased their protein intake as well.

19.12   Treatment

19.12.1   Nutrition support

During episodes of PD peritonitis, appetite may decrease due to nausea and vomiting so it may not always be possible to meet nutritional requirements. Consider using protein-rich sip feeds, which have a higher protein to calorie ratio, rather than standard sip feeds, as these will help replace the large amounts of protein that can be lost. Usually, the amounts lost are approximately 10 g (Young *et al.*, 1987), which is more than the amounts lost via urine in healthy adults. The requirements detailed in Table 19.1 take into account the general increase in protein loss but if patients are not thriving, despite meeting these levels, the patient may benefit from having their protein losses via PD fluid measured.

Some renal units have 1.1% amino acid-based peritoneal dialysis fluids; in small studies, these fluids have been found to offset the losses of protein and amino acids (Kopple *et al.*, 1995; Jones *et al.*, 1998; Tjiong *et al.*, 2005).

Patients on HD can also receive extra calories in the form of intra-dialytic parenteral nutritition (IDPN), but the calories that can be gained is approximately 1000 kcal per session (average of 400 kcal per day). IDPN is not usually used as a first-line treatment of malnutrition, but it can be useful for patients who are refusing any other form of nutritional support (sip feeds or enteral feeds). IDPN is usually given at the venous return during HD and therefore can be an easy method of nutrient delivery. IDPN usually contains very little electrolytes and no vitamins or minerals and therefore may need to be used with caution in patients at risk of refeeding syndrome. If calories and protein are being met with minimal diet, modular feeds (e.g. fat or glucose replacements) and IDPN, then a multivitamin and mineral supplement should be considered.

Most ready-made oral supplements (Fortijuce, Ensure and Resource Shake) are suitable for renal patients but powdered supplements that are made with fresh milk (Complan, Build Up and Scandishake) may have higher potassium and phosphate contents than the pre-made sip feeds. If a patient's oral intake is very poor, then any supplement can be prescribed, since the supplement will replace food they would normally eat, but if supplements are being used to help weight gain, and the patient is eating full meals and snacks, then pre-made sip feeds may be beneficial due to their lower potassium and phosphate content. When counselling patients requiring nutrition support, it is important that the whole team is aware that fluid requirements may be relaxed, as usually fluid allowances given to patients only take the liquids at room temperature into consideration and thus do not include the fluid from solid food. A decreased intake of solid food can therefore enable a larger intake of fluids in the form of supplements if needed.

19.12.2 Achieving good potassium control

Potassium restriction is rarely needed in patients with eGFR >30 unless they are on medications which cause hyperkalaemia, such as ACE inhibitors and angiotensin receptor blockers. Those with GFR values dropping below 30 may need potassium restriction once serum potassium reaches the upper end of the normal range (e.g. above 5 mmol/l). For those whose potassium is within range, review by a dietitian once GFR reaches 30 is beneficial to check that the patient is not taking excessively large amounts of potassium in the form of salt substitutes, juices and other high-potassium foods. Once serum potassium rises above 5.0 mmol/l, it is worth looking at the whole diet and avoiding peaks in potassium intake in any given day.

Ideal plasma potassium levels vary depending on the patient's treatment modality. In the UK those in pre-dialysis and PD should be maintained between 3.5 and 5.5 mmol/l, whereas those on HD may go up to 6.5 mmol/l (Renal Association, 2007). This is because those on HD are less likely to have much residual renal function left and therefore are likely to run a higher potassium level. Patients on haemodialysis seem to tolerate levels slightly higher than the recommended level for non-renal patients.

Some patients, as they are approaching dialysis, may have difficulty maintaining their potassium level below 5.5 mmol/l. If levels are above the recommendation despite good dietary adherence, it is worth discussing with the medical team to what they feel is an appropriate level. It is important that the patient continues as to have a balanced diet. If food groups are being omitted completely (e.g. fruits and vegetables) due to hyperkalaemia, then renal replacement therapy needs to be considered if appropriate.

Potassium can be affected by many factors other than diet: acidosis, which is common in the predialysis stage, can cause potassium to move from the intracellular to the extracellular compartment. Sodium bicarbonate can then be given to reduce potassium. Raised blood osmolality due to severe hyperglycaemia can also raise potassium (Stover, 2006). During renal failure the gut also adapts to remove more potassium and, therefore, once a patient with renal failure becomes constipated they can lose the ability to deplete some potassium via the gut. Gastrointestinal bleeding can also cause hyperkalaemia due to reabsorption of potassium from

Table 19.2 Foods to consider when restricting potassium.

High potassium foods	Lower potassium alternatives
Carbohydrate foods	**Carbohydrate foods**
Potatoes, yam and plantain (1 serving of 120–150 g boiled can be taken)	Rice, pasta, bread, cereals, maize and cornflour
Vegetables	
Pumpkin leaves, calaloo, okra, spinach, pak choi and cerassee	Cabbage, carrots, cho-cho (christophene), courgettes, aubergine, green beans, leeks,
Pulses, if taken in addition to large amounts of meat	cucumber, lettuce, peppers, bean sprouts, peas, broccoli, sweet corn and fresh or tinned
Tomato puree	tomatoes
Boiling potassium containing vegetables enables some potassium to leach out	
Fruits	
Dried fruit, bananas and avocado	Apples, pears, clementines, satsumas, grapes, raspberries and strawberries
	Tinned fruit (drained of juice)
Drinks	
Fruit and vegetable juices	Fruit squashes/cordials/carbonated drinks
Beer, cider, lager and wine	Spirits
Malted drinks, e.g. Horlicks, Ovaltine, Supermalt and Mighty Malt	Tea, herbal (supermarket type)/fruit teas. Coffee – up to 2 cups per day
Miscellaneous	
Salt substitutes (Lo Salt/So Low)	Oil, butter, margarine, sugar, spices and herbs
Kaun/'Rock salt' (Nigerian food tenderiser)	

haemolysed blood cells. Non-dietary reasons for raised potassium should be considered before dietary potassium intake is restricted. Medications such as ACE inhibitors and angiotensin receptor blockers can also cause hyperkalaemia but are unlikely to be stopped due to the beneficial effect these drugs have on blood pressure.

Table 19.2 does not contain any prescriptive amounts, as recommendations depend on the patient's current potassium level and baseline intake. Most patients needing potassium restriction should still be able to consume 4 portions of fruit and vegetables in total. If a patient is requiring further restriction, then other reasons for hyperkalaemia should be considered.

Use of food databases from various countries via the internet should be considered if potassium contents of certain foods are not available, as some patients may be consuming native foods which are not featured in some food composition publications. If unsure about a certain food, it is worth trying to find out which family the fruit or vegetable is related to. This may enable the health care professional to understand how high in potassium the food may be.

19.12.3   Achieving good phosphate control

Hyperphosphataemia

Hyperphosphataemia can occur in patients at stage 4–5 CKD. Hyperphosphataemia can, with time, lead to vascular calcification (Slatopolsky, 2003; Ritz and Gross, 2005) and renal bone disease. Patients with high levels may complain of itching and

Table 19.3 Protein to phosphorus ratio.

Food	Mg phosphorus per g protein
Beef	12.3 mg/g protein
Lamb	9.2 mg/g protein
Pork	7.3 mg/g protein
Chicken	8.8 mg/g protein
Liver	14.3 mg/g protein
Cheese	19.2 mg/g protein
Egg	16 mg/g protein
Sausages	16 mg/g protein

red eyes. Phosphate levels for those on dialysis should be 1.1–1.8 mmol/l and under 1.5 mmol/l for stage 4 patients in the UK (Cassidy *et al.*, 2007).

Patients approaching hyperphosphataemia or those who have increasing parathyroid hormone levels need to have their diet reviewed and if phosphate intake is within recommendations, then a phosphate binder (Table 19.4) may need to be prescribed. Phosphate is mainly found in foods rich in protein. As protein requirements for dialysis patients are high, patients may need phosphate binders to help maintain their phosphate levels (Rufino *et al.*, 1998).

Foods that need to be moderated are those foods with a high phosphorus to protein ratio (i.e. those foods that provide more phosphate per gram of protein), see Table 19.3.

Those on phosphate binders need to generally take them just before a meal containing phosphate (i.e. protein-rich foods). The exception is lanthanum carbonate which is taken post meals to prevent any GI disturbance.

Hypophosphataemia

Hypophosphataemia can also occur, possibly due to malnutrition but also as a result of Fanconi's syndrome. Fanconi's syndrome is a disorder which impairs the function of the proximal tubules. It reduces the reabsorption of certain electrolytes and can be caused by tenofovir. As well as hypophosphataemia, Fanconi's can lead to glycosuria, proteinuria and uricouria, whereas malnutrition will not cause these other symptoms.

Table 19.4 Types of phosphate binder.

Phosphate binder	Pros	Cons
Calcium carbonate	Inexpensive	Risk of raised calcium levels, which can lead to calcification
Calcium acetate	Better binding capacity than calcium carbonate therefore provides less calcium and relatively inexpensive	Large tablet, so difficult to swallow
Aluminium hydroxide	Very good binding and inexpensive	Risk of Al toxicity at high levels
Sevelamer	Non-calcium containing	High pill burden, cost
Lanthanum carbonate	Non-calcium containing	Cost

If hypophosphatemia occurs, the diet needs to be assessed and medication should be reviewed to ensure that the patient is not on a phosphate binder. Even if patients have not been given dietary restrictions, many will pick up information from other patients and members of staff and therefore may be following a low phosphate diet without other health professionals knowing.

19.12.4   Enteral feeding in patients with renal failure

The feeds that can be used in patients with renal failure depend on the patient's fluid balance and blood biochemistry. Patients who have no fluid imbalance or raised potassium and phosphate levels may be on a standard or energy feed. Patients who are on continuous filtration can also be fed with standard feeds. Those on intermittent dialysis with minimal urine output or very fluid overloaded patients may benefit from a low-volume feed.

Refeeding syndrome can occur in people with renal failure but may be more diffi-cult to detect as electrolyte levels may be high, due to renal impairment, when enteral feeding is commenced. These levels can then drop post feeding. When monitoring blood biochemistry in patients on intermittent dialysis, care must be taken to ensure that it is the pre-dialysis bloods that are being monitored. Post-dialysis phosphate and potassium can appear below the normal range but these levels rebound a few hours post HD. It is worth checking urea levels to gain an idea of whether a set of bloods has been taken pre or post dialysis. A sudden drop in urea may indicate the sample has been taken post-dialysis.

19.12.5   Parenteral feeding of patients with renal failure

The indications for parenteral feeding through a dedicated line, in this patient group, is usually due to ileus, malabsorption secondary to intractable vomiting or diarrhoea, or bowel obstructions.

Parenteral feed prescriptions depend on the fluid status and biochemistry of the patient. Patients on haemodialysis or those with poor fluid and electrolyte clearance may need tailored bags, whereas those on continuous filtration can usually manage on standard PN bags. Due to the possible high osmolarity of the PN bags, it should be given via a central line. It must be via a dedicated port and should not be shared with the dialysis port. A triple lumen catheter can be placed to allow HD and PN to be carried out on the same line. Those who have dialysis through a fistula should have a line placed for parenteral nutrition (except IDPN). Irrespective of modality, parenteral nutrition prescriptions for renal failure patients will usually have electrolytes added but it may be in smaller quantities compared to other patient groups. IDPN is used differently and can be used in patients with a functioning gut as a supplement to oral diet and supplements (see Section 19.3.1).

19.12.6   Transplantation

Patients may receive transplants from the cadaveric list or from live donors, assuming they are fit enough to undergo transplantation. From a nutritional point of view, centres are likely to restrict obese people from transplant until they have lost weight. This is due to the increased risks of surgery and also because being obese can shorten the lifespan of the transplant (Meier-Kriesche *et al.*, 2002; Armstrong *et al.*, 2005). Units will vary the criteria but many will not accept people with a BMI >30. Patients may come off the transplant list if they become medically unwell with conditions such as serious infection, cancer or cardiac conditions, as they may not be strong enough to undergo a transplant at that time. These patients may be reactivated on the transplant list once they are medically well. If a patient does not have a living donor, the length of time a patient waits for a suitable transplant can vary. Those from ethnic minorities, e.g. Asians (Jeffrey *et al.*, 2002) and African-Caribbeans tend to wait longer for a suitable match as kidney donations from these groups are low.

Once a patient receives a kidney transplant, electrolyte restrictions for phosphate and potassium can be relaxed. Many people are not aware of this and those that have been on dialysis for many years may find it hard to adjust to the idea of being allowed previously restricted foods. Phosphate levels can drop significantly post transplant and this is thought to be due to increased renal clearance caused by FGF-23 (fibroblast growth factor 23). Some patients may find that their potassium levels may not drop down fully as cyclosporine (immunosuppressive medication) can lead to hyperkalaemia. Only patients with hyperkalaemia problems post transplant need to moderate potassium intake, all others can have an unrestricted diet with respect to potassium.

Post transplant, some patients find that with the relaxation of dietary restrictions and the use of steroids as immunosuppression they gain weight rapidly in the first year. Healthy eating information may, therefore, be particularly beneficial for those with a good appetite post transplant. Steroid induced diabetes is also common post transplant and dietary advice is required for this condition. As the steroids are weaned off, glycaemic control may improve.

Patients with a new transplant are also given food safety advice as they are at increased risk of food poisoning due to the immunosuppression.

19.12.7   Vitamins and minerals in renal failure

Vitamin D

Those with low corrected calcium levels or raised PTH levels may be started on an activated vitamin D therapy. This is because vitamin D is activated via the kidneys and those with renal failure are unlikely to be able to maintain their vitamin D levels. Activated vitamin D (1-alphacalcidol and paricalcitrol) may come in the form of tablets or injections.

Haemoglobin and iron levels

Low ferritin and haemoglobin levels frequently occur in patients with renal failure. This in turn can affect appetite. People with anaemia and renal failure have been found to have more complaints about poor appetite compared to those with renal failure and no anaemia (Bárány *et al.*, 1993). Treatment may include iron, erythropoiesis-stimulating agents or a combination of both. Patients treated with erythropoiesis-stimulating agents may have an increased demand for iron. Oral iron absorption studies have shown that iron absorption is poor in renal patients

(Eschbach *et al.*, 1970; Donnelly *et al.*, 1991; Kooistra *et al.*, 1995). Medications can contribute to this decreased absorption (e.g. phosphate binders) and therefore most units tend to provide iron in the intravenous form (Fishbane *et al.*, 1999). Iron supplementation is usually kept on hold during periods of sepsis due to the concerns that this may exacerbate the infection.

19.12.8   Water-soluble vitamin use

The prescription of water-soluble vitamins in renal units is variable. In the UK 3.7% of renal units prescribe vitamins, while 71% of renal patients are prescribed vitamins in the United States. A recent international study (Fissell *et al.*, 2004) has shown that patients who take water-soluble vitamins are at a significantly lower risk of mortality. Further randomised controlled trials would need to be carried out to prove this, as those who are adherent when it comes to taking vitamin prescriptions may also be more adherent with prescriptions generally, and this may be the explanation for the lower mortality risk. Given the evidence from the international study, it would be worth considering prescribing water-soluble vitamins for those patients who agree to take them, but considerations include adherence and whether increasing the pill burden may have a detrimental effect. People who consume a limited range of foods or those whose weight is being maintained on modular feeds, e.g. fat, glucose and protein supplements, may still benefit from receiving a multivitamin and mineral supplement as opposed to just a water-soluble vitamin. If a multivitamin and mineral supplement is needed, it is wise to avoid ones that provide more than 100% of the recommended daily amount for the various vitamins and minerals, due to the potential risk of toxicity.

19.13   Conclusion

It is recommended that all people living with HIV are screened at baseline to determine glomcrular filtration rate (GFR) and also have urinalysis to ascertain if the patient is proteinuric. People with a higher risk of developing CKD (i.e. those with diabetes, hypertension or vascular disease, as well as those with a CD4 count <200 and a viral load >4000) should be screened annually.

During the early stages of CKD (stages 1–3), potassium and phosphate restriction is not common but good control of diabetes, hypertension and lipid levels can be of benefit to help delay the progression of kidney disease. Clients at stage 4 and 5 renal disease may need dietary advice with regard to electrolyte restriction, i.e. potassium and phosphate, but this is dependent on biochemical levels and also nutritional status. Patients who are struggling to consume adequate amounts may not need dietary restrictions at that stage or may be able to have previous restrictions relaxed until their appetite is resolved. Once clients are consuming adequate amounts, if their biochemical levels, e.g. potassium and phosphate, are approaching the upper levels, then the diet can be reassessed and the patient can be informed of ways to moderate intake. Patients with stage 4 CKD and beyond would benefit from seeing a renal dietitian, in addition to the nutritional support they receive at the genitourinary clinic.

Acknowledgements

This chapter was reviewed by Iain Macdougall, Consultant Nephrologist BSc, MD, FRCP, Renal Department, King's College Hospital NHS Foundation Trust and Frank A Post MD PhD FCP(SA), Clinical Senior Lecturer, King's College London, Honorary Consultant Physician, King's College Hospital.

References

Armstrong KA, Campbell SB, Hawley CM, Johnson DW, Isbel NM. Impact of obesity on renal transplant outcomes. *Nephrology* 2005; **10**(4):405–13.

Bannister DK, Acchiardo SR, Moore LW, Kraus AP. Nutritional effects of peritonitis in continuous ambulatory peritoneal dialysis (CAPD) patients. *J Am Diet Assoc* 1987; **87**(1):53–6.

Barakat MM, Nawab ZM, Yu AW, Lau AH, Ing TS, Daugirdas JT. Hemodynamic effects of intradialytic food ingestion and the effects of caffeine. *J Am Soc Nephrol* 1993; **3**(11):1813–8.

Bárány P, Pettersson E, Konarski-Svensson JK. Long-term effects on quality of life in haemodialysis patients of correction of anaemia with erythropoietin. *Nephrol Dial Transplant* 1993; **8**:426–32.

Blower S, Schwartz EJ, Mills J. Forecasting the future of HIV epidemics: the impact of antiretroviral therapies and imperfect vaccines. *AIDS Rev* 2003; **5**:113–25.

Brook G, Editor. In: Bhagani S, Sweny P, eds. *Guidelines for Kidney Transplantation in Patients with HIV Disease.* London: BHIVA/British Transplant Society, 2005.

Burrowes JD, Larive B, Cockram DB. Effects of dietary intake, appetite, and eating habits on dialysis and non-dialysis treatment days in hemodialysis patients: cross-sectional results From the HEMO study. *J Ren Nutr* 2003; **13**(3):191–8.

CASH. (Consensus Action on Salt and Health), Salt and the black population of African descent, January 2006, Statistics on current salt intake revised September 2008, Blood Pressure Unit, St. George's University Hospital, London.

Cassidy M, Richardson D, Jones C. *Renal Association Clinical Practice Guidelines Module 2 Complications of Chronic Kidney Disease.* Hampshire: Renal Association. 2007.

Donnelly SM, Posen GA, Ali MA. Oral iron absorption in hemodialysis patients treated with erythropoietin. *Clin Invest Med* 1991; **14**:271–6.

Earthman C, Traughber D, Dobratz J, Howell W. Bioimpedance spectroscopy for clinical assessment of fluid distribution and body cell mass. *Nutr Clin Pract* 2007; **22**(4):389–405.

Eschbach JW, Cook JD, Finch CA. Iron absorption in chronic renal disease. *Clin Sci* 1970; **38**:191–6.

Fishbane S, Mittal SK, Maesaka JK. Beneficial effects of iron therapy in renal failure patients on hemodialysis. *Kidney Int* 1999; **55**:S67–70.

Fissell RB, Bragg-Gresham JL, Gillespie BW *et al.* International variation in vitamin prescription and association with mortality in the dialysis outcomes and practice patterns study (DOPPS). *Am J Kidney Dis* 2004; **44**(2):293–9.

Gupta SK, Eustace JA, Winston JA *et al.* Guidelines for the management of chronic kidney disease in HIV infected patients: recommendations of the HIV medicine association of the infectious diseases. *Soc Am Clin Infect Dis* 2005; **40**(11):1559–85.

Herman ES, Klotman PE. HIV-associated nephropathy: epidemiology, pathogenesis, and treatment. *Semin Nephrol* 2003; **23**(2):200–8.

James G, Jackson H. European Guidelines on Nutritional Care of Adult Renal Patients EDTNA/ERCA. Lucerne, Switzerland: European Dialysis and Transplantation Nurses Association/European Renal Care Association. 2002

Jeffrey RF, Woodrow G, Mahler J, Johnson R, Newstead CG. Indo-Asian experience of renal transplantation in Yorkshire: results of a 10-year survey. *Transplantation* 2002; **73**(10):1652–7.

Jones MR, Gehr TW, Burkart JM *et al.* Replacement of amino acid and protein losses with 1.1% amino acid peritoneal dialysis solution. *Perit Dial Int* 1998; **18**(2):210–6.

Kimmel PL, Umana WO, Simmens SJ, Watson J, Bosch JP. Continuous ambulatory peritoneal dialysis and survival of HIV infected patients with end-stage renal disease. *Kidney Int* 1993; **44**:373–8.

Kooistra MP, van Es A, Struyvenberg A, Marx JJM. Low iron absorption in erythropoietin-treated hemodialysis patients. *Abstract J Am Soc Nephrol* 1995; **6**:543.

Kopple JD. Dietary protein and energy requirements in ESRD patients. *Am J Kidney Dis* 1998; **32**(6 Suppl 4):S97–104.

Kopple JD, Bernard D, Messana J *et al*. Treatment of malnourished CAPD patients with an amino acid based dialysate. *Kidney Int* 1995; **47**(4):1148–57.

Lindholm B, Bergstrom J. Protein and amino acid metabolism in patients undergoing continuous ambulatory peritoneal dialysis (CAPD). *Clin Nephrol* 1988; **30**(Suppl 1):S59–63.

Luft FC, Weinberger MH. Heterogeneous responses to changes in dietary salt intake: the salt-sensitivity paradigm. *Am J Clin Nutr* 1997; **65**:612S–7.

McCann L. *Pocket Guide to Nutrition Assessment of the Patient with Chronic Kidney Disease*, 3rd edn. Chapter 3, Hampshire: Renal Association. 2002; 11–2.

Meier-Kriesche H, Herwig-Ulf, Arndorfer JA, Kaplan B. The impact of body mass index on renal transplant outcomes: a significant independent risk factor for graft failure and patient. *Transplantation* 2002; **73**(1):70–4.

Post FA, Campbell LJ, Hamzah L *et al*. Predictors of renal outcome in HIV-associated nephropathy. *Clin Infect Dis* 2008; **46**:1282–9.

Reaich D, Price SR, England BK, Mitch WE. Mechanisms causing muscle loss in chronic renal failure. *Am J Kidney Dis* 1995; **26**(1):242–7.

Renal Association. *Clinical Practice Guidelines for Haemodialysis*, 4th edn. Renal Association, 2007.

Ritz E, Gross ML. Hyperphosphatemia in renal failure. *Blood Purification*. 2005; **23**:6–9.

Rufino M, de Bonis E, Martin M *et al*. Is it possible to control hyperphosphataemia with diet, without inducing protein malnutrition? *Nephrol Dial Transpl* 1998; **13**(Suppl 3):65–7.

Sacks FM, Svetkey LP, Vollmer WM *et al*. Effects on blood pressure of reduced dietary sodium and the dietary approaches to stop hypertension (DASH). *Diet N Engl J Med* 2001; **344**:3–10.

Slatopolsky E. New developments in hyperphosphatemia management. *J Am Soc Nephrol* 2003; **14**:S297–9.

Stover J. Non-dietary causes of hyperkalemia. *Nephrol Nurs J* 2006; **33**(2):221–2.

Tjiong HL, Van Den Berg JW, Wattimena JL *et al*. Dialysate as food: combined amino acid and glucose dialysate improves protein anabolism in renal failure patients on automated peritoneal dialysis. *J Am Soc Nephrol* 2005; **16**(5):1486–93.

Wei A, Burns GC, Williams BA, Mohammed NB, Visintainer P, Sivak SL. Long-term renal survival in HIV-associated nephropathy with angiotensin-converting enzyme inhibition. *Kidney Int* 2003; **64**:1462–71.

Winston JA, Burns GC, Klotman PE. The human immunodeficiency virus (HIV) epidemic and HIV-associated nephropathy. *Semin Nephrol* 1998; **18**(4):373–7.

Young GA, Brownjohn AM, Parsons FM. Protein losses in patients recieiving CAPD. *Nephron* 1987; **45**(3):196–201.

20 The Nutritional Management of Patients Living with HIV and Liver Disease

Tracy Russell and Ruth Westwood

Key Points

- Liver disease is the most frequent cause of non-AIDS-related deaths among people with HIV.
- Treatment for hepatitis C can result in significant weight loss which may lead to malnutrition.
- Malnutrition is a complication of chronic liver disease and there is a direct correlation between the severity of malnutrition and the progression of liver disease.
- Nutritional management should include assessment of cause of malnutrition, nutritional assessment and calculation of nutritional requirements, and provision of optimal nutritional therapies.
- People with untreated hepatitis C who are overweight may benefit from weight reduction programmes to help prevent progression of liver disease.
- Treatment of NAFLD should involve treating the individual parameters of metabolic syndrome by dietary intervention, weight reduction and exercise regimens.

20.1 Introduction

Since the introduction of combination antiretroviral treatment (ART) HIV associated morbidity and mortality has been declining but liver disease has become a major cause of mortality among people with HIV infection (Weber *et al.*, 2006).

Liver disease is classified as acute or chronic. Acute liver disease is a sudden hepatic dysfunction resulting from a hepatocellular necrosis. Hepatic encephalopathy develops within 8 weeks of onset of symptoms such as jaundice and flu-like symptoms. Common causes of acute liver disease among people with HIV include tuberculosis, hepatitis B and C, cytomegalovirus infection and drug toxicity.

In chronic liver disease, liver damage is progressive over many years and becomes irreversible, this results in cirrhosis. Cirrhosis can be compensated (the liver is cirrhotic but there are no signs of liver failure) or decompensated (the liver is cirrhotic and clinical signs associated with liver disease develop such as oedema, ascites, variceal bleeding and steatorrhoea). Causes of chronic liver disease in HIV infection are numerous and often multifactorial. Most common causes include viral hepatitis (B and C), alcohol abuse, intravenous drug use and potential toxic effects associated with prolonged antiretroviral therapy.

High prevalence rates of obesity of 43–51% have been reported in recent studies (Tang *et al.*, 2005; Tedaldi *et al.*, 2006). Obesity is associated with an increasing incidence of non-alcoholic fatty liver disease (NAFLD – fatty inflammation of the liver not related to alcohol intake).

20.2   Hepatitis B, hepatitis C and HIV

The prospective D:A:D. study showed that the most frequent cause of non-AIDS-related death in an HIV population was from causes related to liver disease as follows; 16.9% had active hepatitis B (HBV), 66.1% had active hepatitis C (HCV) and 7.1% had dual viral hepatitis (HBV and HCV) co-infections. There was also evidence of a strong association between immunodeficiency and risk of liver-related mortality (Weber *et al.*, 2006). HBV and HCV infections are commonly seen amongst patients with Human Immunodeficiency Virus Infection (HIV). Approximately 180 million people are infected with HCV and some 350 million people are HBV carriers worldwide (Brook *et al.*, 2005).

There is no comprehensive UK data on HBV and HIV co-infection rates. However, some studies have shown rates of between 6 and 9% depending on area and route of infection (Brook *et al.*, 2005). Prevalence of hepatitis C in the UK population is estimated at 0.4%, but this rate varies by area, population and route of infection. For example, in Scotland it is estimated that 1% of the population is infected (Hepatitis C Action plan for Scotland, Phase I, 2006). Approximately one-third of people with HIV worldwide are co-infected with HCV (WHO, 2006). As with HBV, prevalence varies according to area and route of infection.

Hepatitis C and HIV co-infection may have an adverse effect on progression of HIV. The Swiss cohort study showed co-infection may increase the risk of progression to AIDS or death, and patients are likely to have lower CD4 count rises in response to antiretroviral therapy than patients infected with HIV alone (Grueb *et al.*, 2000).

20.2.1   Transmission routes

The routes of transmission for HBV and HCV are similar to HIV, hence the high rates of co-infection. In the UK the two major risk groups for HCV have been those who have previously received transfusion of infected blood or blood products (prior to 1989) and those sharing drug injection equipment. Recent data has highlighted increased incidences of acute HCV infection associated with unsafe sex practices among men who have sex with men (Danta *et al.*, 2007). In the UK, blood products are no longer a source of HBV/HCV infection due to virus inactivation procedures which were introduced in 1989.

20.2.2   Hepatitis B

Hepatitis B is immunopathic, which means that the immune response to the virus tends to cause most of the liver damage. Co-infection with HIV is accompanied with HBV replication and increased progression to cirrhosis and death (Brook *et al.*, 2005).

The progression of HIV does not seem to be affected when co-infected with hepatitis B, however, there is a higher risk of antiretroviral hepatotoxicity in patients coinfected with HBV compared to HIV alone.

HBV is preventable by vaccine, however, HIV patients tend to respond less well to the vaccine and the response is usually dependent on the degree of immunosuppression as measured by CD4 count. The aim of treatment of HBV is to suppress viral replication and improve liver histology.

Treatment for patients with HBV and HIV co-infection is usually with combinations of nucleoside analogues such as tenofovir and emtricitibine, which are effective against both viruses.

20.2.3 Hepatitis C

HCV usually progresses slowly over a period of years. HCV can present as acute and/or chronic hepatitis. Chronic HCV is defined as ongoing infection 6 months after initial infection. Approximately 80% of patients with acute HCV will develop chronic HCV (WHO, 2000). About 10–20% of patients with chronic HCV will progress to liver cirrhosis and 1–5% to primary hepatocellular carcinoma (HCC) over a period of 20–30 years (WHO, 2000). Co-infection with HCV and HIV generally complicates each disease.

The natural history of HCV infection is accelerated in patients with HIV, with an increased rate of progression to hepatocellular carcinoma (Garcia-Samaniego et al., 2001) and end-stage liver disease compared with HCV mono-infected patients (Graham et al., 2001). Immune restoration with effective HIV antiretroviral therapy may limit HCV liver disease progression (Brau et al., 2006).

HCV may not worsen HIV but may make HIV treatment more complicated. Individuals with HCV are at increased risk of developing hepatotoxicity following treatment with antiretroviral therapy such as Ritonavir or Nevirapine (Powderly, 2004), but the actual risk posed by individual drugs and drug combinations is not clearly understood. Some antiretroviral agents such as zidovudine (AZT) interact with ribavirin and pegylated interferon used to treat hepatitis C, therefore, patients may need to switch drugs prior to undertaking treatment for hepatitis C.

Sustained viral response (SVR), defined as an undetectable level of serum HCV RNA (Ribonucleic acid) 6 months after the end of treatment is the marker of treatment success. Patients with HCV/HIV co-infection generally receive treatment for 48 weeks (SIGN, 2006). Response rates are in the order of 14–60%, depending on the HCV genotype and are poorer than in HCV mono-infected patients (Carrat et al., 2004; Chung et al., 2004; Torriani, 2004).

In addition to liver disease, HCV infection (and its treatment) can be associated with changes in cognitive function, fatigue and depression, decreased quality of life and an increased prevalence of insulin resistance/diabetes mellitus (Lecube et al., 2006). All of these factors can potentially affect both the medical and nutritional management of the patient with HIV/HCV co-infection.

20.2.4 Treatment side effects that may affect nutritional intake

Side effects of pegylated interferon, used in the treatment of hepatitis C and, less commonly, in hepatitis B, can be severe with flu-like symptoms, fatigue, alopecia, nausea (Russo and Fried, 2003), weight loss (Seyam et al., 2005; Lo Re et al., 2007) and depression (Patten and Barbui, 2004). Patients who experience depression should be considered for ongoing psychological and specialist nursing support and treatment with an antidepressant (SIGN, 2006). Side effects may be more common in people with HIV/HCV co-infection compared to HCV alone.

Amount of mean weight loss in HCV mono-infected patients receiving treatment has been reported to be 4–5 kg (Perez-Olmeda *et al.*, 2003), and 8.9–29% loss of original body weight (Manns *et al.*, 2001; Seyam *et al.*, 2005). One study investigating weight loss in HIV/HCV co-infected patients showed a significantly greater amount of weight loss in the co-infected group (76%) compared with both HCV (39%, $p <$ 0.001) and HIV (3%, $p < 0.001$) mono-infected patients (Lo Re *et al.*, 2007).

Because of the significant weight loss experienced in those receiving HCV treatment patients are at risk of developing malnutrition. Poor appetite and weight loss can have a huge impact on ability to continue with treatment of HCV in HIV co-infected individuals. Regular follow-up and support during treatment is essential to prevent malnutrition and help improve adherence to treatment.

Nutritional management of the individual with HBV/HCV and HIV coinfection should be the same as that of other causes of liver disease. It is important to treat the symptoms present, such as nausea and vomiting.

Individuals who do not receive treatment are at risk of progressing to advanced liver disease and cirrhosis. Nutritional management of these patients should be the same as for other forms of liver disease, which is summarised in the next section.

20.3 Nutrition and liver disease

Malnutrition is a complication of chronic liver disease. Protein-energy malnutrition (PEM) is a dietary deficiency of energy and protein resulting in body wasting and is common in chronic liver disease with a prevalence of 27–100%. PEM is an independent risk factor for poor clinical outcome such as increased infection rate, hospital admissions and mortality.

There is a direct correlation between the severity of malnutrition and the progression of liver disease.

Causes of PEM include:

- altered energy metabolism – increasing muscle catabolism with accelerated protein breakdown and reduced protein synthesis
- increased energy expenditure
- reduced oral intake from symptoms such as nausea and vomiting, anorexia, weakness and fatigue.

20.3.1 Nutritional assessment – confounding factors

Nutritional assessment in chronic liver disease is vital to the provision of optimal nutritional support (see Chapter 8, 'Nutritional Screening and Assessment'). Several factors may complicate nutritional assessment in patients with chronic liver disease, as many markers that are usually used are not useful for the prediction of malnutrition in chronic liver disease.

Weight: The presence of ascites or oedema will mask a patient's true dry weight. Dry weight can be calculated as follows: Dry Weight = wet weight – estimated weight of ascites and/or oedema.

Upper-arm anthropometry: It provides one of the most useful methods of assessment in this patient group. Muscle and fat stores can be identified and losses monitored. These measurements are particularly useful when a patient has ascites and/or oedema.

Grip strength (hand-grip dynamometer): This measurement reflects changes in muscle function and is therefore valuable in monitoring the effectiveness in nutritional support.

Laboratory markers: Albumin, pre-albumin, transferin and retinol binding protein are synthesised by the liver and therefore cannot be used to assess nutritional status in liver disease.

20.3.2   Nutritional requirements and support

Nutrition intervention during asymptomatic and compensated stages of liver disease should include the promotion of a healthy balanced diet and achieving weight goals within a normal BMI. Nutritional treatment of chronic liver disease should be based on symptoms present as opposed to the type of liver disease.

Prevention and improvement of PEM is a priority in nutritional management. Nutritional therapy has been shown to improve nutritional status, liver function, reduce complications and prolongue survival (Plauth *et al.*, 2006).

Nutritional guidelines have been formulated for use by health professionals in people with liver disease at various clinical stages (Plauth *et al.*, 2006; Johnson and Bishop, 2007).

Energy and protein requirements have been summarised in Table 20.1.

Energy requirements (EER) can be estimated in several ways, as explained in Table 20.1. Equations are also used, developed by Schofield, which involve estimating basal metabolic rate (BMR) and adding a stress factor and activity factor (see Chapter 8, 'Nutritional Screening and Assessment'). The stress factors used in patients with liver disease are described in Table 20.1.

There is very limited data from research studies of specific nutritional requirements and therapies in people with HIV infection and liver diseases such as hepatitis B, hepatitis C and NAFLD. Further research on this field is required.

20.3.3   Ascites

Ascites is the most common complication of cirrhosis and is defined as excessive fluid accumulation in the peritoneal cavity. Patients with ascites experience anorexia, early satiety, nausea and vomiting. The aim of nutritional treatment is preservation or improvement of nutritional status, meeting protein and energy requirements (as per decompensated cirrhosis). Low sodium diets are not recommended and are likely to restrict oral intake. If a sodium restriction is employed, then a 'No Added Salt' diet should be advised (see Table 20.2). Nutritional support should continue and can be supported by the use of prokinetic agents, sip feeds and, if necessary, enteral feeding with nasojejunal tubes which are well tolerated.

20.3.4   Hepatic encephalopathy

Hepatic encephalopathy (HE) is termed as impaired mental function and abnormal neuromuscular function that occurs as a complication of acute and chronic liver disease. Factors precipitating HE include constipation, bleeding (variceal/

Table 20.1 Energy and protein requirements during clinical stages of liver disease.

Clinical condition	Energy[*]	[†]Nitrogen (N)/protein (P)	Application	Type of feed
Asymptomatic	EER[§]	0.17 g/kg N[§] (1 g/kg P)	Balanced diet aiming to maintain/achieve normal BMI	
Compensated Cirrhosis	25–35 kcal/kg body weight[§] or EER + Stress factor 0–20%[§]	0.19–0.2 g/kg N (1.2–1.3 g/kg P)[§]		
Decompensated Cirrhosis	35–40 kcal/kg body weight[‡] or EER + Stress factor 30–40%[§]	1.2–1.5 g/kg P[‡] 0.25–0.3 g/kg N (1.5–2.0 g/kg P)[§]	Normal food/ONS/TF (PEG associated with higher risk of complications)[‡]	High energy/protein Consider sip feeds containing 20 g protein/200 mls High calorie supplements such as Calogen/Procal can be used to boost energy requirements
Alcoholic Steatohepatitis	35–40 kcal/kg[‡]	1.2–1.5 g/kg[‡]	Normal food/ONS/TF (PEG associated with higher risk of complications)[‡]	High energy/protein[‡] Consider sip feeds containing 20 g protein/200 mls High calorie supplements such as Calogen/Procal can be used to boost energy requirements
Pre Transplantation	As per decompensated cirrhosis[‡]	As per decompensated cirrhosis[‡]	As per decompensated cirrhosis[‡]	As per decompensated cirrhosis[‡]

Condition	Energy	Protein/Nitrogen	Route/Feeding	Notes
Post Transplantation	Initiate nutrition within 12–24 hours post operatively‡ 35–40 kcal/kg body weight‡ or EER + Stress factor 30%§	1.2–1.5 g/kg P‡ 0.25–0.3 g/kg N 1.5–2 g/kg P§	TF – Nasogastric or Jejunostomy for early nutrition‡	High energy/protein‡ Consider sip feeds containing 20 g protein/200 ml High calorie supplements such as Calogen/Procal can be used to boost energy requirements
Acute (Fulminant) liver failure/ventilation	EER + Stress factor 20–30%§	0.2–0.25 g/kg N 1.2–1.5 g/kg P§		
Hepatic Encephalopathy	As per compensated or decompensated	Compensated: 1.2–1.3 g/kg P§ Decompensated: 1.5 g/kg P§	ONS/TF Frequent small meals and a late 50 g carbohydrate/glucose snack	High energy/Protein (up to 100 g protein per day§)

ONS: Oral Nutritional Supplements.
TF: Tube Feed.
PEG: Percutaeneous endoscopic gastrostomy.
BMI: Body Mass Intake.
EER – Estimated Energy Requirements.
N = Nitrogen.
P = Protein.
*If Patient is fluid-overloaded estimate dry body weight.
† Adjust nitrogen requirements for BMI.
‡Plauth et al. (2006).
§Johnson and Bishop (2007).

Table 20.2 No Added Salt.

To restrict sodium to less than 100 mmol/Na/day, the following foods should be avoided:

- Bacon, ham, sausages, and paté
- Tinned fish and meat
- Smoked fish and meat
- Fish and meat pastes
- Tinned and packet soups
- Sauce mixes
- Tinned vegetables
- Bottled sauces and chutneys
- Meat and vegetable extracts and stock cubes
- Salted nuts and crisps
- Soya sauce
- Monosodium glutamate
- Cheese – up to 100 g per week
- Bread – up to 4 slices per day
- A pinch of salt may be used in cooking, but none should be added to food at the table

From Thomas (2007)

gastrointestinal), portosystemic shunting and sepsis. Low protein diets are not recommended in the nutritional management of HE, as encephalopathy can become worse with PEM. The use of branched chain amino acids (BCAA) in patients with HE has been a matter of debate, but in a Cochrane review it was concluded that there was a lack of evidence as to benefits to support the use of BCAAs (Als-Neilson *et al.*, 2003).

Steatorrhoea

Causes of steatorrhoea include a mechanical block in the bilary tract, intrahepatic lesion, or intra- or extrahepatic stricute of the bile duct. Steatorrhoea occurs if secretion of bile is significantly impaired (cholestasis), as fat will not be emulsified and thus lead to excess excretion of fat in stools (excretion of more than 0.3 g/kg/day of fat, although there is no standardised definition).

Steatorrhoea presents as loose, oily/greasy, pale stools, which can be offensive smelling. It can compromise nutritional status and lead to malnutrition in extreme cases. Dietary treatment of steatorrhoea involves alleviating symptoms, preventing weight and muscle mass loss and fat-soluble vitamin deficiencies. Fat reduction should only be advised in patients who regularly report steatorrhoea and have evidence of muscle wasting and weight loss. It is important to determine the degree of fat intolerance on an individual basis.

Patients who have been advised to restrict fat should be educated on energy replacement with the use of carbohydrates and medium-chain triglycerides. The use of oral nutritional supplements may be indicated, especially juice base supplements which contain little fat. If enteral nutrition is necessary, there are MCT-based feeds and low-fat semi-elemental diets available. Note that elemental feeds are not indicated due to their high volume and osmolality.

Patients with chronic steatorrhoea are at risk of fat-soluble vitamin deficiencies (A, D, E and K), therefore supplementation may be necessary (Johnson and Bishop, 2007).

20.3.5   Patterns of eating and carbohydrate snacks

Patients with chronic liver disease may suffer from early satiety and poor appetite, this, along with ongoing muscle catabolism will lead to weight loss and malnutrition. Patients should be encouraged to eat small, frequent, energy-dense snacks throughout the day to prevent periods of fasting and muscle catabolism (Verboeket-van de Venne et al., 1995); this should include an evening snack containing 50 g carbohydrate, which has been shown to increase overnight carbohydrate oxidation rate and decrease the lipid and protein oxidation rate, thus improving nitrogen balance and preventing muscle mass depletion (Miwa et al., 2000).

20.4   Liver transplantation

Due to the improved prognosis of HIV and the high incidence of chronic liver disease in this patient group, there may be an increased need for liver transplantation in patients with HIV infection, particularly in those patients who have causes of chronic liver disease apart from hepatitis C and in whom the post-transplant prognosis is good. Malnutrition has been identified as an area of concern (O'Grady et al., 2005). Post-operative complications and mortality rates are reported in patients who are malnourished pre-operatively (Plauth et al., 2006) Pre-operative nutritional assessment and support when necessary is advised. Following liver transplantation, normal food and/or enteral nutrition should be initiated within 12–24 hours (Plauth et al., 2006).

20.5   Nutritional interventions for hepatitis C

There are published guidelines on nutritional management of hepatitis C mono-infection, which are also applicable for patients with HIV/HCV co-infection (Dietitians of Canada, 2003).

20.5.1   Vitamins and minerals

There is very little evidence to support a role for individual vitamins and minerals in altering the natural history of hepatitis C. There have been a small number of studies in which iron (Iwasa et al., 2002), Vitamin K^2 (Habu et al., 2004) and zinc (Takagi et al., 2001) have been investigated. Many of these studies consisted of small population groups and were not randomised or blind controlled trials. Furthermore they did not take other important, potentially confounding, factors into consideration such as dietary intake. Evidence from further large randomised controlled studies is necessary to demonstrate a beneficial effect of large doses of individual vitamins and minerals in order to support their role in the management of HCV.

Anaemia and low folate: patients are at risk of low iron and folate levels due to increased cell turnover and reduced dietary intake. Low folate levels should be corrected with 5 mg folic acid daily. Erythropoetin is used to treat anaemia induced by ribavirin treatment in patients with hepatitis C. Maintaining adequate iron and folate stores is particularly important for these patients.

20.5.2   Weight

Weight gain in untreated patients

Some studies have shown that being overweight is an independent risk factor for progression of fibrosis (liver scarring) and steatosis (fatty liver) in hepatitis C:

Two studies have show that overweight (BMI ≥ 25 kg/m^2) and obese (BMI ≥ 30 kg/m^2) were found to be independent risk factors for the presence of hepatic steatosis (Hu *et al.*, 2004) and BMI ≥ 25 kg/m^2 was significantly independently associated with rapid fibrosis progression in all patients (Ortiz *et al.*, 2002).

Limited research has shown that implementation of weight reduction programmes may improve the risk factors associated with progression:

Using a single cohort study, Hickman *et al.* (2002) investigated the effect of weight reduction on liver histology and biochemistry in patients with chronic hepatitis C. A 12-week dietary restriction programme was introduced consisting of 55% CHO, 15% protein and 30% fat. The aim of this programme was to promote weekly weight reduction of 0.5 kg. Mean weight reduction in the study group was 5.9 kg and this was associated with a significant reduction in waist circumference and fasting insulin levels. The degree of reduction in steatosis was directly related to the percentage weight loss. Fifty-six per cent of patients who had a reduction in steatosis also showed a reduction in fibrosis.

Patients who are classed as overweight with a BMI ≥ 25 kg/m^2 should be encouraged to explore weight reduction programmes of diet and exercise.

Target weight goals should be discussed and encouraged and ongoing support and advice made available to enable compliance.

Due to the risk of unintentional weight loss during hepatitis C treatment, it is advisable to prevent any planned weight reduction programmes throughout the treatment period unless there is a reason to do so to improve patient's health (SIGN, 2006).

20.5.3   Alcohol

Alcohol intake, even in moderate doses, has been shown to increase progression of liver disease in hepatitis C (SIGN, 2006). It is advisable to abstain from alcohol at all times (SIGN, 2006). Those patients with a high alcohol intake who find it difficult to stop should be advised to limit their alcohol intake. Support is essential from both medical, social and psychological fields (Rockstroh *et al.*, 2008).

20.6   HIV and non-alcoholic fatty liver disease

Non-alcoholic fatty liver disease consists of a spectrum of fatty liver diseases, which range from steatosis (fatty liver) to non-alcoholic steatohepatitis (NASH – fatty inflammation of the liver as a result of NAFLD leading to cirrhosis). NAFLD has been associated with metabolic abnormalities, (characterised by insulin resistance, dyslipidaemia and hypertension) and obesity (Day, 2006). In non-HIV individuals, obesity and diabetes are the two major risk factors associated with NAFLD. The prevalence of NAFLD in the HIV population is unreported. However, individuals with HIV may be at increased risk of developing non-alcoholic fatty liver disease (NAFLD), due to the link with NAFLD and metabolic syndrome. It is not known whether

HIV-associated NAFLD develops as a result of obesity and/or insulin resistance or as a consequence of chronic infection and/or antiretroviral therapy – the latter can have an adverse effect on glucose control, lipid metabolism, body fat redistribution and insulin resistance.

The majority of patients with NAFLD are asymptomatic with diagnosis being made during elevation of persistent plasma liver enzymes, ultrasound or biopsy.

The aim of treatment for NAFLD is the effective management of the metabolic syndrome and associated hypertension, diabetes and dyslipidaemias (see Chapter 10 'The Nutritional Management of Complications Associated with HIV and Antiretroviral Therapy').

Dietary programmes promoting a gradual weight loss, normal glucose and lipid levels should be prescribed, with promotion of increased exercise levels.

20.7   Use of complementary and alternative therapies (CAT) in liver disease

Alternative and complementary therapies are commonly used in the UK, either as a treatment for liver disease or to help relieve the symptoms or treatment side effects (Hanje et al., 2006). Evidence for potential benefits is discussed below. However, these therapies are not without risks, so it is important that we advise our patients to be cautious. These risks include general drug interactions and side effects (see Chapter 16, 'Complementary and Alternative Therapy'), as well as those that induce specific hepatotoxicity (see Table 20.2).

20.7.1   Micronutrient supplements

Therapeutic trials in humans have failed to show any significant benefit for the use of vitamin E as an antioxidant, reducing oxidative damage to liver cells and subsequent fibrogenesis.

Zinc supplements are regularly prescribed for liver cirrhosis, as zinc deficiency in this population group is common. There is interest in the use of zinc supplementation as an adjunct therapy for hepatic encephalopathy, a major complication of cirrhosis. However, results in human RCTs have been mixed and further work is required.

Magnesium deficiency has been linked to the development of insulin resistance seen in NAFLD and NASH, as well as muscle cramps and weakness observed in many types of liver disease. However, few studies have looked at treating patients with chronic liver disease with magnesium supplementation and no human studies have so far looked at the effects of magnesium supplementation on insulin resistance in liver patients (Hanje et al., 2006).

20.7.2   Herbal supplements

Herbal supplements are commonly used among people with liver disease. Examples include milk thistle (Silymarin), liquorice root (Glycyrrhizin) and betaine (from sugar beet). Milk thistle is probably the most popular supplement used by people with liver disease. However, the supplement is poorly absorbed, and content of preparations is highly variable. RCT in humans have again shown mixed results, mainly due to poor study design and compliance issues. There are also interactions with milk thistle and some antiretroviral therapies used to treat HIV, such as the protease inhibitors – Nelfinavir, Ritonavir, Saquinavir and Tipranavir and the NNRTI's – Delavirdine, Efavirenz, Etravirine and Nevirapine.

There has been interest in liquorice root as a hepatoprotective agent. Clinical trials with this supplement have generally been difficult to interpret due to small sample size and poor study design. Most studies indicate that liquorice root may provide clinical benefits in prevention of hepatocellular carcinoma in patients with chronic hepatitis C who do not respond to, or cannot tolerate standard interferon therapy. However, limited studies have failed to show enhanced antiviral effects when used in combination with interferon. Moreover, safety issues with this supplement, limit its widespread use (see Chapter 16, 'Complementary and Alternative Therapy').

Betaine is used as a protective agent against a variety of forms of experimental hepatotoxic agents. Betaine has been used in a pilot study with a small number of NASH patients, and larger studies of its use in NASH are ongoing (Hanje *et al.*, 2006).

To summarise, there is currently no conclusive evidence from clinical trials in humans to support the use of complementary alternative medicines and nutritional treatments as agents in liver disease. However, data is emerging that certain agents may have therapeutic effects. Despite the lack of evidence, some patients will still be keen to take these supplements, so it is important that we provide information on potential side effects and issues concerning product safety (see Box 20.1).

Box 20.1   Selected complementary therapies with reported hepatotoxicity.

Multiple Reported Cases

- Black Cohosh
- Chaparral
- Germander
- Kava Kava (hundreds of cases worldwide)
- LipoKinetix and Ma huang (weight loss)
- Pennyroyal (menthe pulegium)
- Pyrrolizidine alkaloids
- Senna (only with overdoses)
- Skullcap (Scutellaria laterilora)
- Small number of reported cases
- Aristolochia root
- Bajiaolian
- Ascara Sagrada (natural laxative)
- Celandine
- Eternal Life (Chinese herbal remedy)

(*Source*: Hanje *et al.*, 2006)

20.8   Vulnerable groups

Many individuals with HIV and liver disease such as those with chronic alcohol intake or injecting drug use may be vulnerable. It is important to assess the social and food security profile of such patients. Such factors may have an impact on their ability to make use of dietary advice provided.

Alcohol and substance users are a particularly vulnerable group that may experience nutritional deficiencies due to drug-nutrient interactions, chaotic lifestyles, poor dietary intake and low prioritisation for food. Some patients report poor appetite, nausea, vomiting, constipation and reduced saliva production as side effects of drug use.

Injecting drug use is associated with lower weight and fat mass in HIV-positive women (Forrester *et al.*, 2000). Iron-deficiency anaemia appears to be more commonly found among those using intravenous drugs (van der Werf *et al.*, 2000), vitamins C, E and A status has also been reported to be lower (Nazrul Islam *et al.*, 2001).

Diets tend to be high in refined carbohydrates, and lack fruit and vegetables and fibre.

Dentition may be poor due to dietary intake and use of methadone, which is an opiate substitute (however, sugar-free methadone is available).

Poverty can lead to poor nutritional intake. It is important to consider the food security of patients as food availability may be limited due to low income, immigration status and other factors.

Provision of advice on cheap, convenient meals, and the availability of free meals in the locality, is very helpful.

20.9   Conclusion

Although the epidemiology of HIV and liver disease is multifactorial, viral hepatitis appears to be the main cause of mortality in this population group. As individuals infected with HIV are living longer, there is an increased risk of morbidity and mortality from liver-related causes.

To date, there is very limited research in this area of HIV and liver disease. One study has shown that weight loss experienced in an HIV/HCV co-infected group of patients was greater than weight loss that occurred in groups mono-infected with HIV and HCV.

The specific energy, protein and nutritional requirements of liver disease in the HIV group are not known. In the absence of such data, guidelines are available for calculating the nutritional requirements of patients with liver disease, which can be used for patients with HIV and concomitant liver disease. Further research for this population group would be beneficial.

The progression of liver disease can be a slow process with changing medical and nutritional therapies required throughout, depending on symptoms. Prevention of malnutrition is essential. Nutritional therapies should involve nutritional assessment, dietary prescription, ongoing follow-up and support to help individuals meet nutritional requirements and achieve their nutritional goals.

Acknowledgements

This chapter was reviewed by:

Chris Taylor, FRCP, Consultant Physician Sexual Health and HIV, Kings College Hospital NHS Foundation Trust. London

References

Als-Nielsen B, Koretz RL, Gluud LL, Gluud C. Branched-chain amino acids for hepatic encephalopathy. *Cochrane Database Syst Rev* 2003; (1): DOI: 10.1002/14651858.CD001939.

Brau N, Salvatore M, Rios-Bedoya CF *et al*. Slower fibrosis progression in HIV/HCV-coinfected patients with successful HIV suppression using antiretroviral therapy. *J Hepatol* 2006; **44**:47–55.

Brook MG, Gilson R, Wilkins E, BHIVA Hepatitis Coinfection Guideline Committee; British HIV Association. BHIVA guidelines on HIV and chronic hepatitis: coinfection with HIV and hepatitis B virus infection. *HIV Med* 2005; **6**(Suppl 2):84–95.

Carrat F, Bani-Sadr F, Pol S *et al*. Pegylated interferon alfa-2b vs standard interferon alfa-2b, plus ribavirin, for chronic hepatitis C in HIV-infected patients: a randomized controlled trial. *JAMA* 2004; **292**(23):2839–48.

Chung RT, Andersen J, Volberding P *et al*. Peginterferon Alfa-2 a plus ribavirin versus interferon alfa-2 a plus ribavirin for chronic hepatitis C in HIV-coinfected persons. *N Engl J Med* 2004; **351**(5):451–9.

Danta MA, Brown DA, Maghani SB *et al*. Recent Epidemic of acute hepatitis C virus in HIV positive men who have sex with men linked to high risk sexual behaviours. *AIDS* 2007; **21**:983–99.

Day CP. Non alcoholic fatty liver disease: current concepts and management strategies. *Clin Med* 2006; **6**:19–25.

Dietitians of Canada, Hepatitis C: nutrition care, Canadian guidelines for health care providers. *Can J Diet Pract Res*. 2003 Fall;**64**(3):139–41. Available from http://wwwdietitians.ca/resources/HepC_guidelines_March2003.pdf. Accessed 6 June 2010.

Forrester JE, Woods MN, Knox TA, Spiegelman D, Skinner SC, Gorbach SL. Body composition & dietary intake in relation to drug abuse in a cohort of HIV +ve persons. *JAIDS* 2000; **25**(Suppl 1):S43–8.

Garcia-Samaniego J, Rodriguez M, Berenguer J *et al*. Hepatocellular carcinoma in HIV-infected patients with chronic hepatitis C. *Am J Gastroenterol* 2001; **96**:179–83.

Graham CS, Baden LR, Yu E *et al*. Influence of human immunodeficiency virus infection on the course of hepatitis C virus infection: a meta-analysis. *Clin Infect Dis* 2001; **33**(4):562–9.

Grueb G, Ledergerber B, Battegay M *et al*. Clinical progression, survival and immune recovery during antiretroviral therapy in patients with HIV-1 infection and hepatitis C virus coinfection: The Swiss HIV cohort study. *Lancet* 2000; **356**:1800–5.

Habu D, Shiomi S, Tamori A *et al*. Role of vitamin K2 in the development of hepatocellular carcinoma in women with viral cirrhosis of the liver. *JAMA* 2004; **292**(3):358–61.

Hanje AJ, Fortune B, Song M, Hill D, McClain C. The use of selected nutrition supplements and complementary and alternative medicine in liver disease. *Nutr Clin Pract* 2006; **21**:255–72.

Hepatitis C. Action plan for Scotland, Phase I. 2006. //www.scotland.gov.uk/Publications/2006/09/15093626/0. Accessed on 02 June 2008.

Hickman IJ, Clouston AD, Macdonald GA *et al*. Effect of weight reduction on liver histology and biochemistry in patients with chronic hepatitis C. *Gut* 2002; **51**(1):89–94.

Hu KQ, Kyulo NL, Esrailian E *et al*. Overweight and obesity, hepatic steatosis, and progression of chronic hepatitis C: a retrospective study on a large cohort of patients in the United States. *J Hepatol* 2004; **40**(1):147–54.

Iwasa MKM, Ikoma J, Kobayashi Y *et al*. Dietary iron restriction improves aminotransferase levels in chronic hepatitis C patients. *Hepatogastroenterology* 2002; **49**(44):529–31.

Johnson J, Bishop J. Liver and biliary disease. In: Thomas B, Bishop J, eds. *In Manual of Dietetic Practice*, 4th edn. Oxford: Blackwell Publishing, 2007.

Lecube A, Genescà J, Hernández C, Simó R. Glucose abnormalities in patients with hepatitis C virus infection: epidemiology and pathogenesis. *Diabetes Care* 2006; **29**(5):1140–46.

Lo Re V III, Kostman JR, Gross R *et al*. Incidence and risk factors for weight loss during dual HIV/Hepatitis C virus therapy. *J Acquir Immune Defic Syndr* 2007; **44**(3):344–50.

Manns MP, McHutchison JG, Gordon SC *et al*., The International Hepatitis Intervention Therapy Group. Pegylated alpha-2b plus Ribavirin compared with interferon alpha-2b plus Ribavirin for initial treatment of chronic hepatitis C: a randomised trial. *Lancet* 2001; **358**:958–65.

Miwa Y, Shiraki M, Kato M *et al*. Improvement of fuel metabolism by nocturnal energy supplementation in patients with liver cirrhosis. *Hepatol Res* 2000; **18**:184–9.

Nazrul Islam SK, Jahangir Hossain K, Ahsan M. Serum vitamin E, C and A status of the drug addicts undergoing detoxification: influence of drug habit, sexual practice and lifestyle factors. *Eur J Clin Nutr* 2001; 55:1022–7.

O'Grady J, Taylor C, Brook G. Guidelines for liver transplantation in patients with HIV infection: British HIV association. *HIV Med* 2005; 6(Suppl 2):149–53.

Ortiz V, Berenguer M, Rayón JM et al. Contribution of obesity to hepatitis C related fibrosis progression. *Am J Gastroenterol* 2002; 91(9):2408–14.

Patten SB, Barbui C. Drug-induced depression: a systematic review to inform clinical practice. *Psychother Psychosom* 2004; 73(4):207–15.

Perez-Olmeda M, Nunez M, Romero M et al. Pegylated interferon α-2b plus Ribavirin as therapy for chronic hepatitis C in HIV infected patients. *AIDS* 2003; 17:1023–8.

Plauth M, Cabré E, Riggio O, Assis-Camilo M, Pirlich M, Kondrup J. ESPEN guidelines on enteral nutrition: liver disease. *Clin Nutr* 2006; 25:285–94.

Powderly WG. Antiretroviral therapy in patients with hepatitis and HIV: weighing risks and benefits. *Clin Infect Dis* 2004; 38(Suppl 2):S109–13.

Rockstroh JK, Bhagani S, Benhamou Y et al. European AIDS clinical society (EACS) guidelines for the clinical management and treatment of chronic hepatitis B and C coinfection in HIV-infected adults. *HIV Med* 2008; 9:82–8.

Russo M, Fried MW. Side effects of therapy for chronic hepatitis C. *Gastroenterology* 2003; 124(6):1711–9.

Scottish Intercollegiate Guidelines Network, SIGN. Management of Hepatitis C: a national clinical guideline. 2006. Available at http://www.sign.ac.uk/pdf/sign92.pdf. Accessed on 25 June 2008.

Seyam SM, Freshwater DA, O'Donnel K, Mutimer DJ. Weight loss during Pegylated interferon Ribavirin treatment of chronic hepatitis C. *J Viral Hepat* 2005; 12:531–5.

Takagi H, Nagamine T, Abe T et al. Zinc supplementation enhances the response to interferon therapy in patients with chronic hepatitis C. *J Viral Hepat* 2001; 8(5):367–71.

Tang AM, Jacobsen DL, Spiegelman D et al. Increasing risk of 5% or greater unintentional weight loss in a cohort of HIV infected patients, 1995–2003. *J Acquir Immune Defic Syndr* 2005; 40(1):70–76.

Tedaldi EM, Brooks JT, Weidle PJ et al. Increased body mass index does not alter response to initial highly active antiretroviral therapy in HIV-1 infected patients. *J Acquir Immune Defic Syndr* 2006; 43(1):35–41.

Torriani F. Peginterferon Alpha-2 a plus Ribavirin for Chronic Hepatitis C virus infection in HIV-infected patients. *N Engl J Med* 2004; 351(5):438–50.

Van Der Werf MJ, Van Benthem BHB, Van Ameijden EJC. Prevalence, incidence and risk factors of anaemia in HIV-positive and HIV negative drug users. *Addiction* 2000; 95(3):383–92.

Verboeket-van de Venne WPHG, Westerterp KR, van Hoek B, Swart GR. Energy expenditure and substrate metabolism un patients with cirrhosis of the liver: effects of the pattern of food intake. *Gut* 1995; 36(1):110–6.

Weber R, Sabin CA, Friis-Møller N et al. Liver related deaths in persons infected with the human immunodeficiency virus: the D.A.D. study. *Arch Intern Med* 2006; 166(15):1632–41.

World Health organization (WHO). Hepatitis C: Fact sheet no. 164. 2000. Accessed online – http://www.who.int/mediacentre/factsheets/fs164/en/. Accessed on 25 June 2008.

World Health organization (WHO). HIV/HCV Co-infection. 2006. Available at – http://www.euro.who.int/HEN/Syntheses/hepatitisC/20050411_7. Accessed on 15 July 2008.

21 Critical Care, Respiratory and Multi-organ Failure

Sarah Cassimjee

Key Points

- The advent of antiretroviral therapy (ART) has had little or no effect on the number of Intensive Therapy Unit (ITU) admissions amongst HIV-positive patients.
- The main reason for admission of HIV-positive patients to the ITU remains respiratory failure due to opportunistic infection. However, patients are now more likely to be admitted for non-HIV-related disease.
- The optimal nutritional requirements of HIV-positive patients on ITU have yet to be determined.
- HIV patients on ITU with weight loss and wasting are of particular concern, as critically ill patients have an increased risk of undernutrition due to the metabolic response to stress.

21.1 Background/overview

European and North American studies show 5–12% of HIV-positive patients admitted to hospital receive ITU care (Crothers and Huang, 2006). The advent of antiretroviral ART has had little or no effect on the number of ITU admissions in this group. The following points may help explain the reason for this:

- Up to 40% of patients with HIV infection are unaware of their status at the time of ITU admission (Huang *et al.*, 2006).
- Many patients are not on effective ART at the time of admission (Casalino *et al.*, 2004).
- Overall improved survival rates make patients and providers more likely to pursue aggressive life-support measures, which includes ITU admission (Narasimhan *et al.*, 2004).
- There is a growing population of people living with HIV (Narasimhan *et al.*, 2004).

Since the advent of ART, improved survival rates of critically ill HIV-positive patients have been reported in retrospective studies in Europe and North America (Narasimhan *et al.*, 2004; Dickson *et al.*, 2007), but the results of prospective trials are awaited.

The most common reason for admission of HIV-positive patients to ITU is the same as it was before the advent of ART – respiratory failure due to opportunistic

Table 21.1 Common nutritional problems in HIV-positive patients admitted to the ICU.

Problem	Suggestions/Notes
Weight is difficult to interpret	Use weight history and/or MAC. Look for physical signs of undernutrition. Look for the presence of hypermetabolic disease states such as PTB
Energy equations using weight or stress factors may not be accurate	Use equations as a guide, whilst regularly monitoring for over- and underfeeding
The metabolic response to stress alters the way in which our body uses substrates and puts patients at greater risk of undernutrition	Commence feeds as soon as possible Continue to use standard or higher protein feeds Preserving lean mass is not always possible
Various factors affect energy expenditure in the ICU	Check for medication that can affect energy expenditure Check if the patient is on controlled or assisted ventilation
Large amounts of non-nutritional calories, which can change on an hourly basis, can increase energy intake	Take note of large, continuous sources of non-nutritional sources (generally IV Propofol and IV Dextrose) Consider appropriateness of higher protein, concentrated or lower sodium feeds
Reduced gut motility is common in the ITU	Consider the use of prokinetics

infection (OI) (Table 21.1). However, the incidence of this and other HIV-related disease, as a reason for ITU admission, has declined significantly (Casalino *et al.*, 2004; Narasimhan *et al.*, 2004) (see Figure 21.1). Other common reasons for admission in this population include sepsis, CNS dysfunction, GI bleeding and cardiovascular disease.

The evidence base for the optimal nutrition requirements of related critically ill HIV patients is limited. Therefore, when planning nutritional treatment, it is beneficial to make use of data available for other population groups with critical illness and to understand the body's metabolic response to stress.

21.2   Diseases and infections associated with ITU admission

21.2.1   Respiratory failure

Acute respiratory failure still accounts for approximately 25–50% of ITU admissions in this population group. It is frequently caused by bacterial pneumonia (BP) or by the fungal infection *pneumocystis jiroveci* pneumonia (previously called *pneumocystis carinii* pneumonia, and still abbreviated PCP).

21.2.2   Pneumocystis pneumonia (PCP)

In their review of the data, Crothers and Huang (2006) reported that survival rates of HIV-positive patients with PCP in the early 1980s ranged from 0 to 13%. Retrospective studies have showed improved survival rates in the ART era (Morris *et al.*,

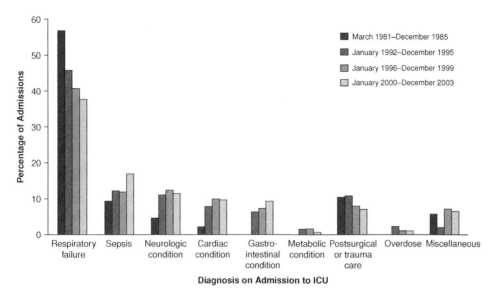

Figure 21.1 Principal diagnosis received by patients with HIV on admission to the medical or surgical ICU at San Francisco General Hospital between 1981 and 2003. The principal diagnosis on admission to the ICU is reported for 86 patients from March 1981 to December 1985,[5] followed by a gap of six years; then for 443 patients (an average of 111 patients per year) from January 1992 to December 1995,[6] for 354 patients (an average of 88 patients per year) from January 1996 to December 1999,[1] and for 328 patients (an average of 82 patients per year) from January 2000 to December 2003. Copyright © [2006] Massachusetts Medical Society. All rights reserved.

2003; Miller *et al.*, 2006; Dickson *et al.*, 2007), although it is not clear if this is due to ART, improvements in the treatment of PCP, or general improvements in the management of respiratory failure and acute respiratory distress syndrome (ARDS) in the ITU. Nevertheless, mortality from PCP remains high.

21.2.3 Bacterial pneumonia (BP)

Community-acquired BP can be caused by bacteria such as *Staphylococcus aureus*. Hospital-acquired pneumonia, most frequently a complication of mechanical ventilation, is also commonly caused by bacteria (Crothers and Huang, 2006).

21.2.4 Other HIV-related causes of respiratory failure

Mycobacterium tuberculosis pneumonia and fungal pneumonias, such as cytomegalovirus (CMV) pneumonia and *Toxoplasma gondii pneumonitis*, have all been associated with respiratory failure in HIV patients as have Karposi's sarcoma (KS), non-Hodgkin lymphoma and lymphocytic interstitial pneumonia (Crothers and Huang, 2006).

Acute respiratory failure unrelated to HIV disease such as exacerbation of asthma accounts for a small percentage of patients (Crothers and Huang, 2006).

21.3   Sepsis and multiple organ dysfunction syndrome (MODS)

In the era of ART, an increasing number of ITU admissions amongst HIV-positive patients have been due to sepsis and, like the general ITU population, this is associated with a high mortality rate (Casalino *et al.*, 2004).

Sepsis is the most common cause of MODS, although MODS can occur in the absence of infection and is known as systemic inflammatory response syndrome.

21.4   Neurological failure

Patients with HIV-related neurological conditions may require ITU admission for intractable seizures or for mechanical ventilation if their neurological complication has resulted in a decreased level of consciousness leading to secondary respiratory failure.

OIs such as *Toxoplasma gondii* can result in mass lesions whilst others such as *Cryptococcus neoformans* can result in meningitis. Other central nervous system (CNS) infections requiring ITU admission include progressive multifocal leukoencephlopathy (PML). In addition, HIV is a neurotropic virus so CNS insult can occur causing peripheral neuropathy, HIV encephalopathy and AIDS dementia, all of which may lead to ITU admission.

21.5   Cardiovascular failure

ART is associated with a number of artherogenic risk factors (Grinspoon and Carr, 2005), which may be contributing to the increase in cardiovascular disease as a reason for ITU admission in HIV-positive patients (see Figure 21.1). A recent study found that 7% of HIV-positive patients admitted to a London ITU were post-cardiac arrest (Dickson *et al.*, 2007).

21.6   Gastrointestinal (GI) failure

HIV-positive patients with GI-related complications may require ITU admission commonly for the treatment of GI Bleeding (Crothers and Huang, 2006). Bleeding is more common in the upper tract and may be due to HIV-related conditions such as KS. Bleeding in the lower tract may be due to HIV-related conditions such as CMV colitis (Chasalani and Wilcox, 1999).

Other HIV-related GI complications requiring ITU admission include peritonitis that can be due to CMV enteritis, bowel perforation, possibly as a result of KS, and hepatic encephalopathy often attributable to hepatitis B or C (HBV or HCV) (Crothers and Huang, 2006).

21.7   Liver failure

Liver failure secondary to HBV or HCV may require ITU admission in HIV-positive patients. Liver failure, lactic acidosis and hepatic steatosis associated with the nucleoside reverse transcriptase inhibitors (NRTIs), especially stavudine (D4T), may also require ITU admission. If necessary, transplant may be considered for patients with liver failure.

21.8   Renal failure

End-stage renal disease secondary to HIV nephropathy, HBV and HCV co-infection, hypertension or diabetes can require ITU admission in HIV-positive patients (Gupta *et al.*, 2005). The management of these patients may include continuous renal replacement therapy and consideration for transplant.

21.9   Medical treatment

The aim of treatment of all patients admitted to the ITU is to preserve life and treat acute life-threatening disorders. There are a number of considerations involved in the treatment of people with HIV in the critical care setting. These include:

21.9.1   Drug interactions

There are numerous potential drug interactions between antiretrovirals and other drugs used in the treatment of HIV and critical care medications.

Some antiretrovirals need to be taken with food and some without. Decreased gut motility or frequent aspiration of stomach contents via an enteral tube may affect the absorption of ART. Frequent interruptions to enteral feeds or 24-hour feeding can also affect absorption of those ARTs that need to be taken with or without food (see Chapter 12, 'Medications, Adherence and Interactions with Food').

21.9.2   Drug hypersensivity

Drug hypersensitivity is an immune-mediated reaction to a drug and is common in HIV-positive patients. It can lead to fever, hypotension and acute interstitial pneumonitis (Crothers and Huang, 2006).

21.9.3   Immune reconstitution inflammatory syndrome (IRIS)

When patients with advanced HIV disease commence antiretroviral treatment, some may experience a paradoxical worsening of disease severity, when the inflammatory response to OIs is increased, e.g. worsening of TB symptoms after commencing ART, leading to the development of ARDS (Crothers and Huang, 2006).

The decision to initiate ART in a critically ill patient would always be considered carefully and the appropriateness of doing so has yet to be examined in a randomised, prospective study.

21.10   Nutritional considerations

21.10.1   Weight

Just as in the general ITU population, traditional measurements of weight and body mass index (BMI) are difficult to interpret as oedema is common (Hall *et al.*, 1992).

HIV-positive patients with wasting may have an accompanying increase in extra-cellular fluid, further increasing fluid weight (Ockenga *et al.*, 2006).

Lastly, HIV-positive patients with ART-associated lipodystrophy may have weight gain or loss depending on the relation between subcutaneous lipoatrophy and intra-abdominal lipohypertrophy making weight difficult to interpret (Ockenga *et al.*, 2006).

21.10.2   Predictive equations

Various energy prediction equations for critically ill patients exist. The ITU population is not homogenous, making research data on the optimal macro/micronutrient requirements difficult to interpret.

21.10.3   The metabolic response to stress

In the critically ill patient, metabolic changes aimed at preserving life result in an often long period of heightened catabolism whereby mass, especially muscle mass, is decreased and protein, fat and carbohydrate utilisation is altered. Trying to compensate for these large losses by providing greater amounts of nutrition does not attenuate nitrogen loss and can actually result in further serious metabolic complications.

The metabolic response to stress can briefly be divided into three stages:

Phase1 – The Ebb Phase: This is the shortest phase (up to 24 hours). There is decrease in metabolism and energy stores are mobilised for use as energy.

Phase 2 – The Flow Catabolic Phase: This phase can last several weeks. There is an increase in metabolism. Protein stores are broken down to release amino acids. Amino acids are used for gluconeogenesis and for the synthesis of acute phase response proteins. This is done in preference to other body proteins such as albumin, so patients will often have a low serum albumin regardless of their nutritional status. Circulating levels of cytokines increase, as they do in HIV wasting, which further increases muscle breakdown and weight loss. In this stage:

- nitrogen loss occurs even if energy balance is attained (Frankenfield *et al.*, 1997)
- weight gain is unlikely until the acute phase/cytokine response is ameliorated by clinical intervention (Woodman, 2007)
- providing large amounts of calories in an attempt to prevent weight loss can increase the stress on the body by inducing the complications of overfeeding (Klein *et al.*, 1998).

Phase 3 – The Flow Anabolic Phase: This phase usually occurs after discharge from the ITU and is characterised by repletion of protein and fat stores.

21.10.4   HIV-related malabsorption

Malabsorption remains a significant cause of HIV-related weight loss (Ockenga *et al.*, 2006) and may be caused by HIV itself or by some bacterial or parasitic OIs. Diarrhoea can also occur if the patient has liver complications or as a short-term side effect of antiretroviral treatment. Fat malabsorption has been shown in many studies.

21.10.5   Non-nutritional energy sources in the ITU

Common non-protein energy (NPE) sources include carbohydrate from intravenous (IV) fluids and fat from IV Propofol, a common sedative that requires a 10% lipid carrier for infusion. Propofol infusions and therefore calories can vary on an hour-to-hour basis and is generally only significant if given in large amounts over a long period of time (Smith and Durman, 2004).

21.10.6   Medication affecting energy expenditure (EE)

Some drugs including Propofol can decrease EE whilst others such as Digoxin can increase EE. Mechanical ventilation can affect EE depending on the setting used (Taylor, 2007).

21.11   Nutritional assessment

It has been established that weight is difficult to interpret in this population. Some suggestions include:

- Ask the patient/family members about any involuntary weight loss or loss of appetite (Chan *et al.*, 1999). This would also help assess if the patient is at risk of the Refeeding Syndrome.
- Measure mid-arm circumference and compare to percentiles (Ravsco *et al.*, 2002).
- Look for physical signs of malnutrition such as temporal wasting (Joliet *et al.*, 1999).
- Look for the presence of disease states such as PTB, which are associated with hypermetabolism and a heightened risk of malnutrition.

21.12   Nutritional requirements

21.12.1   Energy

Indirect calorimetry (IC) is the gold standard for measuring energy expenditure in critically ill patients. However, its use is limited due to poor access to calorimeters and technical and time restraints. Equations are therefore widely used to estimate energy expenditure. To date, no specific equations to estimate the energy expenditure of critically ill HIV-positive patients exist. So equations for the general critical care population are often used.

Equations like the Schofield Equation (see Table 21.2), based on the BMR of healthy subjects, with the addition of an activity factor (usually <10% in ITU) and stress factor can introduce substantial error (Reid, 2007). If using equations based on BMR, factors that affect it should be taken into account such as:

- Is the patient ventilated or non-ventilated?
- Is the patient sedated and, if so, what is the level of sedation?
- Is the patient on other drugs that increase or decrease energy expenditure?

Table 21.2 Equations for estimating basal metabolic rate (Schofield) (DH, 1991).

Females (kcal/day)		Males (kcal/day)	
10–17 years	13.4W + 692	10–17 years	17.7W + 657
18–29 years	14.8W + 487	18–29 years	15.1W + 692
30–59 years	8.3W + 846	30–59 years	11.5W + 873
Females over 60 yrs (Kcal/day)		Males over 60yrs (Kcal/day)*	
60–74 years	9.2W + 687	60–74 years	11.9W + 700
75 years +	9.8W + 624	75 years +	8.3W + 820

W = weight.
Conversion 1 kcal = 4.184 kJ.
*Adapted from DH (1991) and converted from MJ/day to kcal/day.

Amongst other equations, the Ireton-Jones Energy Equations (IJEE) have been recommended as a user-friendly equation for use in critically ill patients (see Table 21.3). The IJEE equation was based on critically ill patients who were predominantly burns and trauma patients, both possible but unlikely reasons for admission of HIV-positive patients to ITU. Recently Frankenfield *et al.* (2007) have questioned the validity of the current IJEE for ventilated patients.

ESPEN Guidelines (2006) recommend the use of 20–25 kcal/kg/day in the acute phase of critical illness or 25–30 kcal/kg/day if the patient is severely undernourished.

When calculating nutritional requirements in the ITU using equations, the clinician should take into account:

- equations are based on weight, something that is often estimated in these patients
- the patient may be on large amounts of NPE calories from drugs.

Equations should be used in conjunction with clinical judgement and careful monitoring.

Overfeeding

Metabolic complications particularly affecting the lungs, liver and kidney can arise from overfeeding patients who are critically ill.

Table 21.3 Ireton-Jones equations (Ireton-Jones and Jones, 2002).

Spontaneously breathing patients
IJEE (s) = 629 − 11 (A) + 25 (W) − 609 (O)

Ventilator dependant patients
IJEE (V) = 1784 − 11 (A) + 5 (W) + 244 (S) + 239 (T) + 804 (B)

s = spontaneously breathing
v = ventilator dependent
A = age (years)
W = body weight (kg)
S = sex (male = 1, female = 0)
T = diagnosis of trauma (present = 1, absent = 0)
B = diagnosis of burn (present = 1, absent = 0)
O = obesity (BMI > 27 kg/m^2)

In their review, Klein *et al.* (1998) concluded the following:

- Excessive fat intake can affect the liver and raise triglyceride levels and cause fat overload.
- Excessive protein can cause azotemia, hypertonic dehydration and metabolic abnormalities by straining the kidneys.
- Excessive carbohydrate can increase blood glucose (BG) and triglyceride levels.
- Lastly, aggressively overfeeding any substrate, but especially carbohydrate, can affect the lungs by causing hypercapnia (high VCO_2 relative to VO_2) and risks prolonging the need for mechanical ventilation. It may also induce the Refeeding Syndrome.

Nutrition plans should include the monitoring of the above, bearing in mind that in the case of BG levels, critically ill patients will often be on strict BG control protocols, so monitoring insulin doses in addition to BG levels may provide greater insight than monitoring BG levels alone.

Hypocaloric feeding

There is increasing evidence to suggest that in the early stages of feeding, the optimal requirements of critically ill patients are low and hypocaloric feeding, where energy content is decreased whilst still providing adequate protein, is generally an accepted short-term nutritional goal in this group (Reid, 2007; Taylor, 2007).

Hypocaloric feeding has only been studied in obese and normal weight patients and its use in underweight patients may be contraindicated (Taylor, 2007). As many patients with HIV infection are admitted to the ITU unaware of their diagnosis and may have untreated, advanced HIV disease with associated wasting, hypocaloric feeding may not be the optimal nutritional goal in this population group. If the risk of metabolic abnormalities is deemed greater than the risk of further depletion of body stores, then short-term hypocaloric feeding may be considered in underweight patients but energy input should be increased as soon as possible to offset/compensate for energy expenditure (Taylor, 2007).

When considering hypocaloric feeding, the clinician should be aware that *unintentional* underfeeding in the ITU tends to be high already due to frequent cessations of feed for procedures, or due to gut motility problems that can prevent the target rate from being met (McClave *et al.*, 1999; Heyland *et al.*, 2004). A prospective 9-month study of five UK ICUs found that due to various reasons, 76% of prescribed feed was received (Adam and Batson, 1997) and Heyland *et al.* (2004) found that only 43% of patients received feeds as prescribed.

21.12.2 Nitrogen requirements

The catabolic phase of the metabolic response to stress results in the breakdown of protein stores. Protein synthesis is also decreased. In stress from traumatic injury, Frankenfield *et al.* (1997) found that achieving energy balance does not attenuate this accelerated nitrogen loss. Furthermore, overfeeding protein can induce further metabolic abnormalities.

In the ITU population, protein requirements are generally 0.2 gN_2/kg/day (Smith and Durman, 2004; Reid, 2007). As with hypocaloric feeding, this may have implications for the severely underweight or wasted patient with HIV infection. ESPEN Guidelines (2006) recommend nitrogen intakes of 0.24 gN_2/kg/day in the acute phase of HIV wasting. These recommendations suggest a range of 0.2–0.24 gN_2/kg/day dependent on the presence of HIV-associated wasting/underweight, although adequate controlled and/or dose-response trials are lacking (Ockenga et al., 2006).

21.12.3   Carbohydrate and fat

The metabolic response to stress is often accompanied by a state of insulin resistance. The exact mechanism is unknown, but Carlson et al. (2001) found a direct correlation between insulin resistance and severity of disease. Hyperglycaemia is known to suppress immune function (in non-HIV infected patients) and stimulate catabolism (Gore et al. 2002). Many ITUs have insulin protocols to maintain strict blood glucose control as tight controls of blood glucose levels have been associated with a reduction in ITU morbidity and mortality (Van den Berghe 2001). However, more recently, the NICE-SUGAR study (a large, international, randomised study) found that more moderate blood glucose control (keeping levels less than 10 mmol/ as opposed to keeping them between 4.5–6 mmol/L) was associated with lower mortality (Finfer et al. 2009). Despite insulin resistance, carbohydrate and fat are well utilised in critical illness (Jeewandan et al., 1991; Taylor 2007).

21.12.4   Nutritional requirements in specific organ failures

The nutrition support of the HIV-positive patient in the ITU should take into account the specific organ failures.

Respiratory failure

It has been established that giving patients on a mechanical ventilator large amounts of calories, especially from carbohydrate, can hamper weaning off the ventilator.

One study showed that patients on controlled ventilation expended significantly less (10%) energy than patients on assisted ventilation (Hoher et al., 2008).

One prospective, double-blind RCT showed that feeds containing omega-3 fatty acids and antioxidants may benefit patients who have developed ARDS (Gadek et al., 1999).

Patients with ARDS may be kept 'dry' through aggressive fluid restriction (Weidman et al., 2006).

Cardiovascular failure

HIV-positive patients admitted with heart failure may be on fluid restrictions.

Neurological failure

HIV-positive patients admitted to the ITU for intractable seizures may be on oral preparations of the anticonvulsant drug Phenytoin, which is best taken during enteral nutrition (EN) breaks (Au Yeung and Enson, 2000).

Patients with neurological failure, from conditions such as PML, may experience dysphagia and, therefore, may require nasogastric feeding after ITU discharge. Consideration of long-term feeding options (e.g. percutaneous endoscopic gastrostomy (PEG)) may be necessary.

GI failure

The decision to initiate enteral feed in a patient with GI bleed is beyond the scope of this chapter and has been described elsewhere (McClave and Chang, 2005).

Reduced gut motility is common in patients in ITU due to reasons such as the administration of sedatives, anaesthesia and muscle relaxants (Reid, 2007). Prokinetics such as Metaclopramide are commonly used to promote gut motility.

Patients with a non-functioning gut in the ITU, e.g. bowel perforation due to KS, should be considered for parenteral nutrition (PN) and Europe-wide guidelines found a reasonable amount of evidence to support the addition of glutamine to these PN bags (MacFie, 2004).

Liver failure

Acute liver failure is a catabolic state and there is a further decrease in the use of nitrogen in this group (Stravitz et al., 2007).

Generally estimated energy requirements are raised: EER + 20–30% stress factor (Johnson and Bishop, 2007). Nitrogen requirements are moderately raised: 0.2–0.25 gN$_2$/kg/day in this group (Johnson and Bishop, 2007).

Electrolyte abnormalities are common, especially if accompanied by renal failure. Patients will often be on fluid restrictions as hyponatraemia may exacerbate cerebral oedema. Patients with ascites may be on sodium restrictions.

Renal failure

Renal Failure in the ITU will often require continuous renal replacement therapy (CRRT), whereby blood is purified via a filter to remove unwanted solutes and water. There are different types of CRRT, which can include dialysate, haemofiltration or a combination of both. In the ITU haemofiltration is most commonly used.

If dialysate is used, it can contain dextrose, which will add to the NPE calories and should be taken into account whilst working out feeding regimens, although the uptake of glucose can be highly variable.

Patients on CRRT will require higher protein intakes to compensate for higher losses and recommendations vary from 0.24–0.4 gN2/kg/day (Reid, 2007) to (+) 10% N$_2$/day (Hartley, 2004).

21.12.5   Vitamin and mineral requirements

Selenium, carotenoids, vitamin E and vitamin C have been investigated in critically ill patients, but at present there is little evidence that they improve outcome (Heyland et al., 2005). Studies looking at micronutrient supplementation in HIV-positive patients did not include patients in the ITU, so until further evidence is produced, the minimum of the reference nutrient intake (RNI) for micronutrients should be the aim, which standard enteral and parenteral regimes should provide when target volumes are met (Department of Health, 1991).

21.13 Nutritional treatments/intervention

21.13.1 Aims of nutritional support

The aim of nutritional support for all patients in the ITU is to minimise nutritional losses (Smith and Durman, 2004).

Providing extra calories for weight gain is generally not an aim at this stage.

21.13.2 Feeding route

Enteral nutrition (EN) is the route of choice in critically ill patients and its benefits over PN have been well documented (Smith and Durman, 2004). Prokinetic drugs or post-pyloric feeding (e.g. nasojejunal feeding) may be recommended if nasogastric feeding is not tolerated (Kreymann et al., 2006). PN may be beneficial in those patients with a non-functional gut.

21.13.3 Choice of feed

Standard, polymeric feeds (1.0–1.2 kcal/ml and approximately 16% protein) are usually appropriate for critically ill patients (Kreymann et al., 2006) and HIV-positive patients (Ockenga et al., 2006). Feeds with soluble fibres may reduce diarrhoea (Spapen et al., 2001).

Patients on fluid restrictions, or those requiring large amounts of calories may benefit from enteral feeds with higher energy contents (1.5–2.0 kcal/ml and approximately 16% protein).

Patients with higher protein requirements may benefit from higher protein feeds (1.25–1.5 kcal/ml and approximately 20% protein). These feeds may also be useful in patients on large amounts of non-nutritional calories.

Low sodium feeds (1.1 mmol sodium/100 ml) may be useful in those patients with hyepernatraemia due to high sodium administration, e.g. Septrin® used in the treatment of PCP is often administered with large amounts of IV saline (150 mmol sodium/L). These feeds may also be useful in patients on sodium restrictions (e.g. patients with ascites) or patients on very strict fluid restrictions (e.g. some patients with ARDS).

MCT-rich feeds may be useful in those patients with HIV-related fat malabsorption (Wanke et al., 1996).

Immune-modulating formulae have been studied extensively in both HIV-positive patients and critically ill patients. To date, evidence fails to support its *general* use in either population (Heyland et al., 2003; Kreymann et al., 2006; Ockenga et al., 2006).

21.14 Early feeding and the use of enteral feeding protocols

Guidelines on the nutritional management of ITU patients often advocate the use of enteral feeding protocols (Heyland et al., 2003; Kreymann et al., 2006). These protocols may vary between institutions, but they generally promote the early (including out of hours), safe and gradual, initiation of EN.

HIV-positive patients who are admitted to such a unit will often be established on nasogastric feeds at the time of nutritional assessment. This can be replaced at the earliest opportunity by a feeding regimen provided by the dietitian, on the basis of individual requirements. Adam and Batson (1997) found that dietetic input on the ITU in conjunction with a feeding protocol increased the delivery of enteral feed.

21.15   Conclusion

There are no known studies investigating the nutritional requirements of a patient who is both critically ill and HIV positive. Similarities (e.g. increased cytokine response contributing to muscle wasting) and differences (e.g. the benefits of hypocaloric feeding in critically ill patients versus the higher calorie requirements of wasted HIV patients/patients with hypermetabolic OI) warrant new studies in this area, especially as the number of HIV-positive patients admitted to the ITU has largely remained the same since the advent of ART.

Current equations used to estimate the nutritional requirements should be used in conjunction with clinical judgement and frequent monitoring. Nutritional treatment of HIV-positive patients in the ITU is governed by the metabolic response to stress and specific organ failures should be taken into consideration when calculating nutritional requirements.

References

Adam S, Batson S. A study of problems associated with the delivery of enteral feed in critically ill patients in five ICU's in the UK. *Intensive Care Med* 1997; **23**:261–6.

Au Yeung SC, Enson MH. Phenytion and enteral feedings: Does the evidence support an interaction? *Ann Pharmacother* 2000; **34**:896–905.

Carlson GL. Insulin resistance and glucose-induced thermogenesis in critical illness. *Proc Nutr Soc* 2001; **60**:381–8.

Casalino E, Wolff M, Ravaud P, Choquet C, Bruneel F, Regnier B. Impact of HAART advent on admission patterns and survival in HIV-infected patients admitted to an intensive care unit. *AIDS* 2004; **8**:1429–33.

Chan S, McCowen KC, Blackburn GL. Nutrition management in the ICU. *Chest* 1999; **115**:145S–148S.

Chasalani N, Wilcox CM. Gastrointestinal haemorrhage in patients with AIDS. *AIDS* 1999; **13**:343–6.

Crothers K, Huang L. Critical care of patients with HIV. 2006. In: HIV In Site Knowledge Base. [online]. Available at http://hivinsite.ucsf.edu/InSite?page=kb-03–03-01. Accessed on 20 June 2007.

Department of Health (DH). *Dietary Reference Values for Food Energy and Nutrients for the United Kingdom*. Report on Health and Social Subjects 41. London: HMSO, 1991.

Dickson SJ, Batson S, Copas AJ, Edwards SG, Singer M, Miller RF. Survival of HIV-infected patients in the intensive care unit in the era of highly active antiretroviral therapy. *Thorax* 2007; **62**. Available at http://thorax.bmj.com/cgi/content/full/32/11/964. Accessed on 01 November 2007.

Finfer S, Chittock DR R, Yu-Shuo Su S, Blair D, Foster D, Dhingra V, Bellomo R, Cook D, Dodek P, Henderson WR, Hebert, PC, Heretier S, Heyland DK, McArthur C, McDonald E, Mitchell I, Myburgh JA, Norton R, Potter J, Robinson BG, Ronco JJ (2009) Intensive versus Conventional glucose control in critically ill patients. *N Engl J Med* 360:1283–1297.

Frankenfield DC, Hise M, Malone A, Russell M, Gradwell E, Compher C. Prediction of resting metabolic rate in critically ill adult patients: results of a systematic review of the evidence. *J Am Diet Assoc* 2007; **107**(9):1552–61.

Frankenfield DC, Smith JS, Cooney RN. Accelerated nitrogen loss after traumatic injury is not attenuated by achievement of energy balance. *J Parenter Enteral Nutr* 1997; **21**:324–9.

Gadek JE, DeMichele SJ, Karlstad MD *et al*. Effect of enteral feeding with eicosapentanoic acid, gamma-linolenic acid, and antioxidants in patients with acute respiratory distress syndrome. Enteral Nutrition in ARDS Study Group. *Crit Care Med* 1999; **27**:1409–20.

Gore DC, Chinkes DH, Hart DW, Wolf SE, Hrerndon DN, Sanford AP. Hyperglycaemia exacerbates muscle protein catabolism in burn-injured patients. *Crit Care Med* 2002; **30**: 2438–42.

Grinspoon S, Carr A. Cardiovascular risk and body-fat abnormalities in HIV-infected adults. *N Engl J Med* 2005; **352**:48–62.

Gupta SK, Eustace JA, Winston JA *et al*. Guidelines for the management of chronic kidney disease in HIV-infected patients: recommendations of the HIV Medicine Association of the Infectious Diseases Society of America. *Clin Infect Dis* 2005; **40**(11):1559–85. [238 references]

Hall I, Pollard BJ, Campbell IT. Daily body weight changes in critical illness. *Proc Nutr Soc* 1992; **51**:126A.

Hartley G. Nutrition in acute renal failure. In: Todorovic VE, Mickelwright A, eds. *A Pocketbook Guide to Clinical Nutrition (Parenteral and Enteral Nutrition Group of The British Dietetic Association)*. The British Dietetic Association Publishing, 2004: 15.1–15.10.

Heyland DK, Dhaliwal R, Day A, Jain M, Drover J. Validation of the Canadian clinical practice guidelines for nutrition support in mechanically ventilated, critically ill adult patients: results of a prospective observational study. *Crit Care Med* 2004; **32**:2260–6.

Heyland DK, Dhaliwal R, Drover JW, Gramlich L, Dodek P Canadian Critical Care Clinical Practice Guidelines Committee. *J Parenter Enteral Nutr* 2003; **27**:355–73.

Heyland DK, Dhaliwal R, Suchner U, Berger MM. Antioxidant nutrients: a systemic review of trace elements and vitamins in the critically ill patient. *Intensive Care Med* 2005; **31**:327–37.

Hoher JA, Zimermann Teixeira PJ, Hertz F, Moreira J da S. A comparison between ventilation modes: how does activity level affect energy expenditure estimates? *J Parenter Enteral Nutr* 2008; **32**(2):176–83.

Huang L, Quartin A, Jones D, Havlir D. Intensive care of patients with HIV infection. *N Engl J Med* 2006; **355**(2):173–81.

Ireton-Jones C, Jones D. Improved equations for predicting energy expenditure in patients: The Ireton-Jones equations. *Nutr Clin Pract* 2002; **17**:29–31.

Jeewandan M, Young D, Schiller W. Obesity and the metabolic response to sever multiple trauma in man. *J Clin Invest* 1991; **87**:262–9.

Johnson J, Bishop J. Liver and Biliary Disease. In: Thomas B, Bishop J, eds. *The Manual of Dietetic Practice*. Kent: Blackwell Publishing, 2007.

Joliet P, Pichard C, Chiolèro R *et al*. Enteral nutrition in intensive care patients: a practical approach. *Intensive Care Med* 1999; **24**:848–59.

Klein CJ, Stanek GS, Wiles CE III. Overfeeding macronutrients to critically ill adults: metabolic complications. *J Am Diet Assoc* 1998; **98**:795–806.

Kreymann KG, Berger MM, Deutz NEP *et al*. ESPEN Guidelines on enteral nutrition. *Clin Nutr* 2006; **25**. [online]. Available at http://intl.elsevierhealth.com/journals/clnu. Accessed on 01 August 2007.

MacFie J. European round table: the use of immunonutrients in the critically ill. *Clin Nutr* 2004; **3**:1426–9.

McClave SA, Chang, W-K. When to feed the patient with gastrointestinal bleeding. *Nutr Clin Pract* 2005; **20**:544–50. Available at http://ncp.sagepub.com/cgi/content/abstract/20/5/544. Accessed on 17 July 2008.

McClave SA, Sexton LK, Spain DA *et al*. Enteral tube feeding in the intensive care unit: factors impeding adequate delivery. *Crit Care Med* 1999; **33**:324–30.

Miller RF, Allen E, Copa A, Singer M, Edwards SG. Improved survival for HIV infected patients with severe Pneumocystis jirovecii pnuemonia is independent of highly active antiretroviral therapy. *Thorax* 2006; **61**:716–21. Available at http://thorax.bmj.com. Accessed on 19 June 2008.

Morris A, Wachter RM, Luce J, Turenre J, Huang L. Improved survival with highly active antiretroviral therapy in HIV-infected patients with severe Pnemocystis carinii pneumonia. *AIDS* 2003; **17**:73–80.

Narasimhan M, Posner AJ, DePalo VA, Mayo PH, Rosen MJ. Intensive care in patients with HIV infection in the era of highly active antiretroviral therapy. *Chest* 2004; 125. Available at http://www.chestjournal.org/cgi/content/full. Accessed on 07 November 2007.

Ockenga J, Grimble R, Jonkers-Schuitema C *et al*. ESPEN Guidelines on enteral nutrition: Wasting in HIV and other chronic infectious diseases. *Clin Nutr* 2006; 25. Available at http://intl.elsevierhealth.com/journals/clnu. Accessed on 01 August 2007.

Ravasco P, Camilo ME, Gouvei-Oliveira A, Adam S, Brum G. A critical approach to nutritional assessment in critically ill patients. *Clin Nutr* 2002; 21(1):73–7.

Reid C. Critical care. In: Thomas B, Bishop J, eds. *The Manual of Dietetic Practice*. Kent: Blackwell Publishing, 2007: 523–36.

Smith, Durman. Nutrition in critical care. In: Todorovic VE, Mickelwright A, eds. *A Pocketbook Guide to Clinical Nutrition (Parenteral and Enteral Nutrition Group of The British Dietetic Association)*. The British Dietetic Association Publishing, 2004: 17.1–17.20.

Spapen H, Diltoer M, van Malderen C, Opdenaker G, Suys E, Huyghens L. Soluble fibre reduces the incidence of diarrhea in septic patients receiving total enteral nutrition: a prospective, double-blind, randomised, and controlled trial. *Clin Nutr* 2001; 20:301–305.

Stravitz RT, Kramer AH, Davern T et al.; the Acute Liver Failure Study Group. Intensive care of patients with acute liver failure: recommendations of the Acute Liver failure Study Group. *Crit Care Med* 2007; 35(11):2498–508.

Taylor S. *Energy and Nitrogen Requirements in Disease States*. London: Smith-Gordan and Company Limited, 2007.

Van den Berghe G, Wouters P, Weekers F, Verwaest C, Bruyninckx F, Schetz M, Vlasselaers D, Ferdinande P, Lauwers P, Bouliin R. Intensive Insulin therapy in the critically ill patients. *New Engl J Med* 2001; 345:1359–1367.

Wanke CA, Plestow D, Degirolami PC, Lambl BB, Merkel K, Akrabawi S. A medium chain triglyceride-based diet in patients with HIV and chronic diarrhea and malabsorption: a prospective, controlled trial. *Nutrition* 1996; 12(11–12):766–71.

Weidman HP, Wheeler AP, Bernard GR *et al*. Comparison of two fluid management strategies in acute lung injury. The National Heart, Lung, and Blood Institute Acute Respiratory Distress Syndrome (ARDS) Clinical Trials Network. *N Eng J Med* 2006; 354:2564–75.

Woodman S. Estimating nutritional requirements. In: Thomas B, Bishop J eds. *The Manual of Dietetic Practice*. Kent: Blackwell Publishing, 2007: 71–79.

22 Nutritional Management of Patients Living with HIV and Cancer

Rachael Donnelly and Rachel Barrett

Key Points

- There is an increased risk of cancer among people living with HIV.
- There are multiple non-AIDS-defining malignancies and three AIDS-defining malignancies; Kaposi's sarcoma, high-grade B-cell non-Hodgkin's lymphoma, and invasive cervical cancer.
- The aims of nutritional support in cancer treatment are to prevent and treat undernutrition, enhance anti-tumour treatment effects, reduce the adverse effects of anti-tumour therapies, and improve the subjective quality of life.
- Early and frequent nutritional assessment should be undertaken throughout the patient's cancer journey.
- Nutritional interventions can range from relaxation of previous dietary advice, provision of oral, enteral, through to parenteral nutritional support.
- Nutritional interventions are vital throughout the cancer journey from diagnosis through to terminal care, encompassing living with and beyond cancer.

22.1 Introduction

Cancer has many definitions, although it is best defined by Brennan (2004) as 'the disordered and uncontrolled growth of cells within a specific organ or tissue type'. Cancer frequently produces secondary growths; these are known as metastasis (Brennan, 2004). It is the metastases that are ultimately the most threatening feature of malignant disease. Its aetiology is multifactorial, but 'lifestyle' factors, particularly diet, smoking and alcohol, are major influences.

Developments in the treatment of cancer have led to substantial improvements in both the management and survival of people with HIV-related cancers. As is the case with treatment of HIV disease, the management of cancer in the UK has evolved enormously within the last 20 years. This is due to advances in both medicine and technology along with the advent of government publications with the aim of improving outcomes in cancer care. In 1995 radical reform of the UK's cancer services were outlined by the publication of the Calman-Hine report, the main recommendation being the management of the care of patients with cancer site-specialist multidisciplinary teams. Since 1999 evidence-based Improving Outcomes Guidance (IOG) reports have been, and continue to be published for the different tumour types commissioned by the National Institute of Clinical Excellence (NICE). These IOGs focus on the need for multidisciplinary team work to ensure high quality diagnosis, treatment and care, along with ensuring effective coordination and continuity of care for patients. These were followed by the NHS Plan (2000a) which presented the government's strategy for investment and reform across the NHS, which gave cancer services high priority. The Cancer Plan (2000) also highlighted the need to continue to improve treatment for cancer patients. The most recent publication, the Cancer Reform Strategy (2007), builds on the progress made since the NHS Cancer Plan and sets a clear direction for cancer services for the next 5 years, including the importance of developing services to support survivorship post-cancer treatment.

22.2 Science of cancer

Formation of cancer in humans is a multi-step process. Defects in regulatory cells that govern normal cell proliferation and homeostasis lead to the development of cancer cells. Hanahan and Weinberg (2000) suggest that there are six essential alterations in cell physiology which together drive malignant growth. These six steps are known as the hallmarks of cancer.

22.2.1 The six hallmarks of cancer (Hanahan and Weinberg, 2000)

1. Self-sufficiency in growth signals: In order for normal cells to proliferate they need growth signals. These growth signals are transmitted into the cell. Cancer cells, however, do not depend upon exogenous growth stimulation but generate their own growth signals. The ability to be independent of external growth signals disrupts a very important mechanism that is usually in place to regulate normal behaviour of cells within a tissue.
2. Insensitivity to antigrowth signals: In normal tissue there are many antigrowth signals that work to maintain tissue homeostasis. Antigrowth signals block cell multiplication. They achieve this by two methods. Cells can be forced into the G_0 phase of the cell replication cycle or they are conditioned so that they give up their proliferation potential. Cancer cells grow by evading antigrowth signals.
3. Evasion of apoptosis (programmed cell death): Apoptosis occurs in normal cells as a way of removing cells that are no longer of use to the human body. Cancer cells have developed the ability to circumvent programmed cell death resulting in their ability to expand not only by proliferating but also by avoiding apoptosis.
4. Limitless replication potential: Many types of human cells are programmed so that the number of times they can replicate is limited. This programming works independently of signalling pathways. Cancer cells disrupt replication programming to enable continued unchecked growth.
5. Sustained angiogenesis: For cells to function and survive they need a supply of oxygen and nutrients. Angiogenesis is the formation of new blood vessels to enable cells in tumours to be supplied with oxygen and nutrients. Cancer cells shift the balance between angiogenesis inducers and inhibitors enabling angiogenesis to be induced and sustained. The development of new blood vessels is a prerequisite for the rapid expansion associated with tumour formation.
6. Tissue invasion and metastasis: Invasion and metastasis are complex processes. Successful invasion and metastasis depends on cells having all the other five hallmarks of cancer.

The ever-increasing understanding of how cancer cells grow and develop is leading to the development of drugs that are targeted at the alteration in cell physiology that dictate malignant growth, e.g. anti-angiogenesis medication.

22.3   Overview of cancer treatments

Cancer treatments are sometimes referred to as cutting, burning and poisoning. These terms relate to the three main treatment modalities namely surgery, radiotherapy and chemotherapy. However, cancer treatment is no longer restricted to just three treatment modalities. Targeted therapy is now hailed as the fourth treatment modality. In addition, palliative and supportive care are also important treatments for the patient with cancer. To provide appropriate nutritional intervention for a patient with cancer it is important to understand the treatment modalities available. It is not possible to provide in-depth information regarding cancer treatments in this chapter, however, an overview of the main treatment modalities is detailed below.

22.3.1   Surgery

Solid tumours have been treated with surgery for more than 100 years (Reed, 2006). Since the publication of the Calman-Hine report (1995), surgical services in the UK have been extensively reconfigured. Certain cancers, e.g. upper gastrointestinal tract, hepato-billary, urology and head and neck are now only treated in cancer centres whilst others, e.g. breast and colorectal are treated in both cancer centres and units. Cancer centres were defined by Calman-Hine (1995) as those which offer expertise in the management of all cancers and only radiotherapy should be undertaken at such an establishment, whereas a cancer unit should manage only the more common cancers, such as lung, breast, and colorectal. The rationale for this is to ensure efficient use of resources and increase expertise with specialist teams dealing with larger caseloads. Surgeons are involved in many areas of cancer treatment. Invariably, surgery is often required for biopsy of suspicious lumps and bumps to help make a diagnosis. Surgeons often deliver the diagnosis and outline the treatment plan. Surgeons are symbolically powerful figures for patients and amidst the fear and emotional chaos caused by diagnosis they are seen as key to survival. Surgery can be both curative and palliative. The most important factor determining the likelihood of cure for patients is the stage of disease at presentation (Reed, 2006). Staging of cancer includes the histological features of the tumour and imaging. Many solid cancers are staged using the Tumour (T) Node (N) Metastasis (M) system. Curative surgical management of cancer varies dependent on the type of cancer treated. Cancers of the upper aero-digestive tract and gastrointestinal tract, as well as urological and gynaecological cancers treated with surgery often have the most impact on nutritional status and the need for dietetic intervention. The impact of surgical resection to the cancer patient is obviously dependent upon the site of the disease and the extent of the surgery. Surgery may also be palliative. Indeed patients treated with surgery who are free of metastases at the time of initial surgery but who subsequently develop metastases in fact underwent palliative surgery at the time of their initial operation (Reed, 2006). However, palliative surgery is often seen as relief of or prevention of distressing symptoms to try to improve quality of life, e.g. internal fixation of a bone with secondary bone disease that is at risk of imminent fracture. Surgery is now rarely used as a single modality treatment. Many patients with solid tumours may now have their disease surgically resected as well as treated with other therapies such as chemotherapy and radiotherapy.

22.3.2   Chemotherapy

Chemotherapy is the use of drugs to treat cancer with the intention of causing regression or destruction of cancer cells (Bhosle and Hall, 2006). Chemotherapy drugs interfere with cell division by causing damage to DNA and/or preventing replication leading to apoptosis (Bhosle and Hall, 2006). Chemotherapy is given systemically ensuring that the anticancer treatment reaches all disease sites including micrometastatic lesions. This is in marked contrast to both surgery and radiotherapy, which only treat the area that they are directed at.

Chemotherapy was first used in the 1940s with the use of chemicals related to mustard gas being used as treatment for leukaemia (Robinson, 1993). Over the last 60 years many more cytotoxic drugs have been developed to treat cancer. Chemotherapy drugs have been developed from plants, e.g. vincristine from the periwinkle flower and paclitaxel from the bark of the pacific yew tree. Platinum-based chemotherapy drugs were developed after an accidental finding of the effect of an electrical current on the mobility of bacteria (Rosenberg et al., 1965).

Chemotherapy may be palliative, curative, adjuvant (given as an adjunct to primary therapy) or neoadjuvant (given before surgery or radiotherapy). Chemotherapy drugs are grouped according to their mechanism of action (Bhosle and Hall, 2006) as outlined in Table 22.1. Drugs that are in the same class can have different side effect profiles and anti-tumour effect.

Chemotherapy drugs are usually given in combination. Single agents are rarely used, as even the most responsive tumours obtain a complete response rate of no more than 20% (Souhami et al., 2002). Drugs with different mechanisms of action are usually combined to ensure independent cell killing by each agent. Tumours often develop resistance to chemotherapy agents. Using them in combination means that cells that are resistant to one drug may still be killed by another in the drug regimen (Souhami et al., 2002).

The maximum dose of chemotherapy drugs is limited by its toxicity in particular haematological toxicity. High dose chemotherapy is used in the management of acute leukaemias and lymphomas (Bhosle and Hall, 2006). Chemotherapy is usually given

Table 22.1   Groups of chemotherapy agents.

Chemotherapy agents	Examples
Alkylating agents	Nitrogen mustard, cisplatin and carboplatin
Antimetabolites	Methotrexate, 5-fluorouracil and capecitabine
Vinca alkaloids	Vincristine and vinblastine
Antibiotics	Epirubicin and doxorubicin
Intercalating agents	Bleomycin
Topoisomerase inhibitors	Irinotecan and etopside
Taxanes	Taxols and taxotere

in cycles every 2, 3 or 4 weeks so that normal cells can recover (Bhosle and Hall, 2006). Chemotherapy is usually given intravenously, although there are now oral chemotherapy agents available, e.g. capecitabine.

Chemotherapy is associated with many side effects. Most side effects are graded from 1 to 4/5 using toxicity scales. Side effects include:

- hair loss
- nausea/vomiting
- diarrhoea/constipation
- sore mouth/ulcers
- taste changes/food aversions
- tiredness/fatigue
- peripheral neuropathy
- myopathy
- infertility
- myelosupression
- secondary malignancies.

Some of the side effects which effect nutritional intake, e.g. nausea and vomiting, are managed with pharmacological agents, such as the anti-emetics granisetron, metoclopramide and cyclizine, as required.

22.3.3 Radiotherapy

Radiotherapy results in cancer cells accumulating damage to their DNA until they are destroyed (Falk, 2006). This treatment is given in fractions, with the fraction-ation having different effects on both tumour and on normal tissue. The number of fractions given is dependent upon a number of factors including the site and stage of disease, and the aim of the treatment, i.e. curative or palliative intent. The dose of radiotherapy is measured in Gray (Gy). The treatment dose is limited by the potential for damage to irreparable surrounding structures and tissue, e.g. spinal cord (Falk, 2006). However, recent advances in radiotherapy has meant that more targeted treatment options are now available to minimise damage to surrounding tissues, i.e. intensity modulated radiotherapy. Radiotherapy is also associated with many side effects; these however, are site-specific as outlined in Table 22.2.

Table 22.2 Side effects of radiotherapy categorised as acute and chronic conditions.

Acute conditions	Chronic conditions
Dysgeusia/hypogeusia	Fibrosis in the treatment field, e.g. lung
Mucositis	Radiation enteritis
Xerostomia	Xerostomia/hypogeusia
Skin irritations	Infertility
Nausea and vomiting	
Diarrhoea	
Fatigue	

22.3.4 Immunotherapy

Immunotherapy is an emerging treatment modality for cancers and these biological treatments rely on the use of the immune system to destroy cancer cells. The main concept being the stimulation of the patient's immune system to attack the malignant cells. There are an increasing number of agents being developed to target malignant disease. These include monoclonal antibodies such as Rituximab (an anti-CD20 antibody) and kinase inhibitors such as Lapatinib.

22.4 Cancers in HIV infection

When compared to the general population, PLHIV are at a significantly greater risk of developing cancer (Cheung *et al.*, 2005). Cancer in this population is also a major cause of both morbidity and mortality (Rabkin, 2001). Spina *et al.* (1999) have suggested that between 30 and 40% of PLHIV will develop a malignancy during the course of their life. At present malignant disease for PLHIV is divided into two categories, AIDS-defining and non-AIDS-defining malignancies.

HIV-infection is associated with three AIDS-defining malignancies: Kaposi's sarcoma, high-grade B-cell NHL and invasive cervical cancer (Bower *et al.*, 2008). Interestingly, these three tumour types have previously been associated in the literature, with a viral aetiology, including human herpes virus 8 (HHV8), human papilloma virus (HPV), and Epstein-Barr virus (EBV) (Grulich *et al.*, 2002) along with declining immune function (Mbulaiteye *et al.*, 2003).

There are a number of non-AIDS defining-malignancies that have been associated with HIV infection. Table 22.3 lists the non-AIDS-defining cancers for which there are both existing and limited data.

Studies have shown that there is a substantially increased risk of non-AIDS defining malignancies in those with an HIV diagnosis (Frisch *et al.*, 2001). However, many of these malignancies have not been shown to be associated with progressive immunosuppression (Mbulaiteye *et al.*, 2003). As a result, other oncogenic mechanisms are likely to be involved in their aetiology, e.g. lifestyle factors. Recent data suggests that the risk of developing a non-AIDS-defining cancer is 60% for those who are HIV positive, versus those who are HIV negative (Bedimo *et al.*, 2007).

22.4.1 Kaposi's sarcoma

Kaposi's sarcoma is an AIDS-defining illness and is the most common tumour type in people with HIV infection (Bower *et al.*, 2008). Kaposi's sarcoma is a rare cancer

Table 22.3 Non-AIDS-defining malignancies.

Existing data	Limited data
Anal cancer	Breast cancer
Hepatocellular cancer	Colon cancer
Hodgkin's disease	Head and neck cancer
Non-small cell lung cancer	Melanoma
Testicular germ cell cancer	Urological cancer

Bower *et al.* (2008).

in the HIV-negative population (Spano *et al.*, 2002) and it usually occurs in older men of Mediterranean descent, people who have undergone organ transplantation or young men in Africa. Kaposi's sarcoma is characterised by purple cutaneous lesions and can also be found in organs such as the lungs and digestive tract.

Management of Kaposi's sarcoma has changed dramatically with the introduction of combination antiretroviral treatment (ART). ART has been associated with a significant reduction in the incidence of Kaposi's sarcoma (Carrieri *et al.*, 2003). Cohort studies have suggested that ART protects against development of Kaposi's sarcoma (Bower *et al.*, 2008).

Treatment for Kaposi's sarcoma can be characterised by either local or systemic therapy. At one time, local therapy consisted of a variety of treatments including radiotherapy, intra-lesional chemotherapy and photodynamic therapy. Many local therapies have now largely been superceded by the introduction of ART (Bower *et al.*, 2008). However, radiotherapy is still used to treat localised Kaposi's sarcoma lesions or for cosmetic reasons.

Systemic treatment consists of ART, cytotoxic chemotherapy and immune therapy. All patients with Kaposi's sarcoma should receive ART (Bower *et al.*, 2008). Bower *et al.* (1999) have shown that ART prolongs the time to treatment failure in Kaposi's sarcoma and Holkova *et al.* (2001) have demonstrated that ART prolongs survival in patients who have had Kaposi's sarcoma treated with chemotherapy. Systemic chemotherapy is usually given to patients with advanced or rapidly progressive disease. The chemotherapy agents of choice are usually liposomal anthracyclines, e.g. liposomal doxorubicin or taxanes, paclitaxel (Bower *et al.*, 2008). The toxicity profiles of these chemotherapy agents rarely cause nutritional problems.

Whilst Kaposi's sarcoma is the most common tumour in patients with HIV infection, it is not associated with nutritional problems when it is confined to the skin. There are no additional nutritional considerations over and above those considered for people with HIV infection as a result of the presence of Kaposi's sarcoma.

22.4.2 Lymphoma

Lymphomas are defined as a diverse group of cancerous tumours of the lymphatic system. The lymphatic system is a part of the immune system that defends the body against disease. There are two main types of lymphoma; non-Hodgkin's lymphoma (NHL) and Hodgkin's lymphoma. Hodgkin's lymphoma (HL) is distinguished from all other types of lymphoma by the presence of a distinctive abnormal lymphocyte called a Reed-Steinberg cell.

HIV-related lymphomas remain a major cause of death in HIV-infected patients despite the advent of ART and its associated reduction in the frequency of opportunistic infections and some other types of cancer (Ribera and Navarro, 2008). The specific types of lymphoma more commonly associated with HIV-infected persons include clinically aggressive B-cell lymphomas, specifically, diffuse large B-cell lymphomas (DLBCL) and Burkitt's or Burkitt's-like lymphomas (BL) (Ratner *et al.*, 2001). The aetiology of lymphomas includes viral infections; specifically the Epstein-Barr virus (EBV), the HIV (AIDS) virus and human T-cell leukaemia/lymphoma virus (HTLV-1) which have all been implicated.

22.4.3   Non-Hodgkin's lymphoma (NHL)

NHL is the most common of all lymphomas that affect PLHIV (Dal Maso and Franceschi, 2003). The incidence of NHL is said to be 100- to 200-fold higher in the HIV-infected than the uninfected population (Ratner *et al.*, 2001). NHL occurs when the body's white blood cells, specifically B-cells, T-cells or NK cells develop abnormally resulting in the development of tumours. Such lymphomas are then defined as either indolent (slow progressing) or aggressive, with indolent lymphomas often being referred to as low-grade and the aggressive as high-grade. In addition, like the majority of cancer types, NHL is staged into four categories otherwise known as the Ann Arbor Staging System. Stage 1 affects only one group of lymph nodes, stage 2 affects two or more lymph node groups on one side of the diaphragm, stage 3 NHL is classified by the involvement of lymph nodes on both sides of the diaphragm and stage 4 by both the involvement of extensive lymph nodes and other organs such as bone marrow, liver and cerebrospinal fluid.

The most common sign of NHL is the existence of swollen lymph nodes. Other symptoms often referred to as B symptoms include fevers, weight loss, fatigue, rectal pain, abnormal pain or vomiting. In addition, those with CNS (central nervous system) lymphoma can develop confusion, loss of memory or speech, changes in personality, seizures, headaches or partial paralysis. However, some of these symptoms could be caused by other HIV-related conditions, although the risk of CNS involvement is increased in HIV-positive individuals (Ratner *et al.*, 2001). Many of those diagnosed with NHL can be treated successfully with chemotherapy agents, radiotherapy, and more recently the addition of monoclonal antibodies as immunotherapy such as Rituximab, as outlined in Table 22.4. However, approximately half of these individuals can relapse within 2 years. Many of these treatment agents are difficult for people to tolerate when the immune system is already compromised. As a result, dose reduction of the chemotherapy may well be considered. In some cases, up to half the regular dose is given to HIV-negative people with NHL. This has been proven to be safer and equally as effective. Those with CNS lymphoma usually receive whole brain radiotherapy and/or intrathecal chemotherapy using methotrexate along with regular chemotherapy since this does not cross the blood-brain barrier.

22.4.4   Burkitt's lymphoma

Burkitt's lymphoma is also rare, accounting for 2 to 5% of all cases of B-cell NHL (Leukaemia Research, 2006) and has also been linked to the presence of EBV. It is an extremely aggressive tumour with a rapid rate of growth consisting of endemic, sporadic and immunodeficiency-associated variants (Blum *et al.*, 2004) and once seen as incurable in adults due to the rapid proliferation rate of cells. It is identified by a distinctive pattern of tumour cells that replicate a starry-sky pattern (Blum *et al.*, 2004). It is usually very responsive to initial chemotherapy but relapses are common. Historically, the application of intensified therapy regimens, such as those given in acute lymphoblastic leukaemia, were often used (Blum *et al.*, 2004), however, in more recent times advances in the management of BL include the use of CODOX-M/IVAC and Hyper-CVAD (Table 22.5), in conjunction with ART for HIV-positive patients (Blum *et al.*, 2004; Bower *et al.*, 2008), but there remains no gold standard therapy as comparative studies have been undertaken (Bower *et al.*, 2008). Due to the high risk of nervous system involvement, it is important that patients should also

Table 22.4 Standard chemotherapy combinations used to treat people with NHL.

Acronym	Chemotherapy agents
CHOP	Cyclophosphamide Doxorubicin Vincristine Prednisolone
R-CHOP	Rituximab (MabThera) Cyclophosphamide Doxorubicin Vincristine Prednisolone
DHAP	Dexamethasone Cisplatin Cytarabine
ESHAP	Etoposide Methylprednisone Cytarabine Cisplatin
Mini-BEAM	Carmustine Etoposide Cytarabine Melphalan
ICE	Ifosfamide Carboplatin Etoposide
–	Chlorambucil (+/– Prednisolone)
–	Fludarabine
FMD	Fludarabine Mitozantrone Dexamethasone
FC	Fludarabine Cyclophosphamide
CVP	Cyclophosphamide Vincristine Prednisolone
R–CVP	Rituximab Cyclophosphamide Vincristine, Prednisolone
PMitCEBO/M	Prednisolone Mitozantrone Cyclophosphamide Etoposide Bleomycin Vincristine (+/– Methotrexate)
GEM-P	Methylprednisolone Gemcitabine Cisplatin

From Sweetenham (2005).

Table 22.5 Standard chemotherapy combinations used to treat people with BL.

Acronym	Chemotherapy agents
CODOX-M/IVAC	Cyclophosphamide
	Vincristine
	Doxorubicin
	Methotrexate/ifosfamide
	Etoposide
	Cytarabine
hyperCVAD	Cyclophosphamide
	Vincristine
	Doxorubicin
	Dexamethasone
	Methotrexate
	Cytarabine

From Bower *et al.* (2008).

receive CNS-directed therapy, such as intrathecal chemotherapy with methotrexate or cytarabine.

22.4.5 Hodgkin's lymphoma

HL accounts for approximately 15% of cases per year and the current trend has been a stable number of cases annually in the UK. HL is roughly twice as common in males, than in females. HL is classified further into five types in two distinct categories; classical Hodgkin's, which incorporates four types including the commoner nodular sclerosing presentation, and nodular lymphocyte predominant. The causes of HL are not specifically known, however, evidence suggests that some cases are linked to specific virus infections, specifically the EBV. HL is more likely to develop in those who are immunosupressed, hence its link with HIV/AIDS. Again like NHL, HL presents with enlarged lymph nodes in the neck, collarbone region, axilla or groin, however, a significant proportion of patients have no obvious symptoms at diagnosis and their disease can be discovered incidentally, i.e. as a result of a routine chest X-ray. It is also staged using the Ann Arbor Staging System. Its management includes chemotherapy with or without radiotherapy as consolidation. Chemotherapy regimens used include two cycles of OEPA with or without COPP, ABVD or ChlVPP chemotherapy plus site-specific radiotherapy as required. Relapsed disease can be managed with further chemotherapy such as ESHAP with or without IVE or gemcitabine, and consideration can also be given to a BEAM autograft or BEAM-Campath allograft where appropriate.

22.5 Nutrition in the management of non-surgical oncology patients

Whilst an improvement in survival due to nutritional interventions has not yet been shown (Arends *et al.*, 2006), unintentional weight loss of $\geq 10\%$ within the previous 6 months signifies substantial nutritional deficit and is a good prognostic indicator of outcome (DeWys *et al.*, 1980). In addition, Mercadante (1998) suggested that up to 20% of patients with cancer die due to the effects of malnutrition, however, this does not consider the additional impact of a diagnosis of HIV.

The aims of nutritional support in the patient with cancer are:

- prevent and treat undernutrition
- enhance anti-tumour treatment effects
- reduce the adverse effects of anti-tumour therapies
- improve the subjective quality of life (QoL) (Arends *et al.*, 2006).

However, the principal aim of nutritional intervention with cancer patients will be to maintain physical strength and optimise nutritional status within the confines of the disease (van Bokhorst-de van der Schueren *et al.*, 1999). Nutritional intervention should also be tailored to meet the needs of the patient and be realistic for them to achieve (Mick *et al.*, 1991). It is well recognised that optimal nutrition improves the efficacy of therapeutic modalities, the clinical course and outcome in cancer patients (Rivadeneira *et al.*, 1998). Numerous studies strongly suggest substantial weight loss >10% leads to adverse consequences, resulting in a reduced response to chemotherapy and radiotherapy, increased morbidity and poor QoL and increased mortality rate (van Bokhorst-de van der Schueren *et al.*, 1997).

22.5.1   Nutritional assessment

All patients with cancer, ideally, should undergo a nutritional assessment at diagnosis, and at regular intervals thereafter in light of both the affects of the tumour itself, and its associated treatments upon nutritional status as already highlighted in this chapter. Assessment pertaining to cancer management should include anthropometric measures (weight history, height, body mass index, hand grip strength and mid-arm circumference), a detailed dietary history, stage of disease, proposed treatment plan and intent and biochemical indices where appropriate, along with current HIV drug treatment regimen. It is vitally important to pay special attention to the details of the treatment plan and intent in order to ensure appropriate and timely nutritional intervention (see Chapter 8, 'Nutritional Screening and Assessment').

22.5.2   Nutritional interventions

Nutritional intervention is dependent upon the patient's tumour type, site and stage of disease, baseline nutritional status, treatment modality and duration, likely side effect profile and curative/palliative intent.

Nutritional interventions can include:

- relaxation of previous dietary advice
- food fortification
- symptom control advice
- consistency modification
- oral nutritional supplements (ONS)
- enteral nutrition (EN)
- parenteral nutrition (PN).

In terms of the healthy eating approach to the lifestyle management of those living with HIV, it is unlikely to be appropriate to continue such diets once cancer has been diagnosed. Whilst the pharmacological management of hyperlipidaemia and diabetes is likely to continue in such patients, relaxation of previous therapeutic diets maybe required in order to minimise further nutritional compromise. Food fortification is often suggested as the first-line nutritional support intervention; however, this may not necessarily be appropriate due to the side effect profiles and the intensity of the treatment regimens. It is important to treat each patient individually in terms of their specific cancer diagnosis and planned treatment. Patients may require more intensive nutritional support methods from the beginning of treatment, over and above traditional food fortification methods, with the early use of oral nutrition support (ONS) and enteral nutrition (EN) being considered. Nutritional support should be administered alongside adequate symptom control and pain relief. This often involves pharmaceutical treatment such as anti-emetics and mouth care agents.

EN is indicated for a patient with cancer if undernutrition is already present, and/or if inadequate food intake is anticipated for more than 7 days. The amount of additional nutrient intake provided should substitute the difference between actual intake and calculated requirements (ASPEN, 2002). It is often questioned whether EN can improve or maintain nutritional status in patients with cancer, although evidence suggests that such interventions in patients who have lost weight as a result of insufficient food intake can reduce the risk of further deterioration of their nutritional status (Arends *et al.*, 2006). However, in patients with cancer cachexia it is extremely difficult to attenuate weight loss due to the overwhelming metabolic influence of the systemic inflammatory response secondary to the presence of a tumour (De Blaauw *et al.*, 1997). In addition, without anti-cancer therapies it is impossible to reverse this metabolic process (Arends *et al.*, 2006).

In terms of nutritional requirements in the patient with cancer, cancer itself does not have a consistent effect on resting energy expenditure since it can remain unchanged, increased or decreased in relation to the predicted energy expenditure (Arends *et al.*, 2006). It has also been suggested that there has been inconsistent information regarding the effect of cancer treatments on energy expenditure and tumour-specific stress factors need to be used with extreme caution. Therefore, regular monitoring of nutritional status of the patient with cancer is essential to ensure that nutritional needs are met.

22.5.3 Developments in nutrition and cancer management

There is no data from controlled studies to suggest routine use of cancer-specific nutritional support products (Arends *et al.*, 2006). Results remain inconclusive regarding the appropriate use of eicosapentanoic acid (EPA)-enriched nutritional supplements. Many patients with HIV-related malignant disease develop haematological cancers, which brings into question the safety aspect of using a substance that has the potential to stimulate the immune system whilst conventional therapy aims to down-regulate the immune system.

The use of pharmaceutical agents to stimulate appetite and promote weight gain in cancer is another controversial subject and has been the focus of much attention in the literature. However, studies are often poor in design, limited in sample size and are often carried out in patients who are being palliated. To date, the following agents have been suggested as appetite stimulants: progestational agents such as megesterol acetate, and corticosteroids, i.e. dexamethasone and prednislone; anti-catabolic agents, i.e. thalidomide (Bruera *et al.*, 1999) and pentoxifylline (Inui, 2002; Laviano *et al.*, 2003); anabolic agents, i.e. hormones such as oxandrolone and flu-oxymesterone (Inui, 2002; Laviano *et al.*, 2003; Giordiano and Jatoi, 2004); and oral supplements of the branched-chain amino acids leucine, isoleucine and valine have been shown to decrease the severity of anorexia in patients with cancer (Inui, 2002). The major active principle of marijuana Δ^9-tetrahydrocannabinol has been licensed for use with palliative patients in two specific preparations, nabilone and dronabinol. These agents are thought to have a tumour-suppressive effect in a number of different tumour types, along with anti-emetic, analgesic and appetite-stimulating properties (Bifulco *et al.*, 2006). In addition, ongoing interest in the role of eicosapentanoeic acid (EPA), an n-3 long-chain polyunsaturated fatty acid found in oily fish and can-cer, suggests it may modulate aspects of the inflammatory response implicated in the metabolic changes associated with weight loss and muscle wasting in cancer patients (Barber, 1998; Gogos *et al.*, 1998; Barber *et al.*, 1999).

In conclusion, as is the case with HIV disease, nutrition has an important role in the management of cancer and its associated treatment modalities. Comprehensive nutritional assessment is necessary to ensure early recognition of malnutrition, as there are an array of factors that affect nutritional status and up to 20% of patients with cancer die as a result of the effect of malnutrition (Mercadante, 1998). Nu-tritional interventions have an important role throughout the course of the disease, from diagnosis through to terminal care (Scott and Hamilton, 1998). The effective implementation of appropriate nutritional interventions should aim to improve qual-ity of life and can enhance the beneficial effects of treatments (Ottery, 1994). With the increasing emphasis on survivorship, which refers to both living with and beyond cancer (Cancer Reform Strategy, 2007), timely and ongoing nutritional interventions will continue to prove vital in this patient group.

References

Arends J, Bodoky G, Bozzetti F *et al.* ESPEN guidelines enteral nutrition: non-surgical oncology. *Clin Nutr* 2006; **25**:245–59.

ASPEN Board of Directors. Clinical guidelines taskforce: nutrition assessment – adults. *J Parent Enteral Nutr* 2002; **26**:9SA–12SA.

Barber MD. The anti-cachectic effect of fatty acids. *Proc Nutr Soc* 1998; **57**:571–6.

Barber MD, Ross JA, Preston T, Shenkin A, Fearon KC. Fish oil-enriched nutritional supplement attenuates progression of the acute-phase response in weight-losing patients with advanced pancreatic cancer. *J Nutr* 1999; **129**:1120–25.

Bedimo RJ, Dunlap M, McGinnis KA, Rodriguez-Barradas M, Justice AC. Incidence of non-AIDS-defining malignancies in HIV-infected vs. non-infected veterans in the ART era: impact of im-munosuppression. Program and abstracts of the 47th Interscience Conference on Antimicrobial Agents and Chemotherapy; September 17–20, 2007; Chicago, IL, 2007. Abstract H-1721.

Bhosle J, Hall G. Principles of cancer treatment by chemotherapy. *Surgery* 2006; **24**:66–9.

Bifulco M, Laezza C, Pisanti S, Gazzerro P. Cannabinoids and cancer: pros and cons of an anti-tumour strategy. *Br J Pharmacol* 2006; **148**:123–35.

Blum KA, Lozanski G, Byrd JC. Adult Burkitt leukaemia and lymphoma. *Blood* 2004; **104**:3009–3020.

Bower M, Collins S, Cottrill C *et al.* BHIVA guidelines on HIV-associated malignancies. *HIV Med* 2008; **9**:336–88.

Bower M, Fox P, Fife K, Gill J, Nelson M, Gazzard B. Highly active anti-retroviral therapy (HARRT) prolongs time to treatment failure in Kaposi's sarcoma. *AIDS* 1999; **13**:2105–11.

Brennan J, Moynihan C. *Cancer in Context: A Practical Guide to Supportive Care.* Oxford: Oxford University Press, 2004.

Bruera E, Neumann CM, Pituskin E, Calder K, Ball G, Hanson J. Thalidomide in patients with cachexia due to terminal cancer: preliminary report. *Ann Oncol* 1999; **10**:857–9.

Calman K, Hine D. *A Policy Framework for Commissioning Cancer Services.* London: HMSO, 1995.

Carrieri M, Pradier C, Piselli P *et al.* Reduced incidence of Kaposi's sarcoma and of systemic non-hodgkin's lymphoma in HIV-infected individuals treated with highly active antiretroviral therapy. *Int J Cancer* 2003; **103**:142–4.

Cheung MC, Pantanowitz L, Dezube BJ. AIDS-related malignancies: emerging challenges in the era of highly active antiretroviral therapy. *Oncologist* 2005; **10**:412–26.

Dal Maso L, Franceschi S. Epidemiology of non-Hodgkin lymphomas and other haemolymphopoietic neoplasms in people with AIDS. *Lancet Oncol* 2003; **4**:110–119.

De Blaauw I, Deutz NEP, von Meyenfeldt MF. Metabolic changes of cancer cachexia – second of two parts. *Clin Nutr* 1997; **16**:223–8.

Department of Health (Calman-Hine Report). A policy framework for commissioning cancer services: a report by the Expert Advisory Group on cancer to the Chief Medical Officers of England and Wales. 1995.

Department of Health. *The NHS Plan: A Plan for Investment, A Plan for Reform.* London: The Stationery Office, 2000a.

Department of Health. *The NHS Cancer Plan: A Plan for Investment, A Plan for Reform.* London: DH, 2000b.

Department of Health. *Cancer Reform Strategy.* London: DH, 2007.

DeWys WD, Begg C, Lavin PT *et al.* Prognostic effect of weight loss prior to chemotherapy in cancer patients. Eastern Co-operative Oncology Group. *Am J Med* 1980; **69**:491–7.

Falk S. Principle of cancer treatment by radiotherapy. *Surgery* 2006; **24**:62–5.

Frisch M, Biggar RJ, Engels EA, Goedart JJ. Association of cancer with AIDS-related immunosuppression in adults. *J Am Med Assoc* 2001; **285**:1736–45.

Giordiano KF, Jatoi A. A synopsis of cancer-related anorexia and weight loss. *Bus Brief: US Oncol Rev* 2004; **1**:1–5.

Gogos CA, Ginopoulos P, Salsa B, Apostolidou E, Zoumbos NC, Kalfarentzos F. Dietary omega-3 polyunsaturated fatty acids plus vitamin E restore immunodeficiency and prolong survival for severely ill patients with generalized malignancy: a randomised control trial. *Cancer* 1998; **82**:395–402.

Grulich AE, Li Y, McDonald A, Correll PKL, Law MG, Kaldor JM. Rates of non-AIDS – defining cancers in people with HIV infection before and after AIDS diagnosis. *AIDS* 2002; **16**:1155–61.

Hanahan D, Weinberg R. The Hallmarks of cancer. *Cell* 2000; **100**:57–70.

Holkova B, Takeshita K, Cheng D *et al.* Effect of highly active antiretroviral therapy on survival in patients with AIDS-associated pulmonary Kaposi's sarcoma treated with chemotherapy. *J Clin Oncol* 2001; **19**:3848–51.

Inui A. Cancer anorexia – cachexia syndrome: current issues in research & management. *CA Cancer J Clin* 2002; **52**:72–91.

Laviano A, Meguid MM, Rossi-Fanelli F. Cancer anorexia: clinical implications, pathogenesis, and therapeutic strategies. *Lancet Oncol* 2003; **4**:686–94.

Leukaemia Research. *Non-Hodgkin's Lymphoma.* London: Leukaemia Research, 2006: 22.

Mbulaiteye SM, Biggar RJ, Goedert JJ, Engels EA. Immune deficiency and risk for malignancy among persons with AIDS. *J Acquir Immune Defic Syndr* 2003; **32**:527–33.

Mercadante S. Parenteral versus enteral nutrition in cancer patients: indications and practice. *Support Care Cancer* 1998; **6**:85–93.

Mick R, Vokes EE, Weichselbaum RR, Panje WR. Prognostic factors in advanced head & neck cancer patients undergoing multi-modality therapy. *Otolaryngol Head Neck Surg* 1991; **105**:62–73.

Ottery FD. Cancer cachexia: prevention, early diagnosis & management. *Cancer Pract* 1994; **2**:123–31.

Rabkin CS. AIDS and cancer in the era of highly active anti-retroviral therapy (ART). *Eur J Cancer* 2001; **37**:1316–9.

Ratner L, Lee J, Tang S *et al.* Chemotherapy for human immunodeficiency virus-associated non hodgkin's lymphoma in combination with highly active antiretroviral therapy. *J Clin Oncol* 2001; **19**:2171–8.

Reed M. Principles of cancer treatment by surgery. *Surgery* 2006; **24**:70–73.

Ribera JM, Navarro JT. Human immunodeficiency virus related non-hodgkin's lymphoma. *Haematologica* 2008; **93**:1129–32.

Rivadeneira DE, Evoy D, Fahey TJ, Lieberman MD, Daly JM. Nutritional support of the cancer patient. *CA Cancer J Clin* 1998; **48**:69–80.

Robinson S. Principles of chemotherapy. *Eur J Cancer Care* 1993; **2**:55–65.

Rosenberg B, Vancamp L, Krigas T. Inhibition of cell division in Escherichia Coli by electrolysis products from a platinum electrode. *Nature* 1965; **13**:698–9.

Scott A, Hamilton K. Nutritional screening: an audit. *Nurs Stand* 1998; **12**:46–7.

Souhami R, Tannock I, Hohenberger P, Horiot J. *Principles of Combination Chemotherapy*. Oxford Textbook of Oncology, 2nd edn. Oxford: Oxford University Press, 2002.

Spano J-P, Atlan D, Breau JL, Farge D. AIDS and non-AIDS relared maligancies: a new vexing challenge in HIV-positive patients Part I: Kaposi's sarcoma, non-Hodgkin's lymphoma, and Hodgkin's lymphoma. *Eur J Intern Med* 2002; **13**:170–79.

Spina M, Vaccher E, Carbone A, Tirelli U. Neoplastic complications of HIV infection. *Ann Oncol* 1999; **10**:1271–86.

Sweetenham JW. Diffuse large B-cell lymphoma: risk stratification and management of relapsed disease. *Hematol Am Soc Hematol Educ Program* 2005; 252–9.

van Bokhorst-de van der Schueren MA, van Leeuwen PAM, Kuik DJ *et al.* The impact of nutritional status on the prognosis of patients with advanced head and neck cancer. *Cancer* 1999; **86**:519–27.

van Bokhorst-de van der Schueren MA, van Leeuwen PA, Sauerwein HP *et al.* Assessment of malnutrition parameters in head and neck cancer and their relation to postoperative complications. *Head Neck* 1997; **19**:419–25.

Section 6
PALLIATIVE, END OF LIFE CARE AND NUTRITION

23 Nutrition and End of Life Care

Vivian Pribram

Key Points

- Although treatment advances have greatly improved prognosis, nutritional management of late stages of progressive illness is an essential aspect of HIV care.
- Reduced oral intake is common and management of this condition includes discussion with patient, relatives and staff and may include artificial nutrition support.
- Due to a lack of evidence it is not known if this treatment improves quality of life or prolongs survival, so it is not possible to define the benefits and harms of this treatment.
- Palliative care is an important part of holistic HIV care throughout the disease trajectory and this includes nutritional management of symptoms.
- In order to provide comprehensive care for patients with HIV at the late stages of progressive illness, nutritional care should be individualised, ethical issues must be considered and the wishes of the patient are paramount.

23.1 Introduction

In regions with good access to antiretroviral treatment (ART), end-of-life issues in HIV infection have become less prominent compared to the early years of the pandemic when HIV was largely a terminal illness with rapid progression. Advances in treatment have restored health, changed lives, and delayed death (Ludwig and Chittenden, 2008). Life expectancy in HIV-infected patients treated with combination antiretroviral therapy increased between 1996 and 2005, although there is considerable variability between subgroups of patients. The average number of years remaining to be lived at age 20 years was found to be about two-thirds of that in the general population in countries included in a collaborative analysis of 14 cohort studies (Antiretroviral Therapy Cohort Collaboration, 2008). Nevertheless, end-of-life issues are still an important consideration in this patient group for a variety of reasons including:

- Although mortality in people with HIV infection continues to decrease as treatment improves, it is still higher than in uninfected people.
- Large numbers of individuals are unaware of their diagnosis, and present only with advanced disease.
- ART is associated with toxicities, side effects and adequate adherence to medication is difficult for many people.

- Lower CD4$^+$ T cell counts on treatment are associated with increased risk of serious non-AIDS conditions such as cancer, liver disease and perhaps cardiovascular disease, and the incidence of these diseases is higher among patients treated for HIV than in age-matched HIV-uninfected people, and the risk of non-AIDS-related morbidity and mortality, including cardiovascular disease, liver disease and cancer, is higher in untreated HIV infection than in treated infection.
- People living with HIV (PLHIV) have increasingly become an ageing population (Harding *et al.*, 2005; Ludwig and Chittenden, 2008; Deeks and Phillips, 2009).

HIV infection continues to be a highly prevalent and rapid killer in low- and middle-income countries, where ART is unavailable to 70–80% of patients for whom it might be beneficial (Ludwig and Chittenden, 2008). There have been many efforts to make HIV medications more available in resource-limited settings by pressuring pharmaceutical manufacturers to reduce prices, permitting production of generic versions of effective therapies and providing funds for drug purchases (Wolf and Lo, 2001).

23.1.1   People living with HIV

Generally, PLHIV have been younger than patients with other diseases (although this is changing in developed countries where there is greater accessibility to ART), and they often are members of marginalised or minority groups. Compared with patients who have malignancies or cardiovascular disease, HIV-infected patients are more likely to have partners, caregivers and family members who are also infected with HIV. They are more likely to have experienced multiple bereavements from HIV within their peer groups (Ludwig and Chittenden, 2008). With the advent of effective ART a number of issues have arisen for patients and providers alike. Some patients who have been long-term survivors have had to re-establish themselves among the living after preparing themselves for death by saying good-byes, leaving work and selling property. When the disease progresses despite ART, patients and providers may feel a sense of failure or anger (Ludwig and Chittenden, 2008).

Some research has shown that traditional markers for disease progression, such as CD4 count and viral load, may not correlate clearly with prognosis in patients with advanced HIV infection, further complicating end-of-life discussions and decision-making. In contrast to the more predictable, consistently worsening disease trajectories seen with terminal cancer, HIV illness can be punctuated by episodes of worsening function (resulting from infection, toxicity or increased symptoms) followed by periods of improvement or symptom-free living that do not necessarily signal a progression of illness (Ludwig and Chittenden, 2008). Added to this, the initiation of effective combination ART has been seen to restore health to many patients who have conditions, such as wasting, chronic diarrhoea or intractable opportunistic infections, that would have predicted death in the pre-ART era. This uncertain disease trajectory underscores the importance of pain, symptom management, good communication, clarification of patients' goals, and advance care planning throughout the course of illness (Ludwig and Chittenden, 2008).

23.2 Palliative care

Palliative care is the active, holistic care of patients with advanced progressive illness with diminishing response to disease-modifying treatment and increasing symptoms. It provides management of pain and other symptoms and also the provision of psychological, social and spiritual support (NICE, 2004). End-of-life care is an important part of palliative care, and usually refers to the care of a person during the last part of their life, from the point at which it has become clear that the person is in a progressive state of decline (Watson *et al.*, 2005). While some interventions, such as artificial nutrition support, may be perfectly appropriate in the earlier palliative phase, it is likely that they would not be appropriate in the last few days of life.

The changing epidemiology of HIV disease in the era of effective ART has resulted in new and evolving roles for palliative care, with a shift from the more conventional HIV palliative care of the 1980s and early 1990s to a greater focus on symptom control in patients who may continue to live for an extended period, or the need for active treatment for one HIV-related condition and palliation for another simultaneously (Harding *et al.*, 2005). Clinical evidence demonstrates that patients with HIV infection require palliative care throughout the disease trajectory in order to:

- control pain and symptoms
- promote adherence through reduction of side effects and toxicity associated with antiretroviral therapy
- manage life-limiting co-morbidities such as cancers and end-stage liver disease and
- provide quality end-of-life care for those whom antiretroviral therapy fails or who are unable to access it (Harding *et al.*, 2005).

Box 23.1 identifies where palliative care can be provided.

Box 23.1   Deciding where palliative care can be provided

- In low HIV seroprevalence countries, palliative care may be a routine part of hospital and clinic care.

In countries with a high burden of HIV infection, palliative care should be part of a comprehensive care and support package, which can be provided in hospitals and clinics or at home by caregivers and relatives. In many settings, HIV-infected people prefer to receive care at home. The provision of palliative care can be augmented significantly by the involvement of family and community caregivers. A mix of psychosocial support, traditional or local remedies, and medicines can be combined to provide palliative care that surpasses that found in many overcrowded or poorly staffed hospitals.

- Wherever palliative care is provided, factors to be assessed include affordability and the presence of community care and support services.
- Developing guidelines and training for palliative care should be specifically included in national guidelines for the clinical management of HIV/AIDS.
- Training on the provision of palliative care should be incorporated into the curriculum for all health care providers.

- Guidelines for home care services should include basic management of palliative care by family members and community volunteers.
- Training courses for family members and community volunteers can be organised and provided by health care workers at the community level.

23.2.1   Symptom management

Studies have consistently documented the under-recognition and under-treatment of pain and other symptoms in patients with AIDS, and have also consistently demonstrated a high prevalence of pain and chronic symptoms, such as fatigue, anorexia/weight loss, nausea/vomiting, dyspnoea and diarrhoea, both in the pre-ART and current eras. Within the narrow biomedical model of care, such symptoms are generally regarded as secondary, or incidental, to the primacy of the infectious disease diagnosis which dictates appropriate pathogen-specific treatment (Selwyn, 2005). Conditions affecting mental health such as depression are also well documented (for a comprehensive discussion of nutritional aspects of symptom management, see Chapters 9 and 15). In the systematic review of patient outcomes, Harding et al. (2005) found home palliative care and inpatient hospice care to significantly improve patient outcomes in the domains of pain and symptom control, anxiety, insight, and spiritual well-being. As with other chronic illnesses, treatment of the underlying condition often constitutes a good basis for symptom management.

23.2.2   Palliative care in resource-limited settings

Access to ART remains a serious issue for palliative care in resource-limited settings. WHO and other international health organisations recognise the importance of adequate pain control, symptom management and psychosocial support as part of the equitable distribution of health resources. Resource-limited communities face a multitude of barriers including overwhelming numbers of patients, underdeveloped health care systems, racial and ethnic disparities in access to health care and limited access to opioids. More training, funding and support are needed to strengthen palliative care programmes being adapted to resource-limited regions. Most notable are those designed on the 'integrated community-based home care' model, utilising community caregivers in home settings. Lastly, there are unique psychosocial challenges to end-of-life care in much of the developing world. Huge numbers of children orphaned by AIDS stress the support systems in place, women in general carry a greater economic burden and also bear most of the responsibility for caregiving, and stigma against PLHIV is rampant (Ludwig and Chittenden, 2008).

23.3   Nutritional care in later stages of progressive illness

Weight change over time is used as an indicator of nutrition excess or inadequacy. A questionnaire sent to physicians in the Netherlands found that less than 2% of physicians followed weights of their patients. If weight loss was noted, it was assumed to be an inevitable result of disease, and no nutrition intervention was initiated. This fatalistic attitude that weight loss is an expected outcome of disease could increase the burden on those attempting to 'replete' severely malnourished patients who have been allowed to lose weight over the course of their disease. Initiation of nutrition interventions early in the course of insidious weight loss could reduce the number of patients who become debilitated and emaciated during the disease treatment and palliative care continuum. Where possible, it is important to avoid symptoms such as severe fatigue, depression and social impairments related to nutrition depletion which can result in a reduced quality of life (QOL) for the patient (Fuhrman and Herrmann, 2006). Expert nutritional therapy can help ensure that the patient is able to retain:

- ability to derive pleasure from food
- physical strength, long enough to fulfil final wishes and ambitions
- some control over the disease process and
- to die with dignity and not as a result of avoidable starvation (Eldridge, 2007).

23.3.1   Oral nutrition support

If the patient is able to manage oral intake, food and fluids should be encouraged with the aim of consuming adequate nutritional intake to meet daily nutritional requirements and maintain weight. Nutrition counselling, use of oral supplements, and regular monitoring of nutritional intake and status, in conjunction with symptom management, can improve nutrient intake and quality of life (QOL) for patients in the later stages of progressive illness (Fuhrman and Herrmann, 2006; also see Chapter 4, 'Paediatric Nutritional Screening, Assessment and Support' and Chapter 7, 'Decreased Nutritional Status and Nutritional Interventions for People Living with HIV'). It is important that eating and drinking are enjoyable experiences while nutritional support measures are not so invasive or unacceptable to the patient that they impair quality of life (Eldridge, 2007). The role of a dietitian includes:

- assessing eating habits
- identifying any nutrition related problems or barriers to food and fluid intake and evaluating their physical and psychological impact
- exploring nutritional concerns held by the patient/partner/relatives
- discussion with patients and carers about dietary goals which are appropriate and achievable and
- integrating these goals into the care plan in a way which is compatible with medical and nursing objectives (Eldridge, 2007).

If weight loss continues, decisions may be made as to whether to continue oral diet as tolerated or initiate either tube feeding (TF) or parenteral nutrition (PN) if physiologically appropriate (Fuhrman and Herrmann, 2006).

Clinicians should focus first on treatment of reversible aetiologies of diminished food intake before progressing to nutrition support. Potential interventions include management of taste changes, pain, nausea, vomiting, dysphagia and constipation, treatment of depression, and alleviation of gastrointestinal dysfunction and obstruction (Fuhrman and Herrmann, 2006).

23.3.2   What is the role of specialised nutrition support in the later stages of progressive illness?

According to 'Standards, Options and Recommendations for Palliative or Terminal Nutrition in Adults with Progressive Cancer', artificial nutrition is contraindicated when life expectancy is less than 3 months, the patient's Karnofsky's index is 50% or less, or World Health Organization (WHO) performance status is >2. Nutrition support is also contraindicated when scientific evidence does not support its use. However, the over-riding contraindication for initiating or continuing nutrition support is when the patient or the patient's surrogate refuses it (Fuhrman and Herrmann, 2006).

Percutaneous endoscopic gastrostomy (PEG) feeding has been shown to be a highly safe and effective method of maintaining adequate nutrition for patients who are unable to ingest sufficient nutrients orally. However, this intervention is regarded as an inappropriate indication in most cases for patients with advanced cancer, end-stage diseases or advanced dementia due to inadequate clinical benefit. Individual benefits from PEG feeding with respect to quality of life is expected to be lower in older patients and patients with complex and severe co-morbidity (Loser et al., 2005). Overall published data support an individualised but critical and restrictive approach to feeding in such patients. Decision-making is still difficult and this needs to be done on an individual basis. Prospective clinical studies have shown that guidelines help to improve the appropriateness of patients' selection and play a pro-active role in decision-making for medically adequate PEG insertion with a consecutively improved outcome (Loser et al., 2005). It is a skill to know when curative or aggressive treatment should be abandoned in favour of the provision of care, comfort, symptom relief and the preservation of dignity (Korner et al., 2006).

23.3.3   Making decisions about artificial nutrition support

If nutritional intake is not adequate, the patient should be involved in decision-making about feeding. Does he or she have capacity to make decisions? If yes, the 'pros and cons' of feeding must be discussed, with a clear explanation of possible outcomes and morbidity. As patients have a right to refuse therapy, respect for their wishes is paramount. Appropriate palliative care must be offered, with offers of oral hydration or nutrients and symptom management. The patient should be able to change his/her mind at any point. If treatment is futile, the doctor has a responsibility to outline this.

The key to determining whether to pursue specialised nutrition support is for the patient, partner/family/carers/advocates and clinician to collectively examine the indications versus contraindications, as well as benefits versus burdens for the nutrition regimen being considered. This mandates an understanding of the patient and family expectations and goals and frequent discussions to reassess the patient's perception of QOL (Fuhrman and Herrmann, 2006). It is also essential to assess the psycho-spiritual impact of undergoing the treatment and what their expectations of artificial nutrition support are (Fuhrman and Herrmann, 2006).

23.4   Ethical and legal considerations

Ethical codes of caring professions include not only minimum standards of behaviour but also ideals, and have been described as the 'collective conscience' of the profession

(Macfie, 2006). Knowing about ethical theories does not automatically mean that we can suddenly resolve all ethical problems easily and wisely. Instead, the most important aspect is to recognise that there *are* ethical issues involved in a particular situation and to ensure that all significant aspects of the case are stated clearly and discussed with all relevant stakeholders.

There is a difference between ethical principles and legal frameworks. The 'law' defends individual rights and liberties and sets minimum standards, below which professional conduct can be regarded as lacking in care, negligent or criminal. It also protects those who lack the capacity to make decisions for themselves and it provides some safeguards and protection for doctors and other professions. An example of this is the principle that no doctor can be obliged to provide treatment which he/she believes to be against the patients' interests or futile. This delicate balance between patients' legal rights and professional judgement has been challenged by legal judgements, particularly in the United States and the UK (Korner *et al.*, 2006).

The law differentiates between oral intake and enteral tube feeding. While tube feeding is clearly considered therapy, oral nutritional supplements can be basic care as well as therapy. Oral nutrition supplements are therapy under certain conditions, e.g. if pharmacological effects should be achieved by specific composition (e.g. branched-chain amino acids (BCAA)). The provision of adequate fluid and nutrients by mouth, including oral nutritional supplements, in most instances, as well as help with eating and drinking where necessary, is regarded by the law as basic care (Korner *et al.*, 2006).

Much of contemporary medical ethics has been based on the work of Beauchamp and Childress. They have developed the use of the four 'prima facie' principles in the field of medicine. These are:

- **autonomy** is the principle of self-determination and involves recognition of patients' rights
- **non-maleficence** is deliberate avoidance of harm
- **beneficence** is the concept that the patient is provided with some form of benefit
- **justice** is the fair and equitable provision of available medical resources to all.

Some of the criticisms levied are that principles can conflict, it is not clear which of the principles should rule, and principles are very general and it is not obvious how they may apply to complex situations (Jonsen, 2005). Advocates of these principles stress that they should be seen, not as precise guides to inform doctors in every circumstance, but as a framework of values that are relevant to ethical debate (MacFie, 2006).

23.4.1 Autonomy

It is well established in law and ethics that adults with capacity have the right to refuse any medical treatment, even if that refusal will result in their death (MacFie, 2006).

For adults who lack the capacity to make decisions for themselves, health professionals should follow a code of practice. In the UK, the Adults with Incapacity (Scotland) Act 2000 and the 2005 Mental Capacity Act (MCA) in England and Wales provide statutory frameworks to empower and protect vulnerable adults who lack capacity to make decisions. The tenet of the MCA and code of practice is that professionals must help patients make as many decisions as possible for themselves (Lyons *et al.*, 2007).

The Acts help clarify who can make decisions and how they should go about this. Through 'advance decisions' patients have the right, within limits, to define in advance the way in which they wish to be treated, should they become incapacitated. Advance decisions (also known as 'Living Wills') are a means for patients to exercise the right to consent to or refuse medical treatment by anticipating a time when they may lose the capacity to make or communicate a decision (Baker *et al.*, 2008). Further information about advance decisions can be obtained via the British Medical Association and in the Mental Capacity Act (see Further Reading and References).

The Mental Capacity Act has five underpinning principles:

A presumption of capacity: Every adult is presumed to have capacity to make their own decisions unless it is established that he or she lacks capacity.

Maximising decision-making capacity: It is important that all practical steps to help people make decisions for themselves have been addressed before anyone concludes that they cannot make their own decisions.

Unwise decisions: Individuals have the right to make decisions that may be seen as eccentric or unwise.

Best interests: Any decision made on behalf of someone lacking capacity must be done or made in their best interests.

Least restrictive approach: Anything done for or on behalf of someone lacking capacity must be achieved in the least restrictive way that is possible (Eldridge, 2007).

Capacity

A patient will lack capacity to consent to a particular intervention if he or she is:

- unable to comprehend and retain information material to the decision, especially as to the consequences of having, or not having, the intervention in question and/or
- unable to use and weigh this information in the decision-making process.

Before making a judgement that a patient lacks capacity, the professional must take all steps reasonable in the circumstances to assist the patient in taking their own decisions (this will clearly not apply if the patient is unconscious). This may involve explaining what is involved in very simple language, using pictures and communication and decision-aids as appropriate. People close to the patient (spouse/partner, family, friends and carers) may often be able to help, as may specialist colleagues such as speech and language therapists or learning disability teams, and independent advocates or supporters.

Capacity is 'decision-specific': a patient may lack capacity to take a particular complex decision, but be quite able to take other more straightforward decisions or parts of decisions (DoH, 2008).

The MCA requires the appointment of an Independent Mental Capacity Advocate (IMCA) where there is no other person available to act as the patient's advocate (usually partner or family member). This does not apply in emergency situations such as when urgent, essential surgery is needed. The role of the IMCA is to observe and ensure that the processes of assessing capacity and making decisions for people who lack capacity are conducted appropriately in accordance with the MCA. They support particularly vulnerable people who lack capacity and who are required to make important decisions about serious and life-changing events. They have the right to see records and documents about an individual, including medical records (Lyons *et al.*, 2007).

Dietitians will need to make assessments of the patient's capacity to consent to routine dietetic interventions during their day-to-day practice and need to be satisfied that capacity has been assessed (Lyons *et al.*, 2007).

Best interest

The goals of providing nutrition support, such as sustaining life or reducing discomfort related to thirst and hunger, must be weighed against the patient's or surrogate's wishes and the potential for benefit versus burden for the patient. Nutrition support provided to patients with terminal illness will not change the course of the patient's clinical outcome or reverse cachexia. Nutrition support should be provided when it is in the best interest of the patient and there are achievable goals associated with the nutrition support (Fuhrman and Herrmann, 2006).

Benefit versus burden

Issues of benefit versus burden frame most discussions of initiating, continuing or discontinuing nutrition support. The interpretation of whether something is a benefit or a burden will depend on the patient's, caregiver's and multidisciplinary team's (MDT) perspectives of the goals for the nutrition therapy. Ongoing evaluation is necessary to determine the effectiveness and benefit of nutrition therapies. According to expert agreement, functional scores, QOL, and patients'/relatives' satisfaction are more appropriate outcomes for decision-making than determinants of nutrition status and complication rates. Valid measures of outcomes exist for patients with cancer, but these same measures have not been validated in other patient populations (Fuhmann and Herrmann, 2006). The placement of an enteral feeding tube may be initiated to achieve several therapeutic goals including increased length of survival, decreased risk of pressure sores, increased comfort and alleviation of symptoms associated with malnutrition including hunger and thirst. However, there is inconclusive evidence to show that tube feeding is effective in achieving such goals (Lyons *et al.*, 2007).

Burdens of nutrition support

Complications of nutrition support and difficulties that may arise as a result of feeding include central access infection, hyperglycemia, aspiration pneumonia, nausea, vomiting and diarrhoea. These symptoms can lead to increased discomfort, morbidity and mortality.

When the end of life is near, nutrition support may not necessarily improve QOL. Constant evaluation of the burdens of therapy is crucial to prevent nutrition support therapy becoming a source of patient discomfort. It may improve QOL for some patients, but health care providers should not assume that nutrition support is 'essential' or necessarily improves the QOL for all dying patients (Fuhrman and Herrmann, 2006). Decisions should be made on the basis of wide-ranging consultation and consideration of individual circumstances.

Best interest decision-making

Members of the health care team or relatives may disagree about the patient's best interests. This may reflect conflicts in religious, ethnic or other value systems, and these must be discussed openly before instigation or withdrawal of therapy.

A patient's best interests are not limited to their best medical interests. Other factors which form part of the best interests' decision include:

- the wishes and beliefs of the patient when competent
- their current wishes
- their general well-being and
- their spiritual and religious welfare.

Two incapacitated patients, whose *physical* condition is identical, may therefore have different best interests (DoH, 2008). However, the issue of physiological futility of treatment remains and no doctor can be forced to give treatment that (s)he deems to be futile.

There is an ethical dilemma, at times, in the management of patients who are confused, semiconscious or have dementia and who may remove or dislodge feeding tubes or lines (MacFie, 2006). These circumstances are not uncommon among patients with HIV due, for example, to opportunistic infections affecting the brain such as progressive multifocal leukoencepahlopathy (PML), cytomegolavirus (CMV), primary CNS lymphoma, cryptococcal meningitis and toxoplasmosis. Use of restraint may be considered a violation of patient freedom, and thereby their autonomy (MacFie, 2006). However, minimal restraint, such as binding hands to prevent removal of feeding tubes to provide life-saving treatment may be justified when a patient lacks capacity. It could be seen to be the case that this may improve autonomy as it may restore the patient to an autonomous state. Clinicians must exercise judgement, compassion and common sense in such situations (MacFie, 2006). It is advisable to consult with the appropriate medical/legal advisor on such restraint matters including placement of nasogastric bridles.

In the UK, when an adult is proven to lack the capacity to take decisions, only a person who has a special legal authorisation (see LPA Section 'Refusal of Treatment') may give or withhold consent on his/her behalf. Family members, friends and partners cannot consent on behalf of a patient if they do not have such authorisation. However, it is always *good practice* to involve such persons in the patient's care, to keep them informed and to treat them with sensitivity (Baker *et al.*, 2008).

Within the multidisciplinary team it is the responsibility of the doctor in charge of the patient's care to make the final decision as to what is deemed futile and what is in the patient's best interests and this requires a clear view of the aims of therapy. Doctors are not obliged to instigate therapies that they believe will do no good (MacFie, 2006). However, where there are doubts about the patient's capacity or best interests, a second opinion and/or High Court approval can also be sought (DoH, 2008).

Refusal of treatment

In the UK a patient may have made a Lasting Power of Attorney (LPA) which may include authority to give or refuse consent to medical treatment or make other health care decisions. In this case, the attorney must be consulted in health care decisions or in deciding what treatment may be in a patient's best interests. Attorneys are likely to require detailed information about treatment options and their consequences from professionals to assist them in this decision-making role. For example, when considering if PEG is in a patient's best interest, a person who is an LPA may require an explanation of:

- the PEG tube and insertion procedures
- the risks and expected benefits
- the impact of treatment, e.g. on quality of life, possible side effects of feeding and infection of the PEG site
- the care of the PEG tube
- the expected goals of PEG feeding, e.g. increased survival, meeting nutritional requirements and weight gain
- alternative options, e.g. nasogastric feeding and
- the consequences of refusing PEG insertion.

If the LPA covers this decision, then the attorney is acting as an agent of the patient and is entitled to all the information relevant to the decision and holds the same responsibility that the patient would have (Lyons *et al.*, 2007).

In a large US study investigating end-of-life discussion and preferences among people with HIV, it was shown that older patients, men, white patients and those with more education and higher income or more advanced illness were more likely to have completed an advance directive. Black and Latino race/ethnicity and low education level were associated with lack of communication about end-of-life issues and not completing an advance directive. The most important factors for of end-of-life discussions and making advance directives were found to be having two or more hospital admissions in the past 6 months, and whether their practitioners discussed advance directives with them (Wenger *et al.*, 2001). When asked about preferences regarding life-extending care or care focused on comfort, study respondents expressed widely divergent opinions (Wenger *et al.*, 2001).

Clinicians must be seen to be transparently honest in their discussions with all concerned. They must not arbitrarily impose their own value systems or preferred biases in feeding modality in the absence of evidence, and they should not make recommendations for treatment or its withdrawal on the basis of resource considerations (MacFie, 2006).

Every endeavour must be made to establish what the patient might have wanted, were she/he able to express a view. The overriding factor must be to do what is in the best interests of the patient. If artificial nutrition is provided, the aims and duration of feeding must be clearly recorded, and frank and open discussion with relatives and other carers is essential (MacFie, 2006).

23.5 Withdrawal of nutrition

In law, withdrawal of artificial nutrition support is regarded in the same way as withholding treatment in the first place – that is, is it in the best interests of the patient, and do the risks outweigh the benefits? Also, it is concerned that autonomy has been preserved and that the patient or legal guardian have been consulted and given approval (Korner *et al.*, 2006).

Decisions concerning nutrition support can be fraught with family conflict. Many patients and families perceive nutrition support as food, with its connotation of love, nurturing and comfort, and may be reluctant to stop nutrition support for fear that they will starve themselves or their loved one to death (Fuhrman and Herrmann, 2006).

There are many misconceptions about the dying process and this includes the belief that lack of appetite and diminished oral intake are causing profound disability and that fluid and nutrition are required. The dying process may include changes such as loss of appetite, decreased oral fluid intake and decreased thirst, increasing weakness and/or fatigue (Alexander *et al.*, 2003).

Nutrition support should contribute to the relief of pain and suffering. When the burden exceeds the benefit, the patient, surrogate, or health care provider can choose to withdraw nutrition support. The withdrawal of nutrition support does not warrant the withdrawal of other comfort measures, including pain medication, hydration, human touch and contact. Meticulous mouth care should be provided, especially when hydration is withdrawn. If hydration is given, the least invasive route should be used (Fuhrman and Herrmann, 2006).

23.6   Implications for practice

In a Cochrane review of medically assisted nutrition for palliative care in adult patients, it was concluded that there are insufficient good quality studies to make any recommendations for practice with regard to the use of medically assisted nutrition in palliative care patients. Clinicians will need to make a decision based on the perceived benefits and harms of medically assisted nutrition in individual patient circumstances, without the benefit of high-quality evidence to guide them. The uncontrolled prospective studies described would suggest that patients with a good performance status and medium- to long-term prognosis (months to years) may benefit from medically assisted nutrition. However, the evidence base to support this at the moment is weak and any intention to use this treatment should be monitored carefully and, ideally, fed into further research (Good *et al.*, 2008). Moreover, these studies did not include population groups of PLHIV. Well-designed studies are needed to determine the benefits and harm of artificial nutrition support for patients in the late stages of progressive illness. Clinical relevant outcomes need to be clearly defined. This includes energy levels, functional status and overall quality of life. It is also important to know the effect of intervention on survival and adverse incidents should be reported so that risks of treatments can be balanced against benefits (Good *et al.*, 2008).

23.7   Conclusion

Although great strides have been made in the treatment of HIV, there is still a long way to go in ensuring access to ART and providing comprehensive care to many PLHIV and their loved ones. As researchers develop more and more treatments for HIV that improve patients' quality of living and extend their lives, it is necessary to remember the importance of pain control, symptom management, excellent communication and psychosocial support from the time of diagnosis to the time of death. Nutritional management of symptoms associated with HIV disease and treatment are essential aspects of care. Patients with HIV/AIDS report needing emotional support, communication and pain control from their physicians, and those patients with advanced illness describe a good death as having pain/symptom control, optimum quality of life, choosing where to die, having control of their treatment and having their spiritual needs addressed (Harding *et al.*, 2005). The study by Wenger *et al.* highlighted patients at high risk of difficult end-of-life decision-making (e.g. intravenous drug users, persons who engage in denial or less positive coping, and those with the least social support as the groups least likely to have an advance directive). Providers of HIV care have an important opportunity to encourage discussions about end-of-life care preferences and decision-making. This is particularly important for the marginalised groups that make up an increasing proportion of the HIV-infected population and who are least likely to have engaged in advance care planning (Wenger *et al.*, 2001).

Within each society, and on a global scale, health care providers must strive to assure access to this kind of comprehensive care for all people living with HIV and other serious illnesses (Ludwig and Chittenden, 2008).

Acknowledgements

This chapter was reviewed by:

Sarah Cox, MBBS, BSc, FRCP, Consultant in Palliative Medicine, Chelsea and Westminster NHS Foundation Trust and Trinity Hospice, Honorary Senior Lecturer Imperial College School of Medicine, London.

Andreas Hiersch, MD, Macmillan Consultant Palliative Medicine, Palliative Care Team, South Downs Health NHS, Brighton.

Mary Poulton, FRCP, MA (ethics), DipGUM, Consultant HIV/GUM Physician, Department of Sexual Health and HIV, Kings College Hospital NHS Foundation Trust, London.

Further reading

0–18 years: guidance for all doctors, General Medical Council, London 2007. Available at: www.gmc-uk.org.

A–Z of ethical Guidance, General Medical Council, London. Available at: http://www.gmc-uk.org/guidance/a_z_guidance/index.asp.

End of Life Care, Department of Health. Available at: http://www.dh.gov.uk/en/Healthcare/IntegratedCare/Endoflifecare/DH_299.

Medical Ethics, British Medical Association (BMA) Website. Available at: http://www.bma.org.uk/ethics/index.jsp.

WHO/CDS/IMAI: Palliative Care: symptom management and end of life care, Integrated Management of Adult and Adolescent Illness, World Health Organization, Geneva, 2004. Available at: http://www.emro.who.int/aiecf/web35.pdf.

WHO, A Community Health Approach to Palliative Care for HIV/AIDS and Cancer Patients in Sub-Saharan Africa, World Health Organization, Geneva. Available at: http://www.who.int/cancer/publications/en/index.html.

References

Alexander CS, Back A, MD, Perrone M. Dying in the Era of HAART, Chapter 24. In: Oneill J, Selwyn PA, Schietinger H, eds. *Medical Care at the End of Life A Clinical Guide on Supportive and Palliative Care for People with HIV/AIDS.* Health Resources Services

Administration, US Department of Health and Human Services, 2003. Available at http://hab.hrsa.gov/tools/palliative/ contents.html. Accessed on 11 May 2009.

Antiretroviral therapy cohort collaboration. Life expectancy of individuals on combination antiretroviral therapy in high-income countries: a collaborative analysis of 14 cohort studies. *Lancet* 2008; **372**(9635):293–9.

Baker A, Jacobs M, Nuckcheddee A, Pohle B. *Trust Strategy and Policy for Consent to Examination or Treatment*. London: King's College Hospital NHS Foundation Trust, 2008.

Deeks S, Phillips A. HIV infection, antiretroviral treatment, ageing, and non-AIDS related morbidity. *BMJ* 2009; **338**:a3172.

Department of Health. *King's College Consent Form 4, Form for Adults Who are Unable to Consent to an Investigation or Treatment*. London: Department of Health, 2008.

Eldridge L. In: Thomas B, Bishop J, eds. *Pallitaive Care and Terminal Illness, Manual of Dietetic Practice*, 4th ed. Oxford: Blackwell Publishing, 2007.

Fuhrman MP, Herrmann VM. Bridging the continuum: nutrition support in palliative and hospice care. *Nutr Clin Pract* 2006; **21**(2):134–41.

Good P, Cavenagh J, Mather M, Ravenscroft P. Medically assisted nutrition for palliative care in adult patients. *Cochrane Database of Systematic Reviews*. 2008; (4):Art. No.:CD006274. DOI: 10.1002/14651858.CD006274.pub2.

Harding R, Karus D, Easterbrook P, Raveis VH, Higginson IJ, Marconi K. Does palliative care improve outcomes for patients with HIV/AIDS? A systematic review of the evidence. *Sex Transm Infect* 2005; **81**(1):5–14.

Jonsen RA. *Bioethics Beyond the Headlines: Who Lives? Who Dies? Who Decides?* Lanham, MD: Rowman and Littlefield Publishers, 2005.

Korner U, Bondolfi A, Buhler E *et al*. Ethical and legal aspects of enteral nutrition, introduction part to the ESPEN guidelines on enteral nutrition. *Clin Nutr* 2006; **25**:196–202. Available at http://intl.elsevierhealth.com/journals/clnu.

Loser C, Aschl G, Hebuterne X *et al*. ESPEN guidelines on artificial enteral nutrition – Percutaneous endoscopic gastrostomy (PEG) consensus statement. *Clin Nutr* 2005; **24**:848–61.

Ludwig A, Chittenden E. In: Peiperl L, Coffey S, Bacon O, Volberding P, eds. *Palliative Care of Patients with HIV, HIV Insite Knowledge Base Chapter, The Comprehensive, On-Line Textbook of HIV Disease from the University of California San Francisco and San Francisco General Hospital*. July 2008 Available at http://hivinsite.ucsf.edu/InSite?page=kb-03-03-05.

Ludwig A, Chittenden E. Palliative Care of Patients with HIV, HIV InSite Knowledge Base Chapter, 2008. Available at http://hivinsite.ucsf.edu/InSite?page=kb-03-03-05. Accessed on 14 May 2010.

Lyons C, Brotherton A, Stanley N, Carrahar NM, Manthorpe J. The mental capacity act 2005: implications for dietetic practice. *J Hum Nutr Diet* 2007; **20**(4):302–10.

MacFie J. Ethics of artificial nutrition medicine. *Nutrition* 2006; **34**(12):548–50.

Mental Capacity Act. (England and Wales) 2005: Code of Practice (2007). London: The Stationery Office, 2005.

National Institute for Clinical Excellence (NICE). *Guidance on Cancer Services: Improving Supportive and Palliative Care for Adults with Cancer*. London: NICE, 2004. Available at www.nice.org.uk.

Selwyn PA, EDITORIAL. Palliative care. *Sex Transm Infect* 2005; **81**:2–3; doi:10.1136/sti.2004.011585.

Watson M, Lucas C, Hoy A, Bank I eds. *Oxford Handbook of Palliative Care*. Oxford: Oxford University Press, 2005.

Wenger NS, Kanouse E Collins L *et al*. End-of-life discussions and preferences among persons with HIV. *JAMA* 2001; **285**(22):2280–87.

Wolf LE, Lo B. Ethical Dimensions of HIV/AIDS, HIV InSite Knowledge Base Chapter August, 2001. The University of California, San Francisco. Available at http://hivinsite.ucsf.edu/InSite?page=kb-08-01-05. Accessed on 14 May 2010.

World Health Organization (WHO). HIV palliative care WHO sites > HIV/AIDS > HIV/AIDS Topics, World Health Organization. Geneva, 2002. Available at http://www.who.int/hiv/topics/palliative/PalliativeCare/en/print.html. Accessed on 11 May 2009.

APPENDICES

Appendix 1
WHO Clinical Staging of HIV/AIDS for Adults and Adolescents

Primary HIV infection
- Asymptomatic
- Acute retroviral syndrome

Clinical stage 1 (mild)
- Asymptomatic
- Persistent generalised lymphadenopathy

Clinical stage 2 (advanced)
- Moderate unexplained weight loss (<10% of presumed or measured body weight)
- Recurrent respiratory infections (sinusitis, tonsillitis, otitis media and pharyngitis)
- Herpes zoster
- Angular cheilitis
- Recurrent oral ulceration
- Papular pruritic eruptions
- Seborrheic dermatitis
- Fungal nail infections

Clinical stage 3 (severe)
- Unexplained severe weight loss (>10% of presumed or measured body weight)
- Unexplained chronic diarrhea for >1 month
- Unexplained persistent fever for >1 month (>37.6°C, intermittent or constant)
- Persistent oral candidiasis (thrush)
- Oral hairy leukoplakia
- Pulmonary tuberculosis (current)
- Severe presumed bacterial infections (e.g. pneumonia, empyema, pyomyositis, bone or joint infection, meningitis and bacteremia)
- Acute necrotizing ulcerative stomatitis, gingivitis or periodontitis
- Unexplained anemia (hemoglobin <8 g/dL)
- Neutropenia (neutrophils <500 cells/μL)
- Chronic thrombocytopenia (platelets <50,000 cells/μL)

Clinical stage 4
- HIV wasting syndrome*
- *Pneumocystis* pneumonia
- Recurrent severe bacterial pneumonia
- Chronic herpes simplex infection (orolabial, genital or anorectal site for >1 month or visceral herpes at any site)
- Esophageal candidiasis (or candidiasis of trachea, bronchi or lungs)
- Extrapulmonary tuberculosis
- Kaposi sarcoma

- Cytomegalovirus infection (retinitis or infection of other organs)
- Central nervous system toxoplasmosis
- HIV encephalopathy
- Cryptococcosis, extrapulmonary (including meningitis)
- Disseminated non-tuberculosis *Mycobacteria* infection
- Progressive multifocal leukoencephalopathy
- Candida of the trachea, bronchi or lungs
- Chronic cryptosporidiosis (with diarrhea)
- Chronic isosporiasis
- Disseminated mycosis (e.g. histoplasmosis, coccidioidomycosis and penicilliosis)
- Recurrent non-typhoidal *Salmonella* bacteremia
- Lymphoma (cerebral or B-cell non-Hodgkin)
- Invasive cervical carcinoma
- Atypical disseminated leishmaniasis
- Symptomatic HIV-associated nephropathy
- Symptomatic HIV-associated cardiomyopathy
- Reactivation of American trypanosomiasis (meningoencephalitis or myocarditis)

*HIV Wasting Syndrome: Wasting syndrome due to HIV (involuntary weight loss >10% of baseline body weight) associated with either chronic diarrhea (≥ 2 loose stools per day ≥ 1 month) or chronic weakness and documented fever ≥ 1 month.

Reprinted from WHO Clinical Staging of HIV/AIDS for Adults and Adolescents, with permission from WHO.

Appendix 2
Weight-for-Height Reference Card (87 cm and above)

Boys' weight (kg)					Height (cm)	Girls' weight (kg)				
−4 SD	−3 SD	−2 SD	−1 SD	Médian		Médian	−1 SD	−2 SD	−3 SD	−4 SD
8.9	9.6	10.4	11.2	12.2	87	11.9	10.9	10.0	9.2	8.4
9.1	9.8	10.6	11.5	12.4	88	12.1	11.1	10.2	9.4	8.6
9.3	10.0	10.8	11.7	12.6	89	12.4	11.4	10.4	9.6	8.3
9.4	10.2	11.0	11.9	12.9	90	12.6	11.6	10.6	9.8	9.0
9.6	10.4	11.2	12.1	13.1	91	12.9	11.8	10.9	10.0	9.1
9.8	10.6	11.4	12.3	13.4	92	13.1	12.0	11.1	10.2	9.3
9.9	10.8	11.6	12.6	13.6	93	13.4	12.3	11.3	10.4	9.5
10.1	11.0	11.8	12.8	13.8	94	13.6	12.5	11.5	10.6	9.7
10.3	11.1	12.0	13.0	14.1	95	13.9	12.7	11.7	10.8	9.8
10.4	11.3	12.2	13.2	14.3	96	14.1	12.9	11.9	10.9	10.0
10.6	11.5	12.4	13.4	14.6	97	14.4	13.2	12.1	11.1	10.2
10.8	11.7	12.6	13.7	14.8	98	14.7	13.4	12.3	11.3	10.4
11.0	11.9	12.9	13.9	15.1	99	14.9	13.7	12.5	11.5	10.5
11.2	12.1	13.1	14.2	15.4	100	15.2	13.9	12.8	11.7	10.7
11.3	12.3	13.3	14.4	15.6	101	15.5	14.2	13.0	12.0	10.9
11.5	12.5	13.6	14.7	15.9	102	15.8	14.5	13.3	12.2	11.1
11.7	12.8	13.8	14,9	16.2	103	16.1	14.7	13.5	12.4	11.3
11.9	13.0	14.0	15.2	16.5	104	16.4	15.0	13.8	12.6	11.5
12.1	13.2	14.3	15.5	16.8	105	16.8	15.3	14.0	12.9	11.8
12.3	13.4	14.5	15.8	17.2	106	17.1	15.6	14.3	13.1	12.0
12.5	13.7	14.8	16.1	17.5	107	17.5	15.9	14.6	13.4	12.2
12.7	13.9	15.1	16.4	17.8	108	17.3	16.3	14.9	13.7	12.4
12.9	14.1	15.3	16.7	18.2	109	18.2	16.6	15.2	13.9	12.7
13.2	14.4	15.6	17.0	18.5	110	18.6	17.0	15.5	14.2	12.9
13.4	14.6	15.9	17.3	18.9	111	19.0	17.3	15.8	14.5	13.2
13.6	14.9	16.2	17.6	19.2	112	19.4	17.7	16.2	14.8	13.5
13.8	15.2	16.5	18.0	19.6	113	19.8	18.0	16.5	15.1	13.7
14.1	15.4	16.8	18.3	20.0	114	20.2	18.4	16.8	15.4	14.0
14.3	15.7	17.1	18.6	20.4	115	20.7	18.8	17.2	15.7	14.3
14.6	16.0	17.4	19.0	20.8	116	21.1	19.2	17.5	16.0	14.5
14.8	16.2	17.7	19.3	21.2	117	21.5	19.6	17.3	16.3	14.8
15.0	16.5	18.0	19.7	21.6	113	22.0	19.9	18.2	16.6	15.1
15.3	16.8	18.3	20.0	22.0	119	22.4	20.3	18.5	16.9	15.4
15.5	17.1	18.6	20.4	22.4	120	22.3	20.7	18.9	17.3	15.6

Appendix 3
Weight-for-Length Reference Card (below 87 cm)

Boys' weight (kg)					Length (cm)	Girls' weight (kg)				
−4 SD	−3 SD	−2 SD	−1 SD	Médian		Médian	−1 SD	−2 SD	−3 SD	−4 SD
1.7	1.9	2.0	2.2	2.4	45	2.5	2.3	2.1	1.9	1.7
1.8	2.0	2.2	2.4	2.6	46	2.6	2.4	2.2	2.0	1.9
2.0	2.1	2.3	2.5	2.8	47	2.8	2.6	2.4	2.2	2.0
2.1	2.3	2.5	2.7	2.9	48	3.0	2.7	2.5	2.3	2.1
2.2	2.4	2.6	2.9	3.1	49	3.2	2.9	2.6	2.4	2.2
2.4	2.6	2.8	3.0	3.3	50	3.4	3.1	2.8	2.6	2.4
2.5	2.7	3.0	3.2	3.5	51	3.6	3.3	3.0	2.8	2.5
2.7	2.9	3.2	3.5	3.8	52	3.8	3.5	3.2	2.9	2.7
2.9	3.1	3.4	3.7	4.0	53	4.0	3.7	3.4	3.1	2.8
3.1	3.3	3.6	3.9	4.3	54	4.3	3.9	3.6	3.3	3.0
3.3	3.6	3.8	4.2	4.5	55	4.5	4.2	3.8	3.5	3.2
3.5	3.8	4.1	4.4	4.8	56	4.8	4.4	4.0	3.7	3.4
3.7	4.0	4.3	4.7	5.1	57	5.1	4.6	4.3	3.9	3.6
3.9	4.3	4.6	5.0	5.4	58	5.4	4.9	4.5	4.1	3.8
4.1	4.5	4.8	5.3	5.7	59	5.6	5.1	4.7	4.3	3.9
4.3	4.7	5.1	5.5	6.0	60	5.9	5.4	4.9	4.5	4.1
4.5	4.9	5.3	5.8	6.3	61	6.1	5.6	5.1	4.7	4.3
4.7	5.1	5.6	6.0	6.5	62	6.4	5.8	5.3	4.9	4.5
4.9	5.3	5.8	6.2	6.8	63	6.6	6.0	5.5	5.1	4.7
5.1	5.5	6.0	6.5	7.0	64	6.9	6.3	5.7	5.3	4.8
5.3	5.7	6.2	6.7	7.3	65	7.1	6.5	5.9	5.5	5.0
5.5	5.9	6.4	6.9	7.5	66	7.3	6.7	6.1	5.6	5.1
5.6	6.1	6.6	7.1	7.7	67	7.5	6.9	6.3	5.8	5.3
5.8	6.3	6.8	7.3	8.0	68	7.7	7.1	6.5	6.0	5.5
6.0	6.5	7.0	7.6	8.2	69	8.0	7.3	6.7	6.1	5.6
6.1	6.6	7.2	7.8	8.4	70	8.2	7.5	6.9	6.3	5.8
6.3	6.8	7.4	8.0	8.6	71	8.4	7.7	7.0	6.5	5.9
6.4	7.0	7.6	8.2	8.9	72	8.6	7.8	7.2	6.6	6.0
6.6	7.2	7.7	8.4	9.1	73	8.8	8.0	7.4	6.8	6.2
6.7	7.3	7.9	8.6	9.3	74	9.0	8.2	7.5	6.9	6.3
6.9	7.5	8.1	8.8	9.5	75	9.1	8.4	7.7	7.1	6.5
7.0	7.6	8.3	8.9	9.7	76	9.3	8.5	7.8	7.2	6.6
7.2	7.8	8.4	9.1	9.9	77	9.5	8.7	8.0	7.4	6.7
7.3	7.9	8.6	9.3	10.1	78	9.7	8.9	8.2	7.5	6.9
7.4	8.1	8.7	9.5	10.3	79	9.9	9.1	8.3	7.7	7.0
7.6	8.2	8.9	9.6	10.4	80	10.1	9.2	8.5	7.8	7.1
7.7	8.4	9.1	9.8	10.6	81	10.3	9.4	8.7	8.0	7.3
7.9	8.5	9.2	10.0	10.8	82	10.5	9.6	8.8	8.1	7.5
8.0	8.7	9.4	10.2	11.0	83	10.7	9.8	9.0	8.3	7.6
8.2	8.9	9.6	10.4	11.3	84	11.0	10.1	9.2	8.5	7.8
8.4	9.1	9.8	10.6	11.5	85	11.2	10.3	9.4	8.7	8.0
8.6	9.3	10.0	10.8	11.7	86	11.5	10.5	9.7	8.9	8.1

Appendix 4
Guidance Table to Identify Target Weight

Guidance table to identity the target weight		Guidance table to identity the target weight	
Weight on admission*	Target weight: 15% weight gain	Weight on admission*	Target weight: 15% weight gain
4.1	4.7	10.7	12.3
4.3	4.9	10.9	12.5
4.5	5.2	11.1	12.8
4.7	5.4	11.3	13.0
4.9	5.6	11.5	13.2
5.1	5.9	11.7	13.5
5.3	6.1	11.9	13.7
5.5	6.3	12.1	13.9
5.7	6.6	12.3	14.1
5.9	6.8	12.5	14.4
6.1	7.0	12.7	14.6
6.3	7.2	12.9	14.8
6.5	7.5	13.1	15.1
6.7	7.7	13.3	15.3
6.9	7.9	13.5	15.5
7.1	8.2	13.7	15.8
7.3	8.4	13.9	16.0
7.5	8.6	14.1	16.2
7.7	8.9	14.3	16.4
7.9	9.1	14.5	16.7
8.1	9.3	14.7	16.9
8.3	9.5	14.9	17.1
8.5	9.8	15.1	17.4.
8.7	10.0	15.3	17.6
8.9	10.2	15.5	17.8
9.1	10.5	15.7	18.1
9.3	10.7	15.9	18.3
9.5	10.9	16.1	18.5
9.7	11.2	16.3	18.7
9.9	11.4	16.5	19.0
10.1	11.6	16.7	19.2
10.3	11.8	16.9	19.4
10.5	12.1	17.1	19.7

*Or weight, free of oedema. *Or weight, free of oedema.

With permission from WHO and UNICEF.

Appendix 5
Basic Steps in Estimating Energy Requirements for Adults

1. Determine appropriate metabolic rate (BMR).

Appendix Table 5.1 Equations for estimating basal metabolic rate (Schofield) (Department of Health 1991).

Females (kcal/day)		Males (kcal/day)	
10–17 years	13.4 W + 692	10–17 years	17.7 W + 657
18–29 years	14.8 W + 487	18–29 years	15.1 W + 692
30–59 years	8.3 W + 846	30–59 years	11.5 W + 873
Females over 60 yrs (kcal/day)		Males over 60 years (kcal/day)*	
60–74 years	9.2 W + 687	60–74 years	11.9 W + 700
75 years +	9.8 W + 624	75 years +	8.3 W + 820

W = weight.
Conversion 1 kcal = 4.184 kJ.
From the Department of Health, 1991. Reproduced under the terms of the Click-Use Licence.

2. Adjust for stress or weight gain/loss: If patient is stressed, add a factor that estimates the increased energy requirements due to disease process (Table 4.2).

Or if an increase or decrease in energy stores is required, add or subtract 400–1000 kcal/day.

Appendix Table 5.2 Stress factors for some clinical conditions.

Condition	Stress factor (% BMR)
Infection	25–45
Intensive care (ventilated)	0–10
Intensive care (septic)	20–60
Lymphoma	0–25
Solid tumours	0–20
Transplantation	20
Surgery (uncomplicated)	5–20
Surgery (complicated)	25–40

With permission from Todorovic and Micklewright (2004) on behalf of the Parenteral and Enteral Nutrition Group, British Dietetic Association.

Note:

- Characteristics of stress response include: elevated temperature, raised white cell count, elevated C-reactive protein (CRP), raised blood urea, and low serum albumin.
- Additional points to consider include fluid-overloaded patients and amputation.

3a. Add a combined factor for activity and diet-induced thermogenesis (DIT).

Appendix Table 5.3 Activity factor for activity: institutionalised patients combined with (DIT).

Activity level	Males and females
Bedbound immobile	+10%
Bedbound mobile/sitting	+15–20%
Mobile on ward	+25%

From the Department of Health, 1991. Reproduced under the terms of the Click-Use Licence.

3b. For patients considered to have activity levels nearer to healthy individuals, a PAL (Physical Activity Level) (Table 4.4) should be added rather than a combined factor for physical activity and DIT. Multiplying the PAL by the BMR gives the actual energy requirements.

Appendix Table 5.4 Calculated physical activity level (PAL) of adults at three levels of occupational and non-occupational activity.

Non-occupational activity	Occupational activity light		Occupational activity moderate		Occupational activity mod/heavy	
	M	F	M	F	M	F
Non-active	1.4	1.4	1.6	1.5	1.7	1.5
Moderately active	1.5	1.5	1.7	1.6	1.8	1.6
Very active	1.6	1.6	1.8	1.7	1.9	1.7

From the Department of Health, 1991. Reproduced under the terms of the Click-Use Licence.

Notes:

1. Further details of these activity levels and examples of lifestyles with different levels of energy demands can be found in various publications (Department of Health, 1991; FAO 2001).
2. Predictive formulae have been developed for obesity.

Appendix 6
NICE Guidelines: What
to Give in Hospital and
the Community

Healthcare professionals who are skilled and trained in nutritional requirements and methods of nutrition support should ensure that the total nutrient intake[1] of people prescribed nutrition support accounts for: **D(GPP)**

- energy, protein, fluid, electrolyte, mineral, micronutrients[2] and fibre needs
- activity levels and the underlying clinical condition – for example, catabolism, and pyrexia
- gastrointestinal tolerance, potential metabolic instability and risk of refeeding problems
- the likely duration of nutrition support.

For people who are not severely ill or injured, nor at risk of refeeding syndrome, the suggested nutritional prescription for total intake[3] should provide all of the following: **D(GPP)**

- 25–35 kcal/kg/day total energy (including that derived from protein[4,5])
- 0.8–1.5 g protein (0.13–0.24 g nitrogen)/kg/day
- 30–35 ml fluid/kg (with allowance for extra losses from drains and fistulae, for example, and extra input from other sources – for example, intravenous drugs) adequate electrolytes, minerals and micronutrients (allowing any pre-existing deficits, excessive losses or increased demands) and fibre, if appropriate.

The prescription should be reviewed according to the person's progress, and care should be taken when: **D(GPP)**

- using food fortification which tends to supplement energy and/or protein without adequate micronutrients and minerals

---

[1] Total intake includes intake from any food, oral fluid, oral nutritional supplements, enteral and/or parenteral nutrition support and intravenous fluid.

[2] The term 'micronutrient' is used throughout to include all essential vitamins and trace elements.

[3] This level may need to be lower in people who are overweight, BMI > 25.

[4] When using parenteral nutrition, it is often necessary to adjust total energy values listed on the manufacturer's information which may not include protein energy values.

[5] (See footnote 4)

- using feeds and supplements that meet full energy and nitrogen needs, as they may not provide adequate micronutrients and minerals when only used in a supplementary role
- using pre-mixed parenteral nutrition bags that have not had tailored additions from pharmacy.

Appendix 7
Basic Steps in Estimation of Nitrogen Requirements for Adults (Source: Elia, 1990)

Appendix Table 7.1 Estimation of nitrogen requirements.

		Nitrogen g/kg/day	
Normal		0.17	(0.14–0.20)
Hypermetabolic	5–25%	0.20	(0.17–0.25)
	25–50%	0.25	(0.20–0.30)
	>50%	0.30	(0.25–0.35)
Depleted		0.30	(0.20–0.40)

With permission from Todorovic and Micklewright (2004) on behalf of the Parenteral and Enteral Nutrition Group, British Dietetic Association.

Note: It is the subject of some debate as to whether there is benefit in providing nitrogen in excess of 0.2 g/kg/day in the critically ill.

For obese individuals:

BMI> 30 kg/m^2: use approximately 75% of the value estimated from weight
BMI> 50 kg/m^2: use approximately 65% of the value estimated from weight.

(Todorovic and Micklewright, 2004)

Appendix 8
Summary of ESPEN Statements: HIV and Nutritional Therapy

Subject	Recommendations	Level of recommendation	Statement number
Indications	Nutritional therapy is indicated when significant weight loss (>5% in 3 months) or a significant loss of body cell mass (>5% in 3 months) has occurred.	B	2.1
	Nutritional therapy should be considered when the BMI is <18.5 kg/m^2.*	C	2.1
	Diarrhoea and/or malabsorption are no contraindication to EN, because:		
	• Diarrhoea does not prevent a positive effect of oral nutritional supplements or tube feeding on nutritional status.	A	2.4
	• Enteral and parenteral nutrition have similar effects in such patients.	A	2.4
	• Enteral nutrition has a positive impact on stool frequency and consistency.	A	2.4
Application	The combination of normal food and enteral nutrition is appropriate in many cases and should be attempted.	C	3.6
	If oral intake is possible, nutritional intervention should be implemented according the following scheme.	C	2.2
	• nutritional counselling • oral nutritional supplements • tube feeding • parenteral nutrition	B	2.2
	Nutritional counselling with oral nutritional supplements, or counselling alone, is equally effective at the beginning of nutritional support and/or for preserving nutritional status.	C	2.2

(*Continued*)

Subject	Recommendations	Level of recommendation	Statement number
	In settings where qualified nutritional counselling cannot be provided, oral nutritional supplements may be indicated in addition to normal food but this should be limited in time.	B	3.2
	Protein intake should achieve 1.2 g/kg bw/day in stable phases of the disease while it may be increased to 1.5 g/kg bw/day during acute illness. Energy requirements are no different from other patient groups.	C	3.2
	In patients with dysphagia, or if oral nutritional supplements are not effective: If normal food intake and optimal use of oral nutritional supplements cannot achieve sufficient energy supply, tube feeding is indicated.	C	2.5
	Drug treatment and enteral nutrition complement each other.		
Route	Use antibiotic prophylaxis during implantation of percutaneous endoscopic gastrostomy (PEG).	A	3.4
Type of formula	Use standard formulae.	B	3.1
	In patients with diarrhoea and severe undernutrition, MCT-containing formulae are advantageous.	A	3.1
	Immune modulating formulae are not recommended.		3.1

From Ockenga et al., 2006, with permission from Elsevier.
ESPEN guidelines are intended to give evidence-based recommendations for the use of enteral nutrition (EN) by means of (ONS) and tube feeding (TF) in HIV-infected patients. They were developed by an interdisciplinary expert group in accordance with officially accepted standards and is based on all relevant publications since 1985. Table 2 contains a summary of recommendations contained in ESPEN Guidelines of HIV and nutritional therapy (Ockenga et al., 2006).

References

Elia M. Artificial nutriton support. *Med Int* 1990; **82**:3392–6.
FAO. Food and Nutrition Technical Report Series, Human Energy Requirements, Report of a Joint WHO/FAO/UNU Expert Consultation, Rome October 2001. Available at ftp://ftp.fao.org/docrep/fao/007/y5686e/y5686e00.pdf.
Todorovic VE, Micklewright A. *A Pocket Guide to Clinical Nutrition*, 3rd edn. On behalf of the Parenteral and Enteral Nutrition Group, British Dietetic Association, 2004.

Appendix 9
Form for Monitoring
Anthropometry Measurements

NAME: _____   D.O.B: _____   HOSPITAL NUMBER: _____   GENDER _____   HEIGHT: _____

Date							
Observer name							
Weight (kg)							
Mid-upper arm circumference (cm)							
Biceps skinfold (mm)							
Triceps skinfold (mm)							
Subscapular skinfold (mm)							
Suprailiac Skinfold (mm)							
Abdominal circumference (cm)							
Chest circumference (cm)							
Hip circumference (cm)							
Mid-thigh circumference (cm)							
Mid-calf circumference (mm)							
Dorsocervical Fat Pad (cm)							

Pribram V, Duncan A, Kings College Hospital and Guy's and St Thomas' NHS Foundation Trusts

Appendix 10
Equations to Calculate Height and Estimation of Height from Ulna Length

10.1 Equations for calculating height from knee height (Chumlea and Guo. 1992; Chumlea et al., 1985, 1994)

Men	18–60 years	Predicted height (cm) = [knee height (cm) x 1.88] + 71.85
	60–90 years	Predicted height (cm) = knee height (cm) x 2.08] +59.01
Women	18–60 years	Predicted height (cm) = [knee height (cm) x 1.87] − [age (years) x 0.06] + 70.25
	60–90 years	Predicted height (cm) = [knee height (cm) x 1.91] − [age (years) x 0.17] + 75.0

10.2 Equations for calculating height from demispan

Men	16–54 years	Predicted height (cm) = [demispan (cm) x 1.3] + 68
	>55 years	Predicted height (cm) = [demispan (cm) x 1.2] + 71
Women	16–54 years	Predicted height (cm) = [demispan (cm) x 1.3] + 62
	>55 years	Predicted height (cm) = [demispan (cm) x 1.2] + 67

10.3 Estimating height from ulna length

Men: Height (m)			Women: Height (m)	
<65 years	>65 years	Ulna length (cm)	<65 years	>65 years
1.94	1.87	32.0	1.84	1.84
1.93	1.86	31.5	1.83	1.83
1.91	1.84	31.0	1.81	1.81
1.89	1.82	30.5	1.80	1.79
1.87	1.81	30.0	1.79	1.78
1.85	1.79	29.5	1.77	1.76
1.84	1.78	29.0	1.76	1.75
1.82	1.76	28.5	1.75	1.73
1.80	1.75	28.0	1.73	1.71
1.78	1.73	27.5	1.72	1.70
1.76	1.71	27.0	1.70	1.68
1.75	1.70	26.5	1.69	1.66
1.73	1.68	26.0	1.68	1.65
1.71	1.67	25.5	1.66	1.63

(Continued)

10.3 (*Continued*)

Men: Height (m)		Ulna length (cm)	Women: Height (m)	
<65 years	>65 years		<65 years	>65 years
1.69	1.65	25.0	1.65	1.61
1.67	1.63	24.5	1.63	1.60
1.66	1.62	24.0	1.62	1.58
1.64	1.60	23.5	1.61	1.56
1.62	1.59	23.0	1.59	1.55
1.60	1.57	22.5	1.58	1.53
1.58	1.56	22.0	1.56	1.52
1.57	1.54	21.5	1.55	1.50
1.55	1.52	21.0	1.54	1.48
1.53	1.51	20.5	1.52	1.47
1.51	1.49	20.0	1.51	1.45
1.49	1.48	19.5	1.50	1.44
1.48	1.46	19.0	1.48	1.42
1.46	1.45	18.5	1.47	1.40

Appendix 11
Mid Upper Arm
Circumference (MUAC)

Age (years)	Mean (cm)	Centile						
		5th	10th	25th	50th	75th	90th	95th
Men								
18–74	31.8	26.4	27.6	29.6	31.7	33.9	36.0	37.3
18–24	30.9	25.7	27.1	28.7	30.7	32.9	35.5	37.4
25–34	30.5	25.3	26.5	28.5	30.7	32.4	34.4	35.5
35–44	32.3	27.0	28.2	30.0	32.0	34.4	36.5	37.6
45–54	32.7	27.8	28.7	30.7	32.7	34.8	36.3	37.1
55–64	32.1	26.7	27.8	30.0	32.0	34.2	36.2	37.6
65–74	31.5	25.6	27.3	29.6	31.7	33.4	35.2	36.6
Women								
18–74	29.4	23.2	24.3	26.2	28.7	31.9	35.2	37.8
18–24	27.0	22.1	23.0	24.5	26.4	28.8	31.7	34.3
25–34	28.6	23.3	24.2	25.7	27.8	30.4	34.1	37.2
35–44	30.0	24.1	25.2	26.8	29.2	32.2	36.2	38.5
45–54	30.7	24.3	25.7	27.5	30.3	32.9	36.8	39.3
55–64	30.7	23.9	25.1	27.7	30.2	33.3	36.3	38.2
65–74	30.1	23.8	25.2	27.4	29.9	32.5	35.3	37.2

Data derived from Bishop *et al.* (1981).

Appendix 12
Mid Arm Muscle Circumference (MAMC)

$$MAMC\ (cm) = MUAC\ (cm) - [TSF\ (mm) \times 0.314]$$

Age (years)	Mean (cm)	Centile						
		5th	10th	25th	50th	75th	90th	95th
Men								
18–74	28.0	23.8	24.8	26.3	27.9	29.6	31.4	32.5
18–24	27.4	23.5	24.4	25.8	27.2	28.9	30.8	32.3
25–34	28.3	24.2	25.3	26.5	28.0	30.0	31.7	32.9
35–44	28.8	25.0	25.6	27.1	28.7	30.3	32.1	33.0
45–54	28.2	24.0	24.9	26.5	28.1	29.8	31.5	32.6
55–64	27.8	22.8	24.4	26.2	27.9	29.6	31.0	31.8
65–74	26.8	22.5	23.7	25.3	26.9	28.5	29.9	30.7
Women								
18–74	22.2	18.4	19.0	20.2	21.8	23.6	25.8	27.4
18–24	20.9	17.7	18.5	19.4	20.6	22.1	23.6	24.9
25–34	21.7	18.3	18.9	20.2	21.4	22.9	24.9	26.6
35–44	22.5	18.5	19.2	20.6	22.0	24.0	26.1	27.4
45–54	22.7	18.8	19.5	20.7	22.2	24.3	26.6	27.8
55–64	22.8	18.6	19.5	20.8	22.6	24.4	26.3	28.1
65–74	22.8	18.6	19.5	20.8	22.5	24.4	26.5	28.1

Appendix 13
Biochemical Reference Ranges

Blood constituent	Range
Albumin	35–45 g/l
Bicarbonate	22–32 mmol/l
Bilirubin	$\leq$17 μmol/l
Calcium	2.25–2.65 mmol/l
Chloride	95–105 mmol/l
Creatinine	40–130 μmol/l
Fasting Glucose	3.0–5.0 mmol/l
Haemoglobin (male)	13.5–17.5 g/dl
Haemoglobin (female)	11.5–15.5 g/dl
Inorganic phosphate	0.8–1.4 mmol/l
Magnesium	0.7–1.0 mmol/l
Osmolality	278–305 mosmol/kg
Potassium	3.5–5.0 mmol/l
Sodium	135–150 mmol/l
Total Protein	60–80 g/l
Urate (Male)	0.25–0.45 mmol/l
Urate (Female)	0.15–0.35 mmol/l
Urea	3.3–6.7 mmol/l

With permission from Vera Todorovic on behalf of the Parenteral and Enteral Nutrition Group, British Dietetic Association (2005).

Appendix 14
Ways to Improve Adherence
to TB Medication

- Fixed-dose combination tablets should be used as part of any TB treatment regimen.
- DOT (directly observed therapy) is when quadruple therapy is given three times a week under full supervision.
- All patients should have a risk assessment for adherence to treatment, and DOT should be considered for patients who have adverse factors on their risk assessment.
- Patients should be involved in treatment decisions.
- Patients should be given a key worker.
- Interventions should be considered following a patient defaulting.
- Pharmacies should make liquids readily available.
- Patient information should be provided in other languages if necessary.
- Using pill alarms as reminders for taking medication (Maartens and Wilkinson, 2007).

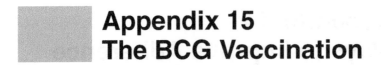

Appendix 15
The BCG Vaccination

In the UK immunisation with BCG is offered to:

- Babies living in areas of the UK where there is a high rate of TB
- Babies whose parents or grandparents have lived in a country with a high rate of TB
- Immigrants to the UK from countries where TB rates are high
- People in high-risk jobs. For example, health workers and prison staff
- Close contacts of people with active TB
- People who intend to live for one month or more in countries with a high TB rate (DOH, 2007).

Index

Note: Page numbers in *italic* indicate figures and those in **boldface** indicate tables.

Printed and bound by CPI Group (UK) Ltd, Croydon, CR0 4YY

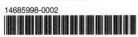